PROCEDURES

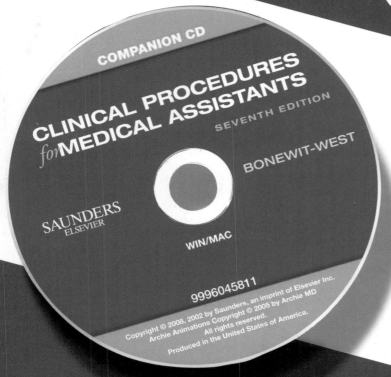

CLINICAL PROCEDURES
for **MEDICAL ASSISTANTS**

evolve

To access your Resources, visit:

http://evolve.elsevier.com/Bonewit/

Evolve® Resources for *Clinical Procedures for Medical Assistants,* **7th Edition** offer the following features:

Resources

- **WebLinks**
  Links to places of interest on the web specific to medical assisting.

- **Content Updates**
  Find out the latest information on relevant issues in the field of medical assisting.

SEVENTH EDITION

CLINICAL PROCEDURES
for MEDICAL ASSISTANTS

KATHY BONEWIT-WEST, BS, MEd

Coordinator and Instructor
Medical Assistant Technology
Hocking College
Nelsonville, Ohio
Former Member, Curriculum Review Board of the American
Association of Medical Assistants

SAUNDERS

ELSEVIER

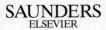

11830 Westline Industrial Drive
St. Louis, Missouri 63146

CLINICAL PROCEDURES FOR MEDICAL ASSISTANTS, SEVENTH EDITION   ISBN: 978-1-4160-3475-9

Previous editions copyrighted 2004, 2000, 1995, 1990, 1984, 1979

Library of Congress Control Number 2007924311

ISBN: 978-1-4160-3475-9

Publisher: Michael S. Ledbetter
Senior Developmental Editor: Melissa K. Boyle
Publishing Services Manager: Pat Joiner-Myers
Project Manager: Jennifer Bertucci
Design Direction: Julia Dummitt
Interior Design: Julia Dummitt

Printed in Canada

Last digit is the print number: 9 8 7 6 5 4 3 2

Contents

CLINICAL PROCEDURES
for MEDICAL ASSISTANTS

The Medical Record

LEARNING OBJECTIVES

Components of the Medical Record

1. List and describe the functions served by the medical record.

2. Identify the information contained in each of the following medical office administrative documents: patient registration record and correspondence.

3. Identify the information contained in each of the following medical office clinical documents: health history report, physical examination report, progress notes, medication record, consultation report, and home health care report.

4. List and describe the information included in each of the following diagnostic procedure documents: electrocardiogram report, Holter monitor report, sigmoidoscopy report, colonoscopy report, spirometry report, radiology report, and diagnostic imaging report.

5. State the purpose of each of the following therapeutic services: physical therapy, occupational therapy, and speech therapy.

6. Identify the information contained in each of the following hospital documents: history and physical report, operative report, discharge summary report, pathology report, and emergency department report.

Consent Documents

1. Identify the information contained in each of the following consent documents: consent to treatment form and release of medical information form.

Medical Record Formats

1. Describe the organization of a source-oriented medical record and a problem-oriented medical record.

2. List and define the four subcategories included in the progress notes of a problem-oriented record (POR).

3. Explain the difference between a paper-based patient record (PPR) and an electronic medical record (EMR).

Health History

1. List and describe the seven parts of the health history.
2. List the guidelines that should be followed in recording the chief complaint.

PROCEDURES

Prepare a medical record for a new patient.

Obtain patient consent for treatment.
Assist a patient in completing a release of medical information form.
Release information according to a completed release of medical information form.

Identify the parts of a source-oriented medical record and a problem-oriented medical record.

Complete or assist the patient in completing a health history form.

Charting

1. List and describe the guidelines to follow to ensure accurate and concise charting.
2. List and describe the types of progress notes that are charted by the medical assistant.
3. List examples of subjective symptoms and objective symptoms.
4. List and describe common symptoms.

Chart the following:
  Procedures
  Administration of medication
  Specimen collection
  Laboratory tests
  Progress notes
  Instructions given to the patient
Obtain and record patient symptoms.

CHAPTER OUTLINE

Introduction to the Medical Record
Components of the Medical Record
Medical Office Administrative Documents
  Patient Registration Record
  Correspondence
Medical Office Clinical Documents
  Health History Report
  Physical Examination Report
  Progress Notes
  Medication Record
  Consultation Report
  Home Health Care Report
Laboratory Documents
  Hematology
  Clinical Chemistry
  Serology
  Urinalysis
  Microbiology
  Parasitology
  Cytology
  Histology
Diagnostic Procedure Documents
  Electrocardiogram Report
  Holter Monitor Report
  Sigmoidoscopy Report
  Colonoscopy Report
  Spirometry Report

  Radiology Report
  Diagnostic Imaging Report
Therapeutic Service Documents
  Physical Therapy
  Occupational Therapy
  Speech Therapy
Hospital Documents
  History and Physical Report
  Operative Report
  Discharge Summary Report
  Pathology Report
  Emergency Department Report
Consent Documents
  Consent to Treatment Form
  Release of Medical Information Form
Medical Record Formats
  Source-Oriented Record
  Problem-Oriented Record
Preparing a Medical Record for a New Patient
  Medical Record Supplies
Taking a Health History
  Components of the Health History
Charting in the Medical Record
  Charting Guidelines
  Charting Progress Notes
  Charting Patient Symptoms
  Other Activities That Need to Be Charted

NATIONAL COMPETENCIES

Clinical Competencies
Patient Care
Perform telephone and in-person screening.
Obtain and record patient history.
Maintain medication and immunization records.

General Competencies
Professional Communications
Respond to and initiate written communications.
Recognize and respond to verbal communications.
Recognize and respond to nonverbal communications.
Demonstrate telephone techniques.

Legal Concepts
Identify and respond to issues of confidentiality.
Perform within legal and ethical boundaries.
Establish and maintain the medical record.
Document appropriately.
Demonstrate knowledge of federal and state health care legislation and regulations.

Patient Instruction
Explain general office policies.

Operational Functions
Use computer software to maintain office systems.

attending physician
charting
consultation report
diagnosis (dye-ag-NOE-sis)
diagnostic procedure
discharge summary report
electronic medical record (EMR)
familial (fah-MIL-yul)
health history report
home health care
informed consent
inpatient
medical impressions

medical record
medical record format
objective symptom
paper-based patient record (PPR)
patient
physical examination
physical examination report
problem
prognosis (prog-NOE-sis)
reverse chronological order
SOAP
subjective symptom
symptom (SIMP-tum)

Introduction to the Medical Record

Medical records are a crucial part of a medical practice. A **medical record** is a written record of the important information regarding a **patient,** including the care of that individual and the progress of his or her condition. A patient is defined as an individual receiving medical care.

The patient's medical record serves many important functions. The physician uses the information in the medical record as a basis for decisions regarding the patient's care and treatment. The medical record documents the results of treatment and the patient's progress. The medical record provides an efficient and effective method by which information can be communicated to authorized personnel in the medical office.

The medical record also serves as a legal document. The law requires that a record be maintained to document the care and treatment being received by a patient. If something goes wrong, good documentation works to protect the physician and the medical staff legally. Incomplete records could be used as evidence in court to show that a patient did not receive the quality of care that meets generally accepted standards.

The medical assistant must always keep in mind that the information contained in a patient's medical record is strictly confidential and must not be read by or discussed with anyone except the physician or medical staff involved with the care of the patient (see *Highlight on the HIPAA Privacy Rule*).

COMPONENTS OF THE MEDICAL RECORD

A medical record consists of numerous documents. Each document in the medical record has a specific function or purpose. Most of these documents are preprinted forms that contain specific information entered by a physician or other health professionals. A large variety of forms are available; the type of form used is based on the specific requirements of each medical office.

Medical record documents can be classified into categories. Each of these categories is outlined in the box on p. 5, along with the specific documents included in each.

It is important that the medical assistant be familiar with each type of document in the medical record. A description of the function or purpose of each type of medical record document follows (by category), along with the specific information that each contains.

MEDICAL OFFICE ADMINISTRATIVE DOCUMENTS

Administrative documents contain information necessary for the efficient (record-keeping) management of the medical office. Medical office administrative documents include the patient registration record and patient-related correspondence.

Patient Registration Record

The patient registration record (Figure 1-1) consists of demographic and billing information. All new patients must complete a patient registration record form. After the patient completes the registration record, the medical assistant enters the information into a computer. This allows the demographic and billing information to be used for numerous computerized functions, such as scheduling appointments, posting patient transactions, and processing patient statements and insurance claims. The original patient registration record is placed in the front of the patient's medical record.

Demographic Information

Demographic information required on a patient registration form includes the following:
- Full name
- Address
- Telephone number (home and work)
- Date of birth
- Gender

OPERATIVE REPORT
ST. MARY'S HOSPITAL

Name: Natalie Boyer

Hospital #: 291734   Room #: OP

Surgeon: Paul Cain, M.D.   Date of Surgery: 1/6/08

Anesthesiologist: John Adams, M.D.   Anesthesia: General

PRE-OP DIAGNOSIS: Abnormal Pap test with history of cervical carcinoma.

POST-OP DIAGNOSIS: Same and awaiting path report.

OPERATION: D&C, laser cone of the cervix.

PROCEDURE: The patient to the operating room, lithotomy position, perineum and vagina were prepped, and moist sterile drape was used. Laser precautions all in place. Bimanual examination revealed a uterus enlarged with a second-degree uterine prolapse. The cervix was dilated. Uterus sounded to around 9 cm. The endocervical canal was dilated and D&C was performed with tissue recovered and submitted to Pathology. The cervix was stained with iodine, and the nonstaining area was identified. The laser was brought in, 50 watts of current were used to remove laser cone, and we submitted that to Pathology. We then vaporized beyond the margins of the cone, 3-4 mm to a depth of 4-5 mm. Hemostasis was adequate. We placed 0 Vicryl figure-of-eight sutures at the 3 and the 9 o'clock positions in the cervix, and then we put Monsel solution on the cervix. Hemostasis adequate. Sponge and needle counts correct times two. The patient tolerated the procedure well, and she returned to the recovery room in stable condition. She will be discharged home when awake and stable on Cipro 250 mg twice a day for a week, Darvocet-N 100, #20 as needed for pain. If she continues to have abnormal Pap tests, we will probably want to do a vaginal hysterectomy.

SURGEON: *Paul Cain, MD*

Paul Cain, MD

Figure 1-9. Operative report.

Pathology Report

A pathology report consists of a macroscopic (gross) and a microscopic description of tissue removed from a patient during surgery or a diagnostic procedure. The report also includes a diagnosis of the patient's condition (Figure 1-11). A pathologist is required to examine the tissue specimen, complete the report, and sign it.

Emergency Department Report

The emergency department report is a record of the significant information obtained during an emergency department visit (Figure 1-12). The report is prepared and signed by the emergency department physician, and a copy is sent to the patient's family physician for the purpose of providing follow-up care. The emergency department report includes the following:
• Date of service
• Patient identification information
• Nature of the illness or injury
• Laboratory or diagnostic test results
• Procedures performed
• Treatment rendered
• Diagnosis
• Condition of the patient at discharge
• Instructions regarding follow-up care

CONSENT DOCUMENTS

Consent forms are legal documents required to perform certain procedures or to release information contained in the patient's medical record.

Consent to Treatment Form

The completion of a consent to treatment form (Procedure 1-1) is required for all surgical operations and nonroutine therapeutic and diagnostic procedures (e.g., sigmoidoscopy) performed in the medical office. The form must be signed by the patient or his or her legally authorized representative and

DISCHARGE SUMMARY

Brennan, Susan
97-32-11
June 18, 2008

ADMISSION DATE: June 14, 2008   **DISCHARGE DATE:**   June 16, 2008

HISTORY OF PRESENT ILLNESS:
This 19-year-old female, nulligravida, was admitted to the hospital on June 14, 2008, with fever of 102°, left lower quadrant pain, vaginal discharge, constipation, and a tender left adnexal mass. Her past history and family history were unremarkable. Present pain had started two to three weeks prior to admission. Her periods were irregular, with latest period starting on May 30, 2008, and lasting for six days. She had taken contraceptive pills in the past but had stopped because she was not sexually active.

PHYSICAL EXAMINATION:
She appeared well developed and well nourished, and in mild distress. The only positive physical findings were limited to the abdomen and pelvis. Her abdomen was mildly distended, and it was tender, especially in the left lower quadrant. At pelvic examination, her cervix was tender on motion, and the uterus was of normal size, retroverted, and somewhat fixed. There was a tender cystic mass about 4-5 cm in the left adnexa. Rectal examination was negative.

PROVISIONAL DIAGNOSIS:
1. Probable pelvic inflammatory disease (PID).
2. Rule out ectopic pregnancy.

LABORATORY DATA ON ADMISSION:
Hgb 10.8, Hct 36.5, WBC 8,100 with 80 segs and 18 lymphs. Sedimentation rate 100 mm in one hour. Sickle cell prep+ (turned out to be a trait). Urinalysis normal. Electrolytes normal. SMA-12 normal. Chest x-ray negative, 2-hour UCG negative.

HOSPITAL COURSE AND TREATMENT:
Initially, she was given cephalothin 2 gm IV q6h, and kanamycin 0.5 gm IM bid. Over the next two days the patient's condition improved. Her pain decreased and her temperature came down to normal in the morning and spiked to 101° in the evening. Repeat CBC showed Hgb 9.8, Hct 33.5. The pregnancy test was negative. She was discharged on June 16, 2008 in good condition. She will be seen in the office in one week.

DISCHARGE DIAGNOSIS:
Pelvic inflammatory disease.

Harold B. Cooper, MD
Harold B. Cooper, MD

Figure 1-10. Discharge summary report. (Modified from Diehl MO, Fordney MT: *Medical transcription: techniques and procedures,* ed 5, Philadelphia, 2003, Saunders.)

must provide written evidence that the patient agrees to the procedure or procedures listed on the form (Figure 1-13).

For the patient's consent to be valid, it must be informed consent. **Informed consent** means that the patient has received the following information before giving consent:
• The nature of the patient's condition
• The nature and purpose of the recommended procedure
• An explanation of risks involved with the procedure
• Alternative treatments or procedures available
• The likely outcome (**prognosis**) of the procedure
• The risks of declining or delaying the procedure

The explanation must be in terms the patient can understand, and the patient should be given an opportunity to ask questions regarding the information.

The consent to treatment form should not be signed until the patient has been provided with all necessary information

COLLEGE HOSPITAL
4567 BROAD AVENUE
WOODLAND HILLS, MD 21532

PATHOLOGY REPORT

Date:	June 20, 2008	Pathology No.:	430211
Patient:	Molly Ramsdale	Room No.:	1308
Physician:	Harold B. Cooper, M.D.		
Specimen Submitted:	Tumor, right axilla		

FINDINGS

GROSS DESCRIPTION: Specimen A consists of an oval mass of yellow fibroadipose tissue measuring 4 x 3 x 2 cm. On cut section, there are some small, soft, pliable areas of gray apparent lymph node alternating with adipose tissue. A frozen section consultation at time of surgery was delivered as NO EVIDENCE OF MALIGNANCY on frozen section, to await permanent section for final diagnosis. Majority of the specimen will be submitted for microscopic examination.

Specimen B consists of an oval mass of yellow soft tissue measuring 2.5 x 2.5 x 1.5 cm. On cut section, there is a thin rim of pink to tan-brown lymphatic tissue and the mid portion appears to be adipose tissue. A pathological consultation at time of surgery was delivered as no suspicious areas noted and to await permanent sections for final diagnosis. The entire specimen will be submitted for microscopic examination.

MICROSCOPIC DESCRIPTION: Specimen A sections show fibroadipose tissue and nine fragments of lymph nodes. The lymph nodes show areas with prominent germinal centers and moderate sinus histiocytosis. There appears to be some increased vascularity and reactive endothelial cells seen. There is no evidence of malignancy.

Specimen B sections show adipose tissue and 5 lymph node fragments. These 5 portions of lymph nodes show reactive changes including sinus histiocytosis. There is no evidence of malignancy.

DIAGNOSIS: A & B: TUMOR, RIGHT AXILLA: SHOWING 14 LYMPH NODE FRAGMENTS WITH REACTIVE CHANGES AND NO EVIDENCE OF MALIGNANCY.

Stanley T. Nason, MD

Stanley T. Nason, MD

Figure 1-11. Pathology report. (Modified from Diehl MO, Fordney MT: *Medical transcription: techniques and procedures,* ed 5, Philadelphia, 2003, Saunders.)

EMERGENCY DEPARTMENT REPORT
CAMDEN CLARK HOSPITAL

Name: ____John Larimer____   DOB: ____2/2/68____

ER Physician: ____John Parsons, MD____   Date: ____7/7/08____

ER Number: ____07398____

Physician: ____James Woods, MD____

NATURE OF ILLNESS/INJURY: This 40-year-old male presents to the Emergency Department complaining of a laceration of the sole of his right foot. Patient cut his foot on a rock 2 days ago and thinks he might have an infection now. Patient also complains of coughing over the past several days.

PHYSICAL EXAMINATION: Temperature 97.4, Pulse 76, Respirations 20, Blood Pressure 120/70. Patient is alert and oriented and is in no acute distress. ENT is normal. Lungs show diffuse rhonchi without crackles or wheezing. Heart has a regular rate and rhythm. Right great toe with marked tenderness with edema and erythema and heat.

DIAGNOSIS: Asthmatic Bronchitis
        Cellulitis, right foot first MTP

TREATMENT: PCMX scrub to right foot. Bacitracin dressing. Tetanus Diphtheria 0.5 cc IM. Biaxin 500 mg bid x 10 days. Guaifenesin with codeine 2 tsp q4h prn. Entex LA,1 bid prn. Debridement of skin flap.

PATIENT INSTRUCTIONS: Patient to follow up with family doctor in 7 days. Discussed bronchospasms with the patient.

James Woods, MD
_____
James Woods, MD

Figure 1-12. Emergency department report.

related to the procedure. The patient's signature must be witnessed; this is usually the responsibility of the medical assistant. *Witnessing a signature* means only that the medical assistant verified the patient's identity and watched the patient sign the form; it *does not* mean that the medical assistant is attesting to the accuracy of the information provided.

The consent to treatment form outlines the details of the discussion with the patient and includes the following information:
- The patient's full name
- Name of the procedure to be performed
- Name of the surgeon
- A statement indicating the patient agrees to receive the procedure
- Acknowledgment that a disclosure of information has been made
- Acknowledgment that all questions were answered in a satisfactory manner

- A statement that no guarantee as to the outcome has been made
- Signature of the patient or his or her legal representative
- Signature of the witness

Release of Medical Information Form

As previously explained in the box entitled *Highlight on the HIPAA Privacy Rule,* a patient's written consent is not required for the use or disclosure of protected health information (PHI) for the purpose of medical treatment, payment, and health care operations (TPO). If a request for protected health information is required for purposes that are not part of TPO, however, a detailed form must be completed, known as a *release of medical information form* (Figure 1-14). If a patient is moving to another state and wants to transfer his or her medical record to a new physician, a release of medical information form must be completed.

(Attach label or complete blanks.)

First name: _____   Last name: _____

Date of Birth: _____ Month _____ Day _____ Year

Account Number: _____

Procedure Consent Form

I, _____ , hereby consent to have

Dr. _____ perform _____ .

I have been fully informed of the following by my physician:

1. The nature of my condition
2. The nature and purpose of the procedure
3. An explanation of risks involved with the procedure
4. Alternative treatments or procedures available
5. The likely results of the procedure
6. The risks involved with declining or delaying the procedure

My physician has offered to answer all questions concerning the proposed procedure.

I am aware that the practice of medicine and surgery is not an exact science, and I acknowledge that no guarantees have been made to me about the results of the procedure.

Patient _____   Date _____
                (or guardian and relationship)

Witnessed _____   Date _____

Figure 1-13. Consent to treatment form.

The release of medical information form must be signed by the patient authorizing the disclosure of his or her PHI (Procedure 1-2). If the patient is a minor, the form must be signed by the parent or legal guardian of the minor. The release of medical information form must stipulate the following:

- The patient's full name and address
- Name of the medical practice releasing the information
- Name of the individual or facility to receive the information
- Specific information to be released
- The purpose of or the need for the information
- Method of release of the information
- Signature of the patient or his or her legal representative
- Date that the consent was signed
- The expiration date of the consent form

Mailed or Faxed Requests for Release of Medical Information

Most medical offices require that the patient come to the office to sign the release of medical information form; however, this may not always be possible. An example is a patient who has moved away and is requesting the transfer of his or her medical records to a new physician. In this instance, a completed and signed release of medical information form may be mailed or faxed to the medical office. The procedure for processing this type of request is outlined at the end of Procedure 1-2.

Text continued on p. 23

RELEASE OF MEDICAL INFORMATION

All information contained in the medical record is confidential, and the release of information is closely controlled. A properly completed and signed authorization form is required for the release of the following information.

PATIENT INFORMATION

Patient Name _____

Address _____   Social Security # _____

City _____ State _____ ZIP _____   Birth date _____/_____/_____

Phone (Home) _____ Work _____

RELEASE FROM:

Name _____

Address _____

City _____ State _____ ZIP_____

RELEASE TO:

Name _____

Address _____

City _____ State _____ ZIP_____

INFORMATION TO BE RELEASED:

1. GENERAL RELEASE:

____Entire Medical Record (excluding protected information)

____Hospital Records only (specify)_____

____Lab Results only (specify) _____

____X-ray Reports only (specify) _____

____Other Records (specify) _____

2. INFORMATION PROTECTED BY STATE/FEDERAL LAW:
If indicated below, I hereby authorize the disclosure and release of information regarding:

____Drug Abuse Diagnosis/Treatment

____Alcoholism Diagnosis/Treatment

____Mental Health Diagnosis/Treatment

____Sexually Transmitted Disease

PURPOSE/NEED FOR INFORMATION:

____Taking records to another doctor

____Moving

____Legal purposes

____Insurance purposes

____Worker's Compensation

____Other/Explain:_____

METHOD OF RELEASE:

____US Mail

____Fax

____Telephone

____To Patient

PATIENT AUTHORIZATION TO RELEASE INFORMATION:

Authorization is valid for 60 days only from the date of my signature. I reserve the right to revoke this authorization at any time prior to 60 days (except for action that has already been taken) by notifying the medical office in writing.

I understand that my records are protected under HIPAA (Health Insurance Portability and Accountability Act) Standards for Privacy of Individually Identifiable Information (45 CFR Parts 160 and 164) unless otherwise permitted by federal law. Any information released or received shall not be further relayed to any other facility or person without my written authorization. I also understand that such information will not be given, sold, transferred, or in any way relayed to any other person or party not specified above without my further written authorization.

I hereby grant authorization to release the information listed above. I certify that this request has been made voluntarily and that the information given above is accurate to the best of my knowledge.

_____   _____
Signature of Patient/Legally Responsible Party   Date

_____   _____
Witness Signature   Date

OFFICE USE ONLY

Information indicated above released on _____
                                          Date

Explanation of information released: _____

_____

Signature and credentials of individual releasing information: _____

Figure 1-14. Release of medical information form.

PROCEDURE **1-1**   Completion of a Consent to Treatment Form

Outcome Complete a consent to treatment form.

Equipment/Supplies

Consent to treatment form

1. **Procedural Step.** Type or print all required information on the consent to treatment form in the spaces provided (e.g., patient's full name, name of the procedure to be performed).
2. **Procedural Step.** Ensure that the physician has had a discussion to give the patient complete information about the procedure to be performed.
   Principle. For the patient's consent to be valid, it must be informed consent.
3. **Procedural Step.** Greet the patient and introduce yourself. Identify the patient the patient by his or her full name and date of birth. Explain the purpose of the consent form to the patient.
4. **Procedural Step.** Give the consent form to the patient, and ask him or her to read it. Ask the patient whether he or she has any questions.
5. **Procedural Step.** Ask the patient to sign the consent form. Witness the patient's signature by signing your name in the appropriate space on the form. Include today's date.
   Principle. Witnessing a signature means only that the medical assistant verified the identity of the patient and watched the patient sign the form; it does not mean that the medical assistant is attesting to the accuracy of the information provided.
6. **Procedural Step.** Provide the patient with a copy of the completed consent form for his or her files.
7. **Procedural Step.** File the original consent to treatment form in the patient's medical record.
   Principle. Maintaining the form provides legal documentation that the patient gave permission for treatment.

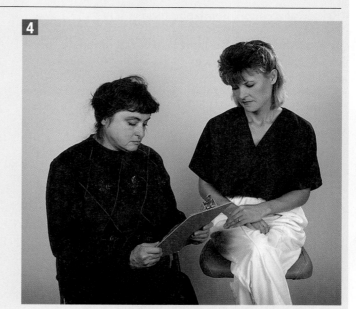

Ask the patient to read the consent form.

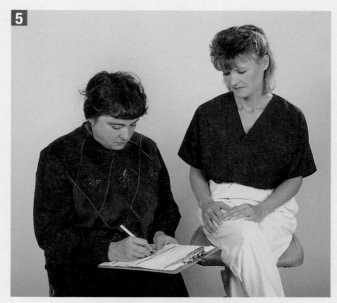

Ask the patient to sign the consent form.

PROCEDURE 1-1

PROCEDURE 1-2   Release of Medical Information

Outcome (1) Assist a patient in the completion of a release of medical information form. (2) Release medical information according to a completed release of medical information form.

Equipment/Supplies

Release of medical information form

1. **Procedural Step.** Greet the patient and introduce yourself. Identify the patient by his or her full name and date of birth. Explain the purpose of the release of medical information form. (*Note:* If you do not recognize the patient, ask him or her to provide photo identification such as a driver's license.)
2. **Procedural Step.** Provide the patient with a release of medical information form, and ask the patient to complete the form. Provide assistance if needed.
   Principle. Information from a patient's medical record can be released only on written authorization of the patient (except when permitted by law).
3. **Procedural Step.** Check to ensure all the requested information on the form has been completed by the patient.
4. **Procedural Step.** Ask the patient to sign the form. Witness the patient's signature by signing your name in the appropriate space on the form. Include today's date. If required by your medical office policy, ask the physician to initial the completed release of medical information form.

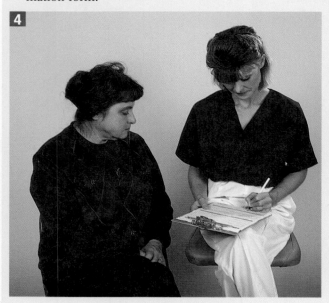

4

Witness the patient's signature.

Principle. To release information, the form must be signed by the patient authorizing the disclosure of medical information.

5. **Procedural Step.** Provide the patient with a copy of the release of medical information form for his or her files.
6. **Procedural Step.** Copy the information requested on the form. Release only the information requested. Include a copy of the completed release form with the medical information.
7. **Procedural Step.** Document what information is being released and the date of its release. Sign the document with your name and credentials.
8. **Procedural Step.** File the original document and the release of medical information form in the patient's medical record.
   Principle. Maintaining the release form provides legal documentation that the patient gave permission for the release of his or her medical information.
9. **Procedural Step.** Send the medical information to the appropriate site according to your medical office policy.

Mailed or Faxed Requests for Release of Medical Information

These steps should be followed when a completed release of medical information form has been mailed or faxed to the medical office:

1. **Procedural Step.** Check the expiration date on the release of medical information form. If the authorization is outdated, a new release form needs to be completed.
2. **Procedural Step.** Verify the authenticity of the signature on the form. This can be accomplished by comparing the patient's signature on the form with the patient's signature in his or her medical record. If you have any doubt as to the authenticity of the signature, do not release the records.
3. **Procedural Step.** Copy the information requested on the form. Release only the information requested. Include a copy of the completed release form with the medical information.
4. **Procedural Step.** Document what information is being released and the date of its release. Sign the document with your name and credentials.
5. **Procedural Step.** File the original document and the release of medical information form in the patient's medical record.
6. **Procedural Step.** Send the medical information according to your medical office policy.

MEDICAL RECORD FORMATS

Most medical offices rely on the use of paper medical records, known as **paper-based patient records (PPRs)**. Although most of the medical record is paper based, some patient data is maintained on the computer; this includes patient registration information and patient charges and payments. As technology advances, some offices are converting to an **electronic medical record (EMR)** for maintaining patient health information. With an electronic medical record, the entire record is stored in a database on the computer, including the health history report and physical examination report, progress notes, laboratory and diagnostic reports, and hospital reports. Because most offices currently use paper-based records, this chapter focuses on the PPR.

The way a PPR is organized is known as its *format*. The two main types of **medical record formats** are the **source-oriented record** and the **problem-oriented record.** Each of these formats is described.

Source-Oriented Record

The source-oriented format is used most often in the medical office for organizing a medical record. The documents in a source-oriented record are organized into sections based on the department, facility, or other source that generated the information (e.g., laboratory, hospital, consultant). Because documents from each source are filed together, it is easier to compare information from laboratory and diagnostic test results, assessments, and treatments.

Each section in a source-oriented record is separated from the other sections by a chart divider. Attached to each divider is a color-coded tab labeled with the title of its section (Figure 1-15). Within each of these sections, the documents are arranged according to date. Most offices use the reverse chronological order to arrange the documents. **Reverse chronological order** means that the most recent document is placed on top or in front of the others, and thus the oldest document is on the bottom or at the end of that section.

The titles that identify each section vary depending on the medical office's preference; however, typical examples include the following:
- History and Physical
- Progress Notes
- Medications
- Laboratory Reports
- ECG
- X-ray Reports
- Consultations
- Rehabilitation Therapy
- Home Health Care
- Hospital Reports
- Insurance
- Consents
- Correspondence
- Miscellaneous

Problem-Oriented Record

The documents in a problem-oriented record (POR), or problem-oriented medical record (POMR), are organized according to the patient's health problems. The advantage of using the POR is that each of the patient's problems can be defined and followed individually. The POR is developed in four stages:
1. Establishing a *database*
2. Compiling a *problem list*
3. Devising a *plan* of action for each problem
4. Following each problem with *progress notes*

Database

The first step in developing a POR is to establish a database. The database consists of a collection of subjective and objective data. These data include the health history report, physical examination report, and results of baseline laboratory and diagnostic tests. The information in the database is used to identify and compile a problem list.

What Would You Do? What Would You *Not* Do?

Case Study 2

Tessa Walsh, her husband, and two children are moving to another state. They will be leaving in 2 days. Tessa calls the office to have their medical records transferred to their new physician. Tessa's daughter has type 1 diabetes, so it is important that this be done as soon as possible. Tessa is quite annoyed to learn that she has to come in and sign a special form. She says that their medical records belong to them. Tessa says that the whole family has been coming there for the past 8 years and is well known by the physician and staff. She says that they have been good patients, have followed the physician's advice, and have always paid their bills on time. Tessa thinks that verbal permission should be enough. She's extremely busy packing and taking care of other moving details and doesn't have a minute to spare. ■

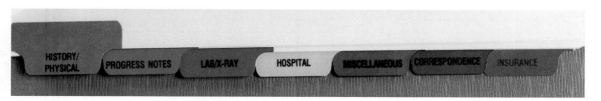

Figure 1-15. Chart dividers in a source-oriented record.

Problem List

The problem list is developed shortly after the database is completed and consists of a list of all of the patient's problems (Figure 1-16). A **problem** is defined as any patient condition that requires observation, diagnosis, management, or patient education. This includes not only medical problems but also psychological and social problems. The problem list is a crucial part of the POR and is always located in the front of the medical record.

The problem list should be thought of as a table of contents for the record. Each problem in the list is numbered and titled. The problem title is stated as a diagnosis, a physiologic finding, a symptom, or an abnormal test result.

All subsequent data (plans and progress notes) added to the medical record are cross-referenced to these numbered problems.

The problem list is modified as needed. If a new problem is identified, it is added to the list and dated accordingly. When a problem is resolved, it is marked as such, and the date is recorded.

Plan

After examining the problem list, the physician develops the third section of the POR. This involves devising a plan of action for further evaluation and treatment of each problem. Each plan begins with a heading that identifies the

---

PATIENT RECORD

Name: Morani, Betty

Number: _____ Blood Type: A+

ALLERGIES/SENSITIVITY: Codeine, Sulfa

Prob. No.	Date	PROBLEM DESCRIPTION	Date Resolved	Index	Prob. No.	Date	PROBLEM DESCRIPTION	Date Resolved	Index
1	10/01	Hypertension - essential		✓					
2	10/01	Diabetes mellitus (mild)		✓					
3	1/04	L. Retinopathy	see below						
4	4/2008	Atherosclerosis with cerebral vascular insuffic.							
5	4/2008	Hearing loss							
6	1/2008	HBP Non-compliance	2/04						
3	1/2008	Bilat. Grade II Retinopathy							

Prob. No.	CONTINUING MEDICATIONS	Start	Stop	Prob. No.	CONTINUING MEDICATIONS	Start	Stop
1	Sinoserp 1 mg. b.i.d.	10/01	10/05				
2	Orinase 0.5 gm. daily	10/01	10/05				
1	Hydrodiuril 50 mg. A.M.	10/05					
2	1500 cal. diet low Na hi K	2/2008					

Periodic Health Examination	Dates	1/04	4/2006				

Figure 1-16. POR problem list. (Courtesy of and modified from Miller Communications, Norwalk, Conn.)

number of the problem, followed by the plan of action for the problem. This may include plans for laboratory and diagnostic tests, medical or surgical treatment, therapy, and patient education.

Progress Notes

The last stage in the development of the POR is the follow-up for each problem, or the progress notes (Figure 1-17). The progress notes begin with the number of a problem and include the following four categories:

Subjective data: Subjective data obtained from the patient

Objective data: Objective data obtained by observation, physical examination, and laboratory and diagnostic tests

Assessment: The physician's interpretation of the current condition based on an analysis of the subjective and objective data

Plan: Proposed treatment for the patient

The acronym for this process is **SOAP,** and the writing of progress notes in this format is called *soaping.* Some physicians who use the source-oriented format have found it advantageous to record progress notes in SOAP format. This structured type of note increases the physician's ability to deal with each problem clearly and to analyze data in an orderly, systematic manner.

PREPARING A MEDICAL RECORD FOR A NEW PATIENT

When a patient comes to the medical office for his or her first visit, a medical record must be prepared for that patient (Procedure 1-3). The method used to prepare the record depends on the following criteria: the format used to organize the record, the filing system, and the type of storage equipment. Most medical offices use the source-oriented format to organize their medical records, the alphabetic filing system to arrange the records, and shelf filing units to store the medical records. Methods used to prepare a medical record are described in the following sections and are based on these criteria.

Medical Record Supplies

Certain supplies are required to prepare a medical record. These supplies are categorized and described next.

File Folders

A file folder is a protective cover made of a heavy material such as manila card stock. A file folder is used to hold medical record documents in an organized format. Flexible metal fasteners are typically used to hold documents in the folder. Folders are available with fasteners located on the top or left side of the folder.

Folders are available with tabs. A tab is a projection extending from a folder and is used to identify its contents. The tab is located on either the side or the top of the folder. A folder with a tab extending across its entire side or top is called a *full cut tab.*

In the medical office, a file folder with a full cut side tab is typically used to prepare a new patient's chart. There are indentations at intervals along the full cut tab to indicate the placement of adhesive labels. This ensures that the labels on all the medical records are affixed at the same place on the file folders.

Folder Labels

Labels to identify the medical record are commercially available in rolls or continuous folded strips for typewriter use. Labels also are available on 8½ × 11–inch sheets for

---

Chart Divider Subject Titles and Documents Typically Filed under Each Title

History and Physical
- Health history
- Physical examination report

Progress Notes
- Progress notes
- Medication record

Laboratory/X-ray
- Hematology report
- Clinical chemistry report
- Serology report
- Urinalysis report
- Microbiology report
- Parasitology report
- Cytology report
- Histology report
- Electrocardiogram report
- Holter monitor report

Laboratory/X-ray—cont'd
- Sigmoidoscopy report
- Colonoscopy report
- Spirometry report
- Radiology report
- Diagnostic imaging report

Hospital
- History and physical report
- Operative report
- Pathology report
- Discharge summary report
- Emergency department report

Correspondence
- Consultation report
- Letter from patient
- Letter from patient's attorney
- Referral letter

Insurance
- Copy of patient's insurance card
- Precertification authorization for hospital admission
- Request for additional information from insurance company

Miscellaneous
- Consent to treatment form
- Release of medical information form
- Home health care report
- Physical therapy report
- Occupational therapy report
- Speech therapy report

PROBLEM-ORIENTED PROGRESS NOTES

Name Jessica Michaels			DOB 9/20/02	Doctor Frank Edwards, MD

DATE	TIME	PROBLEM NUMBER	FORMAT: Problem Number and TITLE: S = Subjective O = Objective A = Assessment P = Plan
11/5/08	9:30 AM	1	S: Mother states that her child has had a runny nose and her throat has been sore for 2 days.
			O: Vital signs: T 98.8 P 96 R 24
			Weight 42 lb.
			General: alert and active. HEENT: sclera clear.
			TMs negative. Positive clear rhinorrhea. Pharynx benign.
			Heart: regular without murmur. Lungs: clear to
			auscultation and percussion. Abdomen: negative
			tenderness. Positive bowel sounds x4. GU: negative
			Neuro: good tone.
			A: Upper respiratory tract infection.
			P: 1. A prescription for Rondec DM, 1/2 tsp q6h prn
			cough and congestion.
			2. Instructed mother to contact office if child does
			not improve.

Figure 1-17. POR SOAP progress notes. (Courtesy of and modified from Briggs, Des Moines, Iowa.)

use with a computer and printer. The most common types of labels used in the medical office include name labels, alphabetic color-coded labels, color-coded year labels, and miscellaneous chart labels.

Chart Dividers

Chart dividers are used to identify each section of the medical record by subject (see Figure 1-15). Chart dividers consist of a heavy material such as manila card stock. Attached to each divider is a color-coded tab labeled with a subject title; the most frequently used subject titles are illustrated in the box on p. 25, along with the documents typically filed under each title.

PROCEDURE **1-3**   Preparing a Medical Record

Outcome Prepare a medical record.

The following procedure outlines the method for preparing a medical record for a new patient using the following organization: a source-oriented format stored in shelf files using a color-coded alphabetic filing system.

Equipment/Supplies

- Patient registration form
- Notice of Privacy Practices (NPP)
- NPP acknowledgment form
- File folder with a full cut side tab
- Metal fasteners
- Name labels

- Color-coded alphabetic bar labels
- Miscellaneous chart labels
- Set of chart dividers
- Blank preprinted forms
- Two-hole punch

1. **Procedural Step.** Greet the patient when he or she arrives at the medical office. Introduce yourself and identify the patient. Verify that the patient is a new patient.
2. **Procedural Step.** Ask the patient to do the following:
   a. Complete a patient registration form.
   b. Read a Notice of Privacy Practices (NPP).
   c. Sign an NPP acknowledgment form.
3. **Procedural Step.** When the patient returns the completed forms, check the patient registration form for accuracy, and make sure that you can read the patient's handwriting. If you have any questions regarding the information on the form, ask the patient for clarification. If required by the medical office policy, ask the patient for his or her insurance card and make a copy of it.
   Principle. A copy of the patient's insurance card is used for third-party billing.
4. **Procedural Step.** Enter the data on the completed registration record into the computer.
5. **Procedural Step.** Assemble supplies needed to prepare the medical record. Type the patient's full name on a name label following these guidelines:
   a. Type the patient's name in transposed order as follows: last name, first name, middle name (or initial).
   b. Type the patient's name two or three typewritten spaces from the left edge of the label and one line down from the top of the label.
   c. Ensure the patient's name is spelled correctly.

Principle. Following these guidelines facilitates the accurate and efficient filing of the patient's medical record.

6. **Procedural Step.** Determine the first two letters of the patient's last name and select the appropriate alphabetic color-coded labels. Attach the color-coded labels to the (full cut) side tab. The labels should be affixed to the folder using the label placement indentations on the tab.
   Principle. Using the label placement indentations ensures that all labels on medical records are affixed at the same place.
7. **Procedural Step.** Affix the name label immediately above the first color-coded alphabetic label.
8. **Procedural Step.** Attach any additional chart labels, such as a year label and miscellaneous chart labels (e.g., allergy, insurance), to the folder according to the office policy.
9. **Procedural Step.** Insert the chart dividers onto the metal fasteners of the file folder.
10. **Procedural Step.** Place the original patient registration form in the front of the medical record. Place the signed NPP acknowledgment form and the copy of the patient's insurance card in the appropriate section of the record.
11. **Procedural Step.** Label preprinted forms to be placed in the record with required information such as the

PROCEDURE 1-3 Preparing a Medical Record—cont'd

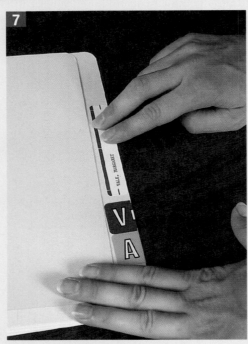

Affix the name label.

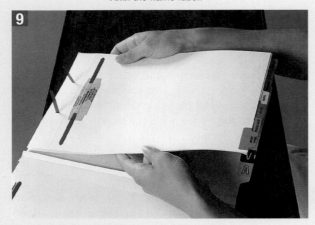

Insert the chart dividers into the metal fasteners.

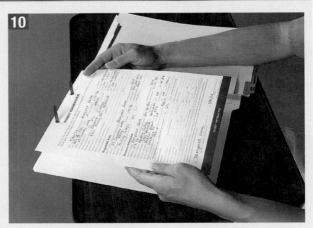

Place the patient registration form in the front of the medical record.

patient's name and date. These forms typically include the medical history form, physical examination form, progress note sheets, and a medication record form. If the forms are not prepunched, the medical assistant must use a two-hole punch to insert two holes into the top or side of the form.

12. **Procedural Step.** Insert each form under its proper chart divider. Refer to the box on p. 25 for a list of chart divider subject titles and documents typically filed under each title.

13. **Procedural Step.** Check the medical record to ensure that it has been prepared properly.

Memories *from* Externship

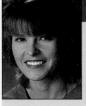

Dawn Bennett: During my externship as a medical assisting student, I was placed in a family practice clinic. I was very nervous my first day, wondering how in the world I would be able to remember everything I had learned in school.

My first patients were an elderly couple. The wife was there for some test results for cancer. I looked at the results, and they were positive. After the physician relayed the results, the husband broke down. He had just lost his granddaughter to a heart attack and his son-in-law to a stroke. You could tell that he just could not bear losing his wife too.

One week later, the elderly man's wife was placed in a nursing home. He came into our office for an appointment. As I was working him up, he was telling me stories about himself and his wife when they were first married. He looked so sad. I sat with him for a few minutes after completing his workup and gave his stories my full attention. As I was leaving the room, a smile came across his face, and he thanked me for listening to him. I realized that working in a physician's office is more than just knowing what I learned in school. Compassion and showing the patients you really do care about them is just as important. I felt good about myself that day. ∎

What Would You Do? What Would You *Not* Do?

Case Study 3

Brett Oberlin is 21 years old and lives at home. He commutes to a local college and is a junior majoring in art education. His mother and father have come to the medical office and ask to see his medical record. The physician is attending a medical conference and will not return for another 4 days. Mr. and Mrs. Oberlin found some medications in Brett's room and looked them up on the Internet. They found out that they are used to treat HIV infection. Brett would not talk to them about the medications and told them he is an adult and it is none of their business. Mr. and Mrs. Oberlin are very concerned about Brett. They also are worried about other members of the family being exposed to HIV. They say that because they are supporting him, they should be allowed to see his record. ■

TAKING A HEALTH HISTORY

The health history is a collection of subjective health data obtained by interviewing the patient and by having the patient complete a preprinted health history form that is then reviewed for completeness by the medical assistant. A thorough history is taken for each new patient, and subsequent office visits (in the form of progress notes) provide information regarding changes in the patient's illness or treatment. A quiet, comfortable room that allows for privacy encourages the patient to communicate honestly and openly. Showing genuine interest in and concern for the patient reduces apprehension and facilitates the collection of data.

Components of the Health History

The health history is taken before the physical examination, providing the physician the opportunity to compare findings. The health history consists of seven parts or sections.

Identification Data

The identification data section is included at the beginning of the health history form to obtain basic demographic data on the patient (Figure 1-18A). The patient completes the identification data section.

Chief Complaint

The chief complaint (CC) identifies the patient's reason for seeking care—that is, the symptom causing the patient the most trouble. The CC is used as a foundation for the more detailed information obtained for the present illness and review of systems sections of the health history. The medical assistant is usually responsible for obtaining the CC from the patient and recording it in the patient's chart. In most offices, this information is recorded on a preprinted, lined form (see Figure 1-18G). Certain guidelines must be followed in obtaining and recording the CC, as follows:

- An open-ended question should be used to elicit the CC from the patient: What seems to be the problem? How can we help you today? What can we do for you today?
- The CC should be limited to one or two symptoms and should refer to a specific, rather than vague, symptom.
- The CC should be recorded concisely and briefly, using the patient's own words as much as possible.
- The duration of the symptom (onset) should be included in the CC.
- The medical assistant should avoid using names of diseases or diagnostic terms to record the CC.

Recording Chief Complaints

The following are correct and incorrect examples of recording chief complaints.

   Correct Examples
- Burning during urination that has lasted for 2 days
- Pain in the shoulder that started 2 weeks ago
- Shortness of breath for the past month
   Incorrect Examples
- Has not felt well for the past 2 weeks (This statement refers to a vague, rather than a specific, complaint.)
- Ear pain and fever (The duration of the symptoms is not listed.)
- Pain upon urination indicative of a urinary tract infection (Names of diseases should not be used to record the chief complaint; the duration of the symptom is not listed.)

Present Illness

The present illness (PI) is an expansion of the chief complaint and includes a full description of the patient's current illness from the time of its onset. The medical assistant is often responsible for completing this section of the health history, which is recorded on the same form as the chief complaint (see Figure 1-18G). To complete this section of the health history, the medical assistant asks the patient questions to obtain a detailed description of the symptom causing the greatest problem. Much skill and practice in asking the proper questions are required to elicit detailed information. A general guide for obtaining further information on symptoms is presented in Procedure 1-4, and a more thorough study for analyzing a symptom is included in the *Study Guide* for students (Chapter 1).

Past History

The past medical history is a review of the patient's past medical status (see Figure 1-18B). Obtaining information on past medical care assists the physician in providing optimal care for the current problem. Most medical offices ask the patient to complete this section of the health history through a checklist type of form. The medical assistant should assist the patient with this section as necessary by offering to answer any questions regarding the information required. The past history includes the following areas:
- Major illnesses
- Childhood diseases

PATIENT HEALTH HISTORY

A **IDENTIFICATION DATA**   Please print the following information.

Today's date _____

Name _____

_____ Male _____ Female

Address _____

_____ Married _____ Separated _____ Divorced _____ Widowed _____ Single

_____

Date of Birth _____

Telephone _____   _____
Home number   Work number

B **PAST HISTORY**

Have you ever had the following: (Circle "no" or "yes", leave blank if uncertain)

Measles _____ no yes	Heart Disease _____ no yes	Diabetes _____ no yes	Hemorrhoids _____ no yes
Mumps _____ no yes	Arthritis _____ no yes	Cancer _____ no yes	Asthma _____ no yes
Chickenpox _____ no yes	Sexually Transmitted no yes Disease	Polio _____ no yes	Allergies _____ no yes
Whooping Cough _____ no yes	Anemia _____ no yes	Glaucoma _____ no yes	Eczema _____ no yes
Scarlet Fever _____ no yes	Bladder Infections _____ no yes	Hernia _____ no yes	AIDS or HIV+ _____ no yes
Diphtheria _____ no yes	Epilepsy _____ no yes	Blood or Plasma _____ no yes Transfusions	Infectious Mono _____ no yes
Pneumonia _____ no yes	Migraine Headaches _____ no yes	Back Trouble _____ no yes	Bronchitis _____ no yes
Rheumatic Fever _____ no yes	Tuberculosis _____ no yes	High Blood _____ no yes Pressure	Mitral Valve Prolapse no yes
Stroke _____ no yes	Ulcer _____ no yes	Thyroid Disease _____ no yes	Any other disease _____ no yes Please list: _____
Hepatitis _____ no yes	Kidney Disease _____ no yes	Bleeding Tendency _____ no yes	_____

MAJOR HOSPITALIZATIONS: If you have ever been hospitalized for any major medical illness or operation, write in your most recent hospitalizations below.

Hospitalizations	Year	Operation or illness	Name of hospital	City and state
1st Hospitalization				
2nd Hospitalization				
3rd Hospitalization				
4th Hospitalization				

TESTS AND IMMUNIZATIONS: Mark an X next to those that you have had.

Tests: Immunizations:

☐ TB Test   ☐ Electrocardiogram   ☐ Influenza

☐ Rectal/Hemoccult   ☐ Chest x-ray   ☐ Hepatitis B

☐ Sigmoidoscopy   ☐ Mammogram   ☐ Tetanus

☐ Colonoscopy   ☐ Pap Test   ☐ MMR

☐ Polio

ALLERGIES: List all allergies (foods, drugs, environment). ☐ None

_____

_____

_____

_____

CURRENT MEDICATIONS: List the following that you are currently taking: Prescription medications, over-the-counter (OTC) medications, vitamin supplements, and herbal supplements. ☐ None

Medication   Frequency

_____

_____

_____

ACCIDENTS/ INJURIES: Describe all serious accidents, severe injuries, head injury, or fractures. Include the date each occurred. ☐ None

Accident/Injury: Date:

_____

_____

_____

_____

Figure 1-18. Health history form.

C FAMILY HISTORY

For each member of your family, follow the purple or blue line across the page and check boxes for:
1. His or her present state of health
2. Any illnesses he or she has had

	Good Health	Poor Health	Deceased	If deceased, write in age and cause of death.	Allergies or Asthma	Diabetes	Heart Disease	Stroke	Cancer	High Blood Pressure	Glaucoma	Arthritis	Ulcer	Kidney Disease	Mental Health Problems	Alcohol/Drug Abuse	Obesity	High Cholesterol	Thyroid Disease
Father:																			
Mother:																			
Brothers/Sisters:																			

D SOCIAL HISTORY

EDUCATION _____ High school _____ College _____ Postgraduate

Occupation _____ Years _____

Previous occupations _____ Years _____

_____ Years _____

Have you ever been exposed to any of the following in your environment?

☐ Excess dust (coal, lime, rock)   ☐ Cleaning fluids/solvents   ☐ Radiation   ☐ Other toxic materials
☐ Sand   ☐ Hair spray   ☐ Insecticides
☐ Chemicals   ☐ Smoke or auto exhaust fumes   ☐ Paints

Please answer the follwing questions by placing an X in the box in front of the word Yes or No, except where you are asked for specific information. This information is obviously highly confidential and will be released to other healthcare professionals or insurance carriers ONLY with your consent.

DIET:
Do you eat a good breakfast? ☐ Yes ☐ No
Do you snack between meals (soft drinks, chips, candy bars)? ☐ Yes ☐ No
Do you eat fresh fruits and vegetables each day? ☐ Yes ☐ No
Do you eat whole grain breads and cereals? ☐ Yes ☐ No
Is your diet high in fat content? ☐ Yes ☐ No
Is your diet high in cholesterol content? ☐ Yes ☐ No
Is your diet high in salt content? ☐ Yes ☐ No
Are you allergic to any foods? ☐ Yes ☐ No
How many glasses of water do you drink each day? _____
How would you describe your overall eating habits? ☐ Excellent ☐ Good ☐ Fair ☐ Poor

PERSONAL HISTORY:
Do you find it hard to make decisions? ☐ Yes ☐ No
Do you find it hard to concentrate or remember? ☐ Yes ☐ No
Do you feel depressed? ☐ Yes ☐ No
Do you have difficulty relaxing? ☐ Yes ☐ No
Do you have a tendency to worry a lot? ☐ Yes ☐ No
Have you gained or lost much weight recently? ☐ Yes ☐ No
Do you lose your temper often? ☐ Yes ☐ No
Are you disturbed by any work or family problems? ☐ Yes ☐ No
Are you having sexual difficulties? ☐ Yes ☐ No
Have you ever considered committing suicide? ☐ Yes ☐ No
Have you ever desired or sought psychiatric help? ☐ Yes ☐ No

EXERCISE:
Do you exercise on a regular basis? ☐ Yes ☐ No
Does your job require strenuous, sustained physical work? ☐ Yes ☐ No

SLEEP PATTERNS:
Do you seem to feel exhausted or fatigued most of the time? ☐ Yes ☐ No
Do you have difficulty either falling asleep or staying asleep? ☐ Yes ☐ No

USE OF TOBACCO/ALCOHOL/CAFFEINE/DRUGS: Amt:
How much do you smoke per day? ☐ Cigarettes __
☐ Don't smoke ☐ Cigars/pipes __
Do you take two or more alcoholic drinks per day? ☐ Yes ☐ No
Do you drink six or more cups of coffee or tea per day? ☐ Yes ☐ No
Are you a regular user of sleeping pills, marijuana, tranquilizers, pain killers, etc? ☐ Yes ☐ No
Have you ever used heroin, cocaine, LSD, PCP, etc? ☐ Yes ☐ No

List any country outside the USA you have visited in the past six months. _____

When did you have your last physical examination? _____

Figure 1-18, cont'd. Health history form.

Continued

PROCEDURE 1-4   Obtaining and Recording Patient Symptoms

Outcome Obtain and record patient symptoms.

Equipment/Supplies

- Medical record of the patient to be interviewed
- Black ink pen

1. **Procedural Step.** Assemble the equipment. Ensure that you have the correct patient's record and a black ink pen for charting patient symptoms.
   Principle. Black ink must be used to provide a permanent record.
2. **Procedural Step.** Go to the waiting room and ask the patient to come back.
3. **Procedural Step.** Escort the patient to a quiet, comfortable room, such as an examination room, that allows for privacy.
   Principle. Patient symptoms should be taken in a room that encourages communication.
4. **Procedural Step.** In a calm and friendly manner, greet the patient and introduce yourself. Identify the patient by his or her full name and date of birth.
   Principle. A warm introduction sets a positive tone for the remainder of the interview.
5. **Procedural Step.** Ask the patient to be seated. You should seat yourself so that you face the patient at a distance of 3 to 4 feet.
   Principle. This type of seating arrangement facilitates open communication.
6. **Procedural Step.** Use good communication skills to interact with the patient. These include the following:
   a. Use the patient's name of choice.
   b. Show genuine interest and concern for the patient.
   c. Maintain appropriate eye contact.
   d. Use terminology the patient can understand.
   e. Listen carefully and attentively to the patient.
   f. Pay attention to the patient's nonverbal messages.
   g. Avoid judgmental comments.
   h. Avoid rushing the patient.
7. **Procedural Step.** Locate the progress note sheet in the patient's medical record. Chart the date and time and the abbreviation for chief complaint (CC).
8. **Procedural Step.** Use an open-ended question to elicit the chief complaint, such as "What seems to be the problem?"
   Principle. An open-ended question allows the patient to verbalize freely.
9. **Procedural Step.** Chart the chief complaint following the charting guidelines outlined on pp. 34–35 and pp. 42–43. In addition, these guidelines should be followed:
   a. Limit the chief complaint to one or two symptoms, and refer to a specific rather than a vague symptom.
   b. Chart the chief complaint concisely and briefly, using the patient's own words as much as possible.
   c. Include the duration of the symptom (onset) in the chief complaint.
   d. Avoid using names of diseases or diagnostic terms to record the chief complaint.
10. **Procedural Step.** Obtain additional information regarding the chief complaint using *what, when,* and *where* questions. Following proper charting guidelines, chart this information after the chief complaint.

What *Questions:*

- What exactly have you been experiencing?
- Does the symptom occur suddenly or gradually?
- Does anything make it worse?

Where *Question:*

- Where is the symptom located?

When *Questions:*

- When did the symptom first occur?
- How long does it last?
- Does anything cause it to occur?
  Principle. This information provides a complete description of the chief complaint.
11. **Procedural Step.** Thank the patient and proceed to the next step in the patient workup. (This usually includes measuring vital signs and height and weight and preparing the patient as needed for the physical examination [see Chapters 4 and 5].)
12. **Procedural Step.** Inform the patient the physician will be with him or her soon.
13. **Procedural Step.** Place the patient's medical record where it can be reviewed by the physician (as designated by the medical office policy).
    Principle. The physician will want to review the patient's medical record before examining the patient.

CHARTING EXAMPLE	
Date	
6/30/08	3:15 p.m. CC: Intense pain in the Ⓛ ear for the past 2 days. Pt states pain is sharp and continuous. Pt noted sl yellow discharge from Ⓛ ear. Fever of 101° F began last night about 9 p.m. Took Tylenol 2 tabs @ 8 a.m.
	—————————— D. Bennett, CMA

Other Activities That Need to Be Charted

Procedures

The medical assistant frequently charts procedures performed on the patient, including vital signs, weight and height, visual acuity, and ear irrigations. Procedures should be charted immediately after being performed; from a legal standpoint, a procedure that is not documented was not performed. In general, the following information should be included: the date and time, the type of procedure, the outcome, and the patient reaction. The specific information to be charted is included with each procedure presented in this text.

CHARTING EXAMPLE	
Date	
6/30/08	9:15 a.m. Irrigated Ⓡ ear c̄ 200 ml of
	normal saline @ 98.6° F. Mod amt of
	cerumen in returned solution. Pt states can
	hear better. —————————D. Bennett, CMA

Procedure.

Administration of Medication

Charting medications administered to the patient is an important responsibility in the medical office. The recording should include the date and time, the name of the medication, the dosage given, the route of administration, the injection site used (for parenteral medication), and any significant observations or patient reactions.

CHARTING EXAMPLE	
Date	
6/30/08	10:15 a.m. Bicillin 900,00 units IM, Ⓛ
	dorsogluteal. ————— D. Bennett, CMA

Administration of medication.

Specimen Collection

Each time a specimen is collected from a patient, the medical assistant should chart the date and time of the collection, the type of specimen, and the area of the body from which the specimen was obtained. If the specimen is to be sent to an outside laboratory for testing, this information also should be charted, including the tests requested, the date the specimen was sent, and where it was sent. In this way, the physician would know that the specimen was collected and sent to the laboratory when test results are not back yet.

CHARTING EXAMPLE	
Date	
6/30/08	1:30 p.m. Venous blood spec collected from Ⓡ
	arm. Sent to Ross Lab for CBC and diff on
	6/30/08 ——————— D. Bennett, CMA
Date	
6/30/08	2:00 p.m. Throat spec collected. Sent to
	Ross Lab for C&S on 6/30/08 ———————
	——————— D. Bennett, CMA

Specimen collection.

Diagnostic Procedures and Laboratory Tests

Diagnostic procedures and laboratory tests ordered for a patient should always be charted in the medical record. If the patient does not undergo the test, documented proof exists that the test was ordered. Charting diagnostic procedures and laboratory tests protects the physician legally and refreshes the physician's memory of the procedures and tests being run on the patient when results are not yet back from the testing facility. Information to include in the charting entry are the date and time, the type of procedure or test ordered, the scheduling date, and where it is being performed.

CHARTING EXAMPLE	
Date	
6/30/08	10:15 a.m. Mammography scheduled for
	7/5/08 at Grant Hospital. ———————
	——————— D. Bennett, CMA
Date	
6/30/08	11:30 a.m. Pt given lab request for GTT at
	Ross Lab. ——————— D. Bennett, CMA

Diagnostic/laboratory tests.

Results of Laboratory Tests

It is usually unnecessary to chart results from laboratory reports returned from outside laboratories because the report itself is filed in the patient's record. In case of a STAT request or critical findings, the test results may be telephoned to the medical office, requiring the medical assistant to record the results on a report form. Careful recording is essential to avoid errors, which could affect the patient's diagnosis. Results of laboratory tests performed by the medical assistant in the office should be charted in the medical record and must include the date and time, name of the test, and test results.

CHARTING EXAMPLE

Date	
6/30/08	8:00 a.m. FBS: 82 mg/dL.———————
	———————————— D. Bennett, CMA
Date	
6/30/08	4:15 p.m. Quick Vue+ Mono Test: neg ———
	———————————— D. Bennett, CMA

Laboratory test results.

Patient Instructions

It often is necessary to relay instructions to a patient regarding medical care (e.g., wound care, cast care, care of sutures). The medical assistant should chart this information, taking care to include the date and time and the type of instructions relayed to the patient. Many medical offices have printed instruction sheets that are given to the patient. The patient is asked to sign a form, which is filed in the patient's record, indicating that he or she has read and understands the instructions (Figure 1-20). The form also should be signed by the medical assistant, who functions as a signature witness. This protects the physician legally in the event that the patient fails to follow the instructions and causes further harm or damage to a body part.

Other areas in which the medical assistant is responsible for charting in the medical record include missed or canceled appointments, telephone calls from patients, medication refills, and changes in medication or dosage by the physician.

CHARTING EXAMPLE

Date	
6/30/08	9:30 a.m. Instructions provided for BSE. Pt
	given a BSE educational brochure. ———
	———————————— D. Bennett, CMA
Date	
6/30/08	10:00 a.m. Explained wound care. Written
	instructions provided. Signed copy in chart.
	To return in 2 days for suture removal. ——
	———————————— D. Bennett, CMA
Date	
6/30/08	10:25 a.m. Provided instructions for applying
	a heating pad to the lower back. —————
	———————————— D. Bennett, CMA

Patient instructions.

CHARTING EXAMPLE

Date	
6/30/08	11:15 a.m. Phoned office. States that
	swelling in the ⓡ ankle is almost gone.
	———————————— D. Bennett, CMA
Date	
6/30/08	1:15 p.m. Missed appointment scheduled for
	6/30/08 @ 1:00 p.m. ——— D. Bennett, CMA

Telephone call and missed appointment.

 *Check out the **Companion CD** bound with the book to access additional interactive activities.*

PATIENT INSTRUCTIONS FOR WOUND CARE

Name of patient: _____

Follow the instructions indicated below for care of your wound:

1. Use ice bag and elevate to reduce swelling and pain. Elevate higher than your heart.
2. You may take aspirin/Tylenol for pain.
3. Keep the dressing clean and dry.
4. Replace the dressing within _____ days.
5. Discard the dressing within _____ days.
6. Cleanse the wound daily as instructed.
7. Stitches should be removed in _____ days.
8. Despite the greatest of care, any wound can become infected. If your wound becomes red or swollen, shows pus or red streaks, or feels more sore instead of less sore, contact the physician **immediately.**

I have received and understand the above instructions:

Patient (or representative): _____

Relationship to patient: _____

Witness: _____   Time and date: _____

Figure 1-20. Instruction sheet for patients.

MEDICAL PRACTICE and the LAW

Documentation can be a deciding factor in a legal case. Everything you do for a patient should be documented in a factual manner in the medical record, or "chart." When a legal issue arises, often several years pass before it comes to trial. If you are involved, you will be asked detailed questions as to your actions on a particular day for a particular patient. Few people have accurate memories for that long. Juries give more credibility to documentation performed at the time of the action than to a memory of years ago.

Ethically, you owe the patient thorough documentation to provide optimal continuity of care. Remember that all patient information is confidential.

Proper charting is a crucial skill for a medical assistant to master. Although proper documentation would not prevent a lawsuit, it might determine the outcome. Pay particular attention to the rules for consents and charting guidelines outlined in this chapter, and follow them to the letter. ■

What Would You Do? What Would You *Not* Do?   RESPONSES

Case Study 1
Page 5
What Did Dawn Do?
- ❑ Listened carefully to Mrs. Celeste and relayed concern through both verbal and nonverbal behavior.
- ❑ Reassured Mrs. Celeste that her information would be kept completely confidential. Explained to Mrs. Celeste that health care professionals are required by law to keep all patient information confidential.
- ❑ Told Mrs. Celeste how important it is to chart information that relates to her health. Explained that the physician must have accurate data to diagnose and treat her. Stressed that certain medications can be harmful to a patient if consumed with alcohol.
- ❑ Gave Mrs. Celeste information (including brochures) on community agencies that could help her. Explained that these agencies are required to maintain confidentiality and encouraged her to contact them.

What Did Dawn Not *Do?*
- ❑ Did not tell Mrs. Celeste to go to a different physician to ensure her information remained private.
- ❑ Did not tell Mrs. Celeste that she needed to stop drinking before it affected her health.

What Would You Do/What Would You *Not* Do? Review Dawn's response and place a checkmark next to the information you included in your response. List the additional information you included in your response.

_____
_____
_____
_____

Case Study 2
Page 23
What Did Dawn Do?
- ❑ Reassured Tessa that she and her family have been good patients and apologized for the inconvenience.
- ❑ Told Tessa that it is against the law to transfer medical records without the patient's written authorization. Explained that the reason for the law is to safeguard a patient's privacy.
- ❑ Asked Tessa if she has a fax machine because the forms could be faxed to her for signing and then faxed back to the office. If not, explained that Tessa and her husband would need to come to the office to sign release forms.

What Did Dawn Not *Do?*
- ❑ Did not get defensive about Tessa being so annoyed.
- ❑ Did not send their medical records to the new physician without the signed release forms.

What Would You Do/What Would You *Not* Do? Review Dawn's response and place a checkmark next to the information you included in your response. List the additional information you included in your response.

_____
_____
_____
_____

Case Study 3
Page 29
What Did Dawn Do?
- ❑ Listened to and empathized with Mr. and Mrs. Oberlin's concerns.

What Would You Do? What Would You *Not* Do?   RESPONSES—cont'd

❑ Told Mr. and Mrs. Oberlin that because Brett is of adult age, it would be against the law to let them see his medical record without his written authorization. Explained that the law is there to protect a patient's right to privacy and just as it protects Brett's right, the law also protects their right so that no one can obtain information from their medical records without their authorization.

❑ Suggested that they talk with Brett again regarding the situation.

What Did Dawn Not Do?

❑ Did not give them any information from Brett's medical record.

What Would You Do/What Would You *Not* Do? Review Dawn's response and place a checkmark next to the information you included in your response. List the additional information you included in your response.

_____

_____

_____

_____

APPLY YOUR KNOWLEDGE

Choose the best answer to each of the following questions.

1. Marcus Westerfield exhibits a positive test result on a Hemoccult fecal occult blood test. Dr. Diagnosis has decided to perform a flexible sigmoidoscopy on Marcus to assist in determining the cause of his bleeding. Marcus must sign a consent to treatment form before undergoing this procedure. Before he signs this form, Dawn Bennett, CMA, must make sure that:
   A. Marcus has sanitized his hands.
   B. A notary public is available to witness Marcus's signature.
   C. Dr. Diagnosis has discussed all aspects of the procedure with Marcus.
   D. Someone is available to drive Marcus home after the procedure.

2. After performing the flexible sigmoidoscopy on Marcus, Dr. Diagnosis dictates the results of the examination. Dawn transcribes the report and files it in Marcus's medical record under this chart divider:
   A. History and Physical.
   B. Laboratory/X-ray.
   C. Hospital.
   D. Progress Notes.

3. Michael Johnson is moving to Michigan. He calls the office and asks Dawn Bennett, CMA, to transfer his medical record to his new physician. Dawn should:
   A. Explain to Michael that his medical record belongs to Dr. Diagnosis and cannot leave the office.
   B. Make a copy of the medical record and send it to Michael.
   C. Tell Michael that the information in a medical record is confidential and cannot be released.
   D. Ask Michael to come into the office and sign a release of medical information form.

4. Eva North, a 52-year-old factory worker, comes to the office complaining of difficulty in breathing and persistent coughing. She smokes 2 packs of cigarettes a day and has tried everything to quit smoking. When taking Eva's symptoms, which of the following would be an appropriate way to communicate with Eva?
   A. Offer Eva some breath mints.
   B. Avoid eye contact so that Eva does not feel embarrassed about coughing so much.
   C. Tell Eva that heavy smoking can damage her alveoli, which can cause emphysema, a chronic obstructive pulmonary disease, and that eventually she may need oxygen therapy.
   D. Observe that Eva is coughing a lot and offer her a glass of water.

Continued

APPLY YOUR KNOWLEDGE—cont'd

5. Patricia McGhee comes to the office, and Dawn Bennett, CMA, escorts her to an examining room. Dawn obtains Patricia's vital signs and asks her what problem has brought her to the office. Patricia describes her symptoms as coughing, running a temperature for 5 days, and shortness of breath. Of the following, which would be the best example of charting Patricia's chief complaint?
   A. CC: Dyspneic, febrile, with cough.
   B. CC: Patricia is sick.
   C. CC: Cough, fever, shortness of breath for 5 days.
   D. CC: Patricia is running a fever and coughing a lot. She is short of breath, especially in the morning. She has been feeling this way for the past 5 days.

6. Dr. Diagnosis wants Dawn to check to see whether Patricia is allergic to penicillin. Dawn would find this information in Patricia's health history under:
   A. Present Illness.
   B. Past History.
   C. Family History.
   D. Social History.

7. Dr. Diagnosis asks Dawn to administer a breathing treatment to Patricia. Which of the following represents the correct method for charting the breathing treatment?
   A. Chart the breathing treatment immediately after administering it.
   B. Use a No. 2 lead pencil to chart the breathing treatment.
   C. Chart the breathing treatment just before administering it.
   D. Have the office manager chart the breathing treatment.

8. Patricia is prescribed medication for pneumonia. Two days later, she calls the office and says she feels sick to her stomach and vomits after taking her medication. Of the following, which would be the best example of charting this information in Patricia's medical record?
   A. 4/2/05 Nausea with medication. D. Bennett, CMA.
   B. 4/2/05 9:00 a.m. Called office. N&V—p taking med. Reported sym to Dr. Diagnosis. D. Bennett, CMA.
   C. 4/2/05 9:00 a.m. N&V probably due to allergic reaction to the medication. Notified Dr. Diagnosis of the problem. D. Bennett, CMA.
   D. 4/2/05 9:00 a.m. Patricia called and said she vomits after taking her medication. I reported this information to Dr. Diagnosis right after he got back from lunch at the Red Lobster. D.B.

9. Inoko Lin comes to the medical office complaining of a skin problem. She is from Japan and is attending college in the United States. Which of the following shows that Dawn Bennett, CMA, is practicing cultural awareness?
   A. Bowing on greeting Inoko Lin.
   B. Speaking loudly so Inoko Lin can understand the conversation.
   C. Asking Inoko Lin how she prefers to be addressed.
   D. Asking Inoko Lin how to make chop suey.

10. Amy Grant is describing her symptoms to Dawn Bennett, CMA. She states that her symptoms include a red, blistery rash; intense itching; nausea; and fatigue. Which of Amy's symptoms is an objective symptom?
    A. Blistery, red rash.
    B. Intense itching.
    C. Nausea.
    D. Fatigue.

CERTIFICATION REVIEW

❑ **The patient registration record** must be completed by all new patients and consists of demographic and billing information.

❑ **The health history** (along with the physical examination and laboratory and diagnostic tests) is used to determine the patient's general state of health, to arrive at a diagnosis and prescribe treatment, and to observe any change in a patient's illness after treatment has been instituted.

❑ **The physical examination report** is a summary of the findings from the physician's assessment of each part of the patient's body.

❑ **The medication record** consists of detailed information relating to a patient's medications and includes one or more of the following categories: prescription medications, over-the-counter (OTC) medications, and medications administered at the medical office.

❑ **A consultation report** is a narrative report of a specialist's opinion about a patient's condition and is based on a review of the patient's medical record and an examination of the patient.

❑ **Home health care** provides medical and nonmedical care in a patient's home or place of residence to minimize the effect of disease or disability.

❑ **A laboratory report** is a report of the analysis or examination of body specimens. Its purpose is to relay the results of laboratory tests to the physician to assist him or her in diagnosing and treating disease.

❑ **A diagnostic procedure report** consists of a narrative description and interpretation of a diagnostic procedure and includes the following reports: electrocardiogram, Holter monitor, sigmoidoscopy, colonoscopy, spirometry, radiology, and diagnostic imaging.

❑ **A therapeutic service report** documents the assessments and treatment designed to restore a patient's ability to function, such as physical therapy, occupational therapy, and speech therapy.

❑ **Hospital documents** are prepared by the attending physician and include the history and physical examination of a hospitalized patient, operative report, discharge summary report, pathology report, and emergency department report.

❑ **A consent to treatment form** is required for all surgical operations and nonroutine diagnostic or therapeutic procedures performed in the medical office. The form must be signed by the patient and provides written evidence that the patient agreed to the procedure(s) listed on the form.

❑ **A release of medical information form** is required to release information that is not part of medical treatment, payment, and health care operations.

❑ **A source-oriented medical record** is organized into sections based on the department, facility, or other source that generated the information. Each section of a source-oriented record is separated from the others by a chart divider labeled with the title of its respective section.

❑ **The documents in a problem-oriented record (POR)** are organized by the patient's specific health problems and include a database, problem list, plan of action for each problem, and progress notes. Progress notes for a POR include four categories: subjective data, objective data, assessment, and plan (SOAP).

❑ **A health history** consists of the following components: identification data, chief complaint, present illness, past history, family history, social history, and review of systems. A health history is taken for each new patient, and subsequent office visits (in the form of progress notes) provide information regarding changes in the patient's illness or treatment.

❑ **Charting** is the process of making written entries about a patient in the medical record. The medical record is a legal document, and the information must be charted as completely and accurately as possible, following established charting guidelines.

❑ **Progress notes** update the medical record with new information each time the patient visits or telephones the medical office. Types of progress notes often charted by the medical assistant include patient symptoms, medical procedures, administration of medication, specimen collection, diagnostic procedures and laboratory tests ordered on a patient, results of laboratory tests, instructions given to the patient regarding medical care, missed or canceled appointments, telephone calls from patients, medication refills, and changes in medication or dosage by the physician.

TERMINOLOGY REVIEW

Attending physician The physician responsible for the care of a hospitalized patient.

Charting The process of making written entries about a patient in the medical record.

Consultation report A narrative report of an opinion about a patient's condition by a practitioner other than the attending physician.

Diagnosis The scientific method of determining and identifying a patient's condition.

Diagnostic procedure A procedure performed to assist in the diagnosis, management, or treatment of a patient's condition.

Discharge summary report A brief summary of the significant events of a patient's hospitalization.

Electronic medical record (EMR) A medical record that is stored on a computer.

Familial Occurring or affecting members of a family more frequently than would be expected by chance.

Health history report A collection of subjective data about a patient.

Home health care The provision of medical and non-medical care in a patient's home or place of residence.

Informed consent Consent given by a patient for a medical procedure after being informed of the nature of his or her condition, the purpose of the procedure, an explanation of risks involved with the procedure, alternative treatments or procedures available, the likely outcome of the procedure, and the risks involved with declining or delaying the procedure.

Inpatient A patient who has been admitted to a hospital for at least one overnight stay.

Medical impressions Conclusions drawn by the physician from an interpretation of data. Other terms for impressions include *provisional diagnosis* and *tentative diagnosis*.

Medical record A written record of the important information regarding a patient, including the care of that individual and the progress of the patient's condition.

Medical record format The way a medical record is organized. The two main types of medical record formats are the source-oriented record and the problem-oriented record.

Objective symptom A symptom that can be observed by an examiner.

Paper-based patient record (PPR) A medical record in paper form.

Patient An individual receiving medical care.

Physical examination An assessment of each part of the patient's body to obtain objective data about the patient that assists in determining the patient's state of health.

Physical examination report A report of the objective findings from the physician's assessment of each body system.

Problem Any condition that requires further observation, diagnosis, management, or patient education.

Prognosis The probable course and outcome of a disease and the prospects for a patient's recovery.

Reverse chronological order Arranging documents with the most recent document on top or in the front, which means that the oldest document is on the bottom or at the back of a section or file.

SOAP format A method of organization for recording progress notes. The SOAP format includes the following categories: subjective data, objective data, assessment, and plan.

Subjective symptom A symptom that is felt by the patient, but is not observable by an examiner.

Symptom Any change in the body or its functioning that indicates the presence of disease.

 ON THE WEB

For Information on Cultural Diversity:

National Geographic Society: www.nationalgeographic.com

U.S. Department of the Interior: Workforce Diversity: www.doi.gov/diversity/workforce

Generations United: www.gu.org

For Information on Communication Assistance:

AT&T Toll-Free Directory: www.tollfree.att.net

U.S. Postal Service Zip Code Access: www.usps.com/zip4/welcome

United Parcel Service: www.ups.com

Federal Express: www.fedex.com

DHL: www.dhl-usa.com

2

Medical Asepsis and the OSHA Standard

LEARNING OBJECTIVES	PROCEDURES
Microorganisms and Medical Asepsis	
1. Define a microorganism and give examples of types of microorganisms.	Handwashing
2. Explain the difference between a nonpathogen and a pathogen.	
3. Define medical asepsis.	
4. List the six basic requirements for growth and multiplication of microorganisms.	
5. Outline the infection process and cycle, including the following:	
Give examples of the means of entry of microorganisms into the body.	
Give examples of the means of transmission of microorganisms from one person to another.	
Give examples of the means of exit of microorganisms from the body.	
List and explain the protective mechanisms the body uses to prevent the entrance of microorganisms.	
6. Explain the difference between resident flora and transient flora.	
7. State when each of the following is performed: handwashing, antiseptic handwashing, and alcohol-based hand rub.	Applying an alcohol-based hand rub
8. Identify medical aseptic practices that should be followed in the medical office.	
9. Explain how proper handwashing helps prevent the transmission of microorganisms.	
10. List examples of when to wear clean disposable gloves.	Application and removal of clean disposable gloves
OSHA Bloodborne Pathogens Standard	
1. Explain the purpose of OSHA.	Adhere to the OSHA Bloodborne Pathogens Standard.
2. Describe the purpose of the Needlestick Safety and Prevention Act.	
3. List and describe the elements that must be included in the OSHA exposure control plan.	
4. Explain the purpose of each of the following OSHA requirements: labeling requirements and sharps injury log.	
5. Define and give examples of each of the following: engineering controls, work practice controls, personal protective equipment, and housekeeping procedures.	
6. Identify the guidelines for use of personal protective equipment.	
Regulated Medical Waste	
1. List examples of medical waste and how to discard each type of waste.	Prepare regulated waste for pickup by an infectious waste service.
2. Explain how to handle and dispose of regulated medical waste.	

Bloodborne Diseases
1. Describe postexposure prophylaxis for hepatitis B.
2. Explain the difference between acute and chronic hepatitis B.
3. Explain the possible effects and consequences of chronic hepatitis C.
4. List and describe the four stages of the AIDS infection cycle.
5. List and describe the AIDS-defining conditions.

CHAPTER OUTLINE

Introduction to Medical Asepsis and the OSHA Standard
Microorganisms and Medical Asepsis
    Growth Requirements for Microorganisms
    Infection Process Cycle
    Protective Mechanisms of the Body
    Medical Asepsis in the Medical Office
OSHA Bloodborne Pathogens Standard
    Purpose of the Standard
    Needlestick Safety and Prevention Act
    OSHA Terminology

    Components of the OSHA Standard
    Control Measures
Regulated Medical Waste
    Handling Regulated Medical Waste
    Disposal of Regulated Medical Waste
Bloodborne Diseases
    Hepatitis B
    Hepatitis C
    Other Forms of Viral Hepatitis
    Acquired Immune Deficiency Syndrome

NATIONAL COMPETENCIES

Clinical Competencies
Fundamental Procedures
Perform handwashing.
Dispose of biohazardous materials.
Practice Standard Precautions.

General Competencies
Legal Concepts
Identify and respond to issues of confidentiality.

Perform within legal and ethical boundaries.
Demonstrate knowledge of federal and state health care legislation and regulations.

Patient Instruction
Identify community resources.

KEY TERMS

aerobe (AIR-obe)
anaerobe (AN-er-obe)
antiseptic
asepsis (ay-SEP-sis)
cilia (SIL-ee-ya)
contaminated (kon-TAM-in-ated)
decontamination (DEE-kon-tam-in-AY-shun)
hand hygiene
infection
medical asepsis
microorganism (MYE-kroe-OR-gan-iz-um)
nonintact (NON-in-takt) skin
nonpathogen (non-PATH-oh-jen)

opportunistic (OP-pore-tune-IS-tik) infection
optimum (OP-tuh-mum) growth temperature
parenteral (pare-EN-ter-al)
pathogen (PATH-oh-jen)
perinatal (pare-ee-NAY-tul)
pH (PEE-AYCH)
postexposure prophylaxis (proe-fil-ACKS-is) (PEP)
regulated medical waste (RMW)
reservoir (REZ-er-vwar) host
resident flora (FLOE-ruh)
susceptible (sus-SEP-tih-bul)
transient (TRAN-zee-ent) flora

Introduction to Medical Asepsis and the OSHA Standard

Medical **asepsis** and **infection** control are crucial in preventing the spread of disease. The medical assistant should always practice good medical aseptic techniques to provide a safe and healthy environment in the medical office. The Occupational Safety and Health Administration (OSHA) Bloodborne Pathogens Standard is important for infection control. This standard is required by the federal government to reduce the exposure of health care employees to infectious diseases. This chapter presents a thorough discussion of medical asepsis, infection control, and the OSHA Bloodborne Pathogens Standard.

MICROORGANISMS AND MEDICAL ASEPSIS

Microorganisms are tiny living plants or animals that cannot be seen with the naked eye, but instead must be viewed with the aid of a microscope. Common types of microorganisms include bacteria, viruses, protozoa, fungi, and animal parasites. Most microorganisms are harmless and do not cause disease. They are termed **nonpathogens.** Other microorganisms, known as **pathogens,** are harmful to the body and can cause disease.

In the medical office, practices must be employed to reduce the number and hinder the transmission of pathogenic microorganisms. These practices are known as medical asepsis. **Medical asepsis** means that an object or area is clean and free from infection. Nonpathogens would still be present on a clean or medically aseptic substance or surface, but all the pathogens would have been eliminated.

Growth Requirements for Microorganisms

For microorganisms to survive, certain growth requirements must be present in the environment, as follows:

1. **Proper nutrition.** Microorganisms that use inorganic or nonliving substances as a source of food are known as *autotrophs.* Microorganisms that use organic or living substances for food are known as *heterotrophs.*
2. **Oxygen.** Most microorganisms need oxygen to grow and multiply and are termed **aerobes.** Other microorganisms, known as **anaerobes,** grow best in the absence of oxygen.
3. **Temperature.** Each microorganism has a temperature at which it grows best, known as the **optimum growth temperature.** Most microorganisms grow best at 98.6°F (37°C), the human body temperature.
4. **Darkness.** Microorganisms grow best in darkness.
5. **Moisture.** Microorganisms need moisture for cell metabolism and to carry away wastes.
6. **pH.** Most microorganisms prefer a neutral pH. If the environment of the microorganisms becomes too acidic or too basic, they die.

If growth requirements are taken away from the environment of microorganisms, they are unable to survive. Eliminating these conditions is one way to reduce the growth and transmission of pathogens in the medical office.

Infection Process Cycle

For a pathogen to survive and produce disease, a continuous cycle must be followed; this is known as the *infection process cycle* (Figure 2-1). If the cycle is broken at any point, the pathogen dies. The medical assistant has a responsibility to help break this cycle in the medical office by practicing good techniques of medical asepsis. These techniques are discussed in the next section.

Protective Mechanisms of the Body

The body has protective mechanisms to help prevent the entrance of pathogens, and these help break the infection process cycle. Protective mechanisms of the body are as follows:

1. The skin is the body's most important defense mechanism; it serves as a protective barrier against the entrance of microorganisms.
2. The mucous membranes of the body, which line the nose and throat and respiratory, gastrointestinal, and genital tracts, help protect the body from invasion by microorganisms.
3. Mucus and cilia in the nose and respiratory tract fight off pathogens. Mucus traps the smaller microorganisms that enter the body, and the hairlike **cilia** constantly beat toward the outside to remove them from the body.
4. Coughing and sneezing help force pathogens from the body.
5. Tears and sweat are secretions that aid in the removal of pathogens from the body.
6. Urine and vaginal secretions are acidic. Pathogens cannot grow in an acidic environment.
7. The stomach secretes hydrochloric acid, which helps in the process of digestion. This acidic environment discourages the growth of pathogens that enter the stomach.

Medical Asepsis in the Medical Office

Hand Hygiene

Hand hygiene refers to the process of cleansing or sanitizing the hands. Hand hygiene is considered the most important medical aseptic practice in the medical office for preventing the spread of infection. Specific techniques for sanitizing the hands in the medical office include the following:

- Handwashing with a detergent soap and water
- Handwashing with an antimicrobial soap and water
- Applying an alcohol-based hand rub

The Centers for Disease Control and Prevention (CDC) issued new recommendations for hand hygiene in health care settings. The purpose of these guidelines is to promote improved hand hygiene practices and to reduce transmission of pathogenic microorganisms to patients and employees in health care settings. The CDC guidelines for hand hygiene as they apply to the medical office are outlined in Box 2-1. They are also discussed further in this section.

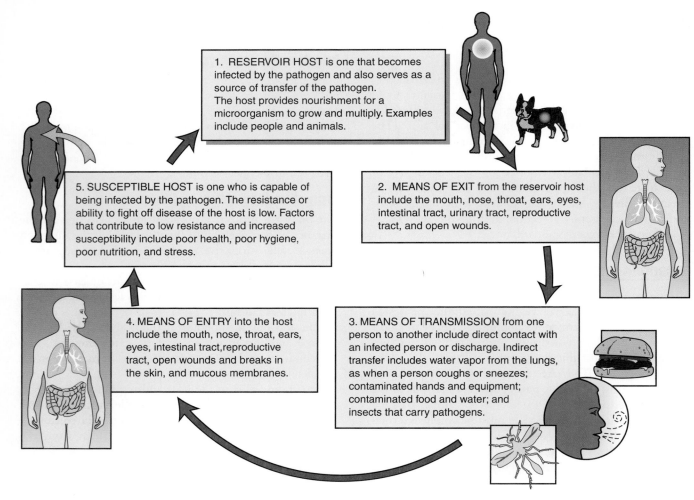

1. RESERVOIR HOST is one that becomes infected by the pathogen and also serves as a source of transfer of the pathogen. The host provides nourishment for a microorganism to grow and multiply. Examples include people and animals.

5. SUSCEPTIBLE HOST is one who is capable of being infected by the pathogen. The resistance or ability to fight off disease of the host is low. Factors that contribute to low resistance and increased susceptibility include poor health, poor hygiene, poor nutrition, and stress.

2. MEANS OF EXIT from the reservoir host include the mouth, nose, throat, ears, eyes, intestinal tract, urinary tract, reproductive tract, and open wounds.

4. MEANS OF ENTRY into the host include the mouth, nose, throat, ears, eyes, intestinal tract, reproductive tract, open wounds and breaks in the skin, and mucous membranes.

3. MEANS OF TRANSMISSION from one person to another include direct contact with an infected person or discharge. Indirect transfer includes water vapor from the lungs, as when a person coughs or sneezes; contaminated hands and equipment; contaminated food and water; and insects that carry pathogens.

Figure 2-1. The infection process cycle.

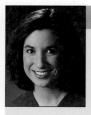

Putting It All into Practice

My Name is Jennifer Hawk, and I work for a large group of physicians in a multispecialty clinic. I work in both the front and back areas of the office. I really enjoy experiencing all of these areas of the office, and I definitely never get bored.

The most interesting experience I have had as a practicing medical assistant is seeing the impact that I make in patients' lives. They rely on you and look to you first for help in their health care situation. You are most often the first person they come into contact with in the office, and they look to you for understanding and empathy. Especially patients who come to your office on a regular basis see you as a kind of family member. They appreciate a familiar face and smile. Most often, you are the individual giving the patient instructions concerning testing they will be having done or medication they will be taking. Patients truly do count on your knowledge and assistance throughout their course of care. I was genuinely surprised at what an impact I could have on others. ■

Resident and Transient Flora

Microorganisms on the hands are classified into the following categories: resident flora and transient flora. **Resident flora** (also known as *normal flora*) normally reside and grow in the epidermis and deeper layers of the skin known as the *dermis*. Resident flora are generally harmless and nonpathogenic. Because resident flora are attached to the deeper skin layers, they are difficult to remove from the skin.

Transient flora live and grow on the superficial skin layers, or epidermis. They are picked up on the hands in the course of daily activities. In the medical office, this may include contact with an infected patient, contaminated equipment, or contaminated surfaces. Transient flora are often pathogenic, but because they are attached loosely to the skin, they can be removed easily with proper handwashing or by applying an alcohol-based hand rub.

Handwashing

Handwashing refers to washing the hands with a detergent soap and water. Detergent soap (commonly known as plain soap) contains agents that help break down and emulsify

BOX 2-1 CDC Guidelines for Hand Hygiene in Health Care Settings

Wash Hands with a Detergent Soap or an Antimicrobial Soap

- When the hands are visibly soiled with dirt or body fluids (e.g., blood, feces, urine, respiratory secretions)
- Before eating
- After using the restroom

Apply an Alcohol-Based Hand Rub (or Wash Hands)

- Before and after patient contact
- Before applying and after removing gloves
- After contact with body fluids or excretions, mucous membranes, nonintact skin, and wound dressings as long as the hands are not visibly soiled
- When moving from a contaminated body site to a clean body site during patient care
- After contact with inanimate objects (e.g., medical equipment) when providing health care to a patient

General Recommendations

- Keep natural nail tips less than ¼-inch long. Avoid wearing artificial nails.
- Do not add soap to a partially empty liquid soap dispenser. The practice of "topping off" dispensers can lead to bacterial contamination of the soap. The correct procedure is either to dispose of an empty dispenser or rinse an empty dispenser thoroughly and then refill it.
- Disposable paper towels are recommended for drying the hands after handwashing. Multiple-use cloth towels are not recommended.
- Use hand lotions or creams to minimize the occurrence of dermatitis associated with frequent handwashing.
- Change gloves during patient care if moving from a contaminated body site to a clean body site.
- Remove gloves after caring for a patient. Do not wear the same pair of gloves for the care of more than one patient.

dirt and oil present on the skin. Soap is used to sanitize the hands through the physical removal of dirt and transient flora. It is important to use adequate friction during handwashing to ensure the removal of all transient flora. Procedure 2-1 outlines the handwashing procedure.

The CDC hand hygiene guidelines recommend that handwashing be performed when the hands are visibly soiled with dirt or body fluids, before eating, and after using the restroom (see Box 2-1). If the hands are not visibly soiled, the CDC recommends that an alcohol-based hand rub be used to sanitize the hands rather than handwashing. This is because repeated handwashing tends to dry out the hands, leading to irritation, chapping, and dermatitis.

Antiseptic Handwashing

Washing the hands with an antimicrobial soap is termed *antiseptic handwashing*. Antimicrobial soaps contain an **antiseptic,** which is an agent that functions to kill or inhibit the growth of microorganisms (Figure 2-2A). Antiseptic handwashing sanitizes the hands through the mechanical scrubbing action and through the action of the antiseptic. Proper handwashing with an antimicrobial soap removes all soil and transient flora from the hands. Most antimicrobial soaps also deposit an antibacterial film on the skin that discourages bacterial growth. Antiseptic handwashing should be performed by the medical assistant before assisting with a minor office surgery. Examples of antiseptics contained in antimicrobial soaps include triclosan, chlorhexidine, hexachlorophene, iodine, and chloroxylenol.

Alcohol-Based Hand Rubs

The CDC guidelines recommend the use of an alcohol-based hand rub for sanitizing the hands when they are not visibly soiled (see Box 2-1). Alcohol-based hand rubs consist of 60% to 90% alcohol (ethanol or isopropanol) and

come in the form of gels, lotions, and foams (Figure 2-2B). Studies have shown that hand rubs are more effective than traditional soap and water handwashing in removing transient flora and reducing bacterial counts on the hands. The advantages that alcohol-based hand rubs offer over traditional handwashing are as follows:

- Alcohol-based hand rubs are usually more accessible than sinks.
- They do not require rinsing; water or hand drying with a towel is not needed.
- Less time is required to perform hand hygiene. It takes 20 to 30 seconds to sanitize the hands with an alcohol-based hand rub compared with 1 to 2 minutes to perform proper handwashing.
- Most alcohol-based hand rubs contain emollients, which help prevent the skin of the hands from overdrying. As the alcohol dries, protective fats and oils remain on the hands.

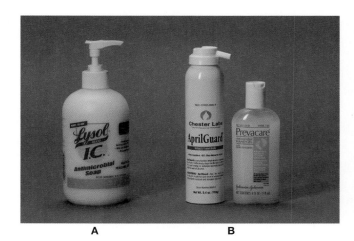

Figure 2-2. **A,** Antimicrobial soap. **B,** Alcohol-based hand rubs.

2. The employer must provide appropriate personal protective equipment at no cost to you. The employer is responsible for ensuring the equipment is available in appropriate sizes, is readily accessible, and is used correctly. In addition, the employer must ensure that the equipment is cleaned, laundered, repaired, replaced, or disposed of as necessary to ensure its effectiveness.

3. Alternatives must be provided for employees who are allergic to the gloves normally provided. Examples of alternatives include hypoallergenic gloves and powderless gloves.

4. If gloves become contaminated, torn, or punctured, replace them as soon as practical.

5. All eye-protection devices must have solid side shields; chin-length face shields, goggles, and glasses with solid side shields are acceptable (Figure 2-7); standard prescription eyeglasses are unacceptable as eye protection.

6. If a garment is penetrated by blood or other potentially infectious materials, it must be removed as soon as possible and placed in an appropriately designated container for washing.

7. All personal protective equipment must be removed before leaving the medical office.

8. When protective equipment is removed, it must be placed in an appropriately designated area or container for storage, washing, decontamination, or disposal.

9. Utility gloves may be decontaminated and reused unless they are cracked, peeling, torn, or punctured or no longer provide barrier protection.

10. If you believe using protective equipment would prevent proper delivery of health care or would pose an increased hazard to your safety or that of a coworker, in extenuating circumstances you may temporarily and briefly decline its use. After such an incident, the circumstances must be investigated to determine whether the situation could be prevented in the future.

Housekeeping

The OSHA standard requires that specific housekeeping procedures be followed to ensure that the work site is maintained in a clean and sanitary condition. The medical office must develop and implement a written schedule for cleaning and decontaminating each area where exposure occurs.

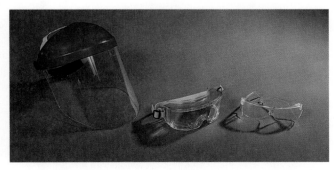

Figure 2-7. Examples of eye-protection devices. *Left,* Face shield; *center,* goggles; *right,* glasses with solid side shields.

What Would You Do? What Would You *Not* Do?

Case Study 2

Tracy Smith is pregnant and is at the medical office to have her blood drawn for a prenatal profile. Tracy says she does not understand why gloves have to be worn when her blood is drawn. She says that it makes her feel like a leper, and she is absolutely sure that she doesn't have any diseases. Tracy says she has been reading information about the hepatitis B vaccine because she knows her baby will be given this vaccine soon after birth. She wants to know why it is recommended that an infant be immunized for hepatitis B. Tracy says that infants are not at risk for contracting hepatitis B because the way it is transmitted is mostly through sexual contact and illegal drug use. ■

The cleaning and decontamination method must be specified for each task and should be based on the type of surface to be cleaned, the type of soil present, and the tasks or procedures being performed in that area. Housekeeping procedures include the following:

1. Clean and decontaminate equipment and work surfaces after completing procedures that involve blood or other potentially infectious materials. Cleaning is accomplished using a detergent soap, and decontamination is performed using an appropriate disinfectant (Figure 2-8).

2. Clean and decontaminate all equipment and work surfaces as soon as possible after exposure to blood or other potentially infectious material. For the decontamination of blood spills, OSHA recommends the use of a 10% solution of sodium hypochlorite (household bleach) in water (1 part bleach to 10 parts water).

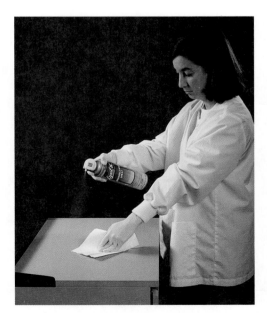

Figure 2-8. Clean and decontaminate work surfaces with an appropriate disinfectant after completing procedures involving blood and other potentially infectious materials.

Highlight on OSHA Bloodborne Pathogens Standard

General Information

The exposure control plan must be made available to OSHA on request.

OSHA inspectors are responsible for determining whether the medical office meets the Bloodborne Pathogens Standard. This is accomplished through a careful review of the exposure control plan, interviews with the medical office employer and employees, and observation of work activities.

Feces, nasal secretions, saliva, sputum, sweat, tears, urine, and vomitus are not considered by OSHA to be potentially infectious material unless they contain blood.

Control Measures

Employees must be trained in the proper use of the following: engineering controls (including safer medical devices), work practice controls, and personal protective equipment.

General work clothes, such as scrubs, uniforms, pants, shirts, and blouses, are not intended to function as protection against a hazard and are not considered personal protective equipment.

Employees are not permitted to launder contaminated clothing at home; it is the employer's responsibility to have contaminated clothing laundered.

If an employee is allergic to the standard latex gloves, the employer must provide a suitable alternative, such as hypoallergenic gloves.

Needlestick Injuries

The CDC estimates that every year 600,000 to 800,000 health care workers in the United States experience needlestick and other sharps injuries, and 1000 of these individuals contract serious infections as a result of these injuries. The CDC estimates that 62% to 88% of sharps injuries can be prevented by the use of safer medical devices.

A wide variety of commercially available safer medical devices have been developed to reduce the risk of needlestick and other sharps injuries.

Safer medical devices that eliminate exposure to the lowest extent feasible must be evaluated and implemented in the health care setting. The lack of injuries on the sharps injury log does *not* exempt the employer from this provision. ∎

---

3. Inspect and decontaminate all reusable receptacles, such as bins, pails, and cans, on a regular basis. If contamination is visible, the item must be cleaned and decontaminated as soon as possible.

4. Do not pick up broken, contaminated glassware with the hands, even if gloves are worn. Use mechanical means, such as a brush and dustpan, tongs, and forceps (Figure 2-9).

5. Protective coverings, such as plastic wrap and aluminum foil, may be used to cover work surfaces or equipment,

but they must be removed or replaced if contamination occurs.

6. Handle contaminated laundry as little as possible and with appropriate personal protective equipment. Place all contaminated laundry in leakproof bags that are properly labeled or color-coded. Contaminated laundry must not be sorted or rinsed at the medical office.

7. If the outside of a biohazard container becomes contaminated, it must be placed in a second suitable container.

8. Biohazard sharps containers (Figure 2-10) must be closable, puncture-resistant, and leakproof. They must bear a biohazard warning label and be color-coded red to

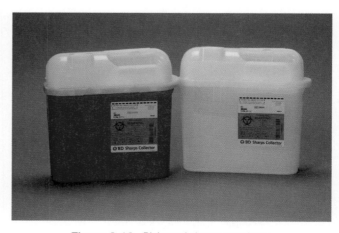

Figure 2-9. Use mechanical means to pick up broken contaminated glass.

Figure 2-10. Biohazard sharps containers.

ensure identification of the contents as hazardous. To ensure effectiveness, the following guidelines must be observed:

- Locate the sharps container as close as possible to the area of use to avoid the hazard of transporting a contaminated needle through the workplace.
- Maintain sharps containers in an upright position to keep liquid and sharps inside.
- Do not reach into the sharps container with your hand.
- Replace sharps containers on a regular basis, and do not allow them to overfill. (It is recommended that sharps containers be replaced when they are three-quarters full.)

Hepatitis B Vaccination

The OSHA standard requires physicians to offer the hepatitis B vaccination series free of charge to all medical office personnel who have occupational exposure. The vaccination must be offered within 10 working days of initial assignment to a position with occupational exposure, unless the following factors exist: (1) The individual has previously received the hepatitis B vaccination series, (2) antibody testing has revealed that the individual is immune to hepatitis B, or (3) the vaccine is contraindicated for medical reasons.

Medical office personnel who decline vaccination must sign a hepatitis B waiver form documenting refusal. This form must be filed in the employee's OSHA record (Figure 2-11). Employees who decline vaccination may request the vaccination later, which the employer must then provide according to the aforementioned criteria.

Universal Precautions

Before the release of the OSHA standard, the CDC issued recommendations for health care workers known as the Universal Precautions. According to the concept of Universal Precautions, all human blood and certain human body fluids are treated as though known to be infectious for HIV, HBV, HCV, and other bloodborne pathogens. The OSHA standard states that the Universal Precautions must be observed; these precautions form the heart of the OSHA standard itself.

REGULATED MEDICAL WASTE

Medical waste is generated in the medical office through the diagnosis, treatment, and immunization of patients. Some of this waste poses a threat to health and safety and is known as **regulated medical waste (RMW).** The OSHA Bloodborne Pathogens Standard defines RMW as follows:

- Any liquid or semiliquid blood or OPIM
- Items contaminated with blood or OPIM that would release these substances in a liquid or semiliquid state if compressed
- Items that are caked with dried blood or OPIM and are capable of releasing these materials during handling
- Contaminated sharps
- Pathologic and microbiologic wastes that contain blood or OPIM

Regulated medical waste must be discarded properly so as not to become a source of transfer of disease. According to the OSHA definition, a dressing saturated with blood is considered RMW and must be discarded in a biohazard bag. A bandage with a spot of blood on it is not considered RMW and can be discarded in a regular waste container.

HEPATITIS B VACCINE REFUSAL

I understand that due to my occupational exposure to blood or other potentially infectious materials, I may be at risk of acquiring hepatitis B virus (HBV) infection. I have been given the opportunity to be vaccinated with hepatitis B vaccine at no charge to myself. However, I decline hepatitis B vaccination at this time. I understand that by declining this vaccine I continue to be at risk of acquiring hepatitis B, a serious disease. If in the future I continue to have occupational exposure to blood or to other potentially infectious materials and I want to be vaccinated with hepatitis B vaccine, I can receive the vaccination series at no charge to me.

_____
Employee Name (printed)

_____   _____
Employee Signature   Date

_____   _____
Witness Signature   Date

Figure 2-11. Hepatitis B vaccine waiver form. This form must be signed by an employee with occupational exposure who declines hepatitis B vaccination.

Highlight on Hepatitis B Vaccine

The hepatitis B vaccine became available in 1982 and is 95% effective in providing immunity.

The hepatitis B vaccine is well tolerated by most patients. The most common side effect is soreness at the injection site, including induration, erythema, and swelling. Occasionally, a low-grade fever, headache, and dizziness occur.

Current data show that the vaccine-induced antibodies may decline over time, but the immune system memory that programs the body to produce these antibodies remains intact indefinitely. Because of this, an individual with declining antibodies is still protected against hepatitis B. At present, the CDC does not recommend a booster dose once an individual has received the initial (three-dose) vaccine series.

The hepatitis B vaccine is recommended for all infants, children, and adolescents who are 18 years old or younger. It also is recommended for adults older than 18 years who are at increased risk for developing hepatitis B. This population includes employees with occupational exposure (e.g., health care workers), hemodialysis patients, hemophiliacs, individuals with multiple sex partners, homosexually active men, injection drug users, and household and sexual contacts of individuals with chronic hepatitis B.

The number of individuals contracting hepatitis B has decreased sharply since the development of the hepatitis B vaccine. As more people become immune to hepatitis B through the immunization of infants, the goal of eliminating hepatitis B in the United States may be realized. ∎

Box 2-2 gives the guidelines for discarding medical waste in the medical office.

Handling Regulated Medical Waste

Regulated medical waste must be handled carefully to prevent an exposure incident. The OSHA Bloodborne Pathogens Standard outlines specific actions to take when handling regulated medical waste, as follows:

1. Separate regulated waste from the general refuse at its point of origin. Disposable items containing regulated medical waste should be placed directly into biohazard containers and not mixed with the regular trash.
2. Ensure that biohazard containers are closable, leakproof, and suitably constructed to contain the contents during handling, storage, and transport. These containers include biohazard bags and sharps containers.
3. To prevent spillage or protrusion of the contents, close the lid of a sharps container before removing it from an examining room. Never open, empty, or clean a contaminated sharps container. If there is a chance of leakage from the sharps container, the medical assistant should place it in a second container that is closable, leakproof, and appropriately labeled or color-coded.
4. Securely close biohazard bags before removing them from an examining room. To provide additional protection, some medical offices double-bag by placing the primary bag inside a second biohazard bag.
5. Transport full biohazard containers to a secured area away from the general public, using personal protective equipment (e.g., gloves).

Disposal of Regulated Medical Waste

Each state is responsible for developing policies for disposal of regulated medical waste. To avoid noncompliance, it is important for the medical assistant to know and understand the specific regulated waste policies and guidelines set forth in his or her state.

Most medical offices use a commercial medical waste service to dispose of regulated medical waste. The service is responsible for picking up and transporting the medical waste to a treatment facility for incineration to destroy pathogens and render it harmless. The waste can then be safely disposed of in a sanitary landfill. Regulated waste treatment facilities must be licensed and hold permits issued by the Environmental Protection Agency (EPA), allowing them to dispose of regulated medical waste.

A series of steps must be followed for preparing and storing regulated medical waste for pickup by the service. Although these steps may vary slightly from state to state, general measures required by most states include the following:

1. Place biohazard bags and sharps containers into a receptacle provided by the medical waste service. The receptacle is usually a cardboard box (Figure 2-12). The box should be securely sealed with packing tape, and a biohazard warning label must appear on two opposite sides of the box.
2. Store the biohazard boxes in a locked room inside the facility or in a locked collection container outside for pickup by the medical waste service. This step is aimed at preventing unauthorized access to items such as needles and syringes. The regulated waste storage area should be labeled with one of the following:
   • "Authorized Personnel Only" sign
   • International biohazard symbol
3. Many states require that a tracking record be completed when the waste is picked up by the medical waste service. The form includes such information as the type and quantity of waste (weighed in pounds) and where it is being sent. The form must be signed by a representative of the medical waste service and the medical office. After the waste has been destroyed at the regulated waste treatment facility, a record documenting its disposal is mailed to the medical office.

BOX 2-2 Guidelines for Discarding Medical Waste in the Medical Office

Regular Waste Container

The following items that have been used for health care *are not* considered regulated medical waste and can be discarded in a covered waste container lined with a regular trash bag.

- Disposable drapes
- Disposable patient gowns
- Examining table paper
- Disposable clean or sterile gloves
- Gauze tinged with blood or other body fluids
- Disposable probe covers for thermometers
- Tongue depressors
- Tissues with respiratory secretions
- Disposable ear speculums
- Empty urine containers
- Urine testing strips
- Disposable diapers
- Feminine hygiene products

Biohazard Sharps Container

The following items are sharps. They *are* considered regulated medical waste and must be discarded in a biohazard sharps container.

- Hypodermic syringes and needles
- Venipuncture needles
- Lancets
- Razor blades
- Scalpel blades
- Suture needles
- Blood tubes
- Capillary pipets
- Microscope slides and coverslips
- Broken glassware

Biohazard Bag Waste Container

The following items *are* considered regulated medical waste. They are not sharps and can be discarded in a covered waste container lined with a biohazard bag.

- Any item saturated or dripping with blood or OPIM (e.g., dressings, gauze, cotton balls, paper towels, and tissues that are saturated or dripping with blood)
- Any item caked with dried blood or OPIM, such as dressings and sutures
- Disposable clean or sterile gloves contaminated with blood or OPIM
- Disposable vaginal speculums and collection devices (swabs, spatulas, brushes)
- Tissue or fluid removed during minor office surgery
- Microbiologic waste, such as specimen cultures and collection devices
- Discarded live and attenuated vaccines

Sanitary Sewer

Disposal of small quantities of blood and other body fluids to the sanitary sewer is considered a safe method of disposing of these waste materials. The following fluids can be carefully poured down a utility sink, drain, or toilet. (*Note:* State regulations may dictate the maximum volume allowable for discharge of blood or body fluids into the sanitary sewer.)

- Blood
- Body excretions such as urine
- Body secretions such as sputum

What Would You Do? What Would You *Not* Do?

Case Study 3

Giles Lee is 45 years old and is at the medical office. Twenty-five years ago, he was in a serious car accident and had to have a blood transfusion. He says that he donated blood for the first time 2 months ago. Last week he received a letter saying that his blood tested positive for hepatitis C and that he should see his physician. Giles says that he must have gotten hepatitis C from the blood transfusion he received when he was 20. He does not understand how that could have happened because the blood supply is tested for these types of diseases. Giles wants to know why he has not had any symptoms. He also wants to know if he can give hepatitis C to his wife and teenage children. ■

BLOODBORNE DISEASES

The biggest threats to health care workers from occupational exposure are HBV, HCV, and HIV. Hepatitis is much easier to transmit than is HIV. After a needlestick exposure to blood infected with HBV, health care workers who are not immune to hepatitis B have a 6% to 30% chance of developing the disease. The risk of infection after a needlestick exposure to blood infected with HCV is approximately 2%. After a needlestick exposure to HIV-infected blood, a health care worker has a 0.3% chance of developing AIDS; he or she has a 0.09% chance of developing AIDS after a mucous membrane exposure.

Hepatitis B

Hepatitis B is an infection of the liver caused by HBV. The most common means of transmitting hepatitis B in the health care setting are blood and blood components, such as serum and plasma.

Health care workers are most likely to contract hepatitis B through needlesticks and cuts with contaminated sharps. The virus also is spread in the health care setting, but less effectively, through blood splashes to the eyes, mouth, and nonintact skin and through body fluids such as semen and vaginal secretions.

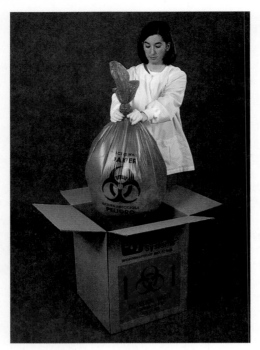

Figure 2-12. Jennifer places a biohazard bag inside a cardboard box in preparation for pickup by the medical waste service.

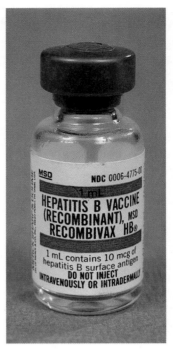

Figure 2-13. Hepatitis B vaccine.

The number of health care workers who contract hepatitis in the workplace has declined dramatically since the development of the OHSA standard and the hepatitis B vaccine. Statistics show that in 1983, there were more than 10,000 health care workers who contracted hepatitis B in the workplace, but by 2001, that number had decreased to less than 400 health care workers. Preventive treatment is available for individuals exposed to hepatitis B who have not been vaccinated.

Postexposure Prophylaxis

Postexposure prophylaxis (PEP) refers to treatment administered to an individual after exposure to an infectious disease to prevent the disease. The PEP for unvaccinated individuals exposed to hepatitis B involves the administration of a passive and an active immunizing agent. It is important to administer both of these agents as soon as possible after an exposure incident—preferably within 24 hours, but no later than 7 days.

The passive immunizing agent provides temporary immunity to hepatitis B, giving the active agent a chance to take effect. The passive agent is hepatitis B immune globulin (HBIG), which contains antibodies that provide immunity to hepatitis B for 1 to 3 months.

The *active immunizing agent* in the hepatitis B vaccine (Figure 2-13) is produced from genetically altered yeast cells; brand names are Recombivax HB and Engerix-B. The hepatitis B vaccine is administered intramuscularly in a series of three doses. The second dose is given 1 month after the first dose, and the third dose is administered 6 months after the first dose (i.e., 0, 1 month, and 6 months). Mild

side effects, such as soreness at the injection site, may occur, but serious reactions to the vaccine are extremely rare.

As previously discussed, the OSHA standard recommends that all health care workers receive the hepatitis B vaccine (an active immunizing agent) as a preventive measure against hepatitis B. After an exposure incident, a medical assistant who has previously been vaccinated probably would not require further treatment, unless laboratory tests reveal that his or her antibody level is low. In this case, a booster dose of the vaccine is recommended.

Acute Viral Hepatitis B

After a person becomes infected, the acute symptoms of hepatitis B usually last 1 to 4 weeks, but it can take 6 months for the patient to recover fully. The symptoms vary greatly in intensity from one individual to another and can range from mild to severe. Approximately one third of people who become infected are asymptomatic and unaware that they have the disease. Another third have relatively mild flulike symptoms that often are mistaken for influenza or similar conditions. The remaining one third of infected patients have such severe symptoms that hospitalization may be required.

The initial symptoms, if present, occur approximately 12 weeks after exposure and include fatigue, headache, loss of appetite, nausea, vomiting, malaise, and muscle and joint pain. In patients with severe acute viral hepatitis, these symptoms progress to abdominal pain, dark urine, and clay-colored stools, followed several days later by jaundice. After the onset of jaundice, the liver enlarges and becomes tender. A small percentage of patients (0.5% to 2% of those infected) develop fulminant hepatitis, which is almost always fatal. Fulminant hepatitis is characterized by a sudden onset of nausea and vomiting, chills, high fever, severe and early jaundice, convulsions, coma, and death as a result of hepatic failure, usually within 10 days of its onset.

There is no specific treatment or drug to treat the acute phase of hepatitis B. Supportive care is prescribed to help the patient's natural defenses overcome the disease. Supportive care includes restricted activity, rest, avoidance of alcohol, a well-balanced diet, adequate fluid intake, and precautionary measures to prevent the disease's spread.

Most patients (90%) are able to clear the virus from their body by producing antibodies that completely destroy the virus. These individuals recover fully and have lifelong immunity to hepatitis B and are not infectious to others.

Chronic Viral Hepatitis B

The remaining 10% of patients with acute viral hepatitis B remain infected and go on to develop chronic hepatitis B. These individuals produce antibodies to hepatitis B, but they are not sufficient to remove the virus from their body. Individuals with chronic hepatitis may or may not experience symptoms; nonetheless, they become carriers of hepatitis B and are capable of transmitting the disease to others. In addition, patients with chronic hepatitis face an increased risk of liver damage, which leaves them vulnerable to diseases such as cirrhosis of the liver and liver cancer. A significant number of these patients (25%) subsequently die from liver failure. In recent years, antiviral drugs have been developed to treat chronic hepatitis. They are effective in removing the virus from approximately 40% of patients infected with chronic hepatitis B.

Hepatitis C

Hepatitis C is an infection of the liver caused by HCV. Currently, no vaccine is available for the prevention of hepatitis C. In the medical office, the most likely means of contracting hepatitis C is through needlesticks and other sharps injuries. The chance of contracting hepatitis C in the health care setting is much lower than that of contracting hepatitis B.

Most individuals with acute hepatitis C have no symptoms; if symptoms do occur, they are mild and flulike. Ap-

proximately 55% to 85% of individuals with acute hepatitis C develop chronic hepatitis C. After 10 to 30 years, about 20% of these individuals develop serious liver disease, including cirrhosis of the liver and cancer of the liver. Ultimately, 1% to 5% of individuals with chronic hepatitis C die from liver failure (see the *Highlight on Viral Hepatitis*). Antiviral drugs also have been developed to treat chronic hepatitis C and are effective in 40% of cases.

Other Forms of Viral Hepatitis

In addition to hepatitis B and C, three other strains that cause viral hepatitis have been identified: hepatitis A, D, and E. Among all strains of hepatitis, hepatitis B poses the greatest threat to health care workers and has already been discussed in detail. Hepatitis A occasionally has been transmitted to health care workers but is not considered a major occupational hazard. In all cases of viral hepatitis, the virus invades the liver and causes inflammation, resulting in similar symptoms. The medical assistant should have a general knowledge of each of the forms of viral hepatitis. Table 2-1 outlines the incubation period, means of transmission, characteristics, onset and symptoms, and prognosis for all strains of viral hepatitis.

Acquired Immune Deficiency Syndrome

Acquired immune deficiency syndrome (AIDS) is a chronic disorder of the immune system that eventually destroys the body's ability to fight off infection. AIDS is caused by a retrovirus known as *human immunodeficiency virus (HIV)*. The following description helps to clarify the difference between these two terms. The virus and the infection itself are known as *HIV*, whereas the term *AIDS* is used to refer to the last stage of HIV infection. Simply put, the terms *HIV infection* and *AIDS* refer to different stages of the same disease.

When HIV gains entrance into the body, it begins to attack and destroy certain white blood cells known as *CD4$^+$ T cells*, which are involved in protecting the body against viral, fungal, and protozoal infections. As more and more CD4$^+$ T cells are destroyed, the immune system is gradually weakened. After a period of time, which may last 10 years or more, the body's immune system becomes so ravaged by the attack that it succumbs to the diseases associated with AIDS.

AIDS is characterized by the presence of severe and life-threatening opportunistic infections and unusual cancers that rarely affect individuals with healthy immune systems. An **opportunistic infection** is an infection that results from a defective immune system that cannot defend itself from pathogens normally found in the environment. Opportunistic infections are extremely difficult to treat because the infection tends to recur quickly after a course of therapy is completed.

Stages of AIDS

The AIDS infection cycle has four stages; however, all stages may not be experienced by every infected individual. These four stages are described next.

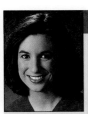

Memories *from* Externship

Jennifer Hawk: As a student, I was extremely nervous to go out on externship. I was so scared to think that I was actually going to be in a medical office setting and would have to put everything I had learned into practice. Would I remember everything? Would I do something wrong and hurt the patient? It was such an overwhelming feeling! But to my relief, I had a very good experience. The office staff was so friendly and helpful to me, and I surprised myself at how easily everything I had learned stayed with me. It was so exciting to see that I was actually functioning as a team member in the health care field. I could not have had better training. ▪

Highlight on Viral Hepatitis

In the United States, there are an estimated 150,000 new cases of hepatitis each year. Approximately 42% of these infections are caused by hepatitis B, 40% are caused by hepatitis A, and 18% are caused by hepatitis C.

Symptoms common to all types of hepatitis include fatigue, nausea, loss of appetite, abdominal pain, and jaundice.

Hepatitis A, B, and C are designated as nationally notifiable diseases by the CDC. When the physician diagnoses a case of hepatitis A, B, or C, a reportable disease form must be completed and filed with the local public health department.

In recent years, antiviral drugs have been developed to treat the chronic forms of hepatitis B and C; however, not all infected individuals are candidates for treatment. These drugs, which must be taken for a prolonged time, are effective in removing the virus from approximately 40% of chronically infected patients.

Hepatitis B

The most common means of transmission of hepatitis B is through sexual contact with an infected individual and by sharing needles for injection drug use with an infected individual. Hepatitis B is not spread by sneezing, coughing, hugging, kissing, casual contact, breastfeeding, food, water, or sharing eating utensils or drinking glasses.

The highest rate of new hepatitis B infections occur in 20- to 49-year-olds. The greatest decline has occurred among children and adolescents as a result of routine hepatitis B immunization.

It is estimated that more than 1.25 million people in the United States are infected with chronic hepatitis B; this means that these individuals are carriers of hepatitis B and capable of transmitting the disease to others. Many of these individuals do not know that they are carriers.

Every year, approximately 5000 Americans die as a result of the long-term consequences of chronic hepatitis B, such as cirrhosis and liver cancer.

Whether or not an HBV-infected individual goes on to develop chronic hepatitis B depends primarily on age. After being infected with acute viral hepatitis B, chronic infection develops in 90% of infants infected by their mothers at birth, 30% of children infected between ages 1 and 5 years, and 6% of individuals infected after age 5 years.

Hepatitis B can survive outside the body in a dried state for at least 1 week and still be capable of causing infection. Examples of surfaces that could harbor dried blood or body fluids infected with HBV include contaminated worktables, equipment, and instruments.

Hepatitis C

Chronic hepatitis C is the most common chronic viral infection in the United States. Approximately 3 million Americans have been diagnosed with chronic hepatitis C, and each year it causes an estimated 10,000 to 12,000 deaths resulting from cirrhosis and liver cancer.

The most common means of transmission of hepatitis C is by sharing needles for injection drug use with an infected individual. Hepatitis C is not spread by casual contact, such as sneezing, coughing, hugging, sharing food or water, or sharing eating utensils or drinking glasses. It is rarely transmitted through sexual contact.

Individuals infected with hepatitis C should not share personal items that may have blood on them with other members of the household (e.g., toothbrushes, nail-grooming equipment, and razors).

Chronic hepatitis C is known as "an epidemic that occurred in the past." Numerous individuals became infected with hepatitis C more than 25 years ago and are now being diagnosed with it. This is because the symptoms of chronic hepatitis C often do not appear until 10 to 30 years after infection, and many times the first symptoms come only with advanced liver disease. Chronic hepatitis C surpasses alcoholism as the leading cause of liver cirrhosis and liver transplantation in the United States.

By 2015, the CDC predicts that there will be a fourfold increase in the number of individuals diagnosed with chronic hepatitis C and a threefold increase in the annual death toll by 2010.

Before 1992, a blood test to determine the presence of hepatitis C did not exist. Because of this, a significant number of people contracted hepatitis C from HCV-infected blood transfusions. The CDC has begun a campaign to encourage people who received blood transfusions before July 1992 to ask their physicians if they should be tested for hepatitis C.

Postexposure prophylaxis with immune globulin is not effective in preventing hepatitis C, and no vaccine exists yet to prevent hepatitis C. Vaccines are difficult to develop for hepatitis C because the virus mutates so frequently. The only way to control the disease is by preventing exposure to the hepatitis C virus. ■

Stage 1: Acute HIV Infection

An individual infected with HIV may first experience a transient flulike illness known as *acute HIV infection*, which occurs 1 to 4 weeks after exposure. Many people do not develop any symptoms, however, when they first become infected with HIV. If they do occur, symptoms of acute HIV infection include fever, sweats, fatigue, loss of appetite, diarrhea, pharyngitis, myalgia, arthralgia, and adenopathy. These symptoms usually disappear within 1 week to 1 month and are often mistaken for symptoms of another viral infection.

Stage 2: Asymptomatic Period

After the early symptoms subside (if they occur at all), the infected individual normally experiences a long incubation period, lasting months to years depending on the individual. During this time, the individual is asymptomatic and looks and feels completely well. Because of this, the individual may not realize the HIV infection is present. The only evidence of HIV infection during this stage is the production by the body of antibodies to HIV that are detectable by blood tests. These HIV antibodies are unable to destroy the virus; however, they are used as a basis for the

Highlight on AIDS

Prevalence

AIDS was first reported in the United States in 1981, but most likely it existed here and in other parts of the world for many years before that. Since 1981, more than 950,000 cases of AIDS have been reported in the United States, and every year 40,000 people in the United States are infected with HIV. Since 1981, there have been an estimated 530,000 deaths in the United States from AIDS.

The epidemic is growing most rapidly among women 25 to 44 years old and minority populations. There also has been an increase in the number of AIDS cases among individuals who are age 50 and over. This increase may be due to the fact that members of this age group do not think of themselves as at risk for contracting AIDS and may not practice safe sex.

Transmission

Scientific evidence shows that HIV is not spread through casual, everyday contact. There is no evidence that HIV is spread by sharing facilities or equipment, such as telephones, computers, food utensils, bedding, doorknobs, and bathrooms. Because HIV is not passed through the air, it is not spread through coughing and sneezing. HIV is also not spread through tears, sweat, shaking hands, hugging, or by donating blood.

Most individuals infected with HIV show no symptoms and may not develop full-blown AIDS for 10 years or more. After infection with HIV, the individual is infected for life.

Women can transmit HIV to their fetuses during pregnancy or birth. Approximately one quarter to one third of pregnant women infected with HIV who are not being treated with antiretroviral drugs pass the infection to their infants. HIV also can be spread to infants through the breast milk of mothers infected with the virus. The CDC recommends that all pregnant women be offered voluntary HIV testing as a routine part of prenatal care.

Worldwide, more than 700,000 infants are infected with HIV each year. If antiretroviral drugs are taken during pregnancy and the infant is delivered by cesarean section, the chance of transmitting HIV to the infant is reduced significantly. In developing countries, such as sub-Saharan Africa, women seldom know their HIV status, and treatment is often unavailable.

Diagnostic Tests

The enzyme immune assay (EIA) test and the enzyme-linked immunosorbent assay (ELISA) test are used as screening tests for the presence of HIV. Because of the possibility of a false-positive result, a second screening test is always performed if a blood specimen tests positive. If the second test also is positive, a more specific test, such as the Western blot test, is performed to confirm the test results. An individual who tests positive for HIV is seropositive.

A negative HIV test is not conclusive for the absence of HIV infection. If an individual has recently been infected with HIV, the antibodies may not have had time to develop. It generally takes 3 to 6 months for the antibodies to appear in the blood.

CDC Definition of AIDS

As scientists have learned more about the disease, the CDC's definition of AIDS has changed several times since the beginning of the AIDS epidemic. The current AIDS definition includes the presence of one or both of the following conditions:

1. HIV positive and a $CD4^+$ T cell count below 200 cells/μL (normal $CD4^+$ T cell count for a healthy individual ranges from 500 to 1500 cells/μL)
2. Presence of one or more AIDS-defining conditions

Treatment

There is no cure for AIDS; there is no vaccine to prevent it. Powerful antiviral drugs have been developed that slow the reproduction of the virus and reduce the viral load in the body. In many patients, these drugs have dramatically delayed HIV from progressing to full-blown AIDS. These drugs can have serious side effects, and they do not prevent the spread of the disease to someone else. Numerous drugs also are available to treat the opportunistic infections and cancers that occur with AIDS. ■

---

test procedure to indicate that the HIV infection is present. Because of the length of time required by the body to develop HIV antibodies, however, these tests may fail to detect HIV for 3 to 6 months after an individual has been infected. Although an infected person may appear perfectly healthy, the virus is very active during this stage destroying $CD4^+$ T cells, which gradually weakens the immune system. Because HIV may be transmitted with or without symptoms, it is during this asymptomatic period that the danger of accidental transmission is greatest.

Stage 3: Symptomatic Period

Before the development of full-blown AIDS, many HIV-infected individuals experience a series of lesser symptoms caused by a weakened immune system. One of the first such symptoms experienced by many people infected with HIV is lymph nodes that remain enlarged for more than 3 months. Other symptoms often experienced months to years before the onset of AIDS include progressive generalized lymphadenopathy, lack of energy, unexplained weight loss, recurrent fevers and sweats, diarrhea, persistent or frequent yeast infections (oral or vaginal), and persistent skin rashes or flaky skin. Some people develop frequent and severe herpes infections that cause mouth, genital, or anal sores or a painful nerve disease known as *shingles*.

Stage 4: AIDS

AIDS is the last stage of the infection cycle that began with HIV infection. As previously described, full-blown AIDS is characterized by the presence of opportunistic infections and unusual cancers known as *AIDS-defining conditions*. They do not usually occur, or produce only mild illness, in individuals with healthy immune systems. A severe and rare type of pneumonia caused by the organism *Pneumocystis*

Text continued on p. 76

Table 2-1 Forms of Viral Hepatitis

	Hepatitis A (HAV)	Hepatitis B (HBV)	Hepatitis C (HCV)	Hepatitis D (HDV)	Hepatitis E (HEV)
Incubation period	2-6 wk	6 wk to 6 mo	2 wk to 6 mo	2 wk to 5 mo	3-6 wk
Means of transmission	Caused by a virus found in the feces of HAV-infected individuals. Transmitted almost exclusively by the fecal-oral route through practices of poor hygiene; also transmitted by the consumption of food and water contaminated with human feces	Caused by a virus found in the blood and certain body fluids of HBV-infected individuals. Transmitted by exposure to contaminated semen and vaginal secretions by personal contact, especially sexual contact; parenteral exposure to contaminated blood and blood components, such as through injecting drugs using contaminated needles and accidental needlestick injuries by health care workers; perinatally from an infected mother to her infant during birth	Caused by a virus found in the blood of HCV-infected individuals. Parenteral exposure to contaminated blood or blood components, primarily from injecting drugs using contaminated needles. It is possible to transmit HCV during intercourse, but it is uncommon	Same as hepatitis B	Fecal-oral route through practices of poor hygiene; consumption of food and water contaminated with feces
Characteristics	Usually occurs in children and young adults, especially in environments of poor sanitation and overcrowding; often a mild disease with symptoms similar to the flu and lasting 1-2 wk; there is a vaccine available to prevent hepatitis A	Symptoms usually last 1-4 wk, but it may be 6 mo before the individual fully recovers; there is a vaccine available to prevent hepatitis B	At risk are individuals who received a blood transfusion before 1992; currently a vaccine does not exist for hepatitis C	Affects only those already infected with hepatitis B; a person who has received the hepatitis B vaccine also is protected from hepatitis D	Rare in the United States; generally seen in developing countries; usually occurs in epidemics rather than sporadic cases

Symptoms	Symptoms include fever, malaise, fatigue, anorexia, nausea, vomiting, and abdominal discomfort, followed in some people by dark urine, clay-colored stools, and mild jaundice	Symptoms include fatigue, headache, loss of appetite, nausea, vomiting, malaise, and muscle and joint pain, followed in some people by dark urine, clay-colored stools, abdominal pain, and jaundice	Symptoms are similar to those of hepatitis B	Occurs as a coinfection or superinfection with hepatitis B and intensifies the symptoms of hepatitis B	Symptoms are similar to those of hepatitis B
Prognosis	Most people recover fully within 6-10 wk and become immune to the virus; rarely fatal; chronic hepatitis does not develop; carrier states do not develop	Most people recover fully and become immune to this disease; some people (10%) go on to develop chronic hepatitis and may develop cirrhosis and liver cancer; these people also are carriers of hepatitis B. Eventually 25% of people with chronic hepatitis B die from liver failure	Approximately 55-85% of people infected with hepatitis C are unable to clear the virus from their body and develop chronic hepatitis, which may lead to liver damage, such as cirrhosis and liver cancer. These people are also carriers of hepatitis C. Eventually 1% to 5% of people with chronic hepatitis C die from liver failure	Frequently leads to chronic hepatitis; high fatality rate (30% of chronic hepatitis patients)	Does not progress to chronic hepatitis; hepatitis E is particularly dangerous if contracted by pregnant women (10-20% fatality rate in these individuals)

BOX 2-3 AIDS-Defining Conditions

Neoplasms

Kaposi Sarcoma

Malignant Neoplasm Kaposi sarcoma is the most common neoplasm occurring in AIDS patients. It is an aggressive tumor that involves multiple body organs, but generally occurs initially on the skin. It is characterized by multiple dark-red or purplish blotches on the skin. The areas of the body most commonly affected are the trunk, arms, head, and neck. Diagnosis of Kaposi sarcoma is made by tissue biopsy. Other body sites commonly affected by this neoplasm are the lymph nodes, the lungs, and the gastrointestinal tract. Kaposi sarcoma is rarely the primary cause of death but does weaken the AIDS patient further, who may die eventually as a result of opportunistic infections.

Opportunistic Infections

Pneumocystis carinii Pneumonia

Protozoa *Pneumocystis carinii* pneumonia (PCP) is the most common opportunistic infection causing death in individuals with AIDS. This protozoan lung infection previously was considered rare and in most instances not fatal. PCP occurs at least once in more than 65% of AIDS patients, and 25% of patients initially infected experience a recurrence. PCP is characterized by moderate-to-severe difficulty in breathing, fever, and a nonproductive cough in the early stages and a productive cough in the later stages of the disease. Death occurs in 30% of PCP-infected patients and is generally caused by acute respiratory failure.

Cytomegalovirus Infection

Virus Cytomegalovirus is a virus that belongs to the herpes virus group and that rarely causes disease in healthy adults. Most AIDS patients have active cytomegalovirus infection. The most common symptoms of its presence in AIDS patients are spots on the retina, which may lead to blindness. This virus also causes pneumonia, esophagitis, and colitis. Specific symptoms include fever, profound fatigue, muscle and joint aches, night sweats, impaired vision, cough, dyspnea, abdominal pain, and diarrhea.

Herpes Simplex 1 and 2

Virus Herpes simplex 1 is spread by contact with oral secretions, and herpes simplex 2 is spread by contact with genital secretions. Herpes simplex causes painful vesicular lesions, usually of the nasopharynx, oral cavity, skin, and genital tract. This virus tends to have periods of latency followed by reactivation of symptoms. In AIDS patients, herpes simplex is apt to cause cervical lymphadenopathy and proctitis.

Mycobacterial Infections

Bacteria Mycobacterial infections are among the most frequent opportunistic infections in AIDS patients. One strain (*Mycobacterium avium* complex) causes fever, fatigue, weight loss, diarrhea, and malabsorption. Another strain (*Mycobacterium tuberculosis*) causes pulmonary tuberculosis, which is not considered an opportunistic infection. In AIDS patients, tuberculosis is characterized by a productive, purulent cough, fever, dyspnea, fatigue, weight loss, and wasting. The AIDS epidemic seems to be causing a resurgence of tuberculosis in the United States. Because tuberculosis is more contagious than most AIDS-defining conditions, it seems to be spreading beyond AIDS patients and into the general population.

Candidiasis

Yeastlike Fungus *Candida albicans* is a fungus that inhabits the oropharynx, large intestine, and skin, causing no harm in individuals with healthy immune systems. Infection with *C. albicans* is often one of the first signs of a weakened immune system in HIV-infected individuals. It is characterized by a white, patchy growth on the mouth, throat, or esophagus (thrush). AIDS patients develop an extremely severe case of candidiasis that makes eating and swallowing difficult and painful. In female AIDS patients, this organism causes severe vaginitis.

Cryptosporidiosis

Protozoa In AIDS patients, this condition usually causes profuse, watery diarrhea along with anorexia, vomiting, fatigue, malaise, and fever. This condition may become chronic, resulting in dehydration and electrolyte imbalance, which lead to weight loss and eventual death.

Toxoplasmosis

Protozoa Toxoplasmosis is one of the most common causes of encephalitis in AIDS patients, resulting in the following symptoms: headache, altered mental state, visual disturbances, cranial nerve palsy, and motor disorders. Toxoplasmosis also may result in infection of the heart, lungs, skin, stomach, abdomen, and testes.

Cryptococcosis

Fungus Cryptococcosis is a common cause of meningitis in AIDS patients and includes chronic symptoms of low-grade fever, malaise, and headaches. Other symptoms manifested after these initial symptoms include photophobia, stiff neck, nausea, vomiting, and seizures.

---

carinii is frequently associated with AIDS patients, as is *Kaposi sarcoma,* a rare type of cancer. Box 2-3 describes these and other AIDS-defining conditions. AIDS is also known to damage the nervous system, which eventually results in varying degrees of dementia and other symptoms. As the HIV infection progresses, the individual becomes overwhelmed by infection and cancer. The body is unable to fight back because of a severely damaged immune sys-

tem, and the patient eventually dies from AIDS-defining conditions.

Transmission of AIDS

Research has shown that HIV is not transmitted through casual contact or even extensive contact such as occurs among family members of AIDS patients. In the general population, HIV is spread primarily through sexual contact

PATIENT TEACHING Acquired Immune Deficiency Syndrome

Teach patients the ways in which AIDS is transmitted.

- Having unprotected sex (vaginal, anal, or oral) with someone who is infected with HIV. The virus is most commonly found in semen, blood, and vaginal secretions.
- Sharing needles for injection drug use with someone who is infected with HIV. This occurs as follows: If an HIV-infected individual uses a needle to pierce his or her skin, there will be a tiny amount of blood left on the needle. If another person uses the same needle, the person will be injecting the HIV-infected blood into his or her body.
- Transmitting in utero. A pregnant woman with HIV can pass it on to her fetus. Infants born with HIV usually develop AIDS by 2 years of age.
- Receiving a blood transfusion or blood products (before 1985) from someone infected with HIV. (In 1985, blood banks began screening blood for AIDS, so this is largely a problem of blood received before then.)
- There is a greater risk of contracting AIDS if you already have another sexually transmitted disease, such as chlamydia, gonorrhea, syphilis, herpes, or bacterial vaginosis.

Teach patients how to prevent AIDS.

- Know your sexual partner(s) and their sexual history and drug use.
- Use a latex condom during sexual intercourse to minimize the risk of infection. HIV cannot pass through the latex if the condom does not break and is used properly. If a lubricant is used with the condom, it should be water based, such as K-Y jelly, because an oil-based lubricant such as petroleum jelly could break down the latex.
- Avoid sexual practices that involve the exchange of body fluids, such as semen or vaginal secretions.
- If you think that you could have HIV, never let your blood, semen, or vaginal fluid enter another person's body.
- Do not share needles for injectable drug use.

Teach patients to recognize the symptoms of AIDS.

- Unexplained fatigue
- Weight loss of 10 to 15 lb in less than 2 months, but without dieting
- Unexplained fever, chills, and sweating at night for more than 2 weeks
- Unexplained swollen glands for more than 1 month
- Unexplained diarrhea or bloody stools for more than 2 weeks
- Unexplained persistent dry cough, shortness of breath, or difficulty in breathing
- White patches on the tongue or mouth that cannot be scraped off

Explain to patients that these symptoms also could be signs of other diseases. If they have any of these symptoms, however, they should consider having an HIV test. The earlier the infection is detected, the earlier treatment can begin that may delay the onset of other symptoms. ■

with an infected person and by sharing drug injection needles with someone who is infected. Untreated HIV-infected women also can transmit the virus to their infants during pregnancy and birth and through their breast milk.

Because HIV is not easily transmitted, the risk to health care workers is low. Since reporting began in 1985, the CDC has received reports of 57 documented cases and 138 possible cases of HIV infection from occupational exposure to health care workers (as of December 2001). Despite the low risk of infection, however, the serious nature of HIV infection warrants the use of the OSHA Bloodborne Pathogens Standard by all health care workers. Because most HIV carriers are asymptomatic and may be unaware of their infection, precautions minimizing the risk of exposure to blood and body fluids should be taken with all patients at all times. The precautions also are recommended as a means of protection against other bloodborne pathogens, such as hepatitis B, hepatitis C, and syphilis.

 *Check out the **Companion CD** bound with the book to access additional interactive activities.*

MEDICAL PRACTICE and the LAW

There are three behaviors that are crucial in protecting yourself from a lawsuit:

1. Establish a rapport. If patients believe that you truly care about them and have their best interests at heart, they rarely sue, even if you make a mistake.
2. Follow all procedures according to your procedures manual. If you do everything right, and the patient has an adverse outcome, you will not likely be found liable.
3. Document everything you do objectively. Lawsuits often come to court years after the incident, and nobody's memory is as good as written documentation. Document only facts, not your opinion. Document the patient's reaction to treatments.

Ethics and Law

Ethics is the highest standard of behavior and is loosely based on the Golden Rule. No law can force you to behave ethically, but most major professions have a written code of ethics, including the American Association of Medical Assistants (AAMA). Ethics uses words such as *should* and *may*. If you are angry with someone, ethically, you should not yell at him or her. This is not against the law, but it is unethical.

Law is the lowest standard of behavior and is enforced by federal, state, and local law enforcement personnel. Laws use words such as *must* and *shall*. If you are angry with someone, le-

MEDICAL PRACTICE *and the* LAW—cont'd

gally, you must not hit him or her. This behavior is illegal, and you could be charged with assault and battery.

Regarding medical asepsis and infection control, you have a duty and a responsibility to protect yourself, your coworkers, and,

most important, your patients. Follow specific guidelines established by OSHA and the CDC to prevent the transmission of pathogens. ■

What Would You Do? What Would You *Not* Do?   RESPONSES

Case Study 1
Page 59
What Did Jennifer Do?
❏ Told Petra that the hand sanitizers (alcohol-based hand rubs) are as good, if not better, than soap and water for removing germs from the hands.
❏ Explained to Petra that an amount of gel equal to the size of a dime should be rubbed on her hands until the gel dries. Told Petra that she did not need to rinse her hands afterward.
❏ Stressed to Petra that hand sanitizers are not designed to remove soil from the hands and that she should wash her hands with soap and water when they are visibly soiled.
❏ Explained that the Centers for Disease Control and Prevention now recommends that hand sanitizers be used in health care settings to help prevent the spread of disease.

What Did Jennifer Not *Do?*
❏ Did not tell Petra that she should switch from soap and water to hand sanitizers.

What Would You Do/What Would You *Not* Do? Review Jennifer's response and place a checkmark next to the information you included in your response. List additional information you included in your response.

_____
_____
_____
_____

Case Study 2
Page 65
What Did Jennifer Do?
❏ Explained to Tracy that a federal agency known as the Occupational Safety and Health Administration (OSHA) requires gloves be worn when drawing a patient's blood in the office. Told her that the office could be fined if they were not worn.
❏ Told Tracy that having her infant immunized for hepatitis B is an investment in her child's future. Explained that her child could come into contact with the virus anytime in his or her life. Stressed that if a young child becomes infected with hepatitis B, the child has a higher risk of developing chronic hepatitis, which can cause serious liver problems later in life.
❏ Gave Tracy a brochure on hepatitis B to take home.

What Did Jennifer Not *Do?*
❏ Did not discourage Tracy from having her baby immunized for hepatitis B.

What Would You Do/What Would You *Not* Do? Review Jennifer's response and place a checkmark next to the information you included in your response. List additional information you included in your response.

_____
_____
_____
_____

Case Study 3
Page 69
What Did Jennifer Do?
❏ Explained to Giles that the blood supply was not tested for hepatitis C until 1992 because a test to detect the presence of hepatitis C was not developed until then.
❏ Told Giles that it is possible for someone to have hepatitis C and not exhibit any symptoms.
❏ Told Giles that he should ask the physician his question about giving hepatitis C to others.

What Did Jennifer Not *Do?*
❏ Did not automatically assume that Giles had hepatitis C because he had not yet been seen by the physician. It would be up to the physician to make a diagnosis of hepatitis C.
❏ Did not tell Giles about the serious complications of hepatitis C. If Giles is diagnosed with hepatitis C, it would be the physician's responsibility to relay this information.

What Would You Do/What Would You *Not* Do? Review Jennifer's response and place a checkmark next to the information you included in your response. List additional information you included in your response.

_____
_____
_____
_____

APPLY YOUR KNOWLEDGE

Choose the best answer to each of the following questions.

1. Jennifer Hawk, CMA, arrives at the medical office and checks to make sure everything is ready to start the day. Jennifer notices that the liquid soap dispenser next to the sink is half empty. Jennifer realizes that she must:
   A. Fill the soap dispenser to the top.
   B. Wait until the soap dispenser is empty before taking any action.
   C. Dump out the remaining soap and refill the dispenser.
   D. Throw away the soap dispenser in the regular trash.

2. Jennifer is washing her hands after using the restroom. Jennifer performs all of the following during the handwashing procedure *except:*
   A. Uses hot water to wash her hands.
   B. Holds her hands lower than her elbows.
   C. Rubs her hands together vigorously as she washes them.
   D. Dries her hands thoroughly with paper towels.

3. Jennifer notices that the back of her right hand is becoming a little irritated. What would be the best action for Jennifer to take?
   A. Not wash her hands until the irritation has healed.
   B. Use only an alcohol-based hand rub until her hand has healed.
   C. Apply hand lotion after washing her hands.
   D. Wear mittens when performing procedures.

4. As Jennifer is pulling on clean disposable gloves, she notices a small tear in the glove of her left hand. Jennifer takes the following action:
   A. Ignores the tear because it is just a small one.
   B. Puts on a second pair of gloves over the first pair.
   C. Applies an alcohol-based hand rub to the gloves.
   D. Takes off the left glove and puts on another one.

5. Jennifer has just removed sutures from a patient's lower leg. She removes her gloves and sees that her hands look clean. Jennifer now performs the following:
   A. Applies an alcohol-based hand rub.
   B. Washes her hands with an antimicrobial soap.
   C. Rinses her hands with a dilute bleach solution.
   D. Charts the procedure in the patient's record.

6. Jennifer is getting ready to eat lunch in the office break room. Before eating, Jennifer should:
   A. Apply an alcohol-based hand rub.
   B. Wash her hands with soap and water.
   C. Put on gloves.
   D. Call the nearest sub shop.

7. Clara Mills has come to the office for a hepatitis B vaccine. Jennifer Hawk, CMA, administers the first dose of the hepatitis B vaccine to Clara. Which of the following statements would *not* be accurate to tell Clara about the hepatitis B vaccine?
   A. You will need a second dose of this vaccine 1 month from now.
   B. You will need a third dose of this vaccine 6 months from now.
   C. You may experience some soreness at the injection site for a few days.
   D. This vaccine will also protect you against hepatitis C.

8. Jennifer Hawk, CMA, has just drawn a blood specimen from a patient, and some blood gets on her glove as she is removing the needle from the patient's arm. Jennifer removes her gloves and discards them in:
   A. A waste container lined with a biohazard bag.
   B. A biohazard sharps container.
   C. A waste container lined with a regular trash bag.
   D. The recycling bin.

9. The medical office is having a meeting to review and update the OSHA exposure control plan. Which of the following statements indicates that this employee does not fully understand the OSHA Bloodborne Pathogens Standard?
   A. A new type of safety syringe is available, and I think we should consider using it.
   B. We need to put a biohazard label on the new refrigerator we just got for storing blood tubes.
   C. We have never had a sharps injury, so we don't need to use safer medical devices.
   D. We need to replace our sharps containers when they are three-quarters full.

10. Jennifer Hawk, CMA, is preparing regulated medical waste for disposal. Jennifer performs all of the following *except:*
   A. Places biohazard bags and sharps containers in a cardboard box.
   B. Ensures there is a biohazard warning label on two opposite sides of the box.
   C. Seals the cardboard box securely with tape.
   D. Places the cardboard box outside for pickup with the regular trash.

CERTIFICATION REVIEW

- **Microorganisms** are tiny living plants or animals that cannot be seen with the naked eye; examples include bacteria, viruses, protozoa, fungi, and animal parasites. Microorganisms that do not cause disease are nonpathogens. Microorganisms that are harmful to the body and can cause disease are pathogens.
- **Medical asepsis** refers to practices that are employed to reduce the number and hinder the transmission of pathogenic microorganisms. Nonpathogens would still be present, but all the pathogens would have been removed.
- **Microorganisms** that use inorganic substances as a source of food are autotrophs; microorganisms that use organic substances for food are heterotrophs. Aerobes are microorganisms that need oxygen to grow and multiply, and anaerobes are microorganisms that grow best in the absence of oxygen.
- **The body has protective mechanisms** to help prevent the invasion of pathogens, which include the following: the skin and mucous membranes, mucus and cilia in the nose and respiratory tract, coughing and sneezing, tears and sweat, urine and vaginal secretions, and hydrochloric acid secreted by the stomach.
- **Hand hygiene** refers to the process of cleaning or sanitizing the hands and is the most important medical aseptic practice for preventing the spread of infection. *Handwashing* refers to washing the hands with a detergent soap; *antiseptic handwashing* refers to washing the hands with an antimicrobial soap. The CDC now recommends that an alcohol-based hand rub be used to sanitize the hands when they are not visibly soiled.
- **Resident flora,** also known as *normal flora,* normally reside and grow in the epidermis and dermis. Resident flora are generally harmless and nonpathogenic. Transient flora live and grow on the superficial skin layers and are picked up in the course of daily activities. Transient flora are often pathogenic but can be removed easily by handwashing or applying an alcohol-based hand rub.
- **OSHA** was established by the federal government to assist employers in providing a safe and healthy working environment for their employees. The OSHA standard must be followed by any employee with occupational exposure, regardless of the place of employment.
- **Occupational exposure** is defined as reasonably anticipated skin, eye, mucous membrane, or parenteral contact with bloodborne pathogens or other potentially infectious materials that may result from the performance of an employee's duties. Bloodborne

pathogens are pathogenic microorganisms in human blood that can cause disease in humans. An exposure incident is a specific eye, mouth, other mucous membrane, nonintact skin, or parenteral contact with blood or other potentially infectious materials that results from an employee's duties.

- **The OSHA standard** requires that the medical office develop a written exposure control plan designed to eliminate or minimize employees' exposure to bloodborne pathogens and other potentially infectious materials. The ECP must be reviewed and updated annually to ensure that it remains current with the latest information eliminating or reducing exposure to bloodborne pathogens.
- **Engineering controls** include all measures that isolate or remove health hazards from the workplace; examples include safer medical devices and biohazard containers. A safer medical device is a device that, based on reasonable judgment, would make an exposure incident involving a contaminated sharp less likely (e.g., sharps with engineered sharps injury protection and needleless systems).
- **Work practice controls** reduce the likelihood of exposure by altering the manner in which a technique is performed and include such practices as bandaging cuts before gloving; sanitizing hands as soon as possible after removing gloves; immediately placing contaminated sharps in a biohazard sharps container; and not eating, drinking, or smoking in areas where you may be exposed to blood or other potentially infectious materials. If exposed to blood or OPIM, perform first aid measures immediately and then report the incident to the physician so that PEP can be instituted.
- **Personal protective equipment** is clothing or equipment that protects an individual from contact with blood or other potentially infectious materials; examples include gloves, chin-length face shields, masks, protective eyewear, laboratory coats, and gowns. The type of protective equipment appropriate for a given task depends on the degree of exposure that is anticipated.
- **Regulated medical waste (RMW)** is waste that may pose a substantial threat to health and safety if exposed to the public. Regulated medical waste must be properly handled and contained in the medical office so as not to become a source of transfer of disease. Regulated medical waste must be disposed of in accordance with all applicable state laws.
- **The biggest threats to health care workers** from occupational exposure are hepatitis B, hepatitis C, and HIV. Hepatitis is an infection of the liver. The most

CERTIFICATION REVIEW—cont'd

common means of transmission of hepatitis in the health care setting are blood and blood products through needlesticks and cuts with contaminated sharps.

❑ **AIDS** is a disorder of the immune system that eventually destroys the body's ability to fight infection. AIDS is characterized by the presence of severe and life-threatening opportunistic infections and unusual cancers. AIDS is caused by HIV, which is transmitted through contaminated body fluids, particularly blood and semen.

TERMINOLOGY REVIEW

Aerobe A microorganism that needs oxygen to live and grow.

Anaerobe A microorganism that grows best in the absence of oxygen.

Antiseptic An agent that inhibits the growth of or kills microorganisms.

Asepsis Free from infection or pathogens; the actions practiced to make and maintain an area or object free from infection or pathogens.

Cilia Slender, hairlike projections that constantly beat toward the outside to remove microorganisms from the body.

Contaminate To soil or to make impure. An aseptic object is contaminated when it touches something that is not clean.

Decontamination The use of physical or chemical means to remove, inactivate, or destroy pathogens on a surface or item to the point where they are no longer capable of transmitting infectious particles; the surface or item is rendered safe for handling, use, or disposal.

Hand hygiene The process of cleansing or sanitizing the hands.

Infection The condition in which the body, or part of it, is invaded by a pathogen.

Medical asepsis Practices that are employed to reduce the number and hinder the transmission of pathogens.

Microorganism A microscopic plant or animal.

Nonintact skin Skin that has a break in the surface. It includes, but is not limited to, abrasions, cuts, hangnails, paper cuts, and burns.

Nonpathogen A microorganism that does not normally produce disease.

Opportunistic infection An infection that results from a defective immune system that cannot defend the body from pathogens normally found in the environment.

Optimum growth temperature The temperature at which an organism grows best.

Parenteral Taken into the body through the piercing of the skin barrier or mucous membranes, such as through needlesticks, human bites, cuts, and abrasions.

Pathogen A disease-producing microorganism.

Perinatal Relating to the period shortly before and after birth.

pH The degree to which a solution is acidic or basic.

Postexposure prophylaxis (PEP) Treatment administered to an individual after exposure to an infectious disease to prevent the disease.

Regulated medical waste (RMW) Medical waste that poses a threat to health and safety.

Reservoir host The organism that becomes infected by a pathogen and serves as a source of transfer of the pathogen to others.

Resident flora Harmless, nonpathogenic microorganisms that normally reside on the skin and usually do not cause disease. Also known as *normal flora*.

Susceptible Easily affected; lacking resistance.

Transient flora Microorganisms that reside on the superficial skin layers and are picked up in the course of daily activities. They are often pathogenic but can be removed easily from the skin by sanitizing the hands.

(see Figure 3-4). Never use steel wool or other abrasives to remove stains because damage could occur to the instrument.

6. **Carefully inspect each instrument for defects and proper working condition.** After cleaning, rinsing, and drying the instrument, it is important to check it for defects and proper working condition as follows:
   - The blades of an instrument should be straight and not bent.
   - The tips of an instrument should approximate tightly and evenly when the instrument is closed.
   - An instrument with a box lock (e.g., hemostatic forceps, needle holders) should move freely but must not be too loose. The pin that holds the box lock together should be flush against the instrument.
   - An instrument with a spring handle (e.g., thumb and tissue forceps) should have sufficient tension to grasp objects tightly.

   - The cutting edge of a sharp instrument should be smooth and devoid of nicks.
   - Scissors should cut cleanly and smoothly. To test for this, the medical assistant should cut into a thin piece of gauze. The scissors are in proper working condition if they cut all the way to the end of the blade without catching on the gauze.

7. **Lubricate hinged instruments.** Lubricate box locks, screw locks, scissor blades, and any other moving part of each instrument. The lubricant makes the instrument function better and last longer. Use a lubricant that can be penetrated by steam, such as a commercial spray lubricant or a lubricant bath (see Figure 3-4). Lubricate after performing the final rinse (and drying of the instrument); otherwise the lubricant would be rinsed off the instrument. Never use industrial oils or silicon sprays. These substances are not steam penetrable and can build up on the instrument, affecting its working condition.

Text continued on p. 95

PROCEDURE 3-1

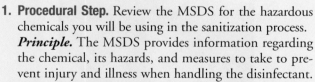

PROCEDURE 3-1   Sanitization of Instruments

Outcome Sanitize instruments.

Equipment/Supplies

- Sink
- Disposable gloves
- Heavy-duty utility gloves
- Contaminated instruments
- EPA-approved chemical disinfectant and MSDS
- Disinfectant container
- Cleaning solution and MSDS

- Basin
- Stiff nylon brush
- Stainless-steel wire brush
- Paper towels
- Cloth towel
- Instrument lubricant

1. **Procedural Step.** Review the MSDS for the hazardous chemicals you will be using in the sanitization process.
   Principle. The MSDS provides information regarding the chemical, its hazards, and measures to take to prevent injury and illness when handling the disinfectant.

2. **Procedural Step.** Apply disposable gloves. Transport the contaminated instruments to the cleaning area as soon as possible after use. The instruments should be carried in a covered basin from the examining room to the cleaning area.
   Principle. Disposable gloves act as a barrier to protect the medical assistant from infectious materials. Transporting contaminated instruments in a covered basin promotes infection control.

3. **Procedural Step.** Apply heavy-duty utility gloves over the disposable gloves.
   Principle. Utility gloves help protect the hands from the irritating effects of chemical solutions.

4. **Procedural Step.** Separate sharp instruments and delicate instruments from other instruments.
   Principle. Separating sharp instruments from others prevents damage to or dulling of the cutting edge of these instruments. Delicate instruments should be separated to protect them from damage.

5. **Procedural Step.** Immediately rinse the instruments thoroughly under warm, not hot, running water (approximately 110°F [44°C]) to remove organic material, such as blood, body fluids, tissue, and other debris.

Continued

PROCEDURE 3-1   Sanitization of Instruments—cont'd

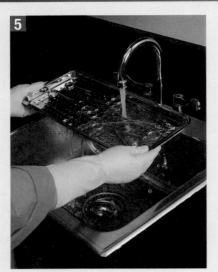

Rinse instruments under warm water to remove organic matter.

Principle. Rinsing the instruments as soon as possible prevents organic material from drying on the instruments, making it difficult to remove later. Hot water may cause coagulation of organic material, making it more difficult to remove.

6. **Procedural Step.** Decontaminate the instruments by disinfecting them in an EPA-approved chemical disinfectant as follows:

   a. Select the proper chemical disinfectant; check the expiration date on the container label.
   b. Observe all personal safety precautions listed on the label of the disinfectant (e.g., wearing safety goggles).
   c. Follow the manufacturer's directions on the label for proper mixing and use of the disinfectant.
   d. Label the plastic or stainless steel disinfecting container with the name of the disinfectant and the date when the disinfectant is no longer effective and must be discarded (reuse life).
   e. Pour the disinfectant into the labeled container and immerse the articles into the disinfectant. Ensure the articles are completely submerged in the disinfectant.
   f. Cover the container that holds the chemical disinfectant.
   g. Disinfect the articles for 10 minutes.

   Principle. Decontaminating the instruments removes pathogenic microorganisms from them, making them safe to handle. A disinfectant past its expiration date loses its potency and should not be used. An EPA-approved disinfectant has been determined by the U.S. Environmental Protection Agency to be effective when used as directed, without causing an unreasonable risk to the public or the environment. The container must be kept covered to prevent the escape of toxic fumes

and to prevent evaporation of the disinfectant, which could change its potency.

7. **Procedural Step.** Clean the instruments. The instruments can be cleaned using the manual method or the ultrasound method as follows:

Manual Method for Cleaning Instruments

   a. Obtain the instrument cleaning solution; check its expiration date.
   b. Observe all personal safety precautions listed on the label of the cleaning agent.
   c. Follow the directions on the manufacturer's label for proper mixing and use of the cleaning agent. The detergent may need to be diluted with water.
   d. Remove the articles from the chemical disinfectant and place them in the basin containing the cleaning solution.
   e. Use a stiff nylon brush to clean the surface of each instrument. Scrub all parts of the instrument thoroughly. Brush delicate instruments carefully to prevent damaging them.
   f. Use a stainless-steel wire brush to clean grooves, crevices, or serrations where contaminants such as blood and tissue may collect.
   g. If there is a stain on the instrument, attempt to remove it using a damp cloth or sponge to which a commercial stain remover has been applied.
   h. Scrub each instrument until it is visibly clean and free from organic material and stains.

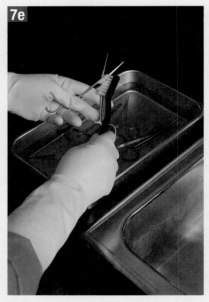

Clean the surface of the instrument with a stiff nylon brush.

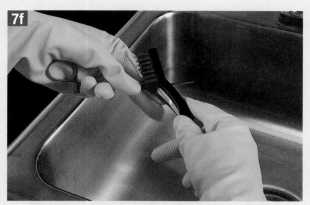

Clean grooves, crevices, or serrations with a wire brush.

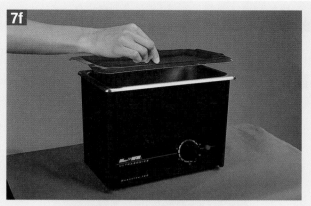

Place the lid on the ultrasonic cleaner.

Principle. A cleaning agent past its expiration date loses its potency and should not be used. Taking appropriate precautions with cleaning agents prevents harm to the medical assistant from hazardous chemicals. All organic material must be removed from the instruments to ensure complete sterilization in the autoclave.

Ultrasound Method for Cleaning Instruments

a. Using a cleaning agent recommended by the manufacturer, prepare the cleaning solution in the ultrasonic cleaner. Observe all personal safety precautions listed on the label.

b. Remove the articles from the chemical disinfectant, and separate instruments made of dissimilar metals, such as stainless steel, aluminum, and bronze.

c. Place the instruments in the ultrasonic cleaner with hinged instruments in an open position.

d. Ensure that sharp instruments do not touch other instruments.

e. Ensure that all instruments are fully submerged in the cleaning solution.

f. Place the lid on the ultrasonic cleaner.

g. Turn on the ultrasonic cleaner, and clean the instruments for the length of time recommended by the manufacturer.

h. After completion of the cleaning cycle, remove the instruments from the machine.

Principle. Taking appropriate precautions with chemical agents prevents harm to the medical assistant from hazardous chemicals. Mixing dissimilar metals together could result in permanent stains on the instruments. Instruments must be completely submerged with hinged instruments in an open position so that the solution can reach all parts of the instrument.

8. Procedural Step. Rinse each instrument thoroughly with warm, not hot, water (110°F [44°C]) for at least 20 to 30 seconds to remove all traces of the detergent. Open and close hinged instruments while rinsing to ensure the solution is completely rinsed out of every part of the instrument.

Principle. Detergent residue left on the instrument could cause stains, which could build up and interfere with the proper functioning of the instrument. Using

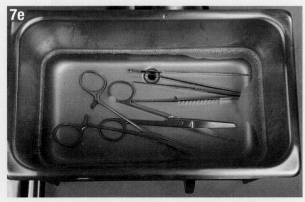

Completely submerge instruments in the cleaning solution.

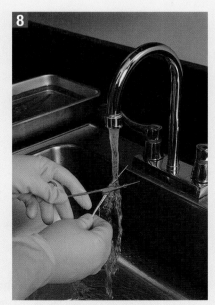

Rinse thoroughly with warm water.

Continued

PROCEDURE 3-1

PROCEDURE **3-1**   Sanitization of Instruments—cont'd

warm water helps to remove the cleaning solution and facilitates the drying process.

9. Procedural Step. Dry each instrument with a paper towel, and place the instrument on a cloth towel for additional air drying.

Principle. If the instrument is not completely dry, stains may occur on the instrument.

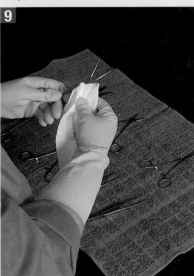

Dry the instrument with a paper towel.

10. Procedural Step. Check each instrument for defects and proper working condition. Scissors should cut all the way to the end of a thin piece of gauze without catching. If defects are noted, or the instrument is not working properly, it must be discarded or sent to the manufacturer for repair.

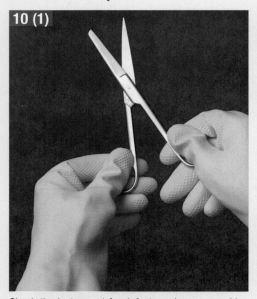

Check the instrument for defects and proper working order.

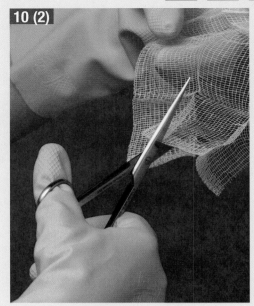

Scissors should cut through gauze without catching.

Principle. Instruments that have defects or are not in proper working condition are unsafe to use on a patient during a medical or surgical procedure.

11. Procedural Step. Lubricate hinged instruments using a steam-penetrable lubricant as follows:
a. Apply the lubricant to a hinged instrument in its open position.
b. Open and close the instrument after applying the lubricant so that it reaches all parts of the hinged area.

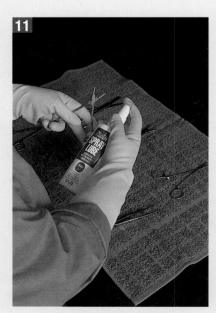

Lubricate hinged instruments.

PROCEDURE 3-1

c. Place the instrument back on the towel, and allow it to drain. Rinsing or wiping are unnecessary.

Principle. Lubricating an instrument makes it function better and last longer.

12. **Procedural Step.** Dispose of the cleaning solution according to the manufacturer's instructions. Remove both sets of gloves, and sanitize your hands.

13. **Procedural Step.** Wrap the instruments and sterilize them in the autoclave according to the medical office policy.

DISINFECTION

Disinfection is the process of destroying pathogenic microorganisms, but it does not kill bacterial spores. Disinfection is accomplished in the medical office through the use of liquid chemical agents that are applied to inanimate objects (Procedure 3-2). Chemical disinfection has been discussed with respect to its role in the sanitization process to decontaminate surgical instruments and make them safe to handle. This section discusses the use of chemical disinfection to disinfect semicritical and noncritical items so that they can be used for patient care.

Levels of Disinfection

Disinfection can be classified according to three levels of disinfection based on killing action.

High-Level Disinfection

High-level disinfection is a process that destroys all microorganisms with the exception of bacterial spores. High-level disinfection is used to disinfect semicritical items. A **semicritical item** is an item that comes in contact with nonintact skin or intact mucous membranes, such as a flexible fiberoptic sigmoidoscope. A frequently used high-level disinfectant is 2% glutaraldehyde (e.g., Cidex, MetriCide). A newer high-level disinfectant that is growing in popularity is Cidex OPA (ortho-phthalaldehyde). Cidex OPA does not contain glutaraldehyde, which means it is less toxic and safer to handle.

Intermediate-Level Disinfection

Intermediate-level disinfection is a process that inactivates tubercle bacilli (the causative agent of tuberculosis), all vegetative bacteria, most viruses, and most fungi, but it does not kill bacterial spores. Intermediate-level disinfection is used to disinfect noncritical items. **Noncritical items** are items that come in contact with intact skin but not mucous membranes, including stethoscopes, blood pressure cuffs, tuning forks, percussion hammers, and crutches. A common intermediate-level disinfectant is isopropyl alcohol, which is frequently used in the form of alcohol wipes.

Low-Level Disinfection

Low-level disinfection is a process that kills most bacteria, some viruses, and some fungi, but it cannot be relied on to kill resistant microorganisms, such as tubercle bacilli, and it cannot kill bacterial spores. Low-level disinfectants typically are used to disinfect surfaces such as examining tables, laboratory countertops, and walls. Low-level disinfectants used in the medical office include sodium hypochlorite (household bleach) and phenolics.

Types of Disinfectants

The disinfectants used most frequently in the medical office are described next. Table 3-1 lists these disinfectants, along with common names and uses for each.

Table 3-1 Disinfectants Used in the Medical Office		
Disinfectant	**Common Names**	**Use in the Medical Office**
Glutaraldehyde	Cidex MetriCide ProCide Omnicide Wavicide	Disinfection of flexible fiberoptic sigmoidoscopes
Alcohol	Isopropyl alcohol	Disinfection of stethoscopes, blood pressure cuffs, tuning forks, and percussion hammers; isopropyl alcohol wipes are used to disinfect rubber stoppers of multiple-dose medication vials
Chlorine and chlorine compounds	Sodium hypochlorite (household bleach)	Recommended by OSHA for decontamination of blood spills
Phenolics	Carbolic acid Hydroxybenzene Phenic acid Phenyl hydroxide Phenylic acid	Disinfection of walls, furniture, floors, and laboratory work surfaces
Quaternary ammonium compounds	Benzalkonium chloride	Disinfection of walls, furniture, floors, and laboratory work surfaces

Glutaraldehyde

Glutaraldehyde is often used as a high-level disinfectant in the medical office. It has a rapid killing action and is not inactivated by the presence of organic material. Because it does not corrode lenses, metal, or rubber, it is the agent of choice for semicritical items that cannot be exposed to heat, such as flexible fiberoptic sigmoidoscopes. Brand names for glutaraldehyde include Cidex and MetriCide.

Glutaraldehyde is highly toxic and can cause harm to the body if not handled properly. When working with glutaraldehyde, the medical assistant must work in an area that is well ventilated. Utility gloves and safety goggles must be worn to protect oneself from the irritating effects of this chemical (Figure 3-5). If the hands or any other part of the body comes in contact with glutaraldehyde, the area should be rinsed thoroughly under running water.

Alcohol

Alcohol is frequently used as a disinfectant in the medical office. The two most common types are *ethyl alcohol* and *isopropyl alcohol.* The disinfecting action of alcohol is increased by the presence of water; a 70% solution of alcohol is recommended. Stronger concentrations (95% to 100%) are not as effective. A disadvantage of alcohol is that it tends to dissolve the cement from around the lenses of instruments.

Ethyl alcohol and isopropyl alcohol provide intermediate- to low-level disinfection and can be used to disinfect stethoscopes, blood pressure cuffs, and percussion hammers. Isopropyl alcohol wipes are used to disinfect small surfaces such as the diaphragm of a stethoscope and rubber stoppers on multiple-dose medication vials.

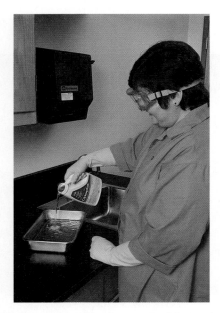

Figure 3-5. Kara wears utility gloves and safety goggles to protect herself from the irritating effects of glutaraldehyde.

What Would You Do? What Would You *Not* Do?

Case Study 2

Alecia Scout brings in her 2-year-old son, Benjamin, for a preschool physical examination. Benjamin is very unhappy and is crying loudly. Mrs. Scout says that Benjamin is upset because she wouldn't let him play with the toys in the waiting room. She is afraid that he will catch a disease from a sick child who has played with the toys. Mrs. Scout is visibly annoyed and says that medical offices should not keep toys in the waiting room because they might spread disease and cause problems for parents who do not want their children to play with the toys. ■

Chlorine and Chlorine Compounds

Chlorine and chlorine compounds are some of the oldest and most used disinfectants. Their most important use is in the chlorination of water. In the medical office, chlorine is used in the form of hypochlorites, such as liquid sodium hypochlorite (household bleach). A 10% solution of household bleach in water inactivates tuberculosis bacteria, hepatitis B and C viruses, human immunodeficiency virus, and many bacteria in 10 minutes at room temperature. Because of this, household bleach is recommended by OSHA for the decontamination of blood spills. A disadvantage of this disinfectant is that it can irritate skin and mucous membranes and is highly corrosive to metal.

Phenolics

Phenolics are used mainly to disinfect walls, furniture, floors, and laboratory work surfaces. This disinfectant is a corrosive poison and tends to be irritating to the eyes and skin. For this reason, eye and skin protective devices should be worn when working with phenolics in the pure form. Many derivatives of phenolics are commonly used and are usually nonirritating, including Lysol and hexachlorophene.

Memories *from* Externship

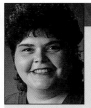

Kara VanDyke: During my externship experience, I was placed in a pediatrician's office. I wanted to go to a pediatric site because I love being around children. One day I was in the examining room with my patient, a 4-year-old boy who was there with his mother. It was standard procedure at this office to take every patient's temperature. I started getting out our electronic thermometer to take his temperature when I noticed he looked a little frightened. He was looking at the thermometer funny, and he said, "Can you do it in my ear?" I said I was sorry but we didn't have that kind of thermometer. I told him I could do it under his arm or under his tongue. His mom looked at him, and he said, "But I want it in my ear." He finally agreed to let me do it under his arm. When I was finished taking his temperature, he smiled and said, "You're the nicest doctor!" ■

Quaternary Ammonium Compounds

The quaternary ammonium compounds are sometimes used in the medical office for the disinfection of noncritical surfaces, such as floors, furniture, and walls.

Guidelines for Disinfection

Certain guidelines should be followed when disinfecting articles with a chemical agent.

Sanitize Articles before Disinfecting Them

The article to be disinfected must first be thoroughly sanitized. As previously described, sanitization includes the following steps: initial rinse, decontamination with a chemical disinfectant, cleaning, rinsing, drying, and checking for working order. It is important to remove all organic matter from the article before it is disinfected. If organic material is still present on the article after it is sanitized, it prevents the chemical disinfectant from reaching the surface of the article to kill microorganisms. In addition, with some disinfectants, organic material can absorb the chemical disinfectant and inactivate it. The article should be thoroughly rinsed of the detergent after cleaning because detergent residue may interfere with the disinfecting process. The article must be completely dry before placing it in the disinfectant because water dilutes the chemical and decreases its effectiveness.

Observe Safety Precautions

The medical assistant should carefully read the MSDS and the container label before using a chemical disinfectant. All safety precautions should be followed when using the chemical to protect against illness or injury from a hazardous chemical.

Properly Prepare and Use the Disinfectant

Products vary substantially among manufacturers; it is important that the manufacturer's directions on preparation, dilution, and use of the chemical disinfectant be followed carefully. The disinfectant should be prepared exactly as indicated on the container label. Some disinfectants are used at their full strength, whereas others require dilution.

Some disinfectants (e.g., glutaraldehyde) require the addition of an activator before they can be used. Preparing the disinfectant properly ensures the destruction of microorganisms. A disinfectant must be applied for a certain length of time to kill microorganisms. The medical assistant must be sure to disinfect for the length of time indicated on the container label.

Properly Store the Disinfectant

Chemical disinfectants should be closed tightly and stored properly under the storage conditions recommended by the manufacturer. Chemical disinfectants lose their potency over time; the medical assistant should strictly adhere to the manufacturer's recommendations for the disinfectant's shelf life, use life, and reuse life. Each of these terms is defined next as it relates to chemical disinfectants.

Shelf life   Shelf life is the length of time a chemical disinfectant may be stored before use and still retain its effectiveness. The shelf life is indicated by an expiration date on the container. The expiration date should always be checked before using the chemical. Outdated disinfectants should not be used.

Use life   Some disinfectants must be combined with another chemical, or activated, before they are used. Use life is the period of time a disinfecting solution is effective after it has been activated. Cidex Plus (Johnson & Johnson) is effective for 28 days after activation. At the end of this time, any chemical remaining in the container must be discarded. When a chemical disinfectant is activated, the date on which it will expire should be written on the label of the container.

Reuse life   Reuse life is the period of time that a disinfecting solution being used and reused remains active. For example, Cidex Plus can be reused for 28 days to disinfect articles after it has been poured into a disinfecting container. At the end of this time, the disinfectant must be discarded. The name of the disinfectant and the date when the disinfectant must be discarded should be written on an adhesive label and affixed to the container into which the disinfectant will be poured.

Text continued on p. 99

PROCEDURE 3-2   Chemical Disinfection of Articles

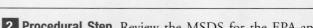
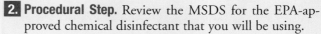

Outcome   Chemically disinfect articles.

Equipment/Supplies

- Sink
- Disposable gloves
- Heavy-duty utility gloves
- Contaminated articles

- EPA-approved chemical disinfectant and MSDS
- Disinfectant container
- Paper towels

---

1. Procedural Step. Sanitize the articles by performing procedural steps 1 through 10 in Procedure 3-1.

2. Procedural Step. Review the MSDS for the EPA-approved chemical disinfectant that you will be using.

Continued

PROCEDURE 3-2

PROCEDURE 3-2   Chemical Disinfection of Articles—cont'd

PROCEDURE 3-2

Principle. The MSDS provides information regarding the chemical disinfectant, its hazards, and measures to take to prevent injury and illness when handling the disinfectant.

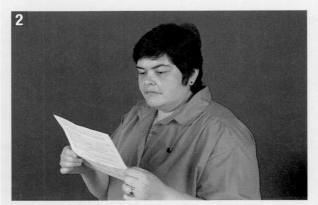

Review the MSDS.

3. **Procedural Step.** Check the expiration date of the chemical disinfectant.

   Principle. A disinfectant past its expiration date loses its potency and should not be used.

4. **Procedural Step.** Observe all personal safety precautions listed on the label. Follow the directions on the manufacturer's label for proper mixing, use, and reuse of the disinfectant. The disinfectant may need to be diluted with distilled water. Label the disinfecting container with the name of the disinfectant and its reuse life expiration date.

   Principle. Taking appropriate precautions with chemical agents prevents harm to the medical assistant from hazardous chemicals. When a disinfectant that is being used and reused reaches its expiration date, it is no longer effective and must be discarded.

5. **Procedural Step.** Immerse the articles in the chemical disinfectant. Ensure that the articles are completely submerged in the disinfectant.

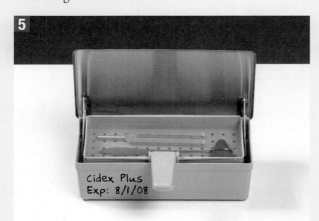

Completely immerse the articles in the disinfectant.

Principle. The articles must be completely submerged to allow the disinfectant to reach all parts of the instrument.

6. **Procedural Step.** Cover the container that holds the chemical disinfectant.

   Principle. The container must be kept covered to prevent the escape of toxic fumes and to prevent evaporation of the disinfectant, which could change its potency.

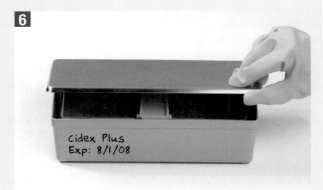

Cover the disinfectant container.

7. **Procedural Step.** Disinfect the articles for the proper length of time as indicated on the label of the container.

   Principle. Proper time requirements must be followed to ensure complete destruction of all microorganisms.

8. **Procedural Step.** Remove the articles from the disinfectant, and rinse them thoroughly. Dry the articles

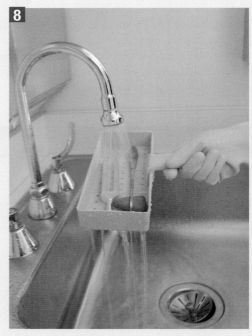

Rinse articles thoroughly to remove the disinfectant.

with paper towels. Dispose of the disinfectant according to the manufacturer's instructions.

Principle. All traces of the chemical disinfectant must be removed to prevent irritation to the patient's tissues. The disinfectant must be disposed of properly to prevent harm to the environment.

9. **Procedural Step.** Remove both sets of gloves, and sanitize your hands.
10. **Procedural Step.** Store the articles according to the medical office policy.

STERILIZATION

Sterilization is the process of destroying all forms of microbial life, including bacterial spores. An item that is sterile is free of all living microorganisms and spores. Sterilization must be used to process all critical items. A **critical item** is an item that comes in contact with sterile tissue or the vascular system.

As previously described, a semicritical item (one that comes in contact with nonintact skin or with intact mucous membranes) can be chemically disinfected using a high-level disinfectant. Most offices prefer instead to sterilize semicritical items in the autoclave (e.g., vaginal specula, nasal specula). The autoclave provides a convenient, efficient, safe, and inexpensive method for destroying microorganisms. Chemical disinfectants are not only more expensive to use, but also are more hazardous and create problems regarding their proper disposal. The exception is any semicritical item that is heat sensitive. Flexible fiberoptic sigmoidoscopes would be damaged by the heat of an autoclave and must be chemically disinfected.

Sterilization Methods

Sterilization involves the use of physical or chemical methods. Each method of sterilization has advantages and disadvantages. The method used to achieve sterility depends primarily on the nature of the item to be sterilized. The most common physical and chemical sterilization methods include the following:

Physical Methods	Chemical Methods
Steam under pressure (autoclave)	Ethylene oxide gas
Hot air (dry heat oven)	Cold sterilization (chemical agents)
Radiation	

The most common method for sterilizing articles in the medical office is steam under pressure using an autoclave. The autoclave is discussed in detail in this chapter; the other methods of sterilization are briefly described.

Autoclave

The autoclave is dependable, efficient, and economical and can be used to sterilize items that are not harmed by moisture or high temperature. Refer to the box *Items Sterilized in the Autoclave* for a list of heat-resistant items that can be sterilized in the autoclave.

Items Sterilized in the Autoclave	
Surgical instruments	Brushes
Medical instruments	Dressings
Minor office surgery trays	Glassware
Liquids	Reusable syringes

An **autoclave** consists of an outer jacket surrounding an inner sterilizing chamber. Under pressure, distilled water is converted to steam, which fills the inner sterilizing chamber. The pressure plays no direct part in killing microorganisms; rather, it functions to attain a higher temperature than could be reached by the steam from boiling water (212°F [100°C]). The cooler, drier air already in the chamber is forced out through the air exhaust valve.

It is important that all the air in the chamber be replaced by steam. When air is present, the temperature in the autoclave is reduced, and a temperature that is adequate for sterilization is not reached. When all the air has been removed, the air exhaust valve seals off the inner chamber, and the temperature in the autoclave begins to increase.

During the sterilization process, the steam penetrates the materials in the sterilizing chamber. The materials are cooler, so the steam condenses into moisture on them, giving up its heat. This heat serves to kill all microorganisms and their spores.

The autoclave is usually operated at approximately 15 pounds of pressure per square inch (psi) at a temperature of 250°F (121°C). Vegetative forms of most microorganisms are killed in a few minutes at temperatures ranging from 130°F to 150°F (54°C to 65°C), but certain bacterial spores can withstand a temperature of 240°F (115°C) for more than 3 hours. No organism, however, can survive direct exposure to saturated steam at 250°F (121°C) for 15 minutes or longer.

The sterilization process using the autoclave is discussed in this section (with the exception of sanitization, which was already presented). The sterilization process consists of the following components:

- Monitoring program
- Sanitizing articles
- Wrapping articles
- Operating the autoclave (autoclave cycle)
- Handling and storing packs
- Maintaining the autoclave

PROCEDURE 3-2

Monitoring Program

To ensure that instruments and supplies are sterile when used, the Centers for Disease Control and Prevention (CDC) recommends that the medical office establish and maintain a monitoring program of the sterilization process. The monitoring program should consist of the following:

1. Written policies and procedures for each step of the sterilization process
2. Sterilization indicators to ensure that minimum sterilizing conditions have been achieved
3. Records for each cycle maintained in an autoclave log (Figure 3-6)

The information that should be recorded for each autoclave cycle includes the following:

- Date and time of the cycle
- Description of the load
- Exposure time
- Exposure temperature
- Results of the sterilization indicator
- Initials of the operator

Some autoclaves have recorders that automatically print out a portion of this information at the end of the cycle (Figure 3-7).

Sterilization Indicators

Materials that are being sterilized must be exposed to steam at a sufficient temperature and for a proper length of time. Sterilization indicators are available to determine the effectiveness of the procedure and to check against improper wrapping of articles, improper loading of the autoclave, and faulty operation of the autoclave.

An article is not considered sterile unless the steam has penetrated to its center; most sterilization indicators are placed in the center of the article. The medical assistant should carefully read the instructions that come with the sterilization indicators. The most reliable indicators check for the attainment of the proper temperature and indicate the duration of the temperature.

If an indicator does not change properly, a problem may be present in the sterilization technique or in the working

AUTOCLAVE LOG						
Date/Time	Description of the Load	Cycle Time (min)	Temperature (° F)	Indicator* (+/–)	Initials	Comments
7/25/08 4:00 PM	Surgical instruments	20	250	—	KV	
7/26/08 3:00 PM	MOS tray setups	30	250	—	KV	

*Indicator Interpretation:
Positive (+): Spores not killed indicating sterilization conditions have not been met.
Negative (–): Spores killed indicating sterilization conditions have been met.

MAINTENANCE: (Indicate date, vendor name, service, etc.)

Figure 3-6. Example of an autoclave log.

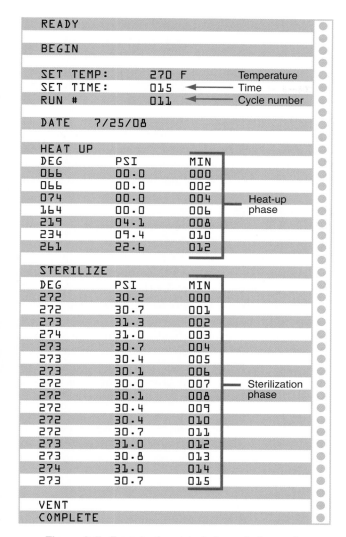

```
READY

BEGIN

SET  TEMP:      270 F      Temperature
SET  TIME:      015  ◄──── Time
RUN #           011  ◄──── Cycle number

DATE    7/25/08

HEAT UP
DEG      PSI       MIN
066      00.0      000
066      00.0      002
074      00.0      004      Heat-up
164      00.0      006      phase
219      04.1      008
234      09.4      010
261      22.6      012

STERILIZE
DEG      PSI       MIN
272      30.2      000
272      30.7      001
273      31.3      002
274      31.0      003
273      30.7      004
273      30.4      005
273      30.1      006
272      30.0      007    ── Sterilization
272      30.1      008       phase
272      30.4      009
272      30.4      010
272      30.7      011
273      31.0      012
273      30.8      013
274      31.0      014
273      30.7      015

VENT
COMPLETE
```

Figure 3-7. Example of a printout of an autoclave cycle.

What Would You Do? What Would You *Not* Do?

Case Study 3

Cassie Augusta is in the examining room and is being prepared for the removal of a sebaceous cyst. Cassie is concerned about the instruments that the physician will be using to perform the procedure. She wants to know if they are "safe." Cassie says that her friend Mackenzie got a tattoo several years ago and developed hepatitis 3 weeks later. Mackenzie thinks she got hepatitis from the instruments that were used for her tattoo procedure. Cassie wants to know if it is possible for an instrument to give someone hepatitis. She says she heard that hepatitis can cause liver cancer and wants to know if this is true. Cassie also wants to know if there is a vaccine to prevent hepatitis. ∎

condition of the autoclave. The manufacturer's guidelines for proper sterilization techniques should be reviewed, and the articles should be resterilized following these guidelines. If the indicator still does not change properly, the autoclave is in need of repair and should not be used until it has been serviced.

Sterilization indicators should be stored in a cool, dry area. Excessive heat or moisture can damage the indicator. The most common sterilization indicators are chemical indicators and biologic indicators, which are described next.

Chemical Indicators

Chemical indicators are impregnated with a **thermolabile** dye that changes color when exposed to the sterilization process. If the chemical reaction of the indicator does not show the expected results, the item may not be sterile and must be resterilized. Chemical indicators include autoclave tape and sterilization strips.

Autoclave Tape. Autoclave tape contains a chemical that changes color if it has been exposed to steam. The tape is available in a variety of colors, can be written on, and is useful for closing and identifying the wrapped article (Figure 3-8). Autoclave tape has some limitations as an indicator. Because it is placed on the outside of the pack, it cannot ensure that steam has penetrated to the center of the pack. It also does not ensure that the item has been sterilized; it merely indicates that an article has been in the autoclave and that a high temperature has been attained.

Sterilization Strips. Sterilization strips are commercially prepared paper or plastic strips that contain a thermolabile dye and that change color when exposed to steam under pressure for a certain length of time (Figure 3-9). Most

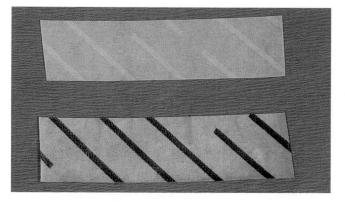

Figure 3-8. Autoclave tape. *Top*, Autoclave tape as it appears before the sterilization process. *Bottom*, Diagonal lines appear on the tape during autoclaving and indicate that the wrapped article has been autoclaved.

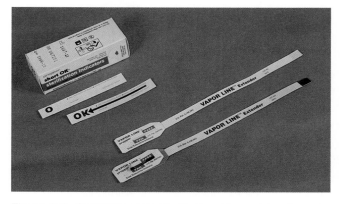

Figure 3-9. Sterilization strips. Sterilization strips contain a thermolabile dye and change color when exposed to steam under pressure for a certain length of time.

sterilization strips are designed to change color after being exposed to a temperature of 250°F (121°C) for 15 minutes. The indicator strip should be placed in the center of the wrapped pack, with the end containing the dye placed in an area of the pack considered to be the hardest for steam to penetrate.

Biologic Indicators

Biologic indicators are the best means available for determining the effectiveness of the sterilization procedure. The CDC recommends that medical office personnel use a biologic indicator to monitor all autoclaves at least once a week.

A biologic indicator is a preparation of living bacterial spores. Biologic indicators are commercially available in the form of dry spore strips in small glassine envelopes. Biologic monitoring of an autoclave requires the use of a preparation of spores of *Bacillus stearothermophilus,* which is a microorganism whose spores are particularly resistant to moist heat.

Each biologic testing unit includes two spore tests that are sterilized and one spore control that is not sterilized (Figure 3-10). The biologic indicator is placed in the center of two wrapped articles. The articles are placed in areas of the autoclave that are the least accessible to steam penetration, such as on the bottom tray of the autoclave, near the front of the autoclave, and in the back of the autoclave.

After the indicators have been exposed to sterilization conditions, they must be processed before the results can be obtained. The two methods for processing results are the in-house method and the mail-in method.

In-House Method. The in-house method involves processing and interpreting the results at the medical office. After sterilization, the processed spores are incubated for 24 to 48 hours. If sterilization conditions have been met, the color or condition of the processed spores is different from those of the control and the spore test is interpreted as negative. If sterilization conditions have not been met, the processed spores and the unprocessed control display the same color or condition and the spore test is interpreted as positive.

Mail-In Method. With this method, the processed bacterial spores and the (unprocessed) control are mailed to a processing laboratory. The test is performed by the laboratory, and the results are returned to the medical office.

If spores are not killed in routine spore tests, the autoclave should be checked immediately for proper use and function, and the spore test should be repeated. If the spore test remains positive, the autoclave should not be used until it is serviced.

Wrapping Articles

Articles to be sterilized in the autoclave first must be thoroughly sanitized (see Procedure 3-1). Next, the articles are prepared for autoclaving by wrapping them. The purpose of wrapping articles is to protect them from recontamination during handling and storage. Articles that are wrapped and handled correctly remain sterile after autoclaving until the package seal is broken.

The wrapping material should be made of a substance that is not affected by the sterilization process and should allow steam to penetrate while preventing contaminants, such as dust, insects, and microorganisms, from entering during handling and storage. It should not tear or puncture easily and should allow the sterilized package to be opened without contamination of the contents. A wrapper should not be used if it is torn or has a hole. Examples of wrapping material used for autoclaving are sterilization paper, sterilization pouches, and muslin.

Sterilization Paper

Sterilization paper is a disposable and inexpensive wrapping material. It consists of square sheets of paper of different sizes (Figure 3-11). The most common sizes (in inches) are 12×12, 15×15, 18×18, 24×24, 30×30, and 36×36. Articles must be wrapped in such a way that they do not become contaminated when the pack is opened. The proper method for wrapping instruments using sterilization paper is outlined in Procedure 3-3. This method of wrapping can be used for all types of instruments and supplies.

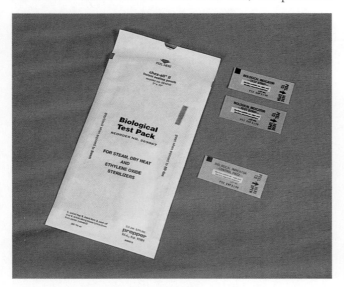

Figure 3-10. Biologic indicator. A biologic indicator includes two spore tests that are sterilized *(top right)* and one spore control that is not sterilized *(bottom right).*

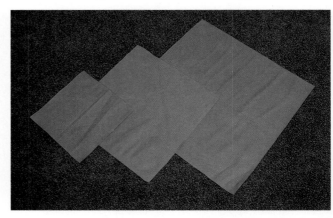

Figure 3-11. Sterilization paper wraps. Sterilization paper consists of square sheets of paper that are available in different sizes.

The disadvantage of sterilization paper is that it is difficult to spread open for removal of the contents. It has a "memory" and tends to flip back easily, so it may not open flat to provide a sterile field. (*Memory* is the ability of a material to retain a specific shape or configuration.) Because sterilization paper is opaque, it is impossible to view the contents of a pack before opening it.

Sterilization Pouches

Sterilization pouches typically consist of a combination of paper and plastic; paper comprises one side of the pouch, and a plastic film comprises the other side (Figure 3-12).

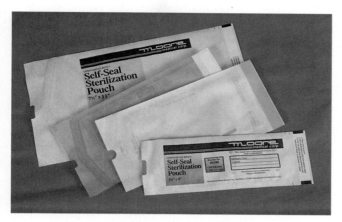

Figure 3-12. Sterilization pouches. Sterilization pouches consist of a combination of paper and plastic and are available in different sizes.

Sterilization pouches are available in different sizes; the most common sizes (in inches) are 3 × 9, 5 × 10, and 7 × 12.

Most pouches have a peel-apart seal on one end that is used later to open the pouch for removal of the sterile item. The other end of the pouch is open and is used to insert the item into the pouch. When the article has been inserted, this end is sealed with heat or adhesive tape. The proper method for wrapping an instrument using a pouch is outlined in Procedure 3-4.

Sterilization pouches provide good visibility of the contents on the plastic side. Most manufacturers include a sterilization indicator on the outside of the pouch. After removing a pouch from the autoclave, the medical assistant should check the indicator for proper color change. If the indicator does not change to the appropriate color (specified by the manufacturer), the contents of the pouch must be resterilized.

Muslin

Muslin is a reusable woven fabric and is available in different sizes. Muslin is flexible and easy to handle and is considered the most economical sterilization wrap because it can be reused. Because of its durability, muslin is frequently used to wrap large packs, such as tray setups for minor office surgery. Muslin is "memory free," so it lies flat when opened. A pack wrapped in muslin may be opened on a table so that the wrapper becomes a sterile field. The procedure for wrapping an article with muslin is the same as that for sterilization paper (see Procedure 3-3).

Text continued on p. 106

PROCEDURE 3-3 Wrapping Instruments Using Paper or Muslin

Outcome Wrap an instrument for autoclaving.

Equipment/Supplies

- Sanitized instrument
- Appropriate-sized wrapping material (sterilization paper or muslin)
- Sterilization indicator strip
- Autoclave tape
- Permanent marker

1. **Procedural Step.** Sanitize your hands.
2. **Procedural Step.** Assemble the equipment. Select the appropriate-sized wrapping material for the instrument being wrapped. Check the expiration date on the sterilization indicator box. If the sterilization strips are outdated, do not use them.
   Principle. Instruments are wrapped so that they are protected from recontamination after they have been sterilized. Outdated strip indicators may not provide accurate test results.
3. **Procedural Step.** Place the wrapping material on a clean, flat surface. Turn the wrap in a diagonal position to your body so that it resembles a diamond shape.

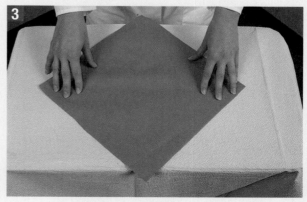

Turn the wrap in a diagonal position.

Continued

4. **Procedural Step.** Place the instrument in the center of the wrapping material with the longest part of the instrument pointing toward the two side corners. If the instrument has a movable joint, place it on the wrap in a slightly open position. If necessary, a gauze square can be used to hold the instrument in an open position.
   Principle. Instruments with movable joints must be in an open position to allow steam to reach all parts of the instrument. If the instrument is in a closed position, heat exposure could cause the instrument to crack at its weakest part, such as the lock area.

5. **Procedural Step.** Place a sterilization indicator in the center of the pack next to the instrument.
   Principle. Sterilization indicators assess the effectiveness of the sterilization process.

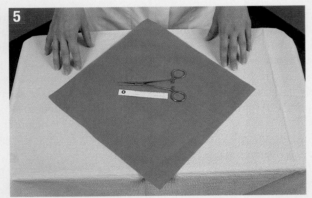

Place a sterilization indicator in the center of the pack next to the instrument.

6. **Procedural Step.** Fold the wrapping material up from the bottom, and double-back a small corner, creating a flap. This flap will later be used to open the sterile pack without contaminating the instrument.

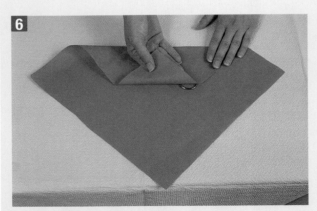

Fold the wrapping material up from the bottom, and double-back a small corner.

7. **Procedural Step.** Fold over one edge of the wrapping material, and double-back the corner.

8. **Procedural Step.** Fold over the other edge of the wrapping material, and double-back the corner.

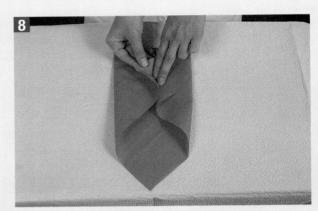

Fold over the other edge of the wrapping material, and double-back the corner.

9. **Procedural Step.** Fold the pack up from the bottom, pull the top flap down, and secure it with autoclave tape. Ensure that the pack is firm enough for handling but loose enough to permit proper circulation of steam.
   Principle. Instruments must be wrapped properly to permit full penetration of steam and to prevent contaminating them when the wrap is opened. Using autoclave tape indicates that the pack has been through the autoclave cycle and prevents mix-ups with packs that have not been processed.

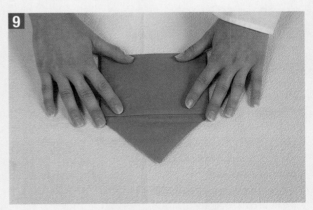

Fold the pack up from the bottom.

10. **Procedural Step.** Label the pack according to its contents. Mark the pack with the date of sterilization and your initials.

Principle. Dating the pack ensures that the most recently sterilized packs are stored in back of previously sterilized packs.

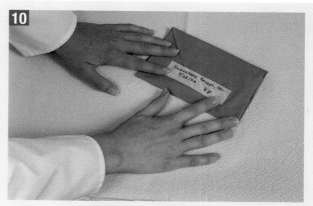

Label and date the pack. Include your initials.

PROCEDURE 3-4   Wrapping Instruments Using a Pouch

Outcome Wrap an instrument for autoclaving.

Equipment/Supplies

- Sanitized instrument
- Appropriate-sized sterilization pouch
- Permanent marker

---

1. **Procedural Step.** Sanitize your hands.

2. **Procedural Step.** Assemble the equipment. Select the appropriate-sized sterilization pouch for the instrument being wrapped. For hinged instruments, use a bag wide enough so that the instrument can be placed in a slightly open position inside the bag.

Principle. Instruments are wrapped so that they are protected from recontamination after they have been sterilized.

3. **Procedural Step.** Place the sterilization pouch on a clean, flat surface.

4. **Procedural Step.** Label the pack according to its contents. Mark the pack with the date of sterilization and your initials.

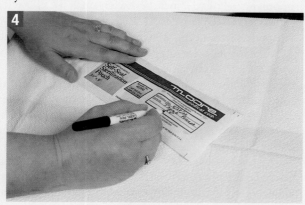

Label and date the pack. Include your initials.

Principle. Dating the pack ensures that the most recently sterilized packs are stored in back of previously sterilized packs.

5. **Procedural Step.** Insert the instrument to be sterilized into the unsealed, open end of the pouch. If the instrument has a movable joint, place it in the pouch in a slightly open position. If necessary, a gauze square can be used to hold the instrument in an open position.

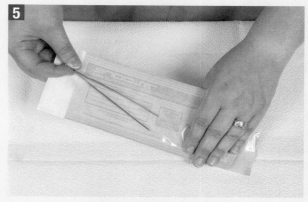

Insert the instrument into the pouch.

6. **Procedural Step.** Seal the open end of the pouch as follows:

Adhesive Closure. Peel off the paper strip located above the perforation to expose the adhesive. Fold

Continued

PROCEDURE 3-4   Wrapping Instruments Using a Pouch—cont'd

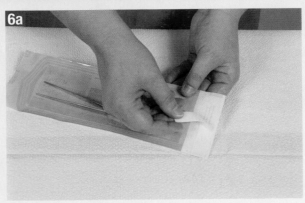

Peel off the paper strip.

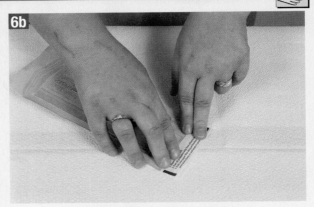

Press firmly to seal the pack.

along the perforation and press firmly to seal the paper to the plastic. Ensure that the seal is secure by running fingers back and forth on both sides of the pouch over the entire sealing area.

Heat Closure. Seal the pouch using a heat-sealing device.

7. **Procedural Step.** Sterilize the pack in the autoclave.

Operating the Autoclave

The autoclave must be operated according to the manufacturer's instructions. The medical assistant should read the operating manual carefully before running the autoclave for the first time. Thereafter, the manual should be kept in an accessible location so that it is available if needed as a reference. Procedure 3-5 outlines a general procedure for sterilizing articles in the autoclave.

The steps involved in achieving sterilization using an autoclave are known as the *autoclave cycle.* Accomplishment of each step varies based on whether the autoclave is operated manually or automatically. Figure 3-13 illustrates the autoclave cycle for manual and automatic autoclave operation.

Guidelines for Autoclave Operation

Location of the Autoclave

The autoclave must be placed on a level surface to ensure that the chamber fills correctly. The front of the autoclave should be near the front of the support surface so that water can be easily drained from the drain tube into a container when the autoclave is being flushed.

Filling the Water Reservoir

Distilled water is used to fill the water reservoir of the autoclave. Normal tap water contains minerals, such as chlorine, which have corrosive effects on the stainless-steel chamber of the autoclave. In addition, using tap water may cause a mineral buildup that can block the air exhaust valve. This causes air pockets, which prevent the temperature from increasing in the autoclave. The water reservoir is filled to the proper level as indicated in the operating manual. An autoclave malfunction may occur if the reservoir is overfilled or if there is not enough water in the reservoir.

Loading the Autoclave

For an item to attain sterility, steam must penetrate every fiber and reach every surface of the item at a required temperature and for a specified time. To accomplish this, all packs must be positioned in the chamber to allow free circulation and penetration of steam. The following guidelines should be followed when loading the autoclave:

1. Small packs are best because steam penetrates them more easily; it takes longer for steam to reach the center of a large pack to ensure sterilization. A pack should be no larger than $12 \times 12 \times 20$ inches.

2. To allow for proper steam penetration, the packs should be packed as loosely as possible inside the autoclave, with approximately 1 to 3 inches between small packs and 2 to 4 inches between large packs. Packs should not be allowed to touch surrounding walls, and at least 1 inch should separate the autoclave trays. Placing the articles too close together retards the flow of steam (Figure 3-14).

3. Jars and glassware should be placed on their sides in the autoclave with their lids removed. If they are placed upright, air may be trapped in them, and they would not be sterilized. Trapped air must flow out and be replaced by steam during the sterilization process (Figure 3-15).

4. Packs that contain layers of fabric, such as dressings, should be placed in a vertical position. Because steam flows from top to bottom, this method allows the steam to penetrate the layers of fabric.

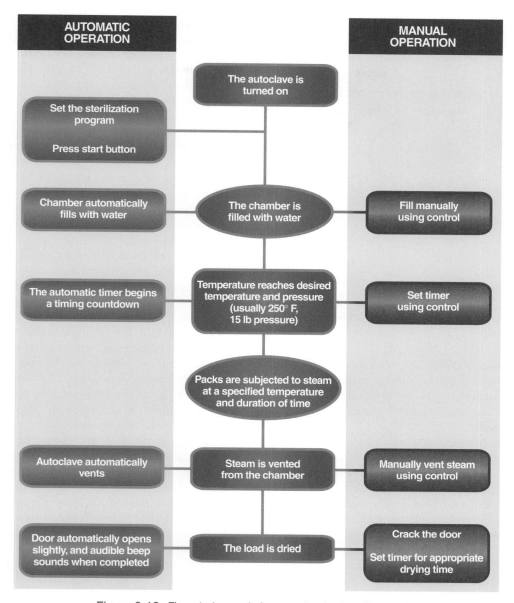

AUTOMATIC OPERATION

MANUAL OPERATION

The autoclave is turned on

Set the sterilization program

Press start button

Chamber automatically fills with water — The chamber is filled with water — Fill manually using control

The automatic timer begins a timing countdown — Temperature reaches desired temperature and pressure (usually 250° F, 15 lb pressure) — Set timer using control

Packs are subjected to steam at a specified temperature and duration of time

Autoclave automatically vents — Steam is vented from the chamber — Manually vent steam using control

Door automatically opens slightly, and audible beep sounds when completed — The load is dried — Crack the door

Set timer for appropriate drying time

Figure 3-13. The autoclave cycle for manual and automatic operation.

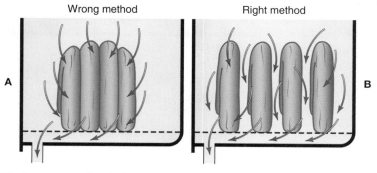

Wrong method   Right method

A   B

Figure 3-14. Arrangement of packs in the autoclave. **A,** Improper arrangement of packs in the autoclave. This arrangement prevents adequate penetration of steam, resulting in failure to sterilize the portions in the center of the mass. **B,** Proper arrangement of packs in the autoclave. The packs are separated from each other, and steam can now permeate each pack quickly and in the much shorter period of exposure needed. (Courtesy of and modified from AMSCO/American Sterilizer Company, Erie, Penn.)

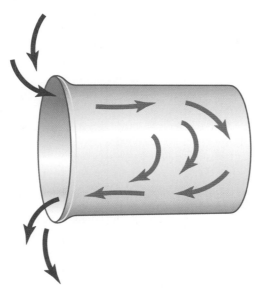

Figure 3-15. Jars and glassware should be placed on their sides in the autoclave with their lids removed. (Courtesy AMSCO/American Sterilizer Company, Erie, Penn.)

5. Sterilization pouches should be positioned on their sides to maximize steam circulation and to facilitate the drying process. Pouches can also be placed on the autoclave tray with the paper side up and the plastic side down.

Timing the Load

The autoclave is operated at approximately 15 psi with a temperature of 250°F (121°C). The length of time required for sterilization varies according to the item that is being sterilized (Table 3-2). Steam can easily reach the surfaces of hard, nonporous items such as unwrapped instruments (e.g., vaginal specula) to kill microorganisms; these items require approximately 15 minutes of sterilization time. A large minor office surgery pack requires a longer sterilization time, about 30 minutes, because more time is needed for steam to penetrate to the center of the pack. Rubber goods may be damaged, however, by exposure to excessive heat. To prevent this, the medical assistant should sterilize rubber items for only the prescribed amount of time.

The sterilizing time should not begin until the desired temperature in the autoclave has been reached. Timing the load is accomplished automatically or manually. Autoclaves with automatic operation begin timing the load automatically when the desired temperature has been reached. With the manual method of operation, the medical assistant must set the timer by hand using a timing control on the front of the autoclave. The medical assistant should not set the timer until the temperature gauge reaches the desired temperature. The articles in the load are not considered sterile unless they have been subjected to steam for the proper length of time at the proper temperature.

Drying the Load

The sterilized articles are moist and must be allowed to dry before they are removed from the autoclave. Microorganisms can move quickly through the moisture on a wet wrap and onto the sterile article inside, resulting in contamination.

When the load has been subjected to steam for the proper length of time and temperature, the chamber must be vented of steam. Venting the chamber permits the pressure in the autoclave to decrease to zero and the chamber to cool, making it safe for the door to be opened. Most autoclaves are designed to vent automatically, which eliminates having to vent them manually.

The door of the autoclave should be opened approximately ½ inch but no more than 1 inch. Opening the door more than 1 inch causes cold air from the outside to rush into the autoclave, resulting in condensation of water on the packs. Cracking the door allows the moisture on the articles to change from a liquid to a vapor and to escape through the crack. The residual heat in the inner chamber also helps to dry the articles. The load should be allowed to dry for 15 to 60 minutes, depending on the type of autoclave and the load. Loads that contain large packs require a longer drying time than loads with smaller

Table 3-2 Minimum Sterilizing Times		
Items (Manual Operation)*	Program (Automatic Operation)†	Time (min at 250°F [121°C])
Unwrapped nonsurgical instruments	Unwrapped	15
Open glass or metal canisters		
Nonsurgical rubber tubing		
Wrapped instruments	Wrapped	20
Fabric or muslin		
Wrapped trays of loose instruments		
Rubber tubing		
Minor office surgery tray setup (wrapped)	Packs	30
Liquids or gels	Liquids	30

*Manual operation: The sterilizing time is selected based on the items being sterilized, as indicated in this column. The sterilizing time is set using the manual timing control when the autoclave has reached a temperature of 250°F (121°C).
†Automatic operation: The sterilization program selected from this column is based on the item being autoclaved. The program is selected by pressing the appropriate program button on the front of the autoclave (i.e., unwrapped, wrapped, packs, liquids). The autoclave automatically begins the proper timing countdown when it reaches 250°F (121°C).

packs. The medical assistant should follow the manufacturer's recommendations for proper drying times of various loads.

Handling and Storing Packs

Sterilized wrapped articles should be handled carefully and as little as possible. If a wrapped article is crushed, compressed, or dropped, the sterility of the contents cannot be assumed, and the pack must be resterilized. This is known as *event-related sterility,* meaning that a sterile pack is considered sterile indefinitely, unless an event occurs that interferes with the sterility of the article.

Sterilized packs should be stored in clean, dry areas that are free from dust, insects, and other sources of contamination. Wrapped articles should be stored with the most recently sterilized articles placed in the back. The medical assistant should thoroughly check each sterilized pack at least twice: before storing it and before using it. If the pack is torn or opened, or if it is wet, it is no longer sterile and must be rewrapped and resterilized.

Maintaining the Autoclave

For the autoclave to work efficiently, it must be maintained properly. The operating manual that accompanies the autoclave provides specific information for the care and maintenance of that type of autoclave.

Safety precautions should be followed when performing maintenance procedures. Before proceeding with preventive maintenance, the autoclave must be cool, the pressure gauge at zero, and the power cord disconnected from the wall socket. Autoclave maintenance is performed on a daily, weekly, and monthly basis as follows:

Daily Maintenance

1. Wipe the outside of the autoclave with a damp cloth and a mild detergent.
2. Wipe the interior of the autoclave and the trays with a damp cloth.
3. Clean the rubber gasket on the door of the autoclave with a damp cloth.
4. Inspect the rubber door gasket for damage that could prevent a good seal.

Weekly Maintenance

1. Wash the inside of the chamber and the trays with a commercial autoclave cleaner according to the manufacturer's instructions, observing all personal safety precautions. This usually involves the following steps: The water reservoir must be drained first. A soft cloth or a soft brush should be used to clean the chamber. Do not use steel wool or a steel brush or other abrasive agents because they can damage the chamber. When the chamber is clean, it should be rinsed thoroughly with distilled water. The chamber must be dried thoroughly and the door left open overnight.
2. Wash the metal shelves with an autoclave cleaner, and rinse them thoroughly with distilled water.

Monthly Maintenance

1. Flush the system to remove any buildup of residue, which could cause corrosion of the chamber lines. Carefully follow the manufacturer's directions in the instruction manual to perform this procedure.
2. Check the air trap jet to ensure it is functioning properly. The air trap jet prevents air pockets from occurring in the chamber, to ensure adequate sterilization.
3. Check the safety valve to ensure it is functioning properly. The safety valve releases pressure in the chamber if it gets too high.

Other Sterilization Methods

In addition to the autoclave, other methods can be used to sterilize articles. These methods are not generally used in the medical office and are discussed only briefly in this chapter.

Dry Heat Oven

Dry heat ovens are used to sterilize articles that cannot be penetrated by steam or may be damaged by it. Dry heat is less corrosive than moist heat for instruments with sharp edges; it does not dull their sharp edges. Oil, petroleum jelly, and powder cannot be penetrated by steam and must be sterilized in a dry heat oven. Moist heat sterilization tends to erode the ground-glass surfaces of reusable syringes, whereas dry heat does not.

Dry heat ovens operate similar to an ordinary cooking oven. A longer exposure period is needed with dry heat because microorganisms and spores are more resistant to dry heat than to moist heat and because dry heat penetrates more slowly and unevenly than moist heat. The most commonly used temperature for dry heat sterilization is 320°F (160°C) for 1 to 2 hours, depending on the article being sterilized. The recommended wrapping material for dry heat sterilization is aluminum foil because it is a good conductor of heat, and it protects against recontamination during handling and storage. Dry heat sterilization indicators are available to determine the effectiveness of the sterilization process.

Ethylene Oxide Gas Sterilization

Ethylene oxide is a colorless gas that is toxic and flammable. It is used to sterilize heat-sensitive items that cannot be sterilized in an autoclave. After items are sterilized with this gas, they must be aerated to remove the toxic residue of the ethylene oxide.

Ethylene oxide sterilization is a more complex and expensive process than steam sterilization. It frequently is used in the medical manufacturing industry for producing prepackaged, presterilized disposable items, such as syringes, sutures, catheters, and surgical packs.

Cold Sterilization

Cold sterilization involves the use of a chemical agent for an extended length of time. Only chemicals that are designated *sterilants* by the U.S. Environmental Protection Agency (EPA) can be used for sterilizing articles. If a chemical agent

PROCEDURE 3-5

holds this status, the word *sterilant* is printed on the front of the container.

The item to be sterilized must be completely submerged in the chemical for a long time (6 to 24 hours depending on the manufacturer's instructions). Prolonged immersion of instruments can damage them. In addition, each time an instrument is added to the instrument container, the clock must be restarted for the entire amount of time. For these reasons, and because this method involves the use of a haz-ardous chemical, cold sterilization should be used only when an autoclave, gas, or a dry heat oven are not indicated or are unavailable.

Radiation

Radiation uses high-energy ionizing radiation to sterilize articles. Medical manufacturers use radiation to sterilize prepackaged surgical equipment and instruments that cannot be sterilized by heat or chemicals.

PROCEDURE 3-5   Sterilizing Articles in the Autoclave

Outcome Sterilize a load of contaminated articles in the autoclave.

Equipment/Supplies

- Autoclave and instruction manual
- Distilled water
- Wrapped articles
- Heat-resistant gloves

1. Procedural Step. Assemble the equipment.

2. Procedural Step. Check the level of water in the autoclave and add distilled water, if needed.
Principle. Water contained in the water reservoir of the autoclave is converted to steam during the sterilization process. Distilled water is used to prevent corrosion of the stainless-steel chamber of the autoclave.

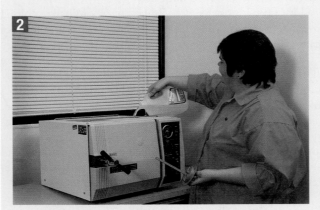

If needed, add distilled water to the autoclave.

3. Procedural Step. Properly load the autoclave following these guidelines:
a. Do not overload the chamber. Small packs should be placed 1 to 3 inches apart, and large packs should be placed 2 to 4 inches apart. The packs should not touch the chamber walls.
b. Ensure that at least 1 inch separates the autoclave trays.
c. Place jars and glassware on their sides.
d. Place dressings in a vertical position.
e. When sterilizing dressings and hard goods together, place dressings on the top shelf and hard goods on the lower shelf.

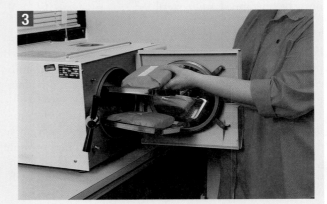

Properly load the autoclave.

f. When using sterilization pouches, set the pouches on their sides to maximize steam circulation and to facilitate drying.
Principle. The autoclave must be loaded properly to ensure adequate steam penetration of all articles.

4. Procedural Step. Operate the autoclave according to the procedure described in the instruction manual. A general procedure for the manual and the automatic methods of operation follows.

Manually Operated Autoclave

a. Determine the sterilizing time for the type of articles being autoclaved (see Table 3-2).
b. Turn on the autoclave.
c. Fill the chamber with water using the appropriate control.
d. Securely close and latch the door of the autoclave.
e. Set the timing control when the temperature gauge reaches the desired temperature (usually 250°F [121°C]). At the end of the steam exposure time, an indicator light usually comes on or a beeper sounds.

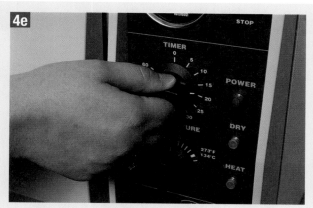
Set the timing control.

f. If the autoclave does not vent automatically, use the appropriate control to release steam from the chamber.

g. Dry the load by cracking open the door approximately ½ inch but no more than 1 inch. Set the drying time using the timing control. The drying time varies between 15 and 60 minutes, depending on the autoclave and the type of load.

Principle. To ensure sterilization, the load should not be timed until the proper temperature has been reached. The sterility of wrapped packs cannot be ensured unless the wrapped articles are allowed to dry fully. Microorganisms can move through the moisture on a wet wrap and contaminate the sterile article inside.

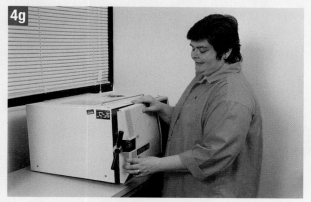
Crack the door to dry the load.

Automatically Operated Autoclave

a. Securely close and latch the door of the autoclave.
b. Turn on the autoclave.
c. Determine the sterilization program according to what is being autoclaved (see Table 3-2). Press the appropriate program button on the front of the autoclave to select the program. Press the start button.
d. Indicators on the front of the autoclave tell you what is happening (automatically) in the autoclave:

Filling Indicator. Lights up when the chamber is filling with water

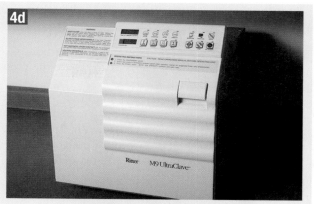
Automatic autoclave buttons and indicators.

Sterilizing Indicator. Lights up during the heat-up and sterilization phases of the cycle
Temperature Display. Digital display of the temperature in the autoclave
Time Display. Digital countdown of the time remaining in the sterilization program
Drying Indicator. Lights up during the drying phase of the cycle
Complete or Ready Indicator. Illuminates when the autoclave has completed the cycle and sterilized articles can be removed from the autoclave

5. Procedural Step. Turn off the autoclave. Wearing heat-resistant gloves, remove the load. Do not touch the inner chamber of the autoclave with your bare hands.

Principle. Heat-resistant gloves protect the medical assistant's hands when the warm packs from the chamber of the autoclave are being removed. The inner chamber of the autoclave is hot and could burn bare skin.

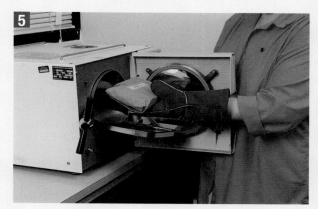
Remove the load with heat-resistant gloves.

6. Procedural Step. Inspect the packs as you take them out of the autoclave. If the packs show any damage, such as holes or tears, the articles should be rewrapped and resterilized.

Continued

PROCEDURE **3-5**   **Sterilizing Articles in the Autoclave—cont'd**

7. Procedural Step. Check the sterilization indicators located on the outside of the pack to ensure the proper response has occurred.

Principle. Autoclave tape only indicates that the article has been through the autoclave cycle; it does not ensure that sterilization has taken place. Sterilization is determined when the pack is opened for use and the sterilization strip indicator in the center of the pack is checked for its proper response.

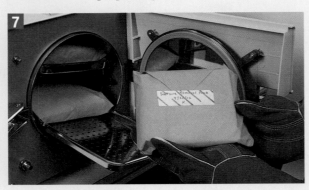
Check the sterilization indicator on the outside of the pack.

8. Procedural Step. Record monitoring information in the autoclave log. Include the date and time of the cycle, a description of the load, the exposure time and temperature. If a biologic indicator has been included in the load, process it according to the medical office policy and record results on the autoclave log.

9. Procedural Step. Store the packs in a clean, dustproof area with the most recently sterilized packs placed behind previously sterilized packs.

10. Procedural Step. Maintain appropriate daily care of the autoclave, following the manufacturer's recommendations. The daily care of the autoclave includes the following:

a. Wipe the outside of the autoclave with a damp cloth and a mild detergent.
b. Wipe the interior of the autoclave and the trays with a damp cloth.
c. Clean the rubber gasket located on the door of the autoclave with a damp cloth.
d. Inspect the rubber door gasket for damage that could prevent a good seal.

Principle. For the autoclave to work efficiently, it must be properly maintained.

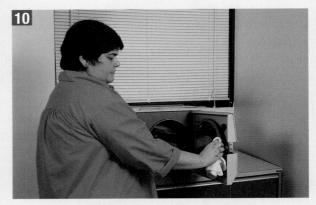
Clean the rubber gasket with a damp cloth.

 *Check out the **Companion CD** bound with the book to access additional interactive activities.*

MEDICAL PRACTICE *and the* LAW

If not performed properly, sterilization and disinfection can adversely affect patients, which can make the medical assistant and other office personnel liable for resultant injuries. Meticulous care must be taken to ensure that all procedures are performed correctly and completely.

Sterilization and disinfection procedures include the use of hazardous chemicals. These chemicals must be stored, used, and disposed of in specific ways mandated by law. The autoclave can be a dangerous machine if it is not used correctly, and it could harm others with hot steam. If you use the autoclave without proper instruction, you could be liable for injuries or accidents resulting from misuse.

Whenever you are dealing with contaminated articles, you have a duty to protect yourself, other employees, patients, and other articles from cross-contamination. ∎

What Would You Do? What Would You *Not* Do? RESPONSES

Case Study 1
Page 86
What Did Kara Do?
❑ Complimented Mrs. Cordera for her concern and efforts to baby-proof her home.
❑ Gave Mrs. Cordera a patient information brochure on baby-proofing the home.
❑ Told Mrs. Cordera that she should assume that all cleaning products are poisonous. Got out a disinfectant container and showed Mrs. Cordera the information on the label that tells what to do in case of an accidental poisoning.
❑ Gave the National Poison Control hotline number (1-800-222-1222) to Mrs. Cordera and told her that was the fastest way to obtain information on what to do in case of an accidental poisoning. Told her to keep this number by her phone.

What Did Kara Not *Do?*
❑ Did not take Mrs. Cordera's question lightly.

What Would You Do/What Would You *Not* Do? Review Kara's response and place a checkmark next to the information you included in your response. List additional information you included in your response.

_____
_____
_____
_____

Case Study 2
Page 96
What Did Kara Do?
❑ Explained to Mrs. Scout that toys are in the waiting room for children to play with to make their visit more comfortable and less stressful.
❑ Reassured Mrs. Scout that the medical office personnel do everything they can to prevent the spread of germs in the office and that the toys are sanitized every day.
❑ Relayed to Mrs. Scout that only toys that can be sanitized are kept in the medical office.
❑ Told Mrs. Scout that her concern would be brought up at the weekly office meeting.

What Did Kara Not *Do?*
❑ Did not get defensive because Mrs. Scout was just being concerned about her child's health.

What Would You Do/What Would You *Not* Do? Review Kara's response and place a checkmark next to the information you included in your response. List additional information you included in your response.

_____
_____
_____
_____

Case Study 3
Page 101
What Did Kara Do?
❑ Told Cassie through verbal and nonverbal behavior that her concern was valid.
❑ Told Cassie that hepatitis can be transmitted through dirty instruments.
❑ Reassured Cassie that all instruments are sterilized in the autoclave, which has special indicators to ensure all germs have been killed.
❑ Gave Cassie a patient information brochure on hepatitis. Told her that individuals with chronic hepatitis can develop liver cancer and that the best way to avoid hepatitis is through measures and behaviors recommended for prevention.
❑ Told Cassie that a vaccine is available to prevent hepatitis B, but not hepatitis C.

What Did Kara Not *Do?*
❑ Did not dismiss her concern about dirty instruments as unimportant.
❑ Did not overly alarm her about the consequences of chronic hepatitis.

What Would You Do/What Would You *Not* Do? Review Kara's response and place a checkmark next to the information you included in your response. List additional information you included in your response.

_____
_____
_____
_____

APPLY YOUR KNOWLEDGE

Choose the best answer to each of the following questions.

1. Kara VanDyke, CMA, is getting ready to sanitize surgical instruments that were used to perform a minor office surgery. Kara performs all of the following steps *except:*
   A. Applies clean disposable gloves.
   B. Applies heavy-duty utility gloves.
   C. Separates sharp and delicate instruments from other instruments.
   D. Rinses the instruments under a stream of hot water.

2. Kara prepares to decontaminate the instruments using Cidex Plus chemical disinfectant. The purpose of decontaminating instruments is to:
   A. Prevent organic material from drying on the instruments.
   B. Remove pathogenic microorganisms from the instruments.
   C. Remove stains from the instruments.
   D. Lubricate the instruments.

3. Kara needs to know what personal protective equipment she should use when working with Cidex Plus. Which of the following would provide her with this information?
   A. The MSDS for Cidex Plus.
   B. The label on the container of Cidex Plus.
   C. Both the MSDS and the container label for Cidex Plus.
   D. Her driver's license.

4. Kara performs the decontamination process. She performs all of the following steps *except:*
   A. Checks the expiration date on the label of the chemical disinfectant.
   B. Completely submerges the instruments in the chemical disinfectant.
   C. Scrubs the instruments with a nylon brush.
   D. Disinfects the instruments for 10 minutes.

5. After the instruments have been decontaminated, Kara prepares to clean them using a commercial instrument cleaner. Kara checks the label of the instrument cleaner to ensure that:
   A. It is low sudsing.
   B. It has an acidic pH.
   C. It destroys bacterial spores.
   D. Four out of five dentists recommend this cleaner.

6. Kara prepares the cleaning solution and places the instruments in the basin that contains the solution. Which of the following does Kara perform to complete the sanitization procedure?
   A. Cleanses the surface of each instrument with a nylon brush.
   B. Rinses each instrument for 20 to 30 seconds.
   C. Checks the working order of each instrument.
   D. Dries the instruments.
   E. All of the above.

7. Kara is preparing to autoclave the surgical instruments that she sanitized. She wraps the instruments in sterilization paper before placing them in the autoclave. The purpose of wrapping articles that are to be sterilized is:
   A. To permit better steam penetration during autoclaving.
   B. To protect the articles from recontamination after autoclaving.
   C. So that they can be given as Christmas gifts.
   D. To protect the instruments from damage.

8. Kara is getting ready to autoclave the wrapped packs of surgical instruments. Which of the following would represent an *error* in technique during the autoclaving process?
   A. Filling the water reserve with tap water.
   B. Loading the autoclave by positioning the packs 1 to 3 inches apart.
   C. Setting the timer when the temperature gauge reaches 250°F.
   D. Ensuring that the sterilized packs are dry before removing them from the autoclave.

9. When Kara removes a pack from the autoclave, she notices the autoclave tape has changed color. She realizes that this indicates that:
   A. The autoclave is functioning properly.
   B. The pack has been exposed to heat.
   C. The pack has been exposed to a temperature of 250°F for 15 minutes.
   D. The pack needs to be rewrapped and run through the autoclave again.

10. Kara properly stores the sterilized packs. Kara performs all of the following steps *except:*
   A. Handles the packs carefully and as little as possible.
   B. Rewraps and resterilizes a pack that is torn.
   C. Places the packs in a clean, dustproof area.
   D. Places the sterilized packs in front of previously sterilized packs.

CERTIFICATION REVIEW

❑ **The Hazard Communication Standard (HCS)** is required by OSHA for any facility that uses or stores hazardous chemicals. Its purpose is to ensure that employees are informed of the hazards associated with chemicals in their workplaces and the precautions to take to protect themselves when working with hazardous chemicals.

❑ **A hazardous chemical** is any chemical that presents a threat to the health and safety of an individual coming into contact with it.

❑ **A hazard communication program** must be developed by employers who use and store hazardous chemicals in their workplace, describing what their facility is doing to meet the requirements of the HCS.

❑ **A hazardous chemical** must contain a label that includes the name of the chemical, manufacturer information, physical and health hazards of the chemical, safety precautions, and storing and handling information.

❑ **A material safety data sheet (MSDS)** provides information regarding the chemical, its hazards, and measures to take to prevent injury and illness when handling the chemical. An MSDS must be kept on file for each hazardous chemical used or stored in the workplace.

❑ **The HCS requires** that employees be provided with information and training regarding hazardous chemicals in the workplace. The training program must be offered at the time of an employee's initial assignment to a work area where hazardous chemicals are present and whenever a new chemical hazard is introduced into the workplace.

❑ **Sanitization** is a process that removes organic material from an article and lowers the number of microorganisms to a safe level. The most frequent items sanitized in the medical office are medical and surgical instruments.

❑ **Instruments can be cleaned** manually or by using an ultrasonic cleaner. The manual method uses a brush, instrument cleaner, and friction to clean instruments. An ultrasonic cleaner uses a cleaning solution and sound waves to clean the instruments. To prevent the formation of a permanent stain, items made of dissimilar metals should not be cleaned together.

❑ **Disinfection** is the process of destroying pathogenic microorganisms; it does not kill bacterial spores. Disinfectants consist of chemical agents that are applied to inanimate objects. The disinfectants used most often in the medical office are glutaraldehyde, alcohol, sodium hypochlorite (household bleach), phenolics, and quaternary ammonium compounds.

❑ **Disinfection can be classified** into the following levels: high, intermediate, and low. High-level disinfection is used to disinfect semicritical items that are heat sensitive, such as flexible fiberoptic sigmoidoscopes. Intermediate-level disinfection is used for noncritical items, such as stethoscopes and blood pressure cuffs. Low-level disinfection is used to disinfect surfaces such as examining tables, countertops, and walls.

❑ **Sterilization** is the process of destroying all forms of microbial life, including bacterial spores. Sterilization must be used for critical items. Critical items are items that come in contact with sterile tissue or the vascular system.

❑ **The autoclave** is used most often in the medical office for sterilization. The autoclave is usually operated at approximately 15 pounds of pressure per square inch at a temperature of 2508°F (1218°C).

❑ **To ensure that instruments and supplies are sterile** when used, a monitoring program should be established in the medical office. This program should include reviewing sterilization policies and procedures, checking the use of sterilization indicators, and maintaining records for each autoclave cycle.

❑ **Sterilization indicators** determine the effectiveness of the sterilization process and include chemical indicators and biologic indicators. Chemical indicators use a thermolabile dye that changes color when exposed to the sterilization process. Biologic indicators are the best indicators available for determining the effectiveness of the sterilization procedure. They consist of a preparation of heat-resistant living bacterial spores.

❑ **The purpose of wrapping articles** for autoclaving is to protect them from recontamination during handling and storage. Examples of wraps commonly used include sterilization paper, sterilization pouches, and muslin.

❑ **The autoclave cycle** refers to the steps involved in achieving sterilization with an autoclave. The autoclave must be loaded properly so that steam can easily penetrate the contents of the load. The length of time for sterilization varies according to the item that is being sterilized. The sterilizing time should not begin until the desired temperature in the autoclave has been reached. To prevent recontamination, articles must be completely dry before they are removed from the autoclave. Sterilized wrapped articles should be handled carefully and as little as possible. They should be stored in a clean, dustproof area. The autoclave should be properly maintained following a daily, weekly, and monthly schedule.

Continued

CERTIFICATION REVIEW—cont'd

❑ **Event-related sterility** means that a sterile pack is considered sterile indefinitely unless an event occurs that interferes with the sterility of the article. If a pack is torn or opened or if it is wet, it is no longer sterile and must be rewrapped and resterilized.

❑ **Other methods that can be used to sterilize articles** include dry heat, ethylene oxide gas, chemical agents, and radiation. Ethylene oxide and radiation are used by the medical manufacturing industry for producing prepackaged and presterilized disposable items.

TERMINOLOGY REVIEW

Antiseptic A substance that kills disease-producing microorganisms but not their spores. An antiseptic is usually applied to living tissue.

Autoclave An apparatus for the sterilization of materials, using steam under pressure.

Contaminate To soil, stain, or pollute; to make impure.

Critical item An item that comes in contact with sterile tissue or the vascular system.

Decontamination The use of physical or chemical means to remove or destroy pathogens on an item so that it is no longer capable of transmitting disease; this makes the item safe to handle.

Detergent An agent that cleanses by emulsifying dirt and oil.

Disinfectant An agent used to destroy pathogenic microorganisms but not their spores. Disinfectants are usually applied to inanimate objects.

Hazardous chemical Any chemical that presents a threat to the health and safety of an individual coming into contact with it.

Incubate To provide proper conditions for growth and development.

Load The articles that are being sterilized.

Material safety data sheet (MSDS) A sheet that provides information regarding a chemical, its hazards, and measures to take to prevent injury and illness when handling the chemical.

Noncritical item An item that comes into contact with intact skin, but not mucous membranes.

Sanitization A process to remove organic matter from an article and to reduce the number of microorganisms to a safe level as determined by public health requirements.

Semicritical item An item that comes into contact with nonintact skin or intact mucous membranes.

Spore A hard, thick-walled capsule formed by some bacteria that contains only the essential parts of the protoplasm of the bacterial cell.

Sterilization The process of destroying all forms of microbial life, including bacterial spores.

Thermolabile Easily affected or changed by heat.

ON THE WEB

For Information on Infection Control in the Health Care Setting:

Centers for Disease Control and Prevention: www.cdc.gov

Environmental Protection Agency: www.epa.gov

National Institute of Environmental Health Sciences: www.niehs.nih.gov

National Institute for Occupational Safety and Health: www.cdc.gov/niosh

Infection Control Today: www.infectioncontroltoday.com

Association for Professionals in Infection Control and Epidemiology: www.apic.com

To Locate a Material Data Safety Sheet:

MSDS-Search: www.msdssearch.com

HazCom: www.hazard.com/msds

4

Vital Signs

NATIONAL COMPETENCIES

Clinical Competencies
Patient Care
Obtain vital signs.
Prepare and maintain examination and treatment areas.

General Competencies
Professional Communications
Recognize and respond to verbal communications.
Recognize and respond to nonverbal communications.

Patient Instruction
Provide instruction for health maintenance and disease prevention.

Operational Functions
Perform routine maintenance of administrative and clinical equipment.

KEY TERMS

adventitious (ad-ven-TISH-us) sounds
afebrile (uh-FEB-ril)
alveolus (al-VEE-uh-lus)
antecubital (AN-tih-CYOO-bi-tul) space
antipyretic (AN-tih-pye-REH-tik)
aorta (ay-OR-tuh)
apnea (AP-nee-uh)
axilla (aks-ILL-uh)
bounding pulse
bradycardia (BRAY-dee-CAR-dee-uh)
bradypnea (BRAY-dip-NEE-uh)
Celsius (SELL-see-us) scale
conduction (kon-DUK-shun)
convection (kon-VEK-shun)
crisis
cyanosis (sye-an-OH-sus)
diastole (dye-AS-toe-lee)
diastolic (DYE-uh-STOL-ik) pressure
dyspnea (DISP-nee-uh)
dysrhythmia (dis-RITH-mee-uh)
eupnea (YOOP-nee-uh)
exhalation (EKS-hal-AY-shun)
Fahrenheit (FAIR-en-hite) scale
febrile (FEH-bril)
fever
frenulum linguae (FREN-yoo-lum LIN-gway)
hyperpnea (HYE-perp-NEE-uh)
hyperpyrexia (HYE-per-pye-REK-see-uh)
hypertension (HYE-per-TEN-shun)

hyperventilation (HYE-per-ven-til-AY-shun)
hypopnea (hye-POP-nee-uh)
hypotension (HYE-poe-TEN-shun)
hypothermia (HYE-poe-THER-mee-uh)
hypoxemia (hye-pok-SEE-mee-uh)
hypoxia (hye-POKS-ee-uh)
inhalation (IN-hal-AY-shun)
intercostal (IN-ter-KOS-tul)
Korotkoff (kuh-ROT-kof) sounds
malaise (mal-AYZE)
manometer (man-OM-uh-ter)
meniscus (men-IS-kus)
orthopnea (orth-OP-nee-uh)
pulse oximeter
pulse oximetry
pulse pressure
pulse rhythm
pulse volume
radiation (RAY-dee-AY-shun)
SaO_2
sphygmomanometer (SFIG-moe-man-OM-uh-ter)
SpO_2
stethoscope (STETH-uh-skope)
systole (SIS-toe-lee)
systolic (sis-TOL-ik) pressure
tachycardia (TAK-ih-KAR-dee-uh)
tachypnea (TAK-ip-NEE-uh)
thready pulse

Introduction to Vital Signs

Vital signs are objective guideposts that provide data to determine a person's state of health. The vital signs include temperature, pulse, respiration (collectively called *TPR*), and blood pressure (BP). Another indicator of a patient's health status is pulse oximetry. Although some physicians order this measurement routinely on all patients as part of the patient workup, most physicians only order this vital sign when the patient complains of respiratory problems (e.g., shortness of breath).

The normal ranges of the vital signs are finely adjusted, and any deviation from normal may indicate disease. During the course of an illness, variations in the vital signs may occur. The medical assistant should be alert to any significant changes and report them to the physician because they indicate a change in the patient's condition. When patients visit the medical office, vital signs are routinely checked to establish each patient's usual state of health and establish baseline measurements against which future measurements can be compared. The medical assistant should have a thorough knowledge of the vital signs and attain proficiency in taking them to ensure accurate findings.

General guidelines that the medical assistant should follow when measuring the vital signs are as follows:

1. Be familiar with the normal ranges for all vital signs. Keep in mind that normal ranges vary based on the different age groups (infant, child, adult, elder).
2. Make sure that all equipment for measuring vital signs is in proper working condition to ensure accurate findings.
3. Eliminate or minimize factors that affect the vital signs, such as exercise, food and beverage consumption, and emotional states.
4. Use an organized approach when measuring the vital signs. If all of the vital signs are ordered, they are usually measured starting with temperature, followed by pulse, respiration, blood pressure, and pulse oximetry.

TEMPERATURE
Regulation of Body Temperature

Body temperature is maintained within a fairly constant range by the hypothalamus, which is located in the brain. The hypothalamus functions as the body's thermostat. It normally allows the body temperature to vary only about 1° to 2° Fahrenheit (F) throughout the day.

Body temperature is maintained through a balance of the heat produced in the body and the heat lost from the body (Figure 4-1). A constant temperature range must be maintained for the body to function properly. When minor changes in the temperature of the body occur, the hypothalamus senses this and makes adjustments as necessary to ensure that the body temperature stays within a normal and safe range. If an individual is playing tennis on a hot day,

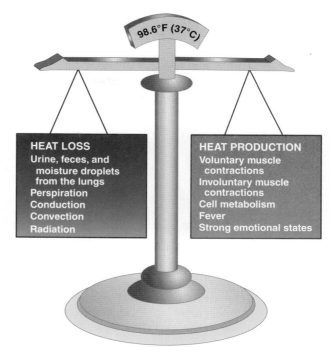

Figure 4-1. Body temperature represents a balance between the heat produced in the body and the heat lost from the body.

the body's heat-cooling mechanism is activated to remove excess heat from the body through perspiration.

Heat Production

Most of the heat produced in the body is through voluntary and involuntary muscle contractions. Voluntary muscle contractions involve the muscles over which a person has control, for example, the moving of legs or arms. Involuntary muscle contractions involve the muscles over which a person has no control; examples are physiologic processes such as digestion, the beating of the heart, and shivering.

Body heat also is produced by cell metabolism. Heat is produced when nutrients are broken down in the cells. Fever and strong emotional states also can increase heat production in the body.

Heat Loss

Heat is lost from the body through the urine and feces and in water vapor from the lungs. Perspiration also contributes to heat loss. Perspiration is the excretion of moisture through the pores of the skin. When the moisture evaporates, heat is released, and the body is cooled.

Radiation, conduction, and convection all cause loss of heat from the body. **Radiation** is the transfer of heat in the form of waves; body heat is continually radiating into cooler surroundings. **Conduction** is the transfer of heat from one object to another by direct contact; heat can be transferred by conduction from the body to a cooler object it touches. **Convection** is the transfer of heat through air

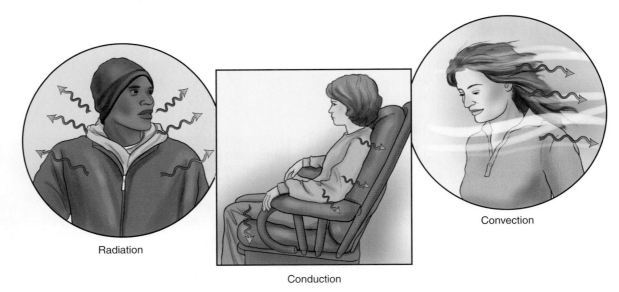

Figure 4-2. Heat loss from the body. With **radiation,** the body gives off heat in the form of waves to the cooler outside air. With **conduction,** the chair becomes warm as heat is transferred from the individual to the chair. With **convection,** air currents move heat away from the body.

currents; cool air currents can cause the body to lose heat. These processes are illustrated in Figure 4-2.

Body Temperature Range

The purpose of measuring body temperature is to establish the patient's baseline temperature and to monitor an abnormally high or low body temperature. The normal body temperature range is 97°F to 99°F (36.1°C to 37.2°C), the average temperature being 98.6°F (37°C). Body temperature is usually recorded using the Fahrenheit system of measurement. Table 4-1 lists comparable Fahrenheit and Celsius temperatures and explains how to convert temperatures from one scale to the other.

Alterations in Body Temperature

A body temperature greater than 100.4°F (38°C) indicates a **fever,** or *pyrexia.* If the body temperature falls between 99°F (37.2°C) and 100.4°F (38°C), it is termed a *low-grade fever.* When an individual has a fever, the heat that the body is producing is greater than the heat the body is losing. A temperature reading greater than 105.8°F (41°C) is known as **hyperpyrexia.** Hyperpyrexia is a serious condition, and a temperature greater than 109.4°F (43°C) is generally fatal.

A body temperature less than 97°F (36.1°C) is classified as subnormal, or **hypothermia.** This means that the heat the body is losing is greater than the heat it is producing. A person usually cannot survive with a temperature less than 93.2°F (34°C). Terms used to describe alterations in body temperature are illustrated in Figure 4-3.

Variations in Body Temperature

During the day-to-day activities of an individual, normal fluctuations occur in the body temperature. The body tem-

Table 4-1 Equivalent Fahrenheit and Celsius Temperatures

Fahrenheit	Celsius
93.2	34
95	35
96.8	36
97.7	36.5
98.6	37
99.5	37.5
100.4	38
101.3	38.5
102.2	39
104	40
105.8	41
107.6	42
109.4	43
111.2	44

Temperature Conversion

1. Celsius to Fahrenheit: To convert Celsius to Fahrenheit, multiply by ⅑⁄₅ and add 32:

$$°F = (°C \times \tfrac{9}{5}) + 32$$

2. Fahrenheit to Celsius: To convert Fahrenheit to Celsius, subtract 32 and multiply by ⅚:

$$°C \times (°F - 32) \times \tfrac{5}{9}$$

perature rarely stays the same throughout the course of a day. The medical assistant should take the following points into consideration when evaluating a patient's temperature.

1. **Age.** Infants and young children normally have a higher body temperature than adults because their

5. Procedural Step. Pull the probe straight up from the cover box. Look at the digital display to see if the thermometer is ready to use.

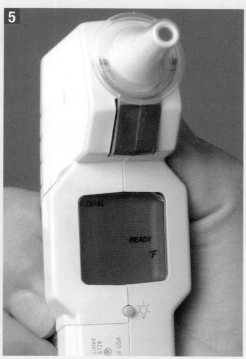

When the thermometer is ready, it displays the word "READY."

6. Procedural Step. Hold the thermometer in your dominant hand. If you are right handed, you should take the temperature in the patient's right ear. If you are left handed, take the temperature in the patient's left ear. *Principle.* Taking the temperature with the dominant hand assists in the proper placement of the probe in the patient's ear.

7. Procedural Step. Straighten the patient's external ear canal with your nondominant hand, as follows:
Adults and Children Older Than 3 Years Old. Gently pull the ear auricle upward and backward.
Children Younger Than 3 Years Old. Gently pull the ear pinna downward and backward.
Principle. Straightening the ear canal allows the probe sensor to obtain a clear picture of the tympanic membrane, resulting in an accurate temperature measurement.

8. Procedural Step. Insert the probe into the patient's ear canal tightly enough to seal the opening, but without causing patient discomfort. Point the tip of the probe toward the opposite temple (approximately midway between the opposite ear and eyebrow). *Principle.* Sealing the ear canal prevents cooler external air from entering the ear, which could result in a falsely low reading. Correct positioning of the probe opti-

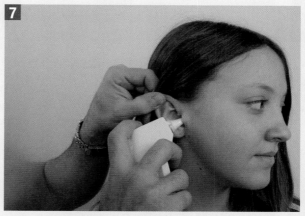

Straighten the canal of adults and children older than 3 years by pulling the ear auricle upward and backward.

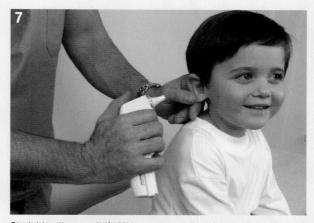

Straighten the canal of children younger than 3 years by pulling the ear auricle downward and backward.

mizes the sensor's view of the tympanic membrane, leading to an accurate temperature reading.

9. Procedural Step. Ask the patient to remain still. Hold the thermometer steady, and depress the activation button. Depending on the brand of the thermometer, perform one of the following:
a. Hold the button down for one full second, and then release it, or
b. Hold down the button down until an audible tone is heard.
Principle. The thermometer cannot take a temperature unless the activation button is depressed for 1 full second. When the button is depressed, the infrared sensor in the probe scans the thermal energy radiated by the tympanic membrane.

10. Procedural Step. Remove the thermometer from the ear canal. Turn the digital display of the thermometer toward you, and read the temperature. Make a mental note of the temperature reading. If the temperature seems to be too low, repeat the procedure to ensure

Continued

PROCEDURE 4-4

that you have used the proper technique. The temperature indicated on this thermometer is 98°F (37.2°C).

Principle. The temperature remains on the display screen until another cover is inserted on the probe. Improper technique can result in a falsely low temperature reading.

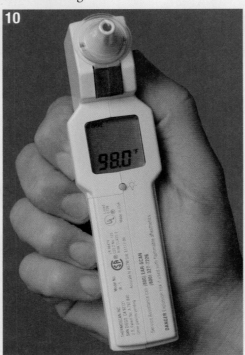

Read the temperature on the digital display.

11. **Procedural Step.** Dispose of the probe cover by ejecting it into a regular waste container.
12. **Procedural Step.** Replace the thermometer in its storage base.
    Principle. The thermometer should be stored in its base to protect the probe lens from damage and dirt.

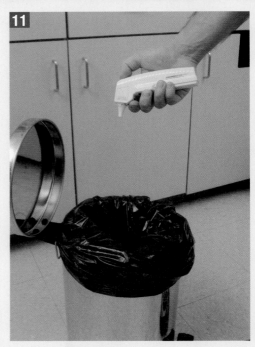

Dispose of the probe cover.

13. **Procedural Step.** Sanitize your hands.
14. **Procedural Step.** Chart the results. Include the date, the time, the aural temperature reading, and which ear was used to take the temperature (AD: right ear; AS: left ear). Using these abbreviations, the physician knows that the temperature was taken through the aural route.

CHARTING EXAMPLE

Date	
10/15/08	3:00 p.m. T: 98° F, AD —S. Martinez, RMA

PROCEDURE 4-5 Measuring Temporal Artery Body Temperature

Outcome Measure temporal artery body temperature.

Equipment/Supplies

- Temporal artery thermometer
- Probe cover
- Antiseptic wipe
- Waste container

1. **Procedural Step.** Sanitize your hands, and assemble the equipment.

2. **Procedural Step.** Greet the patient and introduce yourself. Identify the patient and explain the procedure.

3. **Procedural Step.** Examine the probe lens of the temporal artery thermometer to ensure that the lens is clean and intact.
Principle. A dirty or damaged probe lens could result in a falsely low temperature reading.

4. **Procedural Step.** Place a disposable cover over the probe. If the thermometer does not use disposable covers, clean the probe with an antiseptic wipe and allow it to dry.
Principle. Applying a probe cover or cleaning the probe with an antiseptic wipe provides infection control.

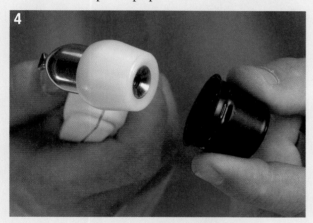

Place a disposable probe cover on the thermometer.

5. **Procedural Step.** Select an appropriate site; the right or left forehead can be used. The site selected should be fully exposed to the environment.
Principle. The temporal artery is located in the center of each side of the forehead, approximately 2 mm below the surface of the skin.

6. **Procedural Step.** Prepare the patient by brushing away any hair that is covering the side of the forehead to be scanned and the area behind the earlobe on the same side.
Principle. Hair covering the area to be measured traps body heat, resulting in a falsely high temperature reading.

7. **Procedural Step.** Hold the thermometer in your dominant hand with your thumb on the scan button.

8. **Procedural Step.** Gently position the probe of the thermometer on the center of the patient's forehead, midway between the eyebrow and the hairline.

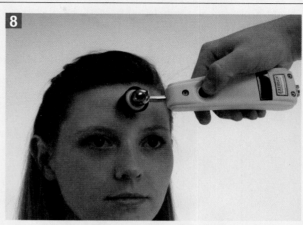

Position the probe on the center of the patient's forehead.

9. **Procedural Step.** Depress the scan button, and keep it depressed for the entire measurement.
Principle: Not keeping the scan button depressed can result in a falsely low temperature reading.

10. **Procedural Step.** Slowly and gently slide the probe straight across the forehead, midway between the eyebrow and the upper hairline. Continue until the hairline is reached. Keep the scan button depressed and the probe flush (flat) against the forehead. During this time, a beeping sound occurs and a red light blinks to indicate a measurement is taking place. Rapid beeping and blinking indicate a rise to a higher temperature. A slow beeping indicates that the thermometer is still scanning but not finding a higher temperature.
Principle. The thermometer continually scans for the peak temperature as long as the scan button is depressed. The probe must be held flat against the

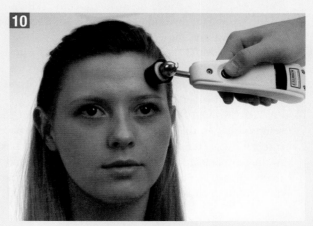

Slowly slide the probe straight across the patient's forehead.

Continued

PROCEDURE 4-5   Measuring Temporal Artery Body Temperature—cont'd

forehead to ensure accurate scanning of the temporal artery.

11. Procedural Step. Keeping the button depressed, lift the probe from the forehead, and gently place the probe behind the earlobe in the soft depression of the neck just below the mastoid process. Hold the probe in place for 1 to 2 seconds.

Principle. Taking the patient's temperature behind the earlobe prevents an error in temperature measurement in the event that the patient is sweating.

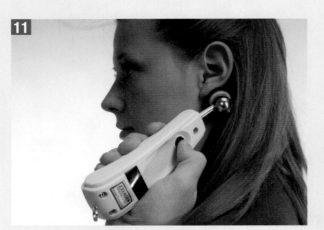

Place the probe behind the ear lobe.

12. Procedural Step. Release the scan button on the digital display, and read the temperature. Make a mental note of the temperature reading (The temperature indicated on this thermometer is 99.1°F [37.3°C]). The reading remains on the display for approximately 15 to 30 seconds after the button is released. The thermometer shuts off automatically after 30 seconds. To turn the thermometer off immediately, press and release the scan button quickly. If the patient's temperature needs to be taken again, wait 60 seconds, or use the opposite side of the forehead.

Principle. Taking a measurement cools the skin, and taking another measurement too soon may result in an inaccurate reading.

13. Procedural Step. Dispose of the probe cover by pushing it off the probe with your thumb and ejecting it into a regular waste container. Wipe the probe with an antiseptic wipe, and allow it to dry.

14. Procedural Step. Sanitize your hands, and chart the results. Include the date, the time, and the temperature reading. The symbol (TA) must be charted next to the temperature reading to tell the physician that a temporal artery reading was taken. Store the thermometer in a clean, dry area.

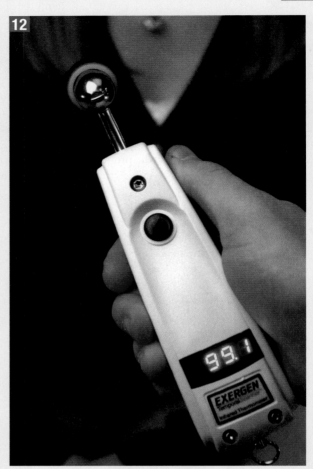

Read the temperature.

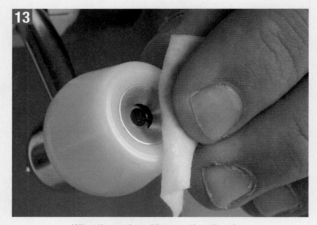

Wipe the probe with an antiseptic wipe.

CHARTING EXAMPLE

Date	
10/15/2008	9:15 a.m. T: 99.1° F(TA)— S. Martinez, RMA

PULSE

Mechanism of the Pulse

When the left ventricle of the heart contracts, blood is forced from the heart into the **aorta,** which is the major trunk of the arterial system of the body. The aorta is already filled with blood and must expand to accept the blood being pushed out of the left ventricle. This creates a pulsating wave that travels from the aorta through the walls of the arterial system. This wave, known as the *pulse,* can be felt as a light tap by an examiner. The pulse rate is measured by counting the number of "taps," or beats per minute. The heart rate can be determined by taking the pulse rate.

Factors Affecting Pulse Rate

Pulse rate can vary depending on many factors. The medical assistant should take each of the following into consideration when measuring pulse:

1. **Age.** The pulse varies inversely with age. As the age increases, the pulse rate gradually decreases. Table 4-4 lists the pulse rates of the various age groups.
2. **Gender.** Women tend to have a slightly faster pulse rate than men.
3. **Physical activity.** Physical activity, such as jogging and swimming, increases the pulse rate temporarily.
4. **Emotional states.** Strong emotional states, such as anxiety, fear, excitement, and anger, temporarily increase the pulse rate.
5. **Metabolism.** Increased body metabolism, such as occurs during pregnancy, increases the pulse rate.
6. **Fever.** Fever increases the pulse rate.
7. **Medications.** Medications may alter the pulse rate. For example, digitalis decreases the pulse rate, and epinephrine increases it.

Pulse Sites

The pulse is felt most strongly when a superficial artery is held against a firm tissue, such as bone. The locations of the sites used for measuring the pulse are shown in Figure 4-10 and are described next.

Radial.   The most common site for measuring the pulse is the radial artery, which is located in a groove on the inner aspect of the wrist just below the thumb. The radial pulse is easily accessible and can be measured with no discomfort to the patient. This site is also used by individuals at home monitoring their own heart rates, such as athletes, patients taking heart medication, and individuals starting an exercise program. The procedure for measuring radial pulse is outlined in Procedure 4-6.

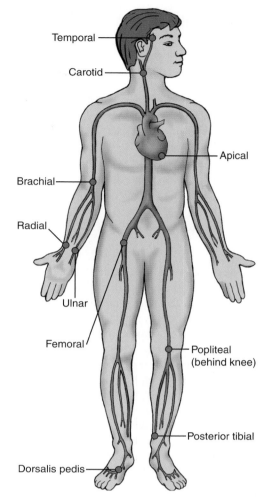

Figure 4-10. Pulse sites.

Table 4-4 Pulse Rates of Various Age Groups		
Age Group	Pulse Range (beats/min)	Average Pulse (beats/min)
Infant (birth to 1 yr)	120-160	140
Toddler (1-3 yr)	90-140	115
Preschool child (3-6 yr)	80-110	95
School-age child (6-12 yr)	75-105	90
Adolescent (12-18 yr)	60-100	80
Adult (after 18th yr)	60-100	80
Adult (after 60th yr)	67-80	74
Well-trained athletes	40-60	50

which the probe is applied. Poor peripheral blood flow may cause the pulse to be so weak that the oximeter cannot obtain a reading. Conditions resulting in poor blood flow include peripheral vascular disease, vasoconstrictor medications, severe hypotension, and hypothermia. In these situations, the medical assistant should try using the earlobe because it is less affected by decreased blood flow. Sometimes patients with cold fingers (but who are not hypothermic) may have enough constriction of the peripheral capillaries that it interferes with obtaining a reading. To solve this problem, the medical assistant should ask the patient to warm his or her fingers by rubbing the hands together. The probe should never be attached to the finger of an arm to which an automatic blood pressure cuff is applied because blood flow to the finger would be cut off when the cuff inflates, resulting in loss of the pulse signal.

4. **Ambient (surrounding) light.** Ambient light shining directly on the probe, such as bright fluorescent light, direct sunlight, or an overhead examination light, may result in an inaccurate reading. This is because some of the ambient light may be picked up by the probe's photodetector and alter the reading. This problem can be corrected by one of the following: turning off the light, moving the patient's hand away from the light source, or covering the probe with an opaque material such as a washcloth.

5. **Patient movement.** Patient movement is a common cause of an inaccurate reading. Motion affects the ability of the light to travel from the LED to the photodetector and prevents the probe from picking up the pulse signal. To avoid this problem, it is important that the medical assistant instruct the patient to remain still and not to move during the procedure. Occasionally, patient movement cannot be eliminated, such as when the patient has tremors of the hands. In these instances, the oxygen saturation level should be measured at a site that is less affected by motion, such as the toe or earlobe.

Pulse Oximeter Care and Maintenance

The pulse oximeter monitor and cable should be cleaned periodically using a damp cloth slightly dampened with a solution of warm water and a disinfectant cleaner. The medical assistant should make sure that the cloth is not too wet to prevent the solution from running into the monitor, which could damage the internal components. The probe should be cleaned periodically with a soft cloth moistened with warm water and a disinfectant cleaner. Cleaning the probe removes dirt and grime that could interfere with proper light transmission, leading to an inaccurate reading. The probe also should be disinfected after each use by wiping it thoroughly with an antiseptic wipe and allowing it to dry. The probe should never be soaked or immersed in a liquid solution because this would damage it. The probe is heat-sensitive and cannot be autoclaved. The pulse oximeter should be stored at room temperature in a dry environment.

Text continued on p. 152

PROCEDURE **4-6**   Measuring Pulse and Respiration

Outcome Measure pulse and respiration.

Equipment/Supplies

• Watch with a second hand

1. **Procedural Step.** Sanitize your hands. Greet the patient and introduce yourself. Identify the patient and explain the procedure. Observe the patient for any signs that might affect the pulse or respiratory rate.
   Principle. Pulse rate can vary according to the factors listed on p. 136.

2. **Procedural Step.** Have the patient sit down. Position the patient's arm in a comfortable position. The forearm should be slightly flexed to relax the muscles and tendons over the pulse site.

   Principle. Relaxed muscles and tendons over the pulse site make it easier to palpate the pulse.

3. **Procedural Step.** Place your three middle fingertips over the radial pulse site. Never use your thumb to take a pulse. The radial pulse is located in a groove on the inner aspect of the wrist just below the thumb.
   Principle. The thumb has a pulse of its own; using the thumb results in a measurement of the medical assistant's pulse and not the patient's pulse.

Continued

PROCEDURE 4-6 Measuring Pulse and Respiration—cont'd

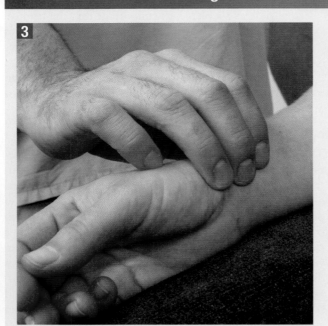

Place the three middle fingers over the radial pulse site.

4. **Procedural Step.** Apply moderate, gentle pressure directly over the site until you feel the pulse. If you cannot feel the pulse, it may be caused by:
   a. Incorrect location of the radial pulse: Move your fingers to a slightly different location in the groove of the wrist until you feel the pulse.
   b. Applying too much pressure or not enough pressure: Vary the depth of your hold until you can feel the pulse.

   Principle. A normal pulse can be felt with moderate pressure. The pulse cannot be felt if not enough pressure is applied, whereas too much pressure applied to the radial artery closes it off, and no pulse is felt.

5. **Procedural Step.** Count the pulse for 30 seconds and make a mental note of this number. Note the rhythm and volume of the pulse. If abnormalities occur in the rhythm or volume, count the pulse for 1 full minute.

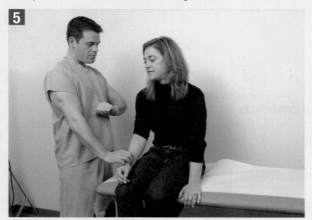

Count the pulse for 30 seconds.

Principle. A longer time ensures an accurate assessment of abnormalities.

6. **Procedural Step.** After taking the pulse, continue to hold three fingers on the patient's wrist with the same amount of pressure, and measure the respirations. This helps to ensure that the patient is unaware that respirations are being monitored.

   Principle. If the patient is aware that respiration is being measured, the breathing may change.

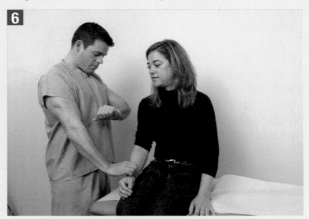

Count the number of respirations for 30 seconds.

7. **Procedural Step.** Observe the rise and fall of the patient's chest as the patient inhales and exhales.

   Principle. One complete respiration includes one inhalation and one exhalation.

8. **Procedural Step.** Count the number of respirations for 30 seconds, and make a mental note of this number; note the rhythm and depth of the respirations. Also observe the patient's color. If abnormalities occur in the rhythm or depth, count the respiratory rate for 1 full minute.

9. **Procedural Step.** Sanitize your hands, and chart the results. If you counted the pulse and respirations for 30 seconds, multiply each of the numbers counted by 2. This will give you the pulse rate and respiratory rate for 1 full minute. Include the date; the time; the pulse rate, rhythm, and volume; and the respiratory rate, rhythm, and depth.

CHARTING EXAMPLE

Date	
10/15/08	2:30 p.m. P: 74. Reg and strong. R: 18.
	Even and reg. —————— S. Martinez, RMA

PROCEDURE 4-6

PROCEDURE 4-7   Measuring Apical Pulse

Outcome Measure apical pulse.

Equipment/Supplies

- Watch with a second hand
- Stethoscope
- Antiseptic wipe

1. **Procedural Step.** Sanitize your hands. Greet the patient and introduce yourself. Identify the patient and explain the procedure. Observe the patient for any signs that might increase or decrease the pulse rate.

2. **Procedural Step.** Assemble the equipment. If the stethoscope's chest piece consists of a diaphragm and a bell, rotate the chest piece to the bell position. Clean the earpieces and chest piece of the stethoscope with an antiseptic wipe.
   Principle. The bell position allows better auscultation of heart sounds. Cleaning the earpieces helps prevent the transmission of microorganisms.

3. **Procedural Step.** Ask the patient to unbutton or remove his or her shirt. Have the patient sit or lie down (supine).
   Principle. A sitting or supine position allows access to the apex of the heart.

4. **Procedural Step.** Warm the chest piece of the stethoscope with your hands. Insert the earpieces of the stethoscope into your ears, with the earpieces directed slightly forward, and place the chest piece over the apex of the patient's heart. The apex of the heart is located in the fifth intercostal space at the junction of the left midclavicular line.
   Principle. Warming the chest piece reduces the discomfort of having a cold object placed on the chest. In addition, a cold chest piece could startle the patient, resulting in an increase in the pulse rate. The earpieces should be directed forward to follow the direction of the ear canal, which facilitates hearing.

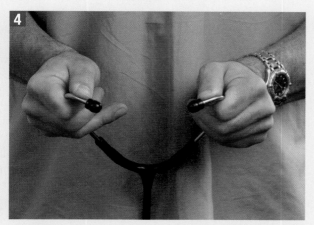

Insert the earpieces into your ears with the earpieces directed slightly forward.

5. **Procedural Step.** Listen for the heartbeat, and count the number of beats for 30 seconds (and multiply by 2) if the rhythm and volume are normal or if the apical pulse is being taken on an infant or child. If abnormalities occur in the rhythm or volume, count the pulse for 1 full minute. You will hear a "lubb-dupp" sound through the stethoscope. This sound is the closing of the heart's valves. Each "lubb-dupp" is counted as one beat.

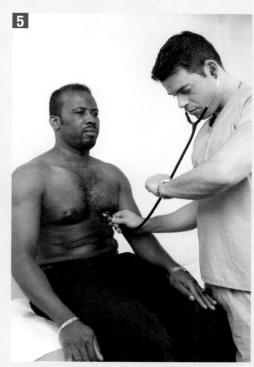

Count the number of beats for 30 seconds, and multiply by 2.

6. **Procedural Step.** Sanitize your hands, and chart the results. Include the date, time, and the apical pulse rate, rhythm, and volume.

7. **Procedural Step.** Clean the earpieces and the chest piece of the stethoscope with an antiseptic wipe.

CHARTING EXAMPLE

Date	
10/15/08	10:15 a.m. AP: 68. Reg and strong._____
	_____ S. Martinez, CMA

PROCEDURE 4-8   Performing Pulse Oximetry

Outcome Perform pulse oximetry.

Equipment/Supplies

- Handheld pulse oximeter
- Reusable finger probe
- Antiseptic wipe

1. Procedural Step. Sanitize your hands.

2. Procedural Step. Assemble the equipment. Handle the probe carefully, and perform the following:
   a. Carefully inspect the probe to ensure it opens and closes smoothly. Inspect the probe windows (LED and photodetector) to ensure they are clean and free of lint.
   b. Disinfect the probe windows and surrounding platforms with an antiseptic wipe, and allow them to dry.

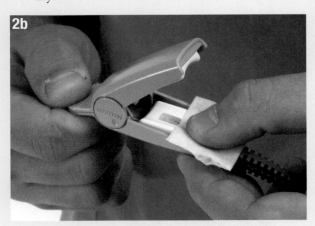

Disinfect the probe with an antiseptic wipe.

   c. If necessary, connect the probe to the cable.
   d. Connect the cable to the monitor by plugging it into the port on the monitor. Do not lift or carry the monitor by the cable.

   Principle. Misuse or improper handling of the probe could damage it. Dirt or lint on the probe windows could interfere with proper light transmission, leading to an inaccurate reading. Cross-contamination between patients is prevented by disinfecting the probe. Lifting the monitor by the cable could damage the cable connections.

3. Procedural Step. Greet the patient and introduce yourself. Identify the patient and explain the procedure. Explain to the patient that the clip-on probe does not hurt and feels similar to a clothespin attached to the finger. If the patient seems fearful, place the probe on your own finger first to reassure the patient it is not painful.

4. Procedural Step. Seat the patient comfortably in a chair with the lower arm firmly supported and the palm facing down.

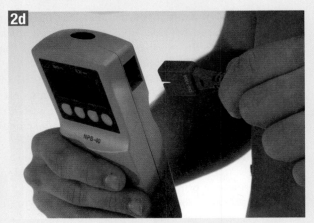

Connect the cable to the monitor by plugging it into the port on the monitor.

   Principle. Supporting the lower arm helps prevent patient movement during the procedure.

5. Procedural Step. Select an appropriate finger to apply the probe. Use the tip of the patient's index, middle, or ring finger. If the patient's fingers are very small or very large, and the probe cannot seem to be aligned properly, use the earlobe to take the measurement. If the patient exhibits tremors of the hands, use the earlobe to obtain the reading.

   Principle. The probe must be applied to a peripheral site with thin skin that is highly vascular. Very small or very large fingers may not allow for proper positioning of the probe on the finger.

6. Procedural Step. Observe the patient's fingernail. If the patient is wearing dark fingernail polish, ask her to remove it with acetone or nail polish remover. If the patient is wearing artificial nails, choose another probe site, such as the toe or earlobe.

   Principle. An opaque coating on the fingernail may interfere with proper light transmission through the finger, leading to an inaccurate reading.

7. Procedural Step. Check to ensure the patient's fingertip is clean. If it is dirty, cleanse the site with soap and water, and allow it to dry. Ensure that the patient's finger is not cold. If it is cold, ask the patient to rub his or her hands together.

   Principle. Oils, dirt, or grime on the finger can interfere with the proper light transmission through the finger, leading to an inaccurate reading. Sometimes patients with cold fingers may have enough constriction of the capillaries that it interferes with obtaining a reading.

8. **Procedural Step.** Ensure that ambient light does not interfere with the measurement. Position the probe securely on the fingertip as follows:

a. Ensure that the probe window is fully covered by placing the finger over the LED window with the fleshy tip of the finger covering the window. The tip of the finger should touch the end of the probe stop.

b. Ensure that the light-emitting diode and the photodetector are aligned opposite to each other.

c. Allow the cable to lay across the back of the hand and parallel to the arm of the patient.

Principle. Ambient light can be picked up by the probe and alter the reading. Proper alignment of the LED and photodetector is necessary for an accurate reading.

9. **Procedural Step.** Instruct the patient to remain still and to breathe normally. Turn on the oximeter by pressing

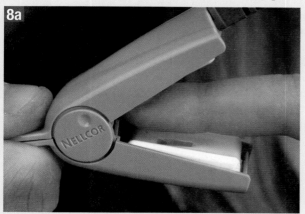

Position the probe securely on the fingertip.

the on/off control. Wait while the oximeter goes through its power-on self-test (POST). If the monitor fails the POST, refer to the troubleshooting section of the user manual for interpretation of the error code and necessary action that should be taken.

Principle. Patient movement may lead to an inaccurate reading. The monitor automatically conducts a POST to ensure it is functioning properly.

10. **Procedural Step.** Allow several seconds for the pulse oximeter to detect the pulse and calculate the oxygen saturation of the blood. Ensure that the pulse strength indicator fluctuates with each pulsation and that the pulse signal is strong. If the oximeter sounds an alarm indicating it was unable to locate a pulse, reposition the probe on the patient's finger, or move the probe to another finger, and perform the procedure again.

Principle. The reading takes several seconds to display. The pulse strength indicator provides a quick assessment of pulse quality. If the oximeter is unable to locate a pulse, it will be unable to obtain a reading.

11. **Procedural Step.** Leave the probe in place until the oximeter displays a reading. Read the oxygen saturation value and pulse rate, and make a mental note of

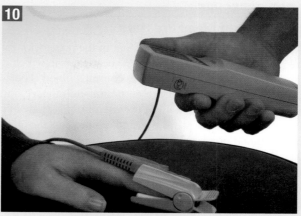

Allow several seconds for the pulse oximeter to detect the pulse.

these readings. On this pulse oximeter, the oxygen saturation reading is 99% and the pulse rate is 69. If the SpO_2 reading is less than 95%, reposition the probe on the finger, and perform the procedure again.

Principle. A low SpO_2 reading may be caused by improper positioning of the probe on the finger.

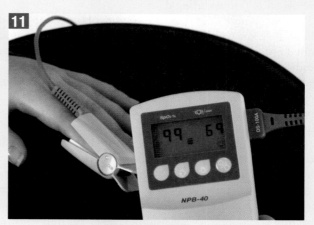

Read the oxygen saturation value and pulse rate.

12. **Procedural Step.** Remove the probe from the patient's finger, and turn off the oximeter.

13. **Procedural Step.** Sanitize your hands, and chart the results. Include the date, the time, the SpO_2 reading, and the pulse rate.

14. **Procedural Step.** Disconnect the cable from the monitor. Disinfect the probe with an antiseptic wipe. Properly store the monitor in a clean, dry area.

CHARTING EXAMPLE

Date	
10/15/2008	2:30 p.m. SpO$_2$: 99%. P: 69. ——— ——————— S. Martinez, RMA

PROCEDURE 4-8

BLOOD PRESSURE

Mechanism of Blood Pressure

Blood pressure (BP) is a measurement of the pressure or force exerted by the blood on the walls of the arteries in which it is contained. Each time the ventricles contract, blood is pushed out of the heart and into the aorta and pulmonary aorta, exerting pressure on the walls of the arteries. This phase in the cardiac cycle is known as **systole,** and it represents the highest point of blood pressure in the body, or the **systolic pressure.** The phase of the cardiac cycle in which the heart relaxes between contractions is referred to as **diastole.** The **diastolic pressure** (recorded during diastole) is lower because the heart is relaxed. Contraction and relaxation of the heart result in two different pressures, systolic and diastolic.

Interpretation of Blood Pressure

Blood pressure measurement is expressed as a fraction. The numerator is the systolic pressure, and the denominator is the diastolic pressure. The standard unit for measuring blood pressure is millimeters of mercury (mm Hg). A blood pressure reading of 110/70 mm Hg means that there was enough force to raise a column of mercury 110 mm during systole and 70 mm during diastole.

Based on guidelines from the National Heart, Lung, and Blood Institute (NHLBI), a blood pressure less than 120/80 mm Hg is classified as normal, whereas a blood pressure reading of 120/80 is classified as *prehypertension.* These guidelines were issued as a result of scientific studies showing that the risk of heart disease begins at a blood pressure reading lower than previously thought. The NHLBI guidelines are outlined in Table 4-7.

Blood pressure should be taken during every office visit to allow the physician to compare the patient's readings over time. This is a good preventive measure in guarding against serious illness. A single blood pressure reading taken on one occasion does not characterize an individual's blood pressure accurately. Several readings, taken on different occasions, provide a good index of an individual's baseline blood pressure.

Blood pressure readings always should be interpreted using a patient's baseline blood pressure. An increase or decrease of 20 to 30 mm Hg in a patient's baseline blood pressure is significant, even if it is still within the normal accepted blood pressure range.

The most common condition that causes an abnormal blood pressure reading is **hypertension.** Hypertension, or high blood pressure, results from excessive pressure on the walls of the arteries. Hypertension is determined by a sustained systolic blood pressure reading of 140 mm Hg or greater or a sustained diastolic reading of 90 mm Hg or greater. See Table 4-7 for the NHLBI classifications for hypertension. **Hypotension,** or low blood pressure, results from reduced pressure on the arterial walls. Hypotension is determined by a blood pressure reading less than 95/60 mm Hg.

Pulse Pressure

The difference between systolic and diastolic pressure is the **pulse pressure.** It is determined by subtracting the smaller number from the larger. If the blood pressure is 110/70 mm Hg, the pulse pressure would be 40 mm Hg. A pulse pressure between 30 and 50 mm Hg is considered to be within normal range.

Factors Affecting Blood Pressure

Blood pressure does not remain at a constant value. Numerous factors may affect it throughout the course of the day. An understanding of these factors helps to ensure an accurate interpretation of blood pressure readings.

1. **Age.** Age is an important consideration when determining whether a patient's blood pressure is normal. As age increases, the blood pressure gradually increases: A 6-year-old child may have a normal reading of 90/60 mm Hg, whereas a young, healthy adult may have a blood pressure reading of 116/76 mm Hg, and it would not be unusual for a 60-year-old man to have a reading of 130/90 mm Hg. As an individual gets older, there is a loss of elasticity in the walls of the blood vessels, causing this increase in pressure to occur. Table 4-8 is a chart of the average optimal blood pressure readings for various age groups.
2. **Gender.** After puberty, women usually have a lower blood pressure than men of the same age. After menopause, women usually have a higher blood pressure than men of the same age.

Table 4-7 Classification of Blood Pressure for Adults Age 18 and Older			
Blood Pressure Classifications	Systolic Blood Pressure (mm Hg)		Diastolic Blood Pressure (mm Hg)
Normal	Less than 120	*and*	Less than 80
Prehypertension*	120-139	*or*	80-89
Hypertension*			
Stage 1	140-159	*or*	90-99
Stage 2	160 or higher	*or*	100 or higher

*Based on the average of two or more properly measured, seated blood pressure readings taken at each of two or more visits.
From National Heart, Lung, and Blood Institute: *Seventh Report of The Joint National Committee on Detection, Evaluation, and Treatment of High Blood Pressure.* Bethesda, MD: NIH Publication No. 03-5231, May, 2003, U.S. Department of Health and Human Services.

Table 4-8 Average Optimal Blood Pressure for Age	
Age	Blood Pressure (mm Hg)
Newborn (6.6 lb)	40 (mean)
1 mo	85/54
1 yr	95/65
6 yr*	105/65
10-13 yr*	110/65
14-17 yr*	120/75
Adult	Less than 120/80

*In children and adolescents, hypertension is defined as blood pressure that is, on repeated measurement, at the 95th percentile or greater adjusted for age, height, and gender (NHBPEP, 1997).
From National High Blood Pressure Education Program (NHBPEP); National Heart, Lung, and Blood Institute; National Institutes of Health: The seventh report of the Joint National Committees on Detection, Evaluation, and Treatment of High Blood Pressure, *JAMA* 239:2560, 2003.

3. **Diurnal variations.** Fluctuations in an individual's blood pressure are normal during the course of a day. When one awakens, the blood pressure is lower as a result of the decreased metabolism and physical activity during sleep. As metabolism and activity increase during the day, the blood pressure rises.

4. **Emotional states.** Strong emotional states, such as anger, fear, and excitement, increase the blood pressure. If the medical assistant observes such a reaction, an attempt should be made to calm the patient before taking blood pressure.

5. **Exercise.** Physical activity temporarily increases the blood pressure. To ensure an accurate reading, a patient who has been involved in physical activity should be given an opportunity to rest for 20 to 30 minutes before blood pressure is measured.

6. **Body position.** The blood pressure of a patient who is in a lying or standing position is usually different from that measured when the patient is sitting. A notation should be made on the patient's chart if the reading was obtained in any position other than sitting, using the following abbreviations: *L* (lying) and *St* (standing).

7. **Medications.** Many medications may increase or decrease the blood pressure. Because of this factor, it is important to record in the patient chart all prescription and over-the-counter medications that the patient is taking.

8. **Other factors.** Other factors that may increase the blood pressure include pain, a recent meal, smoking, and bladder distention.

Assessment of Blood Pressure

The equipment needed to measure blood pressure includes a stethoscope and a sphygmomanometer. The **stethoscope** amplifies sounds produced by the body and allows the medical assistant to hear them.

Stethoscope

The most common type of stethoscope used in the medical office is the acoustic stethoscope. It consists of four parts: earpieces, sidepieces known as *binaurals*, plastic or rubber tubing, and a chest piece (Figure 4-19A).

Stethoscope Chest Piece

There are two types of chest pieces: a *diaphragm,* which is a large, flat disc, and a bell, which has a bowl-shaped appearance (Figure 4-19B). The chest piece of a stethoscope consists of a diaphragm and a bell, or just a diaphragm. If a chest piece consists of a diaphragm and a bell, the medical assistant must ensure the desired piece is rotated into position before use. Failure to do so would not allow the medical assistant to hear sound through the earpieces.

The diaphragm chest piece is more useful for hearing high-pitched sounds, such as lung and bowel sounds, whereas the bell chest piece is more useful for hearing low-pitched sounds, such as those produced by the heart and vascular system. Before using a stethoscope, the medical assistant should ensure that it is in proper working condition.

Sphygmomanometers

The **sphygmomanometer** is an instrument that measures the pressure of blood within an artery. It consists of a **manometer,** an inner inflatable bladder surrounded by a covering known as the *cuff,* and a pressure bulb with a control

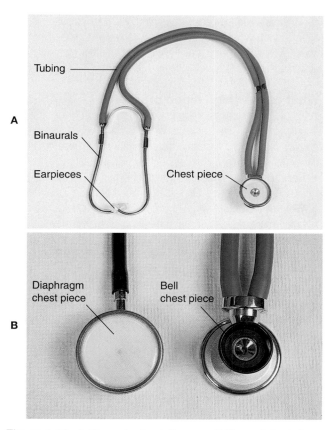

Figure 4-19. **A,** The parts of a stethoscope. **B,** Types of chest pieces.

valve to inflate and deflate the inner bladder. The manometer contains a scale for registering the pressure of the air in the bladder.

The two types of sphygmomanometers are the aneroid and mercury. The *aneroid sphygmomanometer* is lightweight and portable, but the *mercury sphygmomanometer* is more accurate.

Aneroid Sphygmomanometer
The aneroid sphygmomanometer (Figure 4-20) has a manometer gauge with a round scale. The scale is calibrated in millimeters, with a needle that points to the calibrations (Figure 4-21). To ensure an accurate reading, the needle must be positioned initially at zero. The manometer must be placed in the correct position for proper viewing. The

---

PATIENT TEACHING   Hypertension

Answer questions patients have about hypertension.

What is high blood pressure?
Blood pressure is the force of blood against the walls of the arteries. High blood pressure, also called **hypertension,** means the pressure in the arteries is consistently above normal (140/90 mm Hg), resulting in excessive pressure on the walls of the arteries. Hypertension is the most common life-threatening disease among Americans. It is estimated that one in four Americans has high blood pressure. The incidence of hypertension in the United States has increased dramatically as a result of an aging population and increased incidence of obesity.

What are the symptoms of high blood pressure?
Approximately one third of people who have high blood pressure are unaware of it because there are few or no symptoms and, as a result, an individual with hypertension may go undiagnosed for many years. If symptoms do occur, they may include one or more of the following: headaches, dizziness, flushed face, fatigue, epistaxis (nosebleed), excessive perspiration, heart palpitations, frequent urination, and leg claudication (cramping in the legs with walking). The only way to know for sure whether you have high blood pressure is to have it checked regularly.

What causes high blood pressure?
In about 90% of cases, the precise cause of high blood pressure is unknown. This type of hypertension is known as *essential* or *primary hypertension.* Certain factors seem to increase the risk of developing essential hypertension, however, including:
- **Heredity.** A family history of high blood pressure increases an individual's risk of developing high blood pressure.
- **Weight.** Individuals who are overweight or obese are two to six times more likely than the general population to develop high blood pressure.
- **Ethnicity.** Research has shown that more black than white Americans develop high blood pressure.
- **Age.** Blood pressure normally increases as one grows older.
- **Sodium intake.** Sodium, found in salt and processed, canned, and most snack foods, does not cause high blood pressure; however, it can aggravate high blood pressure. Most Americans consume more sodium than they need. The current recommendation is to consume less than 2.4 g (2400 mg) of sodium per day. This is equivalent to 6 g (about 1 teaspoon) of salt.
- **Chronic stress.** Research indicates that people who are under continuous stress tend to develop more heart and circulatory problems than people who are not under stress.

- **Smoking.** Smoking tobacco constricts blood vessels, causing an increase in blood pressure.
- **Alcohol consumption.** Heavy alcohol consumption may increase the blood pressure.

The remaining 10% of individuals with hypertension have *secondary hypertension.* This means that the high blood pressure can be linked to a known cause, which includes chronic kidney disease, adrenal and thyroid disease, narrowing of the aorta, steroid therapy, oral contraceptives, and pre-eclampsia associated with pregnancy.

What can happen if high blood pressure is not treated?
If high blood pressure is not brought under control, it can cause severe damage to vital organs, such as the heart, brain, kidneys, and eyes. This damage can result in a heart attack or heart failure, stroke, kidney damage, or damaged vision. Early detection and treatment of high blood pressure can prevent these complications. High blood pressure is often discovered during a routine medical examination or (less commonly) when an individual experiences one of the complications of hypertension caused by damage to a vital organ.

Can high blood pressure be cured?
Essential hypertension cannot be cured, but many treatments are used to bring it under control. These include lifestyle modifications, such as weight reduction, a healthy diet rich in fruits and vegetables and low in saturated fat, limitation of salt intake, regular aerobic exercise, cessation of smoking, limitation or elimination of alcohol consumption, and stress management. If lifestyle modifications alone are not enough, medications are available for reducing blood pressure, allowing the patient to lead a normal, healthy, active life.

How long will I undergo treatment?
Treatment for essential hypertension is usually lifelong. Even if you feel fine, you'll probably have to continue treatment for the rest of your life to maintain your blood pressure in a healthy range. If you discontinue your diet and lifestyle changes or stop taking your medication, your blood pressure will increase again.

- Encourage patients with hypertension to adhere to the treatment prescribed by the physician. Help patients remember to take their medication by telling them to associate their medication schedule with a daily routine, such as brushing their teeth or having meals.
- Provide the patient with educational materials on high blood pressure available from sources such as the American Heart Association.

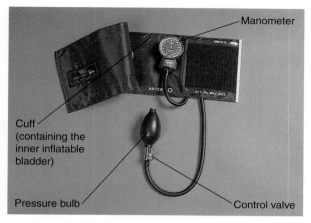

Figure 4-20. The parts of an aneroid sphygmomanometer.

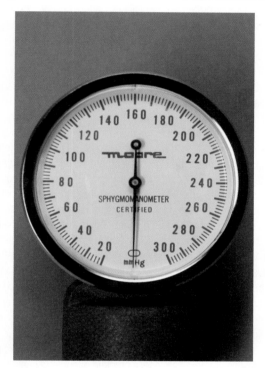

Figure 4-21. The scale of the gauge of an aneroid sphygmomanometer.

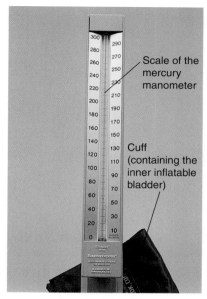

Figure 4-22. The parts of a mercury sphygmomanometer.

medical assistant should be no farther than 3 feet from the scale on the gauge of the manometer, and the manometer should be placed so that it can be viewed directly. At least once a year, an aneroid sphygmomanometer should be recalibrated to ensure its accuracy.

Mercury Sphygmomanometer

The mercury sphygmomanometer (Figure 4-22) has a vertical tube calibrated in millimeters that is filled with mercury. Although more accurate than the aneroid sphygmomanometer, the use of the mercury sphygmomanometer is being discouraged because mercury is a hazardous chemical.

If a mercury manometer is used to measure blood pressure, it must be placed in the correct position for proper

viewing. The medical assistant should be no farther than 3 feet from the scale of the manometer. A portable mercury manometer should be placed on a flat surface so that the mercury column is in a vertical position. The wall model mercury manometer is mounted securely against a wall, placing the mercury column in a vertical position.

The following guidelines must be followed when measuring blood pressure with a mercury sphygmomanometer. Before the blood pressure reading is obtained, the mercury must be even with the zero level at the base of the calibrated tube. Pressure created by inflation of the inner bladder causes the mercury to rise in the tube. The top portion of the mercury column, the **meniscus,** curves slightly upward. The blood pressure should be read at the top of the meniscus, with the eye at the same level as the meniscus of the mercury column.

Cuff Sizes

Blood pressure cuffs come in a variety of sizes and are measured in centimeters (cm) (Figure 4-23). The size of a cuff refers to its inner inflatable bladder, rather than its cloth cover. Table 4-9 lists the types of cuffs available and the size of the inner bladder of each cuff.

Table 4-9 Types of Blood Pressure Cuffs			
Cuff	Bladder Length (cm)	Bladder Width (cm)	Acceptable Circumference (cm)
Child arm	21	8	16-21
Small adult arm	24	10	22-26
Adult arm	30	13	27-34
Large adult arm	38	16	35-44
Adult thigh	42	20	45-52

CERTIFICATION REVIEW—cont'd

- ❑ **A blood pressure** less than 120/80 mm Hg is normal. A single blood pressure reading taken on one occasion does not characterize an individual's blood pressure; several readings must be taken on different occasions.
- ❑ **Hypertension** is excessive pressure on the walls of the arteries and refers to a sustained systolic pressure of 140 mm Hg or greater or a sustained diastolic reading of 90 mm Hg or greater.
- ❑ **Factors that affect blood pressure** are age, gender, diurnal variations, emotional states, exercise, body position, and medication.

TERMINOLOGY REVIEW

Adventitious sounds Abnormal breath sounds.

Afebrile Without fever; the body temperature is normal.

Alveolus A thin-walled air sac of the lungs in which the exchange of oxygen and carbon dioxide takes place.

Antecubital space The space located at the front of the elbow.

Antipyretic An agent that reduces fever.

Aorta The major trunk of the arterial system of the body. The aorta arises from the upper surface of the left ventricle.

Apnea The temporary cessation of breathing.

Axilla The armpit.

Bounding pulse A pulse with an increased volume that feels very strong and full.

Bradycardia An abnormally slow heart rate (less than 60 beats per minute).

Bradypnea An abnormal decrease in the respiratory rate of less than 10 respirations per minute.

Celsius scale A temperature scale on which the freezing point of water is 0° and the boiling point of water is 100°; also called the *centigrade scale.*

Conduction The transfer of energy, such as heat, from one object to another by direct contact.

Convection The transfer of energy, such as heat, through air currents.

Crisis A sudden falling of an elevated body temperature to normal.

Cyanosis A bluish discoloration of the skin and mucous membranes.

Diastole The phase in the cardiac cycle in which the heart relaxes between contractions.

Diastolic pressure The point of lesser pressure on the arterial wall, which is recorded during diastole.

Dyspnea Shortness of breath or difficulty in breathing.

Dysrhythmia An irregular rhythm; also termed *arrhythmia.*

Eupnea Normal respiration. The rate is 16 to 20 respirations per minute, the rhythm is even and regular, and the depth is normal.

Exhalation The act of breathing out.

Fahrenheit scale A temperature scale on which the freezing point of water is 32° and the boiling point of water is 212°.

Febrile Pertaining to fever.

Fever A body temperature that is above normal; synonym for *pyrexia.*

Frenulum linguae The midline fold that connects the undersurface of the tongue with the floor of the mouth.

Hyperpnea An abnormal increase in the rate and depth of respiration.

Hyperpyrexia An extremely high fever.

Hypertension High blood pressure.

Hyperventilation An abnormally fast and deep type of breathing, usually associated with acute anxiety conditions.

Hypopnea An abnormal decrease in the rate and depth of respiration.

Hypotension Low blood pressure.

Hypothermia A body temperature that is below normal.

Hypoxemia A decrease in the oxygen saturation of the blood. Hypoxemia may lead to hypoxia.

Hypoxia A reduction in the oxygen supply to the tissues of the body.

Inhalation The act of breathing in.

Intercostal Between the ribs.

Korotkoff sounds Sounds heard during the measurement of blood pressure that are used to determine the systolic and diastolic blood pressure readings.

Malaise A vague sense of body discomfort, weakness, and fatigue that often marks the onset of a disease and continues through the course of the illness.

Manometer An instrument for measuring pressure.

Meniscus The curved surface on a column of liquid in a tube.

Orthopnea The condition in which breathing is easier when an individual is in a sitting or standing position.

Pulse oximeter A computerized device consisting of a probe and monitor used to measure the oxygen saturation of arterial blood.

Pulse oximetry The use of a pulse oximeter to measure the oxygen saturation of arterial blood.

Pulse pressure The difference between the systolic and diastolic pressures.

Pulse rhythm The time interval between heartbeats.

Continued

TERMINOLOGY REVIEW—cont'd

Pulse volume The strength of the heartbeat.

Radiation The transfer of energy, such as heat, in the form of waves.

SaO$_2$ (saturation of arterial oxygen) Abbreviation for the percentage of hemoglobin that is saturated with oxygen in arterial blood.

SpO$_2$ (saturation of peripheral oxygen) Abbreviation for the percentage of hemoglobin that is saturated with oxygen in arterial blood as measured by a pulse oximeter.

Sphygmomanometer An instrument for measuring arterial blood pressure.

Stethoscope An instrument for amplifying and hearing sounds produced by the body.

Systole The phase in the cardiac cycle in which the ventricles contract, sending blood out of the heart and into the aorta and pulmonary aorta.

Systolic pressure The point of maximum pressure on the arterial walls, which is recorded during systole.

Tachycardia An abnormally fast heart rate (more than 100 beats per minute).

Tachypnea An abnormal increase in the respiratory rate of more than 20 respirations per minute.

Thready pulse A pulse with a decreased volume that feels weak and thin.

ON THE WEB

For Information on Hypertension:

American Heart Association: www.americanheart.org

National Heart, Lung, and Blood Institute: www.nhlbi.nih.gov

Cardiology Channel: www.cardiologychannel.com

Hypertension Education Foundation: www.hypertensionfoundation.org

American Society of Hypertension: www.ash-us.org

Hypertension and Health: www.hypertensionandhealth.com

For Information on Lung Disease:

American Lung Association: www.lungusa.org

Pulmonology Channel: www.pulmonologychannel.com

Lung Cancer Online: www.lungcanceronline.org

5

The Physical Examination

LEARNING OBJECTIVES

Preparation for the Physical Examination
1. Identify the three components of a complete patient examination.
2. List the guidelines that should be followed in preparing the examining room.
3. Identify equipment and instruments used during the physical examination.

Measuring Weight and Height
1. Explain the purpose of measuring weight and height.
2. List the guidelines that should be followed when measuring weight and height.

Positioning and Draping
1. Explain the purpose of positioning and draping.
2. List one use of each patient position.

Assessment of the Patient
1. List and define the four techniques of examining the patient.
2. State an example of the use of each examination technique during the physical examination of a patient.

Assisting the Physician
1. Describe the responsibilities of the medical assistant during the physical examination.

PROCEDURES

Prepare the examining room.
Operate and care for equipment and instruments used during the physical examination, according to the manufacturer's instructions.
Prepare a patient for a physical examination.

Measure weight and height.

Position and drape a patient in each of the following positions:
- Sitting
- Supine
- Prone
- Dorsal recumbent
- Lithotomy
- Sims
- Knee-chest
- Fowler's

Assist the physician during the physical examination of a patient.

CHAPTER OUTLINE

Introduction to the Physical Examination

A complete patient examination consists of three parts: the *health history*, the *physical examination* of each body system, and *laboratory and diagnostic tests*. The physician uses the results to determine the patient's general state of health, to arrive at a diagnosis and prescribe treatment, and to observe any change in a patient's illness after treatment has been instituted.

An important and frequent responsibility of the medical assistant is to assist with a physical examination. Because health-promotion and disease-prevention activities have become an important focus of health care, individuals are becoming more aware of the need for a yearly physical examination to detect early signs of illness and to prevent serious health problems. Also, a physical examination may be a prerequisite for employment, participation in sports, attendance at summer camp, and admission to school. The physical examination is explained in detail in this chapter. Taking the health history, collecting specimens, and performing laboratory and diagnostic tests are discussed in other chapters.

DEFINITION OF TERMS

The medical assistant should know and understand the following terms relating to the patient examination:

Final diagnosis. Often simply called the *diagnosis,* this term refers to the scientific method of determining and identifying a patient's condition through the evaluation of the health history, the physical examination, laboratory tests, and diagnostic procedures. A final diagnosis is crucial because it provides a logical basis for treatment and prognosis.

Clinical diagnosis. The clinical diagnosis is an intermediate step in the determination of a final diagnosis. The clinical diagnosis of a patient's condition is obtained through the evaluation of the health history and the physical examination without the benefit of laboratory or diagnostic tests. Outside laboratories provide a space to specify the clinical diagnosis on the laboratory request form; this information assists the laboratory in correlating the clinical laboratory data and the physician's needs. When the physician has analyzed the test results, a final diagnosis usually can be established.

Differential diagnosis. Two or more diseases may have similar symptoms. The differential diagnosis involves determining which of these diseases is producing the patient's symptoms so that a final diagnosis can be established. For example, streptococcal sore throat and pharyngitis have similar symptoms. A differential diagnosis is made by obtaining a throat specimen and performing a strep test.

Prognosis. The prognosis is the probable course and outcome of a patient's condition and the patient's prospects for recovery.

Risk factor. A risk factor is a physical or behavioral condition that increases the probability that an individual will develop a particular condition; examples are genetic factors, habits, environmental conditions, and physiological conditions. The presence of a risk factor for a certain dis-

Highlight on Health Screening

The chance of developing certain diseases is greater at different ages. Periodic health screening is recommended for the detection and early treatment of disease.

Test or Procedure	Gender	Recommended Frequency
Beginning at age 20 years		
Blood pressure	M & F	Every year
Cholesterol level	M & F	Every 5 years
Blood glucose level	M & F	Every 3-5 years
Breast self-examination	F	Every month
Beginning at the age specified		
Clinical breast examination (by a physician)	F	Every 3 years beginning at age 29, and every year beginning at age 40
Pap test and pelvic examination	F	Begin within 3 years of the onset of vaginal intercourse or at age 21, whichever comes first, then every 1 to 2 years.
Testicular self-examination	M	Every month beginning at age 15
Rectal examination	M & F	Every year beginning at age 40
Fecal occult blood test	M & F	Every year starting at age 50
Sigmoidoscopy	M & F	Every 5 years beginning at age 50
Prostate cancer screening	M	Every year beginning at age 50
Mammography	F	Every year beginning at age 40
Electrocardiogram	M & F	One baseline recording starting at age 40

ease does not mean that the disease will develop; it means only that a person's chances of developing that disease are greater than those of a person without the risk factor. For example, cigarette smoking is a risk factor for developing lung cancer and heart disease. A person who smokes has a higher risk of developing lung cancer than a person who does not or who has stopped smoking.

Acute illness. An acute illness is characterized by symptoms that have a rapid onset, are usually severe and intense, and subside after a relatively short time. In some cases, the acute episode progresses into a chronic illness. Examples of acute illness include influenza, strep throat, and chickenpox.

Chronic illness. A chronic illness is characterized by symptoms that persist for more than 3 months and show little change over a long time. Examples of chronic illness include diabetes mellitus, hypertension, and emphysema.

Therapeutic procedure. A therapeutic procedure is performed to treat a patient's condition with the goal of eliminating it or promoting as much recovery as possible. Examples of therapeutic procedures include the administration of medication, ear and eye irrigations, and therapeutic ultrasound.

Diagnostic procedure. A diagnostic procedure is a procedure performed to assist in the diagnosis of a patient's condition; examples include electrocardiography, x-ray examination, and sigmoidoscopy.

Laboratory testing. Laboratory testing involves the analysis and study of specimens obtained from patients to assist in diagnosing and treating disease.

PREPARATION OF THE EXAMINING ROOM

Proper preparation of the examining room provides a comfortable and healthy environment for the patient and facilitates the physical examination. The following guidelines should be followed in preparing the examining room:

1. Ensure the examining room is free of clutter and well lit.
2. Check the examining rooms daily to ensure there are ample supplies. Restock supplies that are getting low.
3. Empty waste receptacles frequently.
4. Replace biohazard containers as necessary. When removing biohazard containers from the examining room (see Chapter 2), follow the OSHA Bloodborne Pathogens Standard.
5. Make sure the room is well ventilated, and install an air freshener to eliminate odors.
6. Maintain room temperatures that are comfortable not only for a fully clothed individual, but also for an individual who has disrobed.
7. Clean and disinfect examining tables, countertops, and faucets daily.
8. Remove dust and dirt from furniture and towel dispensers.
9. Change the examining table paper after each patient by unrolling a fresh length. Check to ensure there is an ample supply of gowns and drapes ready for use.
10. Ensure that the examining room door is closed during the examination because patient privacy is paramount.
11. Properly clean and prepare equipment, instruments, and supplies that are used for patient examinations so

that they are ready for use by the physician. Table 5-1 lists the equipment and supplies, along with their uses, that may be employed during a physical examination.

12. Check equipment and instruments regularly to verify that they are in proper working condition. This protects the patient from harm caused by faulty equipment.

13. Have the equipment and supplies ready for the examination and arranged for easy access by the physician. The equipment and supplies needed for the physical examination vary according to the type of examination and the physician's preference (Figure 5-1).

14. Know how to operate and care for each piece of equipment and each instrument. The manufacturer includes an operating manual, which should be read carefully and thoroughly and kept available for reference.

PREPARATION OF THE PATIENT

It is the medical assistant's responsibility to prepare the patient for the physical examination. After escorting the patient to the examining room, the medical assistant should identify the patient by his or her name and date of birth. This avoids mistaking one patient for another. If the medical assistant performs a procedure on the wrong patient by mistake, he or she could be held liable. The medical assistant then takes vital signs and measures the weight and height of the patient. The results of these procedures are charted in the patient's medical record.

The medical assistant can reduce a patient's apprehension and embarrassment by addressing the patient by his or her name of choice; by adopting a friendly and supportive attitude; and by speaking clearly, distinctly, and slowly. The medical assistant should explain the purpose of the examination and offer to answer any questions. This also facilitates the physical examination of the patient.

The patient should be asked whether he or she needs to empty the bladder before the examination. An empty bladder makes the examination easier and is more comfortable for the patient. If a urine specimen is needed, the patient is requested to void.

Instructions on disrobing for the examination should be specific so that the patient understands what items of clothing to remove and where to place the clothing. The disrob-

Table 5-1 Equipment and Supplies for the Physical Examination

Item	Description and Purpose
Patient examination gown	Gown made of disposable paper or cloth that provides patient modesty, comfort, and warmth
Drape	A length of disposable paper or cloth to cover patient or parts of patient to provide comfort and warmth and reduce exposure
Sphygmomanometer	Instrument used to measure blood pressure
Stethoscope	Instrument used to auscultate body sounds, such as blood pressure and lung and bowel sounds
Thermometer	Instrument used to measure body temperature
Upright balance scale	Device used to measure weight and height
Otoscope	Lighted instrument with lens, used to examine external ear canal and tympanic membrane
Tuning fork	Small metal instrument consisting of stem and two prongs, used to test hearing acuity
Ophthalmoscope	Lighted instrument with lens, used for examining interior of eye
Tongue depressor	Flat wooden blade used to depress patient's tongue during examination of mouth and pharynx
Antiseptic wipe	Disposable pad saturated with antiseptic, such as alcohol, that is used to cleanse skin
Tape measure	Flexible device calibrated in inches on one side and centimeters on other side, used to measure patient (e.g., diameter of limb, head circumference)
Percussion hammer	Instrument with rubber head, used for testing neurologic reflexes
Speculum	Instrument for opening body orifice or cavity for viewing (e.g., ear speculum, nasal speculum, vaginal speculum)
Disposable gloves	Gloves, usually latex, that are worn only once to provide protection from bloodborne pathogens and other potentially infectious materials
Lubricant	Agent that is applied to physician's gloved hand or to speculum that reduces friction between parts to make insertion easier
Specimen container	Container in which body specimen is placed for transport to laboratory (after it has been labeled)
Tissues	Used for wiping body secretions
Cotton-tipped applicator	Small piece of cotton wrapped around the end of a slender wooden stick, used for collection of specimen from body
Overhead examination light	Light mounted on flexible movable stand to focus light on area for good visibility
Basin	Container in which used instruments are deposited
Biohazard container	Specially made container used for receiving items that contain infectious waste
Waste receptacle	Container for used disposable articles that do not contain infectious waste

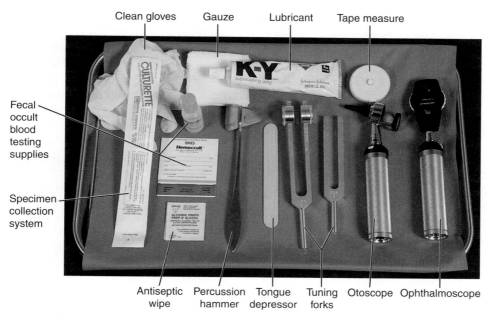

Clean gloves   Gauze   Lubricant   Tape measure

Fecal occult blood testing supplies

Specimen collection system

Antiseptic wipe   Percussion hammer   Tongue depressor   Tuning forks   Otoscope   Ophthalmoscope

Figure 5-1. Common instruments and supplies used for the physical examination.

Highlight on Patient Teaching

The purpose of patient teaching is to help the patient develop habits, attitudes, and skills that enable the individual to maintain and improve his or her own health.

Fact: Patients who are active, informed participants in their health care are more apt to follow the physician's instructions than patients who are passive recipients of medical services.

Action: Provide patients with information on health care. Every patient interaction is an opportunity for teaching.

Fact: Adult learners are goal oriented and performance centered. They need and want information that would assist them in managing and improving their health.

Action: Review the information that you provide to patients, and determine whether it is nice to know or necessary to know. Select subject matter that is practical and useful and relates directly to the patient's needs.

Fact: The more information that is presented, the more the patient is likely to forget. Approximately half of information presented to the patient is forgotten in the first 5 minutes after giving it.

Action: When teaching, use the following pointers to help patients learn and retain information:

- Keep it short and be specific.
- Speak in terms the patient can understand.
- Focus on "how," rather than "why."
- Repeat and reinforce important information.
- Give practical examples, and provide ample time for patient practice.

- Ask for feedback from the patient to determine whether he or she understands the information.
- Provide the patient with written information.

Fact: Each individual has a distinct style of learning and learns best when using his or her preferred learning style. The three main learning styles are reading, listening, and doing. People often use more than one style for learning.

Action: Use a variety of teaching strategies to engage the various learning styles of patients. Examples of teaching strategies include explanations, printed handouts, audiovisual aids, demonstrations, and discussions.

Fact: Only two thirds of patients comply with health care instructions prescribed by the physician. Factors that influence compliance include the patient's adaptation to illness, motivation to change, physical capability, and support systems.

Action: The following help increase patient compliance with prescribed treatment:

- Address the patient by his/her name of choice. (Keep in mind that many patients object to being called by their first name by strangers.)
- Encourage the patient to take an active role in personal health care.
- Help the patient set goals and objectives for change.
- Encourage care and support from family members.
- Make the patient aware of outside resources.
- Give positive reinforcement when the patient makes healthful changes.

5. **Procedural Step.** Ask the patient to move back on the table. As the patient is doing this, pull out the table extension while supporting the patient's lower legs.

6. **Procedural Step.** Ask the patient to lie on his or her back. Provide assistance if needed. Position the drape lengthwise over the patient.

7. **Procedural Step.** Ask the patient to turn onto his or her stomach by rolling toward you. Provide assistance for this step by helping her turn and adjusting the drape to provide modesty.
   Principle. This step prevents the patient from accidentally rolling off the table.

8. **Procedural Step.** Position the patient with the legs together and the head turned to one side. The arms can be placed above the head or alongside the body.

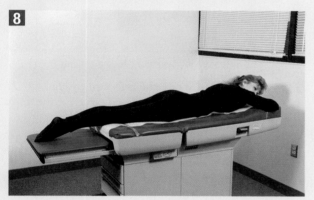

Position the patient's legs together with the head turned to one side.

9. **Procedural Step.** Adjust the drape as needed so that it is positioned lengthwise over the patient to provide warmth and modesty. As the physician examines the patient, move the drape according to the body parts being examined.

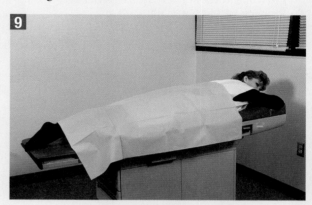

Place a drape lengthwise over the patient.

10. **Procedural Step.** After completion of the examination, ask the patient to turn back over by rolling toward you. Assist the patient into a supine position and then into a sitting position. Slide the table extension back into place while supporting the patient's lower legs.

11. **Procedural Step.** Assist the patient down from the table. Return the footrest to its normal position. Instruct the patient to get dressed. Discard the gown and drape in a waste container.

PROCEDURE 5-5 (side tab)

PROCEDURE 5-5   Dorsal Recumbent Position

Outcome Position and drape a patient in the dorsal recumbent position. The dorsal recumbent position is used to perform vaginal and rectal examinations; to insert a urinary catheter; and to examine the head, neck, chest, and extremities of patients who have difficulty maintaining the supine position. The supine position is an uncomfortable position for patients with respiratory problems, back injury, or lower back pain. Bending the legs (rather than lying flat) is more comfortable for these patients and is easier to maintain.

Equipment/Supplies

- Examining table
- Disposable patient gown
- Disposable patient drape

1. **Procedural Step.** Sanitize your hands. Greet the patient and introduce yourself.

2. **Procedural Step.** Identify the patient and explain the type of examination or procedure that will be performed.

3. **Procedural Step.** Provide the patient with a patient gown. Instruct the patient to remove clothing as appropriate for the type of examination being performed and to put on the patient gown with the opening in front. The disrobing facility should provide privacy, a place to sit, and a place to hang clothing.

4. **Procedural Step.** Pull out the footrest of the examining table, and assist the patient into a sitting position. Place a drape over the patient's thighs and legs.

Continued

5. Procedural Step. Ask the patient to move back on the table. As the patient is doing this, pull out the table extension while supporting the patient's lower legs.

6. Procedural Step. Ask the patient to lie on her back. Provide assistance if needed. The arms can be placed above the head or alongside the body. Position the drape diagonally over the patient.

7. Procedural Step. Ask the patient to bend the knees and place each foot at the edge of the examining table with the soles of the feet flat on the table. Provide assistance during this step. Push in the table extension and the footrest.

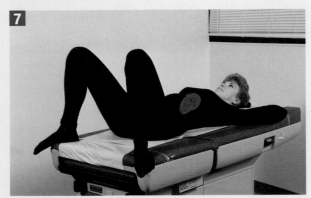

Ask the patient to bend the knees and place each foot at the edge of the examining table.

8. Procedural Step. Adjust the drape as needed to provide the patient with warmth and modesty. The drape should be positioned diagonally, with one corner over the patient's chest and the opposite corner falls between the patient's legs and completely covers the pubic area.

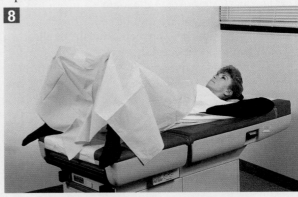

Place a drape diagonally over the patient.

9. Procedural Step. When the physician is ready to examine the genital area, the center corner of the drape is folded back over the abdomen.

10. Procedural Step. After completion of the examination, pull out the footrest and the table extension. Assist the patient into a supine position and then into a sitting position. Slide the table extension back into place while supporting the patient's lower legs.

11. Procedural Step. Assist the patient down from the table. Return the footrest to its normal position. Instruct the patient to get dressed. Discard the gown and drape in a waste container.

PROCEDURE **5-6**   **Lithotomy Position**

Outcome Position and drape a patient in the lithotomy position. The lithotomy position is used for vaginal, pelvic, and rectal examinations. The lithotomy position is the same as the dorsal recumbent position except that the patient's feet are placed in stirrups. The lithotomy position provides maximal exposure to the genital area and facilitates insertion of a vaginal speculum. Because this is an uncomfortable position for the patient to maintain, the patient should not be put into this position until just before the examination.

Equipment/Supplies

- Examining table
- Disposable patient gown
- Disposable patient drape

1. Procedural Step. Sanitize your hands. Greet the patient and introduce yourself.

2. Procedural Step. Identify the patient and explain the type of examination or procedure that will be performed.

3. Procedural Step. Provide the patient with a patient gown. Instruct the patient to remove clothing as appropriate for the type of examination being performed and to put on the patient gown with the opening in front. If the patient is wearing socks, tell her that she may keep them on during the procedure.

The disrobing facility should provide privacy, a place to sit, and a place to hang clothing.

Principle. Socks help to keep the patient's feet warm after they are placed in the metal stirrups.

4. **Procedural Step.** Some medical offices use disposable stirrup covers. If this is the case, apply a cover to each stirrup. Pull out the footrest of the examining table, and assist the patient into a sitting position. Place a drape over the patient's thighs and legs.

Principle. Stirrup covers provide a soft, warm, non-slip surface for the patient's feet.

5. **Procedural Step.** When the physician is ready to examine the patient, ask the patient to move back on the table. As the patient is doing this, pull out the table extension while supporting the patient's lower legs.

6. **Procedural Step.** Ask the patient to lie on the back. Provide assistance if needed. The arms can be placed above the head or alongside the body.

7. **Procedural Step.** Position the drape over the patient to provide warmth and modesty. The drape should be positioned diagonally with one corner over the patient's chest and the opposite corner between the patient's feet.

8. **Procedural Step.** Pull out the stirrups and position them at an angle. Position the stirrups so that they are level with the examining table and pulled out approximately 1 foot from the edge of the table. Check to make sure the stirrups are not too far apart or too close together. Lock the stirrups into place.

Principle. If the stirrups are too far apart, it is uncomfortable for the patient. If the stirrups are too close together, the patient will be unable to move her buttocks to the edge of the table as needed for the exam.

9. **Procedural Step.** Ask the patient to bend the knees and place each foot, one at a time, into a stirrup. Provide assistance during this step. Push in the table extension and the footrest.

10. **Procedural Step.** Instruct the patient to slide the buttocks all the way down to the edge of the examining table and to let her legs fall apart as far as is comfortable.

11. **Procedural Step.** Reposition the drape as needed so that one corner is over the patient's chest and the opposite corner falls between the patient's legs and completely covers the perineal area. When the physician is ready to examine the genital area, the center corner of the drape is pulled up and folded back over the knees.

12. **Procedural Step.** After completion of the examination, pull out the footrest and table extension. Ask the patient to slide the buttocks back from the end of the table. Lift the patient's legs out of the stirrups at the same time, and place them on the table extension (supine position). Remove the stirrup covers and discard them in a waste container. Return the stirrups to their normal position. Assist the patient into a sitting position. Slide the table extension back into place while supporting the patient's lower legs.

Principle. Lifting both the patient's legs out of the stirrups at the same time avoids strain on the back and abdominal muscles.

13. **Procedural Step.** Assist the patient down from the table. Return the footrest to its normal position. Instruct the patient to get dressed. Discard the gown and drape in a waste container.

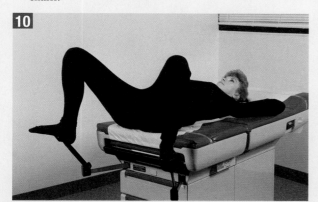

Ask the patient to slide the buttocks to the edge of the table and to rotate the thighs outward.

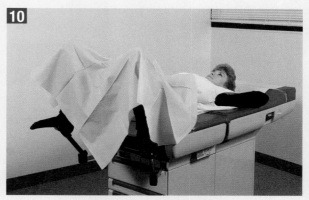

Position the drape diagonally.

PROCEDURE 5-7   Sims Position

Outcome Position and drape a patient in the Sims position. Sims position, also known as the *left lateral position*, is used to examine the vagina and rectum, to measure rectal temperature, to perform a flexible sigmoidoscopy, and to administer an enema.

Equipment/Supplies

- Examining table
- Disposable patient gown
- Disposable patient drape

1. **Procedural Step.** Sanitize your hands. Greet the patient and introduce yourself.
2. **Procedural Step.** Identify the patient and explain the type of examination or procedure that will be performed.
3. **Procedural Step.** Provide the patient with a patient gown. Instruct the patient to remove clothing from the waist down and to put on the patient gown with the opening in back. The disrobing facility should provide privacy, a place to sit, and a place to hang clothing.
4. **Procedural Step.** Pull out the footrest of the examining table, and assist the patient into a sitting position. Place a drape over the patient's thighs and legs.
5. **Procedural Step.** Ask the patient to move back on the table. As the patient is doing this, pull out the table extension while supporting the patient's lower legs.
6. **Procedural Step.** Ask the patient to lie on his or her back. Provide assistance if needed.
7. **Procedural Step.** Position the drape lengthwise over the patient to provide warmth and modesty.
8. **Procedural Step.** Ask the patient to turn onto the left side. Provide assistance during this step to prevent the

patient from accidentally rolling off the table and to adjust the drape to provide modesty. The patient's left arm should be positioned behind the body and the right arm forward with the elbow bent. Assist the patient in flexing the legs. The right leg is flexed sharply, and the left leg is flexed slightly.

9. **Procedural Step.** Adjust the drape as needed. When the physician is ready to examine the patient, a small portion of the drape is folded back to expose the anal area.

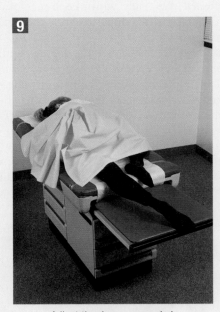

Adjust the drape as needed.

10. **Procedural Step.** After completion of the examination, assist the patient into a supine position and into a sitting position. Slide the table extension back into place while supporting the patient's lower legs.
11. **Procedural Step.** Assist the patient down from the table. Return the footrest to its normal position. Instruct the patient to get dressed. Discard the gown and drape in a waste container.

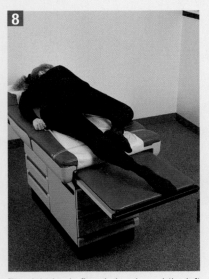

The right leg is flexed sharply, and the left leg is flexed slightly.

PROCEDURE 5-8   Knee-Chest Position

Outcome Position and drape a patient in the knee-chest position. The knee-chest position is used to examine the rectum and to perform a proctoscopic examination because it provides maximal exposure to the rectal area. This is a difficult position to maintain; the patient should not be put into this position until just before the examination.

Equipment/Supplies

- Examining table
- Disposable patient gown
- Disposable patient drape

1. **Procedural Step.** Sanitize your hands. Greet the patient and introduce yourself.
2. **Procedural Step.** Identify the patient and explain the type of examination or procedure that will be performed.
3. **Procedural Step.** Provide the patient with a patient gown. Instruct the patient to remove clothing from the waist down and to put on the gown with the opening in back. The disrobing facility should provide privacy, a place to sit, and a place to hang clothing.
4. **Procedural Step.** Pull out the footrest of the examining table, and assist the patient into a sitting position. Place a drape over the patient's thighs and legs.
5. **Procedural Step.** Ask the patient to move back on the table. As the patient is doing this, pull out the table extension while supporting the patient's lower legs.
6. **Procedural Step.** Assist the patient into the supine position and then into the prone position, making sure to have the patient roll toward you. Position the drape diagonally over the patient to provide warmth and modesty.
7. **Procedural Step.** Ask the patient to bend the arms at the elbows and rest them alongside the head. Ask the patient to elevate the buttocks while keeping the back straight. The patient's head should be turned to one side, and the weight of the body should be supported by the chest. A pillow under the chest can give addi-

tional support and aid relaxation. The knees and lower legs are separated approximately 12 inches.

8. **Procedural Step.** Adjust the drape diagonally as needed with one corner over the patient's back and the opposite corner over the buttocks and falling between the patient's legs. When the physician is ready to examine the patient, a small portion of the drape is folded back to expose the anal area.

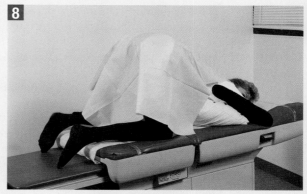

Position the drape diagonally.

9. **Procedural Step.** After completion of the examination, assist the patient into a prone position and then into a supine position. Allow the patient to rest in the supine position before he or she sits up.
   Principle. Patients (especially elderly ones) frequently become dizzy after being in the knee-chest position and should be allowed to rest before they sit up.
10. **Procedural Step.** Assist the patient into a sitting position. Slide the table extension back into place while supporting the patient's lower legs.
11. **Procedural Step.** Assist the patient down from the table. Return the footrest to its normal position. Instruct the patient to get dressed. Discard the gown and drape in a waste container.

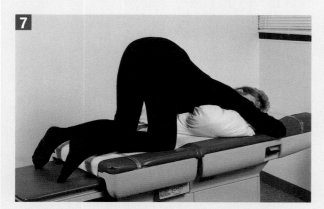

The buttocks are elevated, and the head is turned to one side.

PROCEDURE 5-9   Fowler's Position

Outcome Position and drape a patient in the Fowler's position. Fowler's position is used to examine the upper body of patients with cardiovascular and respiratory problems, such as congestive heart failure, emphysema, and asthma. These patients find it easier to breathe in this position than in a sitting or supine position. This position also is used to draw blood from patients who are likely to faint.

Equipment/Supplies

- Examining table
- Disposable patient gown
- Disposable patient drape

1. **Procedural Step.** Sanitize your hands. Greet the patient and introduce yourself.
2. **Procedural Step.** Identify the patient and explain the type of examination or procedure that will be performed.
3. **Procedural Step.** Provide the patient with a patient gown. Instruct the patient to remove clothing as appropriate for the type of examination being performed and to put on the patient gown with the opening in front. The disrobing facility should provide privacy, a place to sit, and a place to hang clothing.
4. **Procedural Step.** Position the head of the table as follows:
   a. For a semi-Fowler's position, the table should be positioned at a 45-degree angle.
   b. For a full Fowler's position, the table should be positioned at a 90-degree angle.
5. **Procedural Step.** Pull out the footrest of the examining table, and assist the patient into a sitting position. Place a drape over the patient's thighs and legs.
6. **Procedural Step.** Pull out the table extension while supporting the patient's lower legs. Ask the patient to lean back against the table head. Provide assistance during this step.

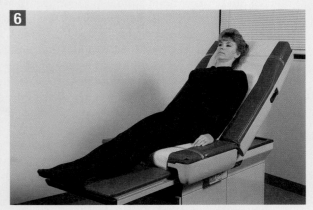

Ask the patient to lean back against the table head.

7. **Procedural Step.** Position the drape lengthwise over the patient to provide warmth and modesty. As the physician examines the patient, move the drape according to the body parts being examined.

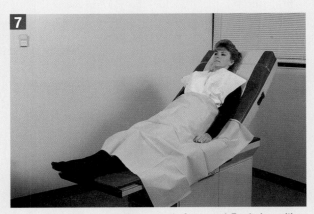

Position the table at a 45-degree angle for a semi-Fowler's position.

8. **Procedural Step.** After completion of the examination, assist the patient into a sitting position. Slide the table extension back into place while supporting the patient's lower legs.
9. **Procedural Step.** Assist the patient down from the table. Instruct the patient to get dressed. Return the head of the table and the footrest to their normal positions. Discard the gown and drape in a waste container.

ASSESSMENT OF THE PATIENT

The extent of patient assessment during the physical examination depends on the purpose of the examination and the patient's condition. A complete physical examination involves a thorough assessment of all the body systems. Table 5-2 outlines the specific assessments included in a complete physical examination. The physician uses an organized and systematic approach in performing a physical examination, starting with the patient's head and proceeding toward the feet. Using this type of approach facilitates the examination process and requires the fewest position changes by the patient. The physician notes the results of the physical examination in the patient's medical record. Figure 5-6 is an example of a preprinted form for this purpose.

Patients who exhibit symptoms of illness usually require only selected portions of the physical examination. A patient who comes to the medical office with the symptoms of bronchitis usually does not require a complete physical examination; rather, the physician examines the body system that is most likely to be associated with the symptoms. Four assessment techniques are used to obtain information during the physical examination: inspection, palpation, percussion, and auscultation.

Inspection

Inspection involves observation of the patient for any signs of disease, and of the four assessment techniques, it is the one most frequently used. Good lighting, either natural or artificial, is important for effective observation. The patient's color, speech, deformities, skin condition (e.g., rashes, scars, and warts), body contour and symmetry, orientation to the surroundings, body movements, and anxiety level are assessed through inspection. The medical assistant should develop a high level of detailed observational skills to assist the physician in assessing physical characteristics.

Palpation

Palpation is the examination of the body using the sense of touch (Figure 5-7). The physician uses palpation to determine the placement and size of organs; the presence of

lumps; and the existence of pain, swelling, or tenderness. Examining the breasts and taking the pulse are performed by palpation. Palpation often helps verify data obtained by inspection. The patient's verbal and facial expressions also are observed during palpation to assist in the detection of abnormalities.

The two types of palpation, light and deep, are categorized by the amount of pressure applied. *Light palpation* of structures is performed to determine areas of tenderness. The fingertips are placed on the part to be examined and are gently depressed approximately one half inch. *Deep palpation* is used to examine the condition of organs such as those in the abdomen. Two hands are used for deep palpation. One hand is used to support the body from below, and the other hand is used to press over the area to be palpated. Deep palpation is used by the physician to perform a bimanual pelvic examination.

Text continued on p. 196

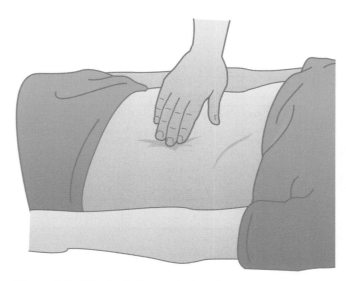

Figure 5-7. Palpation is the examination of the body using the sense of touch.

Memories *from* Externship

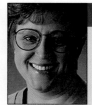

Hope Fauber: During my externship at a student health center at a 4-year college, I was responsible for working up patients for gynecologic examinations. The two-piece drapes had the top opening in the front and the bottom opening in the back. After explaining this to an Asian student who spoke very little English, I noticed that she had the openings opposite of what I had explained. I explained again, with words and gestures, that she needed to reverse the openings. To my surprise, she stood up, turned around in a circle, and sat down! ■

What Would You Do? What Would You *Not* Do?

Case Study 3

Ben-Yi Sun has brought his father, Chang-Yi Sun, to the medical office. Chang-Yi Sun is 76 years old and lives with Ben-Yi and his family. Because there is a large Asian population in the community, the medical office personnel have learned two things about the Asian culture: (1) They are brought up to respect elders, and elders are always considered first, and (2) Asians have a great respect for harmony. If they do not understand something, they may not admit it to avoid disrupting harmony. Ben-Yi Sun speaks very good English, but his father understands only a few words of English. Chang-Yi Sun has been diagnosed with hypertension, and he needs education about going on a low-sodium diet. He also needs instructions on taking his blood pressure at home and recording the results. ■

PHYSICAL EXAMINATION

INSTRUCTIONS:
(WNL) Within Normal Limits
(POS) Positive findings (X) Omitted

1. GENERAL

a. Posture _____
b. Gait _____
c. Speech _____
d. Appearance _____
e. Emotion _____

2. HEAD

a. Hair _____
b. Masses _____
c. Shape _____
d. Bruits _____
e. Tenderness _____
f. Sinus _____
g. Articulations _____

3. EYES

a. Lids R ___ L ___   f. Pupils R ___ L ___
b. Sclera R ___ L ___   g. Fundi R ___ L ___
c. Conjunctiva R ___ L ___   h. Light R ___ L ___
d. Muscles R ___ L ___   i. Bruits R ___ L ___
e. Cornea R ___ L ___
j. Accommodation R ___ L ___

4. EARS

a. Pinna R ___ L ___
b. Canal R ___ L ___
c. Drum R ___ L ___
d. Weber _____
e. Rinne _____

5. NOSE

a. Septum _____
b. Mucosa R ___ L ___
c. Obstruction _____

6. MOUTH/THROAT

a. Lips ___   f. Teeth ___
b. Breath ___   g. Dentures ___
c. Tongue ___   h. Caries ___
d. Pharynx ___   i. Larynx ___
e. Tonsils ___   j. Floor ___

7. NECK

a. Thyroid _____   d. Nodes R ___ L ___
b. Trachea _____   e. Bruits R ___ L ___
c. Veins _____   f. Carotid R ___ L ___

8. LUNGS

a. Chest _____   e. Bruits _____
b. Symmetry _____   f. Sounds _____
c. Diaphragm _____   g. Fremitus _____
d. Rubs _____

9. HEART

a. PMI ___   e. Rub ___
b. Rate ___   f. Murmur ___
c. Rhythm ___   g. Palpation ___
d. Thrill ___

10. BREASTS

a. Nodes R ___ L ___
b. Nipple R ___ L ___
c. Areolae R ___ L ___
d. Symmetry _____
e. Discharge _____

11. ABDOMEN

a. Sounds _____   e. Hernia R ___ L ___
b. Masses _____   f. Bruits R ___ L ___
c. Tenderness _____   g. Femoral R ___ L ___
d. Organs _____   h. Ing. nodes R ___ L ___

12. MUSCULOSKELETAL

a. Cervical _____
b. Thoracic _____
c. Lumbar _____
d. Sacral _____
e. Pelvic _____
f. Rib cage _____

13. FEMALE GENITALS

a. Labia _____   e. Cervix _____
b. Bartholin _____   f. Uterus _____
gland   g. Adnexa
c. Urethra   R ___ L
d. Vagina _____   h. Pap smear
done _____

14. MALE GENITALS

a. Penis _____   e. Scars _____
b. Scrotum _____   f. Meatus _____
c. Testicles _____   g. Epididymis _____
d. Discharge _____

15. RECTAL

a. Masses _____   f. Fissure _____
b. Anus _____   g. Hemorrhoids _____
c. Sphincter _____   h. Sigmoid _____
d. Prostate _____   ___cm.
e. Pilonidal _____   i. Mucosa _____
j. Other _____

16. SKIN

a. Scars _____
b. Marks _____
c. Texture _____
d. Sweat _____
e. Color _____
f. Ulcers _____

17. NEUROLOGICAL

	Strength*	Reflex**
a. Biceps	R ___ L ___	R ___ L ___
b. Triceps	R ___ L ___	R ___ L ___
c. Knee	R ___ L ___	R ___ L ___
d. Ankle	R ___ L ___	R ___ L ___

e. Romberg _____   i. Coordination _____
f. Babinsky _____   j. Tremor _____
g. Cranial N _____   k. Vibratory _____
h. Sensory _____

18. EXTREMITIES

a. Range of Motion
Shoulder _____   Knee _____
Elbow _____   Ankle _____
Wrist _____   Hand _____
Hip _____   Foot _____
Phalanges _____

b. General UR ___ UL ___ LR ___ LL ___
c. Muscular UR ___ UL ___ LR ___ LL ___
d. Bruits UR ___ UL ___ LR ___ LL ___
e. Edema UR ___ UL ___ LR ___ LL ___
f. Varicosities UR ___ UL ___ LR ___ LL ___

*When testing strength use grades:
Weak (W); Normal (N); Strong (S)

**When testing reflexes use:
Absent (A); Present (P); Brisk (B)

Signature _____

Figure 5-6. A preprinted form for recording the results of the physical examination.

Table 5-2 Physician Assessment during the Physical Examination

Body Structure	Assessment	Normal Findings	Abnormal Findings
General appearance	Observation of body build, posture, gait	Good posture and balance Steady gait	Poor posture or balance Unsteady, irregular, or staggering gait
	Determination of weight and height	Weight within ideal range	Patient is overweight or underweight
	Observation of hygiene and grooming	Good hygiene and grooming	Poor hygiene and grooming
	Observation for signs of illness	No signs of illness	Obvious signs of illness
	Observation of attitude, emotional state, mood	Patient speaks clearly and is cooperative	Patient is uncooperative, withdrawn, incoherent, negative, or hostile
Skin	Inspection of skin for color, vascularity, lesions	Smooth, supple, free of blemishes No unusual color	Blisters, wounds, lesions, rashes, swelling Unusual skin color (e.g., flushing, cyanosis, jaundice, or pallor)
	Palpation of temperature, moisture, turgor, texture	Warm to touch	Rough, dry, flaky skin Poor skin turgor
Head and neck	Inspection of size, shape, contour of head	Round head with prominences in front and back	Head is asymmetric or of unusual size
	Inspection of hair and scalp	Hair is resilient, evenly distributed, and not excessively dry or oily	Loss of hair Scaliness or dryness of scalp Presence of lice or other parasites
	Palpation of head and neck	No lumps, swelling, tenderness, or lesions of head or neck	Lumps, swelling, tenderness, or lesions of head or neck
Eyes	Evaluation of visual acuity and color vision	Good visual ability with or without glasses or contact lenses Appropriate color perception	Poor visual acuity or blindness Color blindness
	Evaluation of visual field	No visual field loss	Gaps in field of vision
	Inspection of eyelids and eyeballs	Eyes are bright	Dull or glossy eyes
	Inspection of conjunctiva	Pink mucous membranes	Inflamed mucous membranes Excessive tearing Drainage from eyes
	Inspection of eye movements	Eyes move equally in all directions	Drooping eyelids Uncoordinated eye movements
	Tests for pupillary reaction using penlight	Pupils are black, are equal in size, react appropriately to light	Dilated, constricted, or unequal pupils
	Inspection of internal eye structures using ophthalmoscope	Reddish-pink retina, even caliber, intact retinal blood vessels	Cloudy lens or narrowed blood vessels
Ears	Test for hearing using tuning fork or audiometer	Good hearing ability	Limited hearing or deafness
	Inspection of size, shape, symmetry of ears	Ears are symmetric and proportionate to head	Ears are asymmetric and not proportionate to the head

Continued

Table 5-2 Physician Assessment during the Physical Examination—cont'd

Body Structure	Assessment	Normal Findings	Abnormal Findings
Ears—cont'd	Inspection of external ear canal and tympanic membrane using an otoscope	Cerumen is soft and easily removed No drainage or discomfort Skin of ear canal is intact, pink, warm, and slightly moist Tympanic membrane is pearly gray and semi-transparent	Lesions, redness, or swelling of external ear canal Drainage from ear Pain when ear is moved Impacted cerumen Tympanic membrane is red, bulging, or perforated
Nose	Inspection of size, shape, symmetry of nose	Nose is symmetric, straight, not tender	Nose is asymmetric, deformed, flaring, or tender
	Inspection of nostrils using nasal speculum	Septum is intact and midline Nasal mucosa is moist and pink	Deviation or perforation of septum Redness, swelling, polyps, or discharge Nostrils are obstructed
	Test for sense of smell	Correct or very few incorrect responses to odors	Absent, decreased, exaggerated, or unequal responses to test substances
Mouth and pharynx	Inspection of lips for contour, color, texture	Pink, moist, soft, smooth lips	Pallor, cyanosis, blisters, swelling, cracking, excessive dryness of lips
	Inspection of mucosa	Pink, moist mucous membranes	Pale or dry mucosa with ulcers or abrasions
	Inspection of gums and palate	Smooth, pink, moist, firm gums Hard palate is firm and white Soft palate is pink and cushiony	Gums are red, bleeding, swollen, tender, spongy, or receding
	Inspection of teeth	Smooth, white enamel; regularly spaced teeth or well-fitting dentures	Missing or loose teeth, dental caries, poor-fitting dentures
	Inspection of tongue	Moist, pink, slightly rough-surfaced tongue	Tongue is dry, furry, smooth, red, or ulcerated
	Inspection of pharynx	Pink and smooth pharynx Tonsils are pink and normal in size Gag reflex is present	Pharynx is red, swollen, or ulcerated Tonsils are red or swollen Absent gag reflex
Arms and hands	Inspection of hands and arms for general appearance	Firm, strong muscles Normal range of motion in joints	Muscle weakness, lack of control or coordination Restricted range of motion
	Palpation of arm muscles	Good muscle control and coordination	
	Palpation for tenderness or lumps	No tenderness or lumps	Tenderness or lumps of hands or arms
	Inspection of fingernails	Colorless nail plate with a convex curve Smooth nail texture	Indentation, infection, brittleness, thickening, or angulation of nails Cyanosis or pallor of nails
Chest and lungs	Inspection of size and shape of chest	Chest is symmetric	Abnormal chest contour
	Assessment of respiratory rate, rhythm, depth	Normal respiratory rate, rhythm, depth	Labored, slow, rapid, or irregular respirations

Table 5-2 Physician Assessment during the Physical Examination—cont'd

Body Structure	Assessment	Normal Findings	Abnormal Findings
Chest and lungs—cont'd	Percussion of chest		
	Auscultation of breath sounds	Normal breath sounds No cough	Flat or dull lung sounds Noisy breath sounds Productive or nonproductive cough
	Palpation of ribs	No tenderness of ribs	Tenderness of ribs
Heart	Auscultation of heart sounds	Normal heart sounds	Irregular heartbeats or murmur
	Auscultation of apical pulse, rate, rhythm, volume	Regular, strong heartbeats	Rates slower or more rapid than normal
	Palpation of peripheral pulses	Palpable peripheral pulses	Weak or absent peripheral pulses
	Auscultation of blood pressure	Blood pressure within normal range for age	Low or high blood pressure
	Assessment of peripheral vascular perfusion	Skin is pink, resilient, moist	Cyanosis, pallor, edema
		Immediate return of color to nail beds	Poor capillary filling in nail beds
	Electrocardiogram to assess heart function	Normal heart function	Abnormal electrocardiogram
Breasts	Inspection of size, symmetry, contour	Breasts are round, smooth, symmetric	Retraction, dimpling, redness, or swelling of breasts
	Inspection of nipple	Nipples are round and equal in size, are similar in color, appear soft and smooth Areola is round and pink	Bleeding, cracking, discharge, or inversion of nipples
	Palpation of breasts and axillary lymph nodes	No lumps or tenderness of breasts or axillary lymph nodes	Lumps or tenderness of breasts or axillary lymph nodes
Abdomen	Inspection of contour, symmetry, skin condition, integrity	Symmetric contour Unblemished skin Soft abdomen	Asymmetric contour Rash or other skin lesions Abdominal distention
	Auscultation of bowel sounds	Active bowel sounds	Increased, diminished, or absent bowel sounds
	Percussion to assess underlying organs	Normal position and size of liver and spleen	Tenderness or lumps Enlarged liver or spleen
	Palpation of underlying organs, tenderness, lumps		
Genitalia and rectum	*Male*		
	Inspection of penis and urethra	Penis is smooth	Ulceration or discharge from penis
	Inspection of scrotum and palpation of testes	Testicles are smooth, firm, and movable within scrotal sac Scrotum is symmetric	Lumps or tenderness of scrotum, testes, or prostate gland
	Palpation of rectum and prostate gland	Increased pigmentation in anal area Good anal sphincter tone	Enlarged prostate gland Hemorrhoids or relaxed anal sphincter
	Stool specimen to test for occult blood	Absence of occult blood in stool	Occult blood in stool
	Female		
	Inspection of external genitalia	External genitalia are smooth and without lesions	Ulceration or redness or swelling of external genitalia

Continued

Table 5-2 Physician Assessment during the Physical Examination—cont'd

Body Structure	Assessment	Normal Findings	Abnormal Findings
Genitalia and rectum—cont'd *Female*—cont'd	Inspection of vagina and cervix using vaginal speculum	Vaginal mucosa is pink and moist Cervix is pink and smooth	Lacerations, tenderness, redness, or discharge from vagina or cervix
	Specimen collection from vagina and cervix for Pap test	Pap test is normal	Pap test is abnormal
	Bimanual pelvic examination	No tenderness or lumps of uterus and ovaries	Tenderness or lumps of uterus and ovaries
	Palpation of rectum	Good anal sphincter tone	Hemorrhoids or relaxed anal sphincter
	Stool specimen to test for occult blood	Increased pigmentation in anal area	Occult blood in stool
Lower extremities	Inspection of legs for general appearance and palpation of legs	Firm, strong muscles Normal range of motion in joints	Muscle weakness, lack of control or coordination Restricted range of motion Tenderness or lumps Limp or foot dragging during walking
	Inspection of toenails	Smooth nail texture	Indentation, infection, brittleness, thickening, or angulation of nails
Neurologic	Determination of mental status and level of consciousness	Alert and responds appropriately Oriented to person, place, and time	Responds inappropriately Disoriented
	Determination of sense of pain and touch	Normal response to pain and touch	Diminished or absent response to stimuli
	Use of percussion hammer to test reflexes	Normal reflexes	Abnormal or absent reflexes

Percussion

Percussion involves tapping the patient with the fingers and listening to the sounds produced to determine the size, density, and location of organs. This technique is often used to examine the lungs and abdomen.

The fingertips are used to produce a sound vibration similar to that of tapping a drumstick on a drum. The nondominant hand is placed directly on the area to be assessed, with the fingers slightly separated. The dominant hand is used to strike the joint of the middle finger placed on the patient to produce the sound vibration (Figure 5-8). Structures that are dense, such as the liver, spleen, and heart, produce a dull sound. Empty or air-filled structures, such as the lungs, produce a hollow sound. Any condition that changes the density of an organ or tissue, such as fluid in the lungs, would change the quality of the sound.

Auscultation

Auscultation is an examination technique that involves listening with a stethoscope to the sounds produced within the body. This technique is used to listen to the heart and lungs or to measure blood pressure. Environmental noise interferes with effective auscultation of body sounds and should be minimized. The diaphragm of the stethoscope chest piece is used to assess high-pitched sounds, such as lung and bowel sounds; the bell of the stethoscope chest piece is used to assess low-pitched sounds, such as those produced by the heart and vascular system. The chest piece should be cleaned with an antiseptic wipe and warmed with the hands before being placed on the patient.

ASSISTING THE PHYSICIAN

During the patient assessment, the medical assistant should assist the physician as required. This includes helping the patient change positions for the physician's examination of the different parts of the body, handing the physician instruments and supplies, and reassuring the patient to reduce apprehension. When the examina-

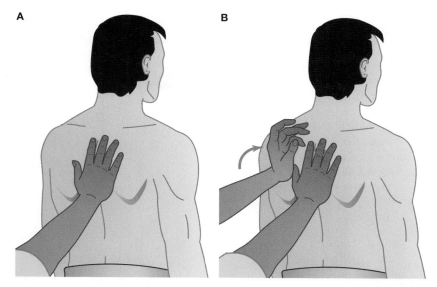

Figure 5-8. Percussion involves tapping the patient with the fingers. **A,** The nondominant hand is placed directly on the area to be assessed, with the fingers slightly separated. **B,** The fingers of the dominant hand are used to strike the joint of the middle finger to produce a sound vibration.

PROCEDURE 5-10

tion is completed, the medical assistant should assist the patient off the examining table and provide additional information if needed, such as scheduling a return visit or patient education to promote wellness. Procedure 5-10 describes the procedure for assisting with the physical examination.

PROCEDURE 5-10   Assisting with the Physical Examination

Outcome Prepare the patient and assist with a physical examination.

Equipment/Supplies

- Examining table
- Equipment for the type of examination to be performed

1. **Procedural Step.** Prepare the examining room. Ensure that the room is clean, free of clutter, and well lit and that the room temperature is comfortable for the patient.
2. **Procedural Step.** Sanitize your hands.
3. **Procedural Step.** Assemble the equipment according to the type of examination to be performed and the physician's preference. Arrange the instruments and supplies in a neat and orderly manner on a table or tray. Do not allow one item to lay on top of another.
4. **Procedural Step.** Obtain the patient's medical record. Go to the waiting room and ask the patient to come back to the examining room.
5. **Procedural Step.** Escort the patient to the examining room.

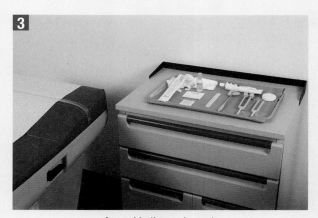

Assemble the equipment.

bright sunlight, may change the appearance of shades of color on the plates, leading to inaccurate test results.

The medical assistant is responsible for performing the color vision test and recording results in the patient's chart. The physician assesses the results to determine whether the patient has a deficiency in color vision.

The Ishihara test consists of 14 color plates. Plates 1 through 11 are used to conduct the basic test, and plates 12, 13, and 14 are used to assess further patients who exhibit a red-green color deficiency. It is unnecessary to include these plates (12, 13, and 14) in the test of patients who exhibit normal color vision. In interpreting the results, if 10 or more plates are read correctly, the patient's color vision is considered normal. If 7 or fewer of the 11 Ishihara plates are read correctly, the patient is identified as having a color vision deficiency. It would be unusual for the medical assistant to obtain results in which the patient read 8 or 9 plates correctly. The test is structured so that a patient with a color vision defect generally does not read 8 or 9 plates correctly and the rest incorrectly.

If a defect in color vision is detected, the patient is referred for additional assessment of color vision to an ophthalmologist or optometrist, who would use more precise color vision tests. The procedure for assessing color vision using the Ishihara color plates is outlined in Procedure 6-2.

Text continued on p. 214

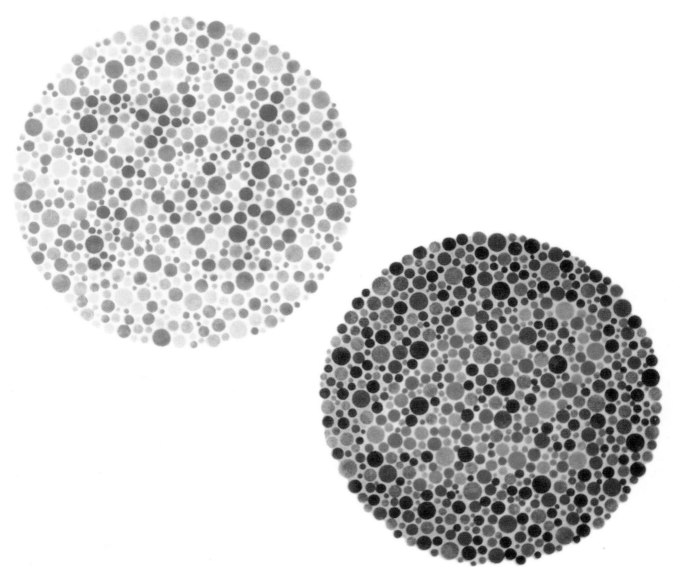

Figure 6-7. Ishihara color plates. Polychromatic plates. In the *upper figure,* a person with normal color vision reads 74, but a person with red-green color blindness reads 21. In the *lower figure,* a red-blind person (protanope) reads 2, but a green-blind person (deuteranope) reads 4. A normal-vision person reads 42. Reproduced plates are not good for testing for color deficiency. (From Ishihara J: *Tests for color blindness,* Tokyo, 1920, Kanehara.)

PROCEDURE 6-1   Assessing Distance Visual Acuity—Snellen Chart

Outcome Assess distance visual acuity.

Equipment/Supplies

- Snellen eye chart
- Eye occluder
- Antiseptic wipe

1. **Procedural Step.** Sanitize your hands.
2. **Procedural Step.** Assemble the equipment. Perform the test in a well-lit room that is free of distractions. Wipe the eye occluder with an antiseptic wipe, and allow it to dry completely.
   Principle. The eye occluder should be disinfected before use.
3. **Procedural Step.** Greet the patient and introduce yourself. Identify the patient and explain the procedure. Tell the patient that he or she will be asked to read several lines of letters. The patient should not have an opportunity to study or memorize the letters before beginning the test.
4. **Procedural Step.** Determine whether the patient wears contact lenses or glasses (other than reading glasses). If the patient wears such aids, he or she should be told to keep them on during the test.
5. **Procedural Step.** Ask the patient to stand on the marked line located 20 feet from the chart.
6. **Procedural Step.** Position the center of the Snellen chart at the patient's eye level. Stand next to the chart during the test to indicate to the patient the line to be identified.
   Principle. Ensure that the chart is at the patient's eye level rather than your eye level, to provide the most accurate results.
7. **Procedural Step.** Test the acuity of each eye separately. Measure the visual acuity of the right eye first.
   Principle. The medical assistant should establish a pattern of beginning with the same eye (traditionally the right eye) every time the test is performed. This helps to reduce errors during the recording of results.
8. **Procedural Step.** Ask the patient to cover the left eye with the eye occluder. If the patient wears eyeglasses, tell him or her to place the occluder in front of the glasses gently to prevent the glasses from being moved out of their normal position. Instruct the patient to keep the left eye open. During the test, the medical assistant should check to make sure the patient is keeping the left eye open.
   Principle. Eyeglasses moved out of normal position may lead to inaccurate test results. Keeping the left eye open prevents squinting of the right eye, which temporarily improves vision, leading to inaccurate test results.

9. **Procedural Step.** Instruct the patient not to squint during the test because squinting temporarily improves vision. Ask the patient to identify orally one line at a time on the Snellen chart, starting with the 20/70 line (or a line that is several lines above the 20/20 line).
   Principle. It is best to start at a line above the 20/20 line to give the patient a chance to gain confidence and to become familiar with the test procedure.
10. **Procedural Step.** If the patient is able to read the 20/70 line, proceed down the chart until reaching the smallest line of letters the patient can read. If the patient is unable to read the 20/70 line, proceed up the chart until the smallest line of letters the patient can read is reached.
11. **Procedural Step.** While the patient is reading the letters, observe him or her for unusual symptoms, such as squinting, tilting of the head, or watering of the eyes.
    Principle. These symptoms may indicate that the patient is having difficulty identifying the letters.
12. **Procedural Step.** Jot down the numbers next to the smallest line of letters that the patient is able to read. If one or two letters are missed, record the visual acuity with a minus sign next to the bottom number, along with the number of letters missed. If more than two letters are missed, the previous line is recorded.
13. **Procedural Step.** Ask the patient to cover the right eye with the eye occluder and to keep the right eye open. Measure the visual acuity in the left eye as de-

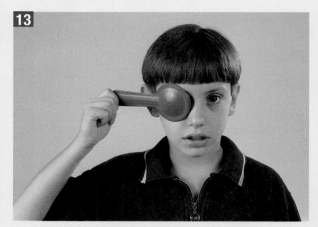

Ask the patient to cover the right eye and to keep the left eye open.

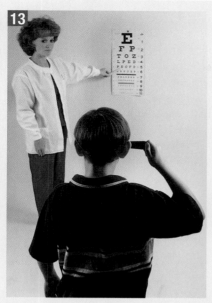

Ask the patient to identify one line at a time.

scribed in steps 8 through 10. During the test, check to make sure the patient is keeping the right eye open.

Principle. Keeping the right eye open prevents squinting of the left eye.

14. **Procedural Step.** Chart the procedure. Include the date and time, the name of the test (Snellen test), the visual acuity results, and any unusual symptoms the patient exhibited during the test. Also chart whether the patient was wearing corrective lenses during the test. Use the following abbreviations: s̄c without correction or c̄c with correction.

    Latin abbreviations are used to record visual acuity. The abbreviation for the right eye is OD *(oculus dexter),* the abbreviation for the left eye is OS *(oculus sinister),* and the abbreviation for both eyes is OU *(oculus uterque).*

15. **Procedural Step.** Disinfect the eye occluder with an antiseptic wipe, and sanitize your hands.

CHARTING EXAMPLE	
Date	
11/5/08	3:30 p.m. Snellen test, s̄c: OD 20/20-1.
	OS 20/25. Exhibited squinting, OD. —————
	————————————— C. Lindner, CMA

PROCEDURE 6-2   Assessing Color Vision—Ishihara Test

Outcome Assess color vision.

Equipment/Supplies

- Ishihara book
- Cotton swab

1. **Procedural Step.** Sanitize your hands. Assemble the equipment.
2. **Procedural Step.** Conduct the test in a quiet room illuminated by natural daylight.
   Principle. Using unnatural light may change the appearance of the shades of color on the plates, leading to inaccurate test results.
3. **Procedural Step.** Greet the patient and introduce yourself. Identify the patient and explain the procedure. Using the first (practice) plate as an example, instruct the patient to identify orally numbers formed by colored dots. Tell the patient that 3 seconds will be given to identify each plate.
   Principle. The first plate is designed to be read correctly by all individuals and is used to explain the procedure to the patient.
4. **Procedural Step.** Hold the first color plate 30 inches (75 cm) from the patient, at a right angle to the pa-

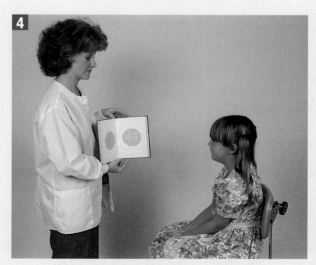

Hold the color plate 30 inches from the patient.

Continued

PROCEDURE 6-2   Assessing Color Vision—Ishihara Test—cont'd

tient's line of vision. The patient should keep both eyes open during the test.

5. **Procedural Step.** Ask the patient to identify the number on the plate. If the plate consists of a traceable winding colored line, ask the patient to trace the line using a cotton swab or the eraser end of a pencil. The patient's finger should not be used to make the tracing.
Principle. The patient's finger should not be used to trace the line because soiled fingers can degrade the plate over time.

6. **Procedural Step.** Record results after each plate. Continue until the patient has viewed all the plates. To record the color vision results, use the plate identification number and the number given by the patient. If the patient is unable to identify a number, the mark "X" should be recorded to indicate that the patient could not read the plate. Examples:
Plate 5: 21 This means the patient read the number 21 on plate 5.
Plate 6: X This means the patient could not identify a number on plate 6.
Plate 11: Traceable This means that the patient correctly traced a winding line on plate 11.

7. **Procedural Step.** Complete the charting entry. Include the date and time, the name of the test (Ishihara test), and any unusual symptoms the patient exhibited during the test, such as squinting or rubbing the eyes.

8. **Procedural Step.** Return the Ishihara book to its proper place. The book of color plates must be stored in a closed position to protect it from light.
Principle. Exposing the plates to excessive and unnecessary light results in fading of the color.

CHARTING EXAMPLE		
Plate No.	Normal Person	Results
1	12	12
2	8	8
3	5	5
4	29	29
5	74	74
6	7	7
7	45	45
8	2	2
9	X	X
10	16	16
11	Traceable	Traceable
11/6/08	10:00 a.m.	
	C. Lindner, CMA	

EYE IRRIGATION

An eye irrigation involves washing the eye with a flowing solution. Eye irrigations are performed for the following purposes: to cleanse the eye by washing away foreign particles, ocular discharges, or harmful chemicals; to relieve inflammation through the application of heat; and to apply an antiseptic solution. Procedure 6-3 shows how to perform an eye irrigation.

EYE INSTILLATION

An eye instillation involves the dropping of a liquid into the lower conjunctival sac of the eye. Eye instillations are performed to treat eye infections (with medication), to soothe an irritated eye, to dilate the pupil, and to anesthetize the eye during an eye examination or treatment. Medication to be instilled in the eye may come in the form of a liquid, as ophthalmic drops, or as an ophthalmic ointment. The eye drops

What Would You Do? What Would You *Not* Do?

Case Study 2

Peter Mitchell comes in with his 5-year-old son, Clive. Clive is diagnosed with conjunctivitis, and the physician prescribes Polytrim ophthalmic suspension. Mr. Mitchell says that Clive does not cooperate very well when having drops put in his eyes and asks for any ideas that might make it less of an ordeal. Mr. Mitchell has 7-year-old twin girls at home and wants to know what can be done so they don't get pink eye. He asks if it would be all right to instill the drops in the twins' eyes as a preventive measure. ■

are usually dispensed in a flexible plastic container with an attached dropper. Eye ointment is dispensed in a small metal tube with a small tip for applying the medication. Procedure 6-4 shows how to perform an eye instillation.

Text continued on p. 219

PATIENT TEACHING   Conjunctivitis

Answer questions patients have about conjunctivitis.

What is conjunctivitis?

Conjunctivitis, often referred to as *pink eye*, is an inflammation of the conjunctiva. The conjunctiva is a thin transparent membrane that covers the white of the eye. Conjunctivitis occurs when the conjunctiva becomes infected with a bacterium or virus. Other causes of conjunctivitis include allergies; the prolonged use of contact lenses; and irritation from wind, dust, and smoke. Conjunctivitis is almost always harmless and clears up by itself within 2 weeks. If it is caused by a bacterium, the physician may prescribe antibiotic eye drops or ointment.

What are the symptoms of conjunctivitis?

Most types of conjunctivitis are relatively painless. The eye is red or pink because of irritation, and there is a feeling of sandiness or grittiness in the eye. A discharge is usually present, which dries at night when the eyes are closed. This may cause the eyelids to be stuck together in the morning. Other symptoms include tearing, itching, and sensitivity of the eye to light.

Is conjunctivitis contagious?

Conjunctivitis caused by a virus or bacterium is highly contagious. It can be spread easily from one eye to another and throughout a family or classroom in a matter of days.

How can we avoid spreading conjunctivitis?

The following measures help prevent the spread of conjunctivitis:

- Avoid touching or rubbing the infected eye, which can spread the infection to the other eye or other people.
- Sanitize your hands frequently with soap, particularly after touching the eyes or face.
- Do not share washcloths, towels, or pillows with anyone.
- Do not wear contact lenses or eye makeup until the conjunctivitis is completely gone.
- Discard eye makeup that is used while you are infected to prevent reinfection.
- Encourage the patient to practice techniques that prevent the spread of conjunctivitis.
- If the physician has prescribed eye medication, teach the patient (or parent) the proper procedure for performing an eye instillation.
- Give the patient educational materials on conjunctivitis. ∎

PROCEDURE 6-3

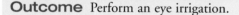

PROCEDURE 6-3   Performing an Eye Irrigation

Outcome   Perform an eye irrigation.

Equipment/Supplies

- Disposable gloves (nonpowdered)
- Irrigating solution
- Solution basin
- Bath thermometer

- Disposable rubber bulb syringe
- Basin
- Moisture-resistant towel
- Gauze pads

1. **Procedural Step.** Sanitize your hands.
2. **Procedural Step.** Assemble the equipment. If both eyes are to be irrigated, two sets of equipment must be used to prevent cross-infection from one eye to the other. Normal saline is generally used to irrigate the eye. Perform the following:
   a. Carefully check the label of the irrigating solution three times to make sure you have the correct solution. The first time is after you remove the solution container from the shelf. Compare the label of the solution container with the physician's instructions. Normal saline is generally used to irrigate the eye.

   b. Check the expiration date of the solution.
   c. Warm the irrigating solution to body temperature (98.6°F [37°C]) by placing the solution container in a basin of warm water. Use a bath thermometer to make sure the temperature of the water used to warm the solution does not exceed body temperature.
   d. Check the solution label a second time before pouring the solution.
   e. Pour the solution as follows:
   Palm the label of the container and remove the cap. Place the cap on a flat surface with the open end up.

Continued

PROCEDURE 6-3   Performing an Eye Irrigation—cont'd

Pour the solution into the basin and replace the cap without contaminating it. Cover the basin to keep the solution warm.

f. Check the solution label a third time before returning the container to its storage area.

Principle. The solution label should be carefully checked three times to prevent an error. Outdated solutions may produce undesirable effects and should be discarded. If the solution is too cold or too warm, it will be uncomfortable for the patient. Palming the label prevents solution from dripping on the label and obscuring it or loosening the label. Placing the cap open end up prevents contamination.

3. **Procedural Step.** Greet the patient and introduce yourself. Identify the patient and explain the procedure and of the irrigation. If the patient wears glasses or contact lenses, ask him or her to remove them.

4. **Procedural Step.** Position the patient. The patient may be placed in a sitting or lying position. Place a moisture-resistant towel on the patient's shoulder to protect the patient's clothing. Position a basin tightly against the patient's cheek under the affected eye to catch the irrigating solution, and ask the patient to hold it in place. Ask the patient to tilt the head in the direction of the affected eye.

Principle. The patient is positioned so that the solution flows away from the unaffected eye to prevent cross-infection.

5. **Procedural Step.** Apply nonpowdered gloves. Cleanse the eyelids from inner to outer canthus with a moistened gauze pad to remove any discharge or debris on the lids. The inner canthus is the inner junction of the eyelids next to the nose. The outer canthus is the junction of the eyelids farthest from the nose. Normal saline or the solution ordered for the irrigation may be used. Discard the gauze pad after each wipe.

Principle. Nonpowdered gloves avoid irritation of the patient's eye with powder that may have gotten on the outside of the glove. The eyelids should be clean to

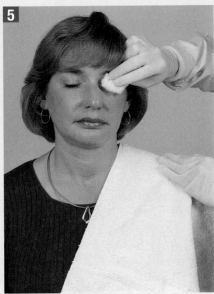

Cleanse the eyelids from inner to outer canthus.

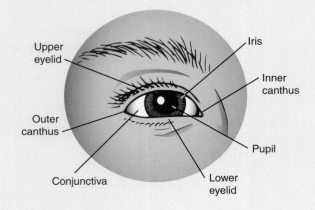

prevent foreign particles from entering the eye during the irrigation. Cleansing from inner to outer canthus prevents cross-infection.

6. **Procedural Step.** Fill the irrigating syringe with the solution by squeezing the bulb and slowly releasing it until the desired amount of solution enters the bulb. Instruct the patient to keep both eyes open and to find a focal point in the room and focus on it.

Principle. Looking at a focal point helps the patient keep the irrigated eye open during the procedure.

7. **Procedural Step.** Separate the eyelids with the index finger and thumb to expose the lower conjunctiva and to hold the upper eyelid open.

Principle. The medical assistant must hold the eye open during the procedure because the patient will have a tendency to close it.

8. **Procedural Step.** Hold the tip of the syringe approximately 1 inch above the eye. Gently release the solution onto the eye at the inner canthus. This allows the solution to flow over the eye at a moderate rate from the inner to the outer canthus. Direct the solution to the lower conjunctiva. To prevent injury, do not allow the tip of the syringe to touch the eye.

Principle. The solution flows away from the unaffected eye to prevent cross-infection. The cornea is sensitive and can be harmed easily. The irrigating solution must be directed to the lower conjunctiva to prevent injury to the cornea.

9. **Procedural Step.** Refill the syringe, and continue irrigating until the desired results have been obtained

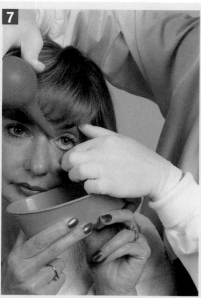

7

Separate the eyelids, and hold the tip of the syringe 1 inch above the eye.

or all the solution is used, depending on the purpose of the irrigation.

10. **Procedural Step.** Dry the eyelids from inner to outer canthus with a gauze pad.

11. **Procedural Step.** Remove the gloves, and sanitize your hands.

12. **Procedural Step.** Chart the procedure. Include the following: the date and time; which eye was irrigated; the type, strength, and amount of solution used; and any significant observations and patient reactions. Use one of these abbreviations to indicate which eye was irrigated:

OU—Both eyes
OD—Right eye
OS—Left eye

13. **Procedural Step.** Remove reusable equipment to a work area for sanitization, sterilization or disinfection as required by the medical office policy.

CHARTING EXAMPLE

Date	
11/5/08	10:30 a.m. Irrigated OS $\bar{c}$ sterile saline @
	98.6° F. No complaints of discomfort.
	—————————————— C. Lindner, CMA

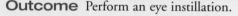

PROCEDURE 6-4   Performing an Eye Instillation

Outcome Perform an eye instillation.

Equipment/Supplies

- Disposable gloves (nonpowdered)
- Ophthalmic drops or ophthalmic ointment as ordered by the physician
- Tissues
- Gauze pads

1. **Procedural Step.** Sanitize your hands.
2. **Procedural Step.** Assemble the equipment, and perform the following:
   a. Check the drug label three times to make sure you have the correct medication. The first time should be when you remove the medication from the shelf. The medication label must bear the word *ophthalmic.*
   b. Check the medication label a second time against the physician's instructions. Also check the dosage ordered by the physician.
   c. Check the expiration date.
   d. Check the medication label a third time before the cap is removed to instill the medication.
   Principle. The drug label should be carefully checked three times to prevent a medication error. Medication not bearing the word *ophthalmic* must never be placed in the eye because it could injure the eye. An outdated

medication may produce undesirable effects and should be discarded.

3. **Procedural Step.** Greet the patient and introduce yourself. Identify the patient and explain the procedure and purpose of the instillation. If the patient wears glasses or contact lenses, ask him or her to remove them.
4. **Procedural Step.** Help the patient into a sitting or supine position.
5. **Procedural Step.** Apply nonpowdered gloves. Prepare the medication. **Eye drops:** If the medication requires mixing, shake the container well. Check the medication label for the third time, and remove the cap from the container. **Eye ointment:** Check the medication label for the third time, and remove the cap from the tip of the tube.
   Principle. Nonpowdered gloves avoid irritation of the patient's eyes with powder that may have gotten on the outside of the gloves.

Continued

PROCEDURE 6-4

6. **Procedural Step.** Ask the patient to look up at the ceiling, and expose the lower conjunctival sac by using the fingers of the nondominant hand placed over a tissue. The fingers should be placed on the patient's cheekbone just below the eye, and the skin of the cheek should be drawn gently downward.
Principle. Looking up helps keep the patient from blinking when the drops are instilled.

7. **Procedural Step.** Insert the medication. **Eye drops:** Invert the container and hold the tip of the dropper approximately ½ inch above the eye sac. Do not allow the dropper to touch the eye or any other surface. Gently squeeze the container and place the correct number of eye drops in the center of the lower conjunctival sac. Never place the drops directly on the

eyeball. Replace the cap on the container. **Eye ointment:** Gently squeeze the tube and place a thin ribbon of ointment along the length of the lower conjunctival sac from inner to outer canthus. Be careful not to touch the tip of the ointment tube to the eye or any other surface. Discontinue the ribbon by twisting the tube. Replace the cap on the tube.
Principle. Touching the dropper or tip of the tube to the eye (or other surfaces) could injure the eye and contaminate the medication. Placing the medication in the conjunctival sac, rather than directly on the eyeball, is more comfortable for the patient.

8. **Procedural Step.** Ask the patient to close his or her eyes gently and move the eyeballs. Instruct the patient not to shut the eyes tight or to blink and to keep the eyes closed for 1 to 2 minutes. Tell the patient that the instillation may blur the vision temporarily.
Principle. Moving the eyeballs helps distribute the medication over the entire eye. Keeping the eyes closed allows the medication to be absorbed. If the eyes are shut tightly or if the patient blinks, the drops or ointment may be pushed out of the eye.

9. **Procedural Step.** Dry the eyelid from inner to outer canthus with a gauze pad to remove excess medication.

10. **Procedural Step.** Remove the gloves, and sanitize your hands.

11. **Procedural Step.** Chart the procedure. The medication dosage for eye drops is recorded in the number of drops instilled. The abbreviation for drop is *gtt;* for drops, *gtts.* The number of drops must be recorded in Roman numerals (i.e.; i, ii) following the *gtt* abbreviation. The recording should include the date and time, the name and strength of the medication, the number of drops or amount of ointment, which eye received the instillation, your observations, and the patient's reaction.

12. **Procedural Step.** Return the medication to its proper storage area.

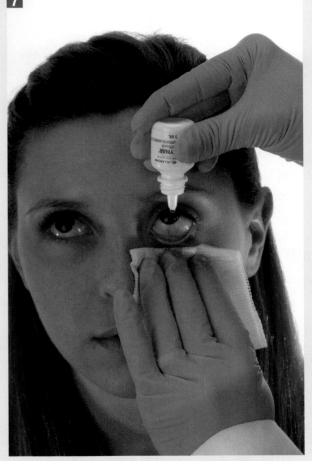

7

Ask the patient to look up, and insert the medication.

CHARTING EXAMPLE	
Date	
11/5/08	2:30 p.m. Atropine sulfate, 1% gtts ii OU.
	Pt states a temporary blurring of vision. ——
	—————————— C. Lindner, CMA

THE EAR

STRUCTURE OF THE EAR

The ear functions in hearing and in maintaining equilibrium. It consists of three divisions: the *external ear,* the *middle ear,* and the *inner ear.* The structures in the ear are illustrated in Figure 6-8 and described next.

The external ear is composed of the auricle (or pinna) and the external auditory canal, also known as the *external ear canal.* The opening into this canal is the *external auditory meatus.*

The *auricle* is a flap of cartilage covered with skin that projects from the side of the head. Its function is to receive and collect sound waves and to direct them toward the external auditory canal.

The *external auditory canal* is approximately 1 inch long in an adult and extends from the auricle to the tympanic membrane. It is lined with skin that contains fine hairs, nerve endings, and glands. The glands secrete earwax, or **cerumen,** which lubricates and protects the ear canal. The canal has an S-shaped curve as it leads inward. The canal must be straightened during an examination with an otoscope, an ear instillation or irrigation, or aural temperature measurement.

The **tympanic membrane** is at the end of the external auditory canal. It is a pearly gray, semitransparent membrane that receives sound waves.

The middle ear is an air-filled cavity that contains three small bones, or *ossicles:* the malleus, the incus, and the stapes. The *eustachian tube* connects the middle ear to the nasophar-

ynx. Air pressure between the external atmosphere and the middle ear is stabilized through the eustachian tube.

The inner ear contains the *cochlea,* which is the essential organ of hearing. The *semicircular canals* also are located in the inner ear and help to maintain equilibrium.

ASSESSMENT OF HEARING ACUITY

The assessment of hearing acuity is an integral part of a complete physical examination. It is possible for an individual to have a hearing loss and not be aware of it. Early detection and treatment of hearing problems help prevent permanent hearing loss.

What Would You Do? | What Would You *Not* Do?

Case Study 3

Willow Basil brings in her 6-year-old daughter, Jade. For the past 3 days, Jade has been running a fever and has had persistent pain and hearing loss in her left ear. Mrs. Basil practices alternative medicine and uses prescription medications as little as possible. She says that she has been trying herbal therapy and aromatherapy to make Jade better, but it does not seem to be helping. Jade is diagnosed with acute otitis media, and the physician prescribes amoxicillin for 10 days. Mrs. Basil wants to know if she has to give Jade the amoxicillin for the entire 10 days. She asks if she can stop using it when Jade starts feeling better. Mrs. Basil also wants to know if the ear infection will cause a permanent problem with Jade's hearing. ■

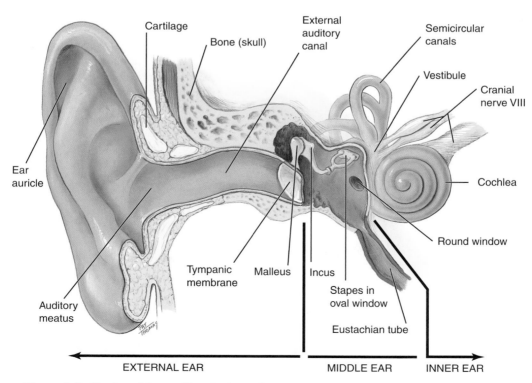

Figure 6-8. Structure of the ear. (From Applegate EJ: *The anatomy and physiology learning system,* ed 2, Philadelphia, 2000, Saunders.)

An individual with normal hearing should be able to hear the frequencies of normal speech, which range from 300 to 4000 Hz (hertz, or cycles per second) at a normal sound intensity. Patients who exhibit hearing loss are referred to an otolaryngologist or an audiologist for further evaluation.

Types of Hearing Loss

There are three types of hearing loss: conductive, sensorineural, and mixed. *Conductive hearing loss* is the most common and results when there is a physical interference with the normal conduction of sound waves through the external and middle ear. Because of the interference, the amount of sound reaching the inner ear is less than normal, resulting in hearing impairment. Conductive loss in the external ear may be caused by an obstruction in the external ear canal, such as impacted cerumen, swelling from external otitis (swimmer's ear), foreign bodies, and benign growths such as polyps. Conductive loss in the middle ear may be caused by serous otitis media (fluid in the middle ear) or acute otitis media (infection in the middle ear), a perforated tympanic membrane, or otosclerosis. The cause of conductive hearing loss often can be detected by examining the external ear canal with an otoscope. Hearing is frequently restored by removing the obstruction (e.g., impacted cerumen) or treating the disorder (e.g., serous otitis media).

Sensorineural hearing loss results from damage to the inner ear or auditory nerve. With this type of hearing loss, the sound is conducted normally through the outer and middle ear structures, but because of a problem with the perception of sound waves, a hearing deficit occurs. Specific causes of sensorineural loss include hereditary factors, intense noise exposure over time, tumors, degenerative changes from the normal aging process, ototoxicity caused by certain medications and infectious diseases, such as measles, mumps, and meningitis. *Mixed hearing loss* is a combination of conductive and sensorineural loss.

Hearing Acuity Tests

Numerous tests can be used to assess hearing acuity. Tests range from the simple gross screening test to qualitative tests using a tuning fork to highly specific quantitative tests using an audiometer. It is important to test only one ear at a time because a hearing deficit can exist in one ear only. The ear not being tested should be blocked by an earplug or masked. *Masking* involves the presentation of sound (usually noise) to the ear not being tested so that the patient's response is based only on hearing in the ear being tested.

Gross Screening Test

The gross hearing test is a simple and quick screening test used to identify a large hearing impairment. The physician performs the screening test during the physical examination. Hearing is assessed by asking the patient to repeat a simple word or series of numbers whispered from a distance of 1 to 2 feet from the ear. When a hearing loss is discovered, a tuning fork or audiometer is used for a more precise assessment of hearing.

Tuning Fork Tests

Tuning fork tests provide a general assessment of hearing acuity and may be part of the physical examination. A tuning fork with a frequency of 512 Hz or 1024 Hz is generally used because these frequencies fall within the range of normal speech. The Weber and Rinne tests are the tuning fork tests most commonly performed by the physician; they are used to identify conductive and sensorineural hearing loss.

The *Weber test* is a useful assessment of hearing loss when one ear hears better than the other. The tuning fork is set in vibration, and the base of the fork is placed on the center of the patient's head. The patient is asked to indicate where the sound is heard best. A patient with normal hearing would hear the sound equally in both ears or in the center of the head. Figure 6-9 illustrates the Weber test and describes the interpretation of results.

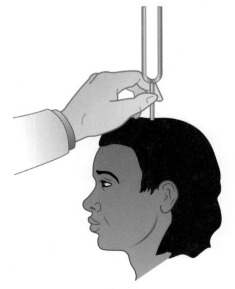

Normal Hearing
The patient hears the sound equally in both ears or in the center of the head.

Conductive Hearing Loss
The patient hears the sound better in the problem ear.

Sensorineural Hearing Loss
The patient does not hear the sound as well in the problem ear.

Figure 6-9. Weber test.

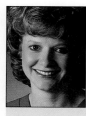

Memories *from* Externship

Cammie Lindner: There is one characteristic that is shared by all patients. I first noticed this during my externships, and it does not seem to matter what type of practice it is. Patients like to feel special and to be treated that way. They like consistency in their physician and in the office staff, in seeing familiar faces. This is especially hard during externship. The time spent is too short to truly get to know the patients, but it is a great learning experience.

It is important to observe the staff and patient communication and interaction skills. By doing this, you can decide which ones you admire and those that you do not wish to copy. The following are just a few of the guidelines that have helped me: (1) Call patients by name, and be sure that they know your name. (2) Follow through with what you have told a patient you will do, and keep them updated if circumstances change. (3) Smile and do not let one patient's negative attitude interfere with your care of others. (4) Take time to listen.

When you do begin your career, it does not take long to get into a routine and to start knowing your patients. When patients see a familiar face, they are more willing to share information that can contribute to improved communication and good health care. ∎

The *Rinne test* compares the duration of sound perception by air conduction with that of bone conduction. The tuning fork is set in vibration, and the base of the fork is placed against the bone of the mastoid process. The patient is instructed to indicate when the sound is no longer heard. The prongs of the fork (still vibrating) are placed in the air about 1 inch from the opening of the patient's ear canal, and the patient indicates when the sound is no longer heard. An individual with normal hearing is able to hear the sound at least twice as long through air conduction as through bone conduction. Figure 6-10 illustrates the Rinne test and describes the interpretation of results.

Audiometry

Audiometry is the measurement of hearing acuity using a special instrument called an **audiometer.** An audiometer quantitatively measures hearing for the various frequencies of sound waves. Audiometry is a more specific hearing acuity test because it provides information on how extensive a hearing loss is and which frequencies are involved. It is important that the test be conducted in a quiet room because outside noise may affect the results, especially in the lower frequencies. The patient wears headphones placed snugly over the ears (Figure 6-11). The audiometer delivers a single frequency at a time at specific intensities, starting with low-frequency tones of 250 to 500 Hz and

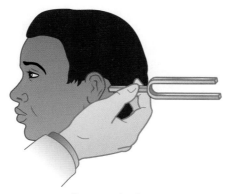

Bone conduction

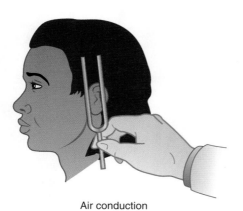

Air conduction

Normal Hearing
The patient hears the sound at least twice as long through air conduction as through bone conduction.

Conductive Hearing Loss
The patient hears the sound longer by bone conduction than by air conduction.

Sensorineural Hearing Loss
The sound is reduced. The patient will also hear the sound longer through air conduction than through bone conduction but not twice as long.

Figure 6-10. Rinne test.

7

Physical Agents to Promote Tissue Healing

LEARNING OBJECTIVES

Local Application of Heat and Cold
1. State examples of moist and dry applications of heat and cold.
2. State the factors to consider when applying heat and cold.
3. List the effects of local application of heat, and state reasons for applying heat.
4. List the effects of local application of cold, and state reasons for applying cold.

Therapeutic Ultrasound
1. Describe the general use of therapeutic ultrasound.
2. Explain the purpose of the ultrasound coupling agent.

Casts
1. List reasons for applying a cast.
2. Identify the advantages and disadvantages of synthetic casts.
3. Explain the purpose of each step in the cast application procedure.

Splints and Braces
1. Describe a splint and explain its use.
2. Explain the purpose of a brace.

Ambulatory Aids
1. List factors that are taken into consideration when ambulatory aids are prescribed.
2. Explain the difference between an axillary crutch and a forearm crutch.
3. State conditions that may result when axillary crutches are not fitted properly.
4. List the guidelines that should be followed by the patient to ensure safe use of crutches.
5. State the use of each of the following crutch gaits: four-point gait, two-point gait, three-point gait, swing-to gait, and swing-through gait.
6. List and describe the three types of canes.
7. Identify the patient conditions that warrant the use of a cane or walker.

PROCEDURES

Apply each of the following heat treatments:
    Heating pad
    Hot soak
    Hot compress
    Chemical hot pack
Apply each of the following cold treatments:
    Ice bag
    Cold compress
    Chemical cold pack

Administer an ultrasound treatment.

Assist with the application of a cast.
Assist with the removal of a cast.
Instruct a patient in proper cast care.

Apply a splint following the manufacturer's instructions.
Apply a brace following the manufacturer's instructions.

Measure a patient for axillary crutches.
Instruct a patient in the proper use of crutches.
Instruct a patient in the proper procedure for each of the following crutch gaits:
    Four-point
    Two-point
    Three-point
    Swing-to
    Swing-through
Instruct a patient in the use of a cane.
Instruct a patient in the proper use of a walker.

NATIONAL COMPETENCIES

Clinical Competencies

Patient Care
Prepare and maintain examination and treatment areas.
Prepare patient for and assist with procedures, treatments, and minor office surgery.

General Competencies

Patient Instructions
Instruct individuals according to their needs.
Provide instruction for health maintenance and disease prevention.

KEY TERMS

ambulation (AM-byoo-LAY-shun)
ambulatory
brace
compress (KOM-press)
edema (uh-DEE-muh)
erythema (err-uh-THEE-muh)
exudate (EKS-oo-date)
long arm cast
long leg cast

maceration (mass-er-AY-shun)
orthopedist (OR-thoe-PEE-dist)
short arm cast
short leg cast
soak
splint
sprain
strain
suppuration (SUP-er-AY-shun)

Introduction to Tissue Healing

Physical agents are often employed in the medical office to promote tissue healing for individuals who experience a disability as a result of injury, disease, or loss of a body part. Physical agents are used therapeutically to improve circulation, provide support, and promote the return of motion so that the individual can perform the activities of daily living. Physical agents frequently used in the medical office include heat and cold applied locally; therapeutic ultrasound; casts; and ambulatory aids, such as crutches, canes, and walkers.

LOCAL APPLICATION OF HEAT AND COLD

The application of heat and cold is used therapeutically to treat conditions such as infection and trauma. The medical assistant may be responsible for applying various forms of heat and cold at the medical office or for instructing patients in the proper procedure for applying heat or cold at home. The medical assistant should have a basic under-

standing of the physiologic effects of heat and cold on the body and possible adverse reactions if they are not administered correctly.

Heat and cold can be applied in moist or dry forms. The common applications of dry and moist heat and cold are as follows:

1. *Dry heat:* heating pad, chemical hot pack
2. *Moist heat:* hot soak, hot compress
3. *Dry cold:* ice bag, chemical cold pack
4. *Moist cold:* cold compress

Heat and cold are applied for short periods (generally 15 to 30 minutes) to produce the desired therapeutic results. The application may be repeated at time intervals specified by the physician. Prolonged application of heat or cold is not recommended because it can result in adverse secondary effects. The type of heat or cold application used for a particular condition depends on the purpose of the application, the location and condition of the affected area, and the age and general health of the patient. The physician instructs the medical assistant to apply a heat or cold treatment based on these factors.

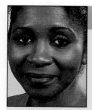

Putting It All into Practice

My Name is Marlyne Cooper, and I am a certified medical assistant. I work in a community health center. My primary responsibilities are to take patients back to the examination rooms and to prepare them for procedures and treatments. I take the patient's chief complaint and the health history. I greet each patient in a kind and calm way. This helps put the patient at ease before the physician goes into the examining room.

I once worked in a private office with a small waiting room and narrow hall. One of my regular patients was a healthy young 20-year-old man who was confined to a wheelchair by a spinal injury from an automobile accident. He had great difficulty maneuvering his motorized chair in tight spaces, and he felt embarrassed and conspicuous sitting in the middle of the waiting room. I began bringing him through the larger back door into the physician's office, directly into an examination room. Talking about things we had in common, such as an interest in sports and movies, made him feel more at ease. By making the situation as easy as possible for him, he was able to keep his dignity and not draw attention to his special needs. ■

Heat and cold receptors in the skin readily adapt to changes in temperature, eventually resulting in diminished heat or cold sensations. The temperature actually remains the same and is providing the intended therapeutic effects. The patient, not perceiving the same degree of temperature, may want to increase the intensity of the application, however, without realizing the inherent dangers. Excessive heat or cold could result in tissue damage. A common example of this situation is a patient who turns up the setting of a heating pad from medium to high when the heating pad no longer feels warm. The medical assistant should fully explain to the patient the necessity of maintaining a safe temperature range during the application.

Factors Affecting the Application of Heat and Cold

Before applying heat or cold, certain factors must be taken into consideration to prevent unfavorable reactions, such as tissue necrosis. The temperature may need to be adjusted based on the following conditions:

1. **The age of the patient.** Young children and elderly patients tend to be more sensitive to the application of heat or cold.
2. **Location of the application.** Certain areas of the body are more sensitive to the application of heat or cold, especially thin areas of the skin and areas that are usually covered by clothing, such as the chest, back, and abdomen. The skin on the hands and face is not as sensitive and is better able to tolerate temperature change. Broken skin, such as is found with an open wound, is more

sensitive to heat and cold and is more prone to tissue damage.

3. **Impaired circulation.** Patients with impaired circulation tend to be more sensitive to heat and cold. This impairment may be at the site of the application or may be a systemic problem involving the entire body that is a result of certain conditions, such as peripheral vascular disease, diabetes mellitus, or congestive heart failure.
4. **Impaired sensation.** Patients with impaired sensation, such as diabetic patients, must be watched carefully because tissue damage may occur from the application of heat or cold without the patient's awareness.
5. **Individual tolerance to change in temperature.** Some individuals cannot tolerate temperature change as easily as others.

The medical assistant should observe the area to which the heat or cold has been applied before, during, and after the treatment for signs indicating that a modification of temperature is needed. Prolonged erythema or paleness, pain, swelling, and blisters should be reported to the physician. The medical assistant also should ask the patient whether the application feels comfortable or is too hot or too cold.

Heat

Local Effects of Heat

The application of moderate heat to a localized area of the body for a short time (approximately 15 to 30 minutes) produces *dilation,* or an increase in diameter, of the blood vessels in the area as the body tries to rid itself of excess heat (Figure 7-1). This results in an increased blood supply to the area, and tissue metabolism increases. Nutrients and oxygen are provided to the cells at a faster rate, and wastes and toxins are carried away faster. The skin in the area becomes warm and exhibits erythema. **Erythema** is the reddening of the skin caused by dilation of superficial blood vessels in the skin.

These physiologic effects of moderate heat applied to a localized area promote healing. Prolonged application of heat (more than 1 hour) produces secondary effects, however, that reverse this healing process. Blood vessels constrict, and blood supply to the area decreases. The medical assistant must be careful to apply heat for the length of time specified by the physician.

Purpose of Applying Heat

Heat functions in relieving pain, congestion, muscle spasms, and inflammation. Conditions for which the local application of heat is often prescribed are low back pain, arthritis, menstrual cramping, and localized abscesses.

Heat promotes muscle relaxation and is often used for the relief of pain caused by excessive contraction of muscle fibers. **Edema,** or swelling, in the tissues can be reduced through the application of heat because the increased blood supply functions to increase the absorption of fluid from the tissues through the lymphatic system.

Heat, usually in the form of a hot **compress,** can be used to soften exudates. An **exudate** is a discharge produced by

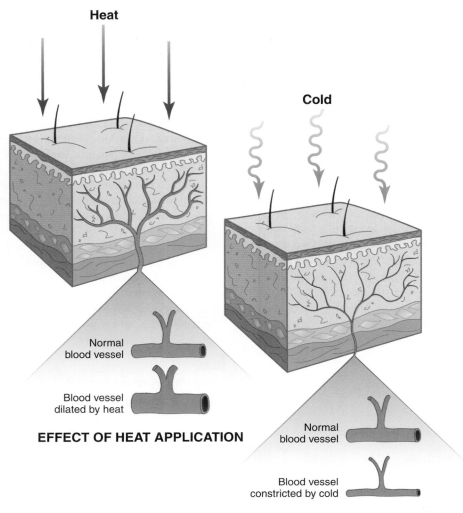

Figure 7-1. Effects of the local application of heat and cold. (From Wood LA, Rambo BJ: *Nursing skills for allied health services,* vol 2, Philadelphia, 1980, Saunders.)

the body's tissues. Exudates may sometimes form a hard crust over an area and require removal. Heat also increases **suppuration,** or the process of pus formation, to help in the relief of inflammation by breaking down infected tissues. Heat is not recommended, however, for the initial treatment of acute inflammation or trauma.

Type of Heat Applications
The most common type of heat applications are described next, including the conditions they are often used to treat.

Heating Pad
The electric heating pad consists of a network of wires that function to convert electric energy into heat to provide a constant and even heat application. The wires must not be bent or crushed. This could damage the pad, resulting in overheating of parts of the pad and leading to burns or fire. Pins must not be inserted in the pad as a means of securing it; if a pin comes in contact with a wire, an electric shock could result. To prevent electric hazards, heating pads should not be used over areas that contain moisture, such as wet dressings. Heating pads are often used to relieve pain and muscle spasms.

Hot Soak
A soak is the direct immersion of a body part in water or a medicated solution. A soak can be applied to an extremity or a part of the torso. Hot soaks are used to cleanse open wounds, increase suppuration, increase the blood supply to

an area to hasten the healing process, and apply a medicated solution to an area.

Hot Compress

A hot compress is a soft, moist, absorbent cloth, such as a washcloth, that is immersed in a warm solution and applied to a body part. Hot compresses are used to increase suppuration, to improve circulation to a body part to aid in healing, to promote drainage from infection, and to soften exudates. Applying a hot compress to an open wound requires the use of sterile technique.

Chemical Hot Pack

Chemical hot packs are available in a variety of sizes and shapes. When activated, they provide a specific degree of heat for a specific period of time (usually 30 to 60 minutes), as indicated on the package label. A chemical hot pack consists of a vinyl bag containing calcium chloride crystals and a smaller bag (encased in the vinyl bag) containing water. Pressure is applied with the hands to break the inner bag. The water in the inner bag combines with the calcium chloride crystals to produce heat. After using the pack, it should be discarded in an appropriate receptacle. Chemical hot packs should be stored at room temperature and are used as an alternative to a heating pad to relieve pain and muscle spasms.

Procedures 7-1, 7-2, 7-3, and 7-6 (see later) present proper application of heat with a heating pad, a hot soak, a hot compress, and a chemical hot pack.

Cold

Local Effects of Cold

The application of moderate cold to a localized area produces *constriction,* or a decrease in diameter, of blood vessels in the area as the body attempts to prevent heat loss (see Figure 7-1). This constriction leads to decreased blood supply to the area. Tissue metabolism decreases, less oxygen is used, and fewer wastes accumulate. The skin becomes cool and pale. Prolonged application of cold (more than 1 hour) has a reverse secondary effect. Blood vessels dilate, and there is an increase in tissue metabolism. To prevent secondary

What Would You Do? What Would You *Not* Do?

Case Study 1
Aaron Collins is at the office. Aaron recently helped a friend move, and the next day he developed intense pain in his lower back. To alleviate the pain, he slept on a heating pad, but when he woke up, his back was red and blistered. Aaron says he turned the setting on the heating pad to high because his back was hurting so much and he thought that it would help his back feel better sooner. Aaron wants to know the best way to apply heat using a heating pad. He also wants to know what he can do to prevent low back pain in the future. ■

effects, the medical assistant must apply cold for the recommended length of time only.

Purpose of Applying Cold

The application of moderate cold for a short time is used to prevent edema. Cold may be applied immediately after an individual has suffered direct trauma, such as a bruise, minor burn, **sprain, strain,** joint injury, or fracture. The cold limits the accumulation of fluid in the body tissues by constricting blood vessels and reducing the leakage of fluid into the tissues. Through the constriction of peripheral blood vessels, cold can be used to control bleeding. Cold temporarily relieves pain because of its anesthetic, or numbing, effect, which reduces stimulation of the pain receptors. Cold also slows the movement of blood and tissue fluids in the affected area, resulting in less pressure against pain receptors and therefore less pain. In the early stages of an infection, the local application of cold inhibits the activity of microorganisms. In this way, suppuration is decreased and inflammation is reduced. Cold applications should always be placed in a protective covering because applying cold directly to the skin could result in a skin burn.

Types of Cold Applications
Ice Bag
An ice bag consists of a waterproof bag with a screw-on cap. Before use, it must be filled with small pieces of ice and placed in a protective covering. Ice bags are used to prevent swelling, control bleeding, and relieve pain and inflammation.

Cold Compress
A cold compress is a soft, moist, absorbent cloth, such as a washcloth, that is immersed in a cold solution and applied to a body part. Cold compresses are used to relieve pain and inflammation and to treat conditions such as headaches, injury to the eyes, and pain after tooth extraction.

Chemical Cold Pack
Chemical cold packs are available in a variety of sizes and shapes. When activated, they provide a specific degree of coldness for a specific period of time (usually 30 to 60 minutes), as indicated on the package label. Most cold packs consist of a vinyl bag of ammonium nitrate crystals. Enclosed in this bag is a smaller vinyl bag of water. The cold pack is activated by applying pressure until the inner bag ruptures. This releases the water into the larger bag, and a chemical reaction occurs between the crystals and water, producing coldness. These packs are disposable, and when the coldness diminishes, they should be discarded in an appropriate receptacle. Chemical cold packs should be stored at room temperature. They are used as an alternative to ice bags for the local application of cold to prevent swelling, control bleeding, and relieve pain and inflammation.

Procedures 7-4, 7-5, and 7-6 present proper application of cold with an ice bag, a cold compress, and a chemical cold pack.

Text continued on p. 243

PROCEDURE **7-1**   Applying a Heating Pad

Outcome   Apply a heating pad.

Equipment/Supplies

• Heating pad with a protective covering

1. **Procedural Step.** Sanitize your hands.
2. **Procedural Step.** Assemble the equipment.
3. **Procedural Step.** Greet the patient and introduce yourself. Identify the patient and explain the procedure. Explain the purpose of the application (e.g., to relieve pain).
4. **Procedural Step.** Place the heating pad in the protective covering.
   Principle. The protective covering provides more comfort for the patient and absorbs perspiration.

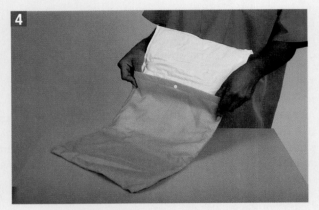

Place the heating pad in a protective covering.

5. **Procedural Step.** Connect the plug to an electric outlet. Set the selector switch at the proper setting, as designated by the physician (usually low or medium).
6. **Procedural Step.** Place the heating pad on the patient's affected body area. Ask the patient how the temperature feels. The heating pad should feel warm but not uncomfortable.

7. **Procedural Step.** Instruct the patient not to lie on the pad or turn the control higher to prevent burns.
   Principle. Lying on the pad causes heat to accumulate and burn the patient. The patient's heat receptors eventually become adjusted to the temperature change, resulting in a decreased heat sensation, and the patient may be tempted to increase the temperature. Turning the control higher results in excessive heat on the patient's skin, which could burn the patient.
8. **Procedural Step.** Check the patient periodically for signs of an increase or decrease in redness or swelling, and ask the patient whether the site is painful. Administer the treatment for the proper length of time as designated by the physician.
9. **Procedural Step.** Sanitize your hands, and chart the procedure. Include the date and time, method of heat application (heating pad), temperature setting of the pad, location and duration of the application, appearance of the application site, and patient's reaction. Also, chart any instructions provided to the patient on applying a heating pad at home.
10. **Procedural Step.** Properly care for equipment, and return it to its storage location.

CHARTING EXAMPLE

Date	
12/10/08	10:15 a.m. Heating pad on medium setting applied to lower back x 20 min. Area appears pink following application. Pt states a relief of pain and better mobility. Provided instructions on the application of a heating pad at home. —————— M. Cooper, CMA

PROCEDURE **7-2**   Applying a Hot Soak

Outcome   Apply a hot soak.

Equipment/Supplies

• Soaking solution ordered by the physician
• Bath thermometer
• Basin
• Bath towels

1. **Procedural Step.** Sanitize your hands.
2. **Procedural Step.** Assemble the equipment. Check the label on the solution container to make sure you have the correct solution as ordered by the physician. Place the solution containers in a basin of warm water. Warm the soaking solution to a temperature between 105°F to 110°F (41°C to 44°C).

3. **Procedural Step.** Greet the patient and introduce yourself. Identify the patient and explain the procedure. Explain the purpose of the application (e.g., to apply a medicated solution).

4. **Procedural Step.** Fill the basin one-third to two-thirds full with the warmed soaking solution.

5. **Procedural Step.** Check the temperature of the solution with a bath thermometer. The temperature for an adult should be 105°F to 110°F (41°C to 44°C).

6. **Procedural Step.** Assist the patient into a comfortable position to avoid fatigue and muscle strain. Pad the side of the basin with a towel for the patient's comfort.

7. **Procedural Step.** Slowly and gradually immerse the patient's affected body part in the solution. Ask the patient how the temperature feels.
Principle. The affected body part should become accustomed to the change in temperature gradually.

8. **Procedural Step.** Test the temperature of the solution frequently. To keep the solution at a constant tem-

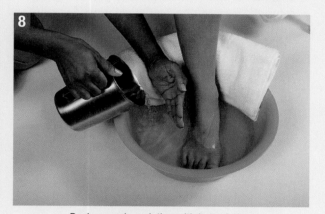

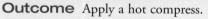
Replace cooler solution with hot solution.

perature, remove cooler fluid every 5 minutes, and replace it with hot solution. Pour the hot solution in near the edge of the basin by placing your hand between the patient and the solution. Stir the solution as you pour.
Principle. The solution should be added away from the patient's body part to prevent splashing hot fluid on the patient. Stirring in the solution helps distribute the heat and keep the temperature constant.

9. **Procedural Step.** Check the patient's skin periodically for signs of an increase or decrease in redness or swelling, and ask the patient whether the site is painful. Apply the hot soak for the proper length of time as designated by the physician (usually 15 to 20 minutes).

10. **Procedural Step.** Dry the affected part completely and gently.

11. **Procedural Step.** Sanitize your hands, and chart the procedure. Include the date and time, method of heat application (hot soak), name and strength of the solution, temperature of the soak, location and duration of the application, appearance of the application site, and patient's reaction.

12. **Procedural Step.** Properly care for equipment, and return it to its storage location.

PROCEDURE 7-2

CHARTING EXAMPLE	
Date	
12/12/08	1:15 p.m. Normal saline hot soak @ 105° F
	applied to Ⓡ ankle x 20 min. Area appears
	pink following application. Pt states less
	stiffness in ankle. ———— M. Cooper, CMA

PROCEDURE 7-3   Applying a Hot Compress

Outcome Apply a hot compress.

Equipment/Supplies

- Solution ordered by the physician
- Bath thermometer
- Basin
- Washcloths
- Waterproof covering
- Towel

1. **Procedural Step.** Sanitize your hands.
2. **Procedural Step.** Assemble the equipment. Check the label on the solution container to make sure you have the correct solution as ordered by the physician. Place the solution containers in a basin of warm water. Warm the soaking solution to a temperature between 105°F to 110°F (41°C to 44°C).

3. **Procedural Step.** Greet the patient and introduce yourself. Identify the patient and explain the procedure. Explain the purpose of the application (e.g., to soften an exudate).
4. **Procedural Step.** Fill the basin half full with warmed solution. Check the temperature of the solution with the bath thermometer. The temperature for an adult should be 105°F to 110°F (41°C to 44°C).

Continued

PROCEDURE 7-3   Applying a Hot Compress—cont'd

5. Procedural Step. Completely immerse the compress in the solution. Wring the compress to remove excess moisture. The compress should be wet but not dripping. Apply it lightly at first to the affected site to allow the patient to become used to the heat gradually. You may want to cover the compress with a waterproof cover to help hold in the heat. Ask the patient how the temperature feels. The compress should be as hot as the patient can comfortably tolerate.
Principle. The waterproof cover prevents cool air currents from coming into contact with the compress and reduces the number of times the compress needs to be changed.

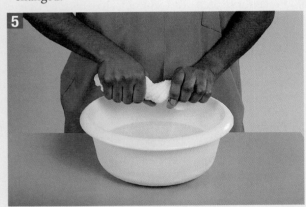

Wring out the compress.

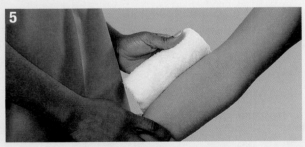

Apply the compress to the affected site.

6. Procedural Step. Place additional compresses in the solution so that they are ready for use.
7. Procedural Step. Repeat the application of the compress every 2 to 3 minutes for the duration of time specified by the physician (usually 15 to 20 minutes). Check the patient's skin periodically for signs of an increase or decrease in redness or swelling, and ask the patient whether the site is painful.
8. Procedural Step. Check the temperature of the solution periodically. Remove cooler fluid and replace it with hot solution if needed. Administer the treatment for the proper length of time as designated by the physician.
9. Procedural Step. Dry the affected part thoroughly and gently.
10. Procedural Step. Sanitize your hands, and chart the procedure. Include the date and time, method of heat application (hot compress), name and strength of the solution, temperature of the solution, location and duration of the application, appearance of the application site, and patient's reaction.
11. Procedural Step. Properly care for equipment, and return it to its storage location.

CHARTING EXAMPLE	
Date	
12/20/08	10:30 a.m. Normal saline hot compress @ 110° F applied to Ⓡ forearm x 20 min. No complaints of discomfort. — M. Cooper, CMA

PROCEDURE 7-4   Applying an Ice Bag

Outcome Apply an ice bag.

Equipment/Supplies

- Ice bag with a protective covering
- Small pieces of ice (ice chips or crushed ice)

1. Procedural Step. Sanitize your hands.
2. Procedural Step. Assemble the equipment.
3. Procedural Step. Greet the patient and introduce yourself. Identify the patient and explain the procedure.

Explain the purpose of applying the ice bag (e.g., to prevent swelling).
4. Procedural Step. Check the ice bag for leakage.

Principle. A leaking bag would get the patient wet and cause chilling.

5. **Procedural Step.** Fill the bag one half to two thirds full with small pieces of ice.
   Principle. Small pieces of ice work better than large pieces because they reduce the air spaces in the bag, resulting in better conduction of cold. In addition, small pieces of ice allow the bag to mold better to the body area.

6. **Procedural Step.** Expel air from the bag by squeezing the empty top half of the bag together and screwing on the stopper.
   Principle. Air is a poor conductor of cold and makes it difficult to mold the ice bag to the body area.

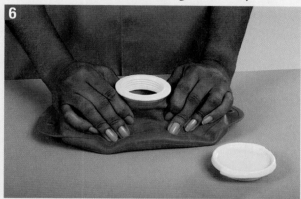

Expel air from the bag.

7. **Procedural Step.** Place the bag in the protective covering.
   Principle. The protective covering provides for patient comfort and absorbs the moisture that condenses on the outside of the bag.

8. **Procedural Step.** Place the bag on the patient's affected body area. Ask the patient how the temperature feels. The application of ice is usually uncomfortable, but most patients tolerate it when they know how much benefit may be derived from it.

Principle. Individuals vary in their ability to tolerate cold.

9. **Procedural Step.** Check the patient's skin periodically for signs of an increase or decrease in redness or swelling, and ask the patient whether the site is painful. If extreme paleness and numbness or a mottled blue appearance occurs at the application site, remove the bag, and notify the physician.

10. **Procedural Step.** Refill the bag with ice as necessary, and change the protective covering if needed. Administer the treatment for the proper length of time, as designated by the physician (usually until the area feels numb, approximately 15 to 30 minutes).

11. **Procedural Step.** Sanitize your hands, and chart the procedure. Include the date and time, method of cold application (ice bag), location and duration of the application, appearance of the application site, and patient's reaction. Also, chart any instructions provided to the patient on applying an ice bag at home.

12. **Procedural Step.** Properly care for the ice bag. Dispose of or launder the protective covering as required. Cleanse the ice bag with a warm detergent solution, rinse thoroughly, and dry by hanging the bag upside down with the top removed. Store the bag by screwing on the stopper, leaving air inside to prevent the sides from sticking together.

CHARTING EXAMPLE

Date	
12/22/08	11:30 a.m. Ice bag applied to ⓡ knee x 20 min. Pt complained of slight discomfort during the application. Area appears less swollen following application. Provided instructions on the application of an ice bag at home. ——————— M. Cooper, CMA

PROCEDURE 7-5   Applying a Cold Compress

Outcome Apply a cold compress.

Equipment/Supplies

- Ice cubes
- Basin
- Washcloths

- Towel
- Ice bag

---

1. **Procedural Step.** Sanitize your hands.
2. **Procedural Step.** Assemble the equipment. Check the label on the solution container to make sure you have the correct solution as ordered by the physician.

3. **Procedural Step.** Greet the patient and introduce yourself. Identify the patient and explain the procedure. Explain the purpose of the application (e.g., to treat an eye injury).

Continued

PROCEDURE 7-5   **Applying a Cold Compress—cont'd**

4. Procedural Step. Place large ice cubes in the basin. Add the solution until the basin is half full.

Principle. Using larger pieces of ice prevents them from sticking to the compress and slows the rate at which they melt in the solution.

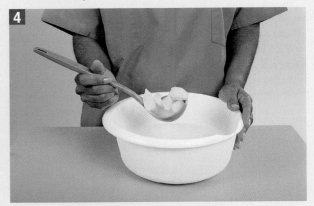

Place large ice cubes in the basin.

5. Procedural Step. Completely immerse the compress in the solution. Wring the compress to rid it of excess moisture. The compress should be wet but not dripping. Apply it lightly at first to the affected site to allow the patient to become used to the cold gradually. The compress can be covered with an ice bag to help keep it cold and to reduce the number of times it needs to be changed. Ask the patient how the temperature feels.

6. Procedural Step. Place additional compresses in the solution to be ready for use.

7. Procedural Step. Repeat the application of the compress every 2 to 3 minutes for the duration of time specified by the physician (usually 15 to 20 minutes). Check the patient's skin periodically for signs of an increase or decrease in redness or swelling, and ask the patient whether the site is painful.

8. Procedural Step. Add ice if needed to keep the solution cold. Administer the treatment for the proper length of time designated by the physician.

9. Procedural Step. Thoroughly dry the affected part.

10. Procedural Step. Sanitize your hands, and chart the procedure. Include the date and time, method of cold application (cold compress), location and duration of the application, appearance of the application site, and patient's reaction.

11. Procedural Step. Properly care for equipment, and return it to its storage location.

CHARTING EXAMPLE	
Date	
12/27/08	9:15 a.m. Normal saline cold compress
	applied to bridge of nose x 15 min. Nose
	appears less swollen following application.
	Tolerated application well. — M. Cooper, CMA

see DVD

PROCEDURE 7-6   **Applying a Chemical Pack**

Outcome Apply a chemical cold pack and a chemical hot pack.

The procedure for applying a chemical cold or hot pack is as follows:

1. Procedural Step. Shake the crystals to the bottom of the bag.

2. Procedural Step. Squeeze the bag firmly with your hands to break the inner water bag.

3. Procedural Step. Shake the bag vigorously to mix the contents.

4. Procedural Step. Cover the bag with a protective covering.

5. Procedural Step. Apply the bag to the affected area. Check the patient's skin periodically.

6. Procedural Step. Administer the treatment for the proper length of time.

7. Procedural Step. Discard the bag in an appropriate receptacle.

8. Procedural Step. Sanitize your hands and chart the procedure. Include the date and time, method of applica-

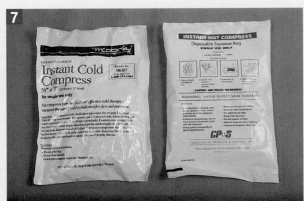

Chemical packs.

tion (chemical cold or hot pack), location and duration of the application, appearance of the application site, and the patient's reaction.

THERAPEUTIC ULTRASOUND

Therapeutic ultrasound uses high-frequency sound waves as a penetrating, deep-heating agent for the soft tissues of the body, such as tendons and muscles. Many physicians use ultrasound in the medical office for the local application of heat to treat musculoskeletal disorders.

The beneficial physiologic effects of ultrasound result primarily from the deep heat produced in the tissues and include reduction of edema, breakup of exudates, increased cellular metabolism, relief of pain, and micromassage. The physician may order ultrasound to treat musculoskeletal conditions, including sprains, joint contractures, neuritis, arthritis, edema, synovitis, scar tissue, bursitis, fibrositis, strains, and dislocations. Therapeutic ultrasound must not be used over the eyeball, over malignant tumors, directly over the spinal cord, over the heart or brain, over reproductive organs including a pregnant uterus, or over areas of impaired sensation or inadequate circulation. The medical assistant is responsible for performing the ultrasound treatment, which includes preparing the patient, operating the machine, and administering the treatment.

Parts of the Ultrasound Machine

The ultrasound machine consists of two main parts: the generator and the transducer. The *generator* is located in the main unit of the machine, which also contains the controls to operate the machine. The *transducer* is a crystal inserted between two electrodes; it is located in a device called the *applicator head* or *sound head*. The applicator

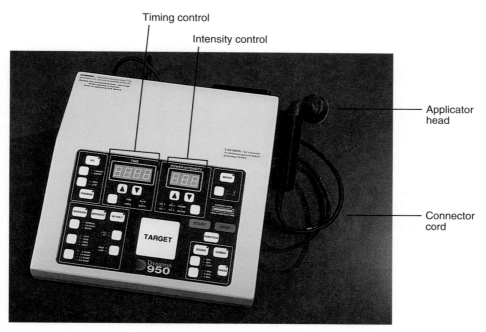

Figure 7-2. The parts of an ultrasound machine.

PATIENT TEACHING **Low Back Pain**

Answer questions patients have about low back pain.

What causes low back pain?
Low back pain is one of the most common health problems in the United States. Approximately 80% of Americans are affected by low back pain at some time during their life. The most frequent cause of low back pain is poor posture and poor body mechanics, which strain the muscles and ligaments that support the back. Other causes include physical inactivity, excessive body weight, disc damage, osteoarthritis, and congenital deformities.

How might the physician treat low back pain?
To treat low back pain caused by strain, the physician might prescribe bed rest, local application of heat or cold, massage, medications, back manipulation, use of back-supporting devices, deep-heating treatments such as ultrasound, and exercises to strengthen the supporting structures of the back and prevent the back pain from recurring or becoming chronic.

What can be done to prevent low back pain?
Most cases of low back pain can be prevented by practicing good posture and body mechanics.
- Encourage patients to follow practices that prevent strain to the lower back.
- Teach the patient the procedure for the local application of heat or cold as prescribed by the physician.
- Provide the patient with a sheet that describes and illustrates the correct way to perform back exercises prescribed by the physician.
- Provide the patient with educational materials on low back pain. ■

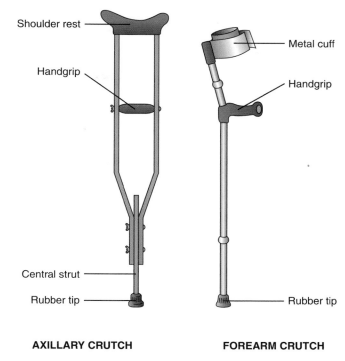

Figure 7-12. Types of crutches.

orthopedic surgery. It also may be prescribed for a long-term condition, such as paralysis, deformity, and permanent weakness of the lower extremities.

Crutches

Crutches are artificial supports that consist of wood or tubular aluminum. They are used for patients who require assistance in walking as a result of disease, injury, or birth defects of the lower extremities. Crutches function by removing weight from the legs and transferring it to the arms. The two main crutch types are the axillary crutch and the forearm crutch (Figure 7-12). The axillary and the forearm crutch require rubber tips, which increase the surface tension to prevent the crutches from slipping on the floor.

The *axillary crutch* is used most frequently and is made of wood or tubular aluminum. This type of crutch has a shoulder rest and handgrips and extends from the ground almost to the patient's axilla.

The *forearm crutch,* also known as a *Lofstrand crutch,* consists of a single adjustable tube of aluminum that extends to the forearm. A metal cuff attached to the crutch fits securely around the patient's forearm, and a handgrip covered with rubber extends from the crutch for weight bearing. The metal cuff and the handgrip stabilize the patient's wrists to make walking safer and easier. One advantage of the forearm crutch is that the individual can release the handgrip, enabling use of the hand, while the metal cuff holds the crutch in place. Individuals who are paraplegic or have cerebral palsy use the forearm crutch most often.

Axillary Crutch Measurement

The patient must be measured for axillary crutches to ensure the correct crutch length and the proper placement of the handgrip. Incorrectly fitted crutches increase the patient's risk of developing back pain, nerve damage, and injuries to the axillae and palms of the hands. Procedure 7-8 presents the correct way to measure a patient for axillary crutches.

If the crutches are too long, the shoulder rests exert pressure on the patient's axillae. This can injure the radial nerve in the brachial plexus, which eventually may lead to *crutch palsy,* a condition of muscular weakness in the forearm, wrist, and hand. In addition, crutches that are too long force the patient's shoulders forward, preventing the patient from pushing his or her body off the ground. Crutches that are too short force the patient to be bent over and uncomfortable, also making them awkward to use. If the handgrips are too low, pressure is put on the patient's axillae, whereas handgrips that are too high are awkward.

Wooden crutches are made with bolts and wing nuts, which allow proper adjustment of the length and handgrip level. Aluminum crutches consist of aluminum tubes. Spring-loaded pushbuttons on an inner tube "pop out" into holes on an outer tube to allow proper adjustment of the crutch length.

Crutch Guidelines

It is important that the patient receive specific guidelines to ensure safety while using crutches, to prevent injuries and falls. The medical assistant is responsible for instructing the patient in the following guidelines:

1. Wear well-fitting flat shoes with firm, nonskid soles to provide good traction and stability.
2. Use correct posture to prevent strain on muscles and joints and to maintain proper body balance.
3. Support your weight with your hands on the handgrips and the axillary pads pressing against the sides of the rib cage. The body weight should not be supported by the axillae because pressure on the axillae may cause crutch palsy.
4. Look ahead when walking, rather than down at your feet.
5. Be aware of the surface on which you are walking. It should be clean, flat, dry, and well lighted. Throw rugs and objects serving as obstacles should temporarily be removed from your environment to prevent falls.
6. Keep the crutches about 4 to 6 inches out from the side of your feet when walking to prevent obstruction of the pathway for the feet.
7. Take steps by moving the crutches forward a safe and comfortable distance, preferably 6 inches. When first learning to use the crutches, take small steps rather than large ones. Do not move forward more than 12 to 15 inches with each step. A greater distance might cause the crutches to slide forward and you to lose your balance.
8. Report tingling or numbness in the upper body to the physician. You might be using the crutches incorrectly, or they might be the wrong size for you.
9. Extra padding can be added to the shoulder rests of your crutches to make them more comfortable. If you do this, ensure that the extra padding does not press against your axillae, but rather against your lateral rib cage. The handgrips also can be padded for increased comfort.

10. To prevent slipping, keep the crutch tips dry to maintain their surface friction. If they become wet, dry them completely before use.
11. Inspect the crutch tips regularly. They should be securely attached. If the crutch tips are worn down, they should be replaced with tips of the proper size.
12. For wooden crutches, periodically check the wing nuts holding the central strut and handgrips in place to ensure that they are tight.

Crutch Gaits

The type of crutch gait used depends on the amount of weight the patient is able to support with one or both legs and the patient's physical condition and muscular coordination. The patient should learn a fast and a slow gait. The faster gait is used for making speed in open areas, and the slower one is used in crowded places. In addition, learning more than one gait reduces patient fatigue because a different combination of muscles is used for each gait. Procedure 7-9 provides guidelines and charts for use in instructing the patient on how to walk with crutches.

Canes

A cane is a lightweight, easily movable device made of wood or aluminum with a rubber tip and is used to help provide balance and support. Canes are generally used by patients who have weakness on one side of the body, such as patients with hemiparesis, joint disabilities, or defects of the neuromuscular system. The three main types of canes are the *standard cane,* the *tripod cane,* and the *quad cane* (Figure 7-13). The standard cane provides the least amount of support and is used by patients who require only slight assistance in walking. The tripod and quad canes have three and four legs, respectively, a bent shaft, and a T-shaped handle with grips. They are easier to hold and provide greater stability than a standard cane because of the wider base of support. In addi-

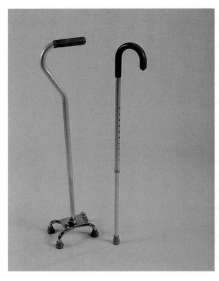

Figure 7-13. Examples of a quad cane *(left)* and a standard cane *(right).* (Courtesy 3M Health Care, St. Paul, Minn.)

tion, multilegged canes are able to stand alone, which frees the arms when the patient is getting up from a chair. The disadvantage of a multilegged cane is that it is bulkier and more difficult to move.

A cane is held on the side of the body that is opposite to the side that needs support. The cane length must be properly adjusted to ensure optimal stability. The cane handle should be approximately level with the greater trochanter, and the elbow should be flexed at a 25- to 30-degree angle. The patient should be instructed to stand erect and not lean on the cane to ensure good balance. Procedure 7-10 presents guidelines on instructing the patient on how to walk with a cane.

Walkers

A walker is an ambulatory aid consisting of an aluminum frame with handgrips and four widely placed legs with rubber suction tips and one open side (Figure 7-14). A walker is light and easily movable. Walkers are available with wheels that facilitate movement of the walker. They are also available with a fold-up feature that allows them to be easily transported in a vehicle. For proper ambulation, the walker should extend from the ground to approximately the level of the patient's hip joint. Procedure 7-11 presents guidelines on instructing the patient on how to walk with a walker.

Walkers are used most often by geriatric patients with weakness or balance problems. Walkers also are used during the healing process for patients who have had knee or hip joint replacement surgery. These patients need more help with balance and walking than can be provided by crutches or a cane. Because of its wide base, a walker provides the patient with a great amount of stability and security. Disadvantages of a walker include a slow pace and difficulty in maneuvering the walker in a small room.

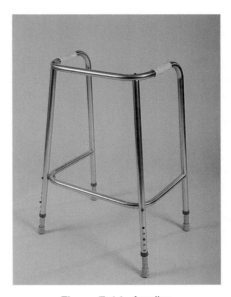

Figure 7-14. A walker.

What Would You Do? What Would You *Not* Do?

Case Study 3

Thaddeus Bernard calls the office. Thaddeus fractured the femur of his left leg in a skiing accident 2 weeks ago. The physician applied a long leg fiberglass cast, and Thaddeus was properly fitted with aluminum crutches. Thaddeus says that he is having some problems with his crutches. He is complaining of weakness in his forearms and hands and some tingling and numbness in his fingers. He also says that he has bruises under his arms. Thaddeus says that after he got home, his crutches didn't seem to fit right, so he readjusted them. Thaddeus is getting ready to return to college and wants to know the best way to carry his books while using crutches. ■

PROCEDURE 7-8 Measuring for Axillary Crutches

Outcome Measure an individual for axillary crutches.

Determining Crutch Length

For you to determine crutch length correctly, the patient must wear shoes while being measured. The measurement can be taken while the patient is standing.

1. **Procedural Step.** Ask the patient to stand erect.
2. **Procedural Step.** Position the crutches with the crutch tips at a distance of 2 inches (5 cm) in front of and 4 to 6 inches (15 cm) to the side of each foot. (The large dots in the figure represent crutch tips.)
3. **Procedural Step.** Adjust the crutch length so that the shoulder rests are approximately 1½ to 2 inches (about 2 finger-widths) below the axilla.

Wooden Crutches. The length of the crutch is adjusted by removing the bolt and wing nut and sliding the central strut (support piece) at the bottom upward or downward as necessary to attain the proper length. The strut is secured by replacing the bolt and securely fastening the wing nut.

Tubular Aluminum Crutches. The length of the crutch is adjusted by pressing the spring-loaded push-

Continued

PROCEDURE 7-8 Measuring for Axillary Crutches—cont'd

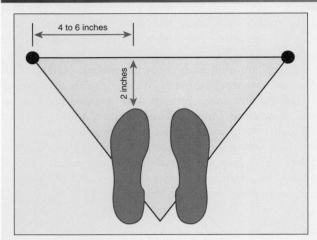

Position for measuring for crutches.

button with your thumb and sliding the outer tube upward or downward as necessary to attain the proper length. The spring-loaded button on the inner tube should be allowed to "pop out" into the appropriate hole on the outer tube.

Handgrip Positioning

When the crutch length has been adjusted, the correct placement of the handgrips must be determined.

1. **Procedural Step.** Ask the patient to stand erect with a crutch under each arm and to support his or her weight by the handgrips.
2. **Procedural Step.** Adjust the handgrips on the crutches so that the patient's elbow is flexed to an angle of ap-

proximately 30 degrees. The handgrip level is adjusted by removing the bolt and wing nut and sliding the handgrip upward or downward, as required. The handgrip is secured by replacing the bolt and tightly fastening the wing nut. The angle of elbow flexion can be verified using a measuring device known as a *goniometer*. A *goniometer* is an instrument that measures the angle of a joint.

3. **Procedural Step.** Check the fit of the crutches. If the crutches are measured correctly, the medical assistant should be able to insert two fingers between the top of the crutch and the axilla when the patient is standing erect with the crutches under the arms.

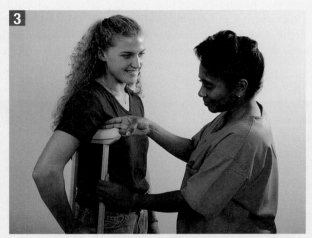

Insert two fingers between the top of the crutch and the axilla.

PROCEDURE **7-9**   Instructing a Patient in Crutch Gaits

Outcome Instruct a patient in the following crutch gaits: four-point, two-point, three-point, swing-to, and swing-through.

Tripod Position

The tripod position is the basic crutch stance used before crutch walking. It provides a wide base of support and enhances stability and balance.

Instruct the patient in the tripod position as follows:

1. **Procedural Step.** Stand erect, and face straight ahead.
2. **Procedural Step.** Place the tips of the crutches 4 to 6 inches (15 cm) in front of the feet and 4 to 6 inches (10 to 15 cm) to the side of each foot. (The large dots in the figure represent crutch tips.)

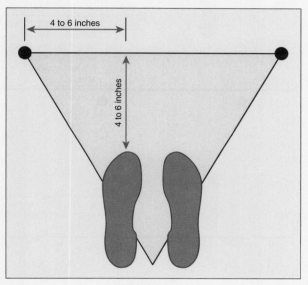

Tripod position.

Four-Point Gait

The four-point gait is a basic and slow gait. To use this gait, the patient must be able to bear considerable weight on both legs. The four-point gait is the most stable and safest of the crutch gaits because it provides at least three points of support at all times. It is used most often by patients who have leg muscle weakness or spasticity, poor muscular coordination or balance, or degenerative leg joint disease. Instruct the patient in the procedure for the four-point gait following the steps in the accompanying figure.

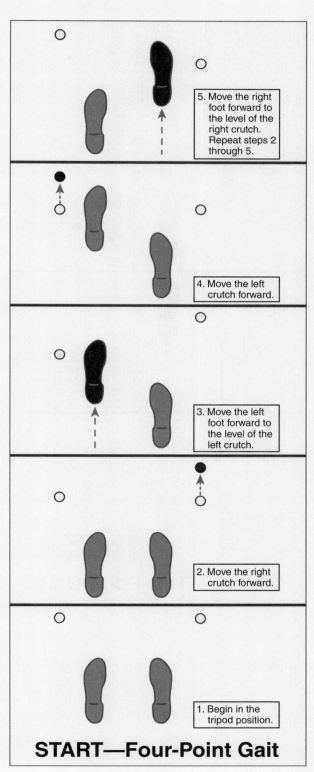

5. Move the right foot forward to the level of the right crutch. Repeat steps 2 through 5.

4. Move the left crutch forward.

3. Move the left foot forward to the level of the left crutch.

2. Move the right crutch forward.

1. Begin in the tripod position.

START—Four-Point Gait

Continued

PROCEDURE 7-9

PROCEDURE **7-9** Instructing a Patient in Crutch Gaits—cont'd

Two-Point Gait

The two-point gait is similar to, but faster than, the four-point gait. This gait requires more balance because only two points support the body at one time. The two-point gait is used when the patient is capable of partial weight bearing on each foot and has good muscular coordination. Instruct the patient in the procedure for the two-point gait following the steps in the accompanying figure.

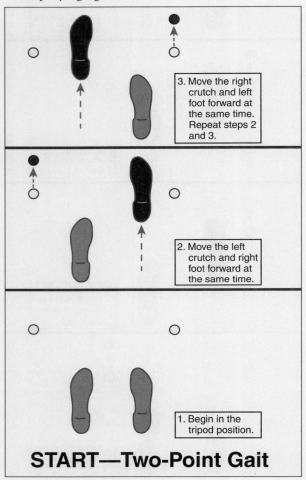

3. Move the right crutch and left foot forward at the same time. Repeat steps 2 and 3.

2. Move the left crutch and right foot forward at the same time.

1. Begin in the tripod position.

START—Two-Point Gait

Three-Point Gait

The three-point gait is used by patients who cannot bear weight on one leg. The patient must be able to support his or her full weight on the unaffected leg. With this gait, the crutches and the unaffected leg alternately bear the patient's weight. This gait is used most often by amputees without a prosthesis, patients with musculoskeletal or soft tissue trauma to a lower extremity (e.g., fracture, sprain), patients with acute leg

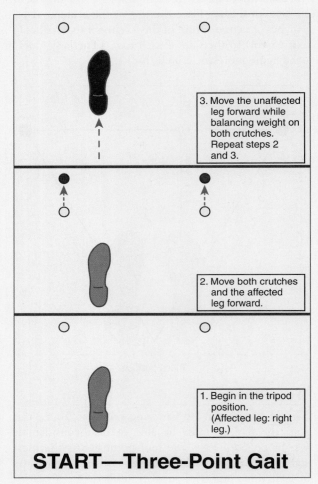

3. Move the unaffected leg forward while balancing weight on both crutches. Repeat steps 2 and 3.

2. Move both crutches and the affected leg forward.

1. Begin in the tripod position. (Affected leg: right leg.)

START—Three-Point Gait

PROCEDURE 7-9

inflammation, and patients who have had recent leg surgery. To use this gait, the patient must have good muscular coordination and arm strength. Instruct the patient in the procedure for the three-point gait, following the steps in the accompanying figure.

Swing Gaits

The swing gaits include the swing-to gait and the swing-through gait and are used by patients with severe lower extremity disabilities, such as paralysis, and by patients who wear supporting braces on their legs.

Instruct the patient in the procedure for the swing-to and the swing-through crutch gaits, following the steps in the accompanying figures.

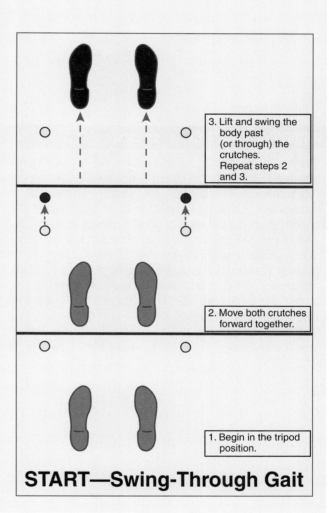

3. Lift and swing the body to the crutches. Repeat steps 2 and 3.

2. Move both crutches forward together.

1. Begin in the tripod position.

START—Swing-To Gait

3. Lift and swing the body past (or through) the crutches. Repeat steps 2 and 3.

2. Move both crutches forward together.

1. Begin in the tripod position.

START—Swing-Through Gait

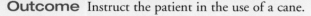

PROCEDURE **7-10**　Instructing a Patient in Use of a Cane

Outcome Instruct the patient in the use of a cane.

1. **Procedural Step.** Hold the cane on the strong side of the body (i.e., in the hand opposite the affected extremity).
2. **Procedural Step.** Place the tip of the cane 4 to 6 inches to the side of the foot.
3. **Procedural Step.** Move the cane forward approximately 12 inches (1 foot).
4. **Procedural Step.** Move the affected leg forward to the level of the cane.

5. **Procedural Step.** Move the strong leg forward and ahead of the cane and weak leg.
6. **Procedural Step.** Repeat steps 3 through 5.

Note: The cane and the affected leg can be moved forward simultaneously (steps 3 and 4); however, the patient has less support with this method.

PROCEDURE 7-11   Instructing a Patient in Use of a Walker

Outcome Instruct the patient in the use of a walker.

1. **Procedural Step.** Pick up the walker, and move it forward approximately 6 inches.
2. **Procedural Step.** Move the right foot and then the left foot up to the walker.

3. **Procedural Step.** Repeat steps 1 and 2.

*Check out the **Companion CD** bound with the book to access additional interactive activities.*

MEDICAL PRACTICE *and the* **LAW**

The procedures described in this chapter deal with the goal of returning full function to an injured area. Sometimes, despite correct treatment, full function does not return. This problem can become a legal issue if the patient believes he or she should have healed fully or cannot return to work. To protect yourself, follow each procedure to the letter, and record the patient's progress (or lack of progress) carefully in the medical record. Sometimes the patient is involved in insurance fraud and falsely complains of pain or impaired function to continue receiving disability benefits. If you suspect this is the case, objectively document the functions you have seen the patient perform.

The application of heat and cold must be performed precisely to maximize effectiveness of the treatment without injury to the patient. Failure to follow procedures correctly or to obtain the correct temperature could leave you legally liable.

The ultrasound machine, if used incorrectly, can burn the patient. To protect yourself and benefit the patient, keep the applicator head moving at all times, and keep adequate coupling agent on the skin at all times.

Ambulatory aids used correctly can help the patient regain mobility. If crutches are used improperly, the patient could fall or develop nerve or other injuries. When instructing about ambulation aid use, allow enough time for the patient to give a return demonstration, and send home written instructions in case the patient forgets what was taught. ■

What Would You Do? What Would You *Not* Do? RESPONSES

Case Study 1
Page 237
What Did Marlyne Do?
- ❑ Empathized with Aaron for being in so much pain.
- ❑ Explained to Aaron that he should never sleep on a heating pad because the heat builds up and causes the type of burn he experienced.
- ❑ Explained to Aaron that it is best to apply heat for 15 to 30 minutes at a time with the pad set no higher than the medium setting. Told him the pad may not feel warm after his body gets used to it, but that it is still helping him. Told Aaron that the high setting could burn his skin.
- ❑ Told Aaron how to prevent low back pain by using good body mechanics, especially during lifting.

What Did Marlyne Not *Do?*
- ❑ Did not critcize Aaron for sleeping on the heating pad or turning the pad to the high setting.

What Would You Do?/What Would You *Not* Do? Review Marlyne's response and place a checkmark next to the information you included in your response. List the additional information you included in your response.

_____
_____
_____
_____

Case Study 2
Page 251
What Did Marlyne Do?
- ❑ Reassured Christina that the medical staff are there to help her, and she should never hesitate to call when she needs information or is having a problem.
- ❑ Asked Christina what she did to try to make her arm feel better, and recorded this information in her chart. Checked with the physician to determine whether he wanted to see Christina.
- ❑ Reeducated Christina in proper cast care instructions over the phone and mailed her another cast care instruction sheet.
- ❑ Explained to Christina how to dry her cast properly by first blotting it and then using a hair dryer. Told her that if she is unable to dry her cast completely, she will need to come in to have it replaced.
- ❑ Explained to Christina that the physician applied the type of cast that would best treat her injury and help her to heal.

What Did Marlyne Not *Do?*
- ❑ Did not criticize Christina for waiting so long to call the office.
- ❑ Did not tell Christina it would be a good idea for her to have a "removable cast."

What Would You Do/What Would You *Not* Do? Review Marlyne's response and place a checkmark next to the information you included in your response. List the additional information you included in your response.

_____
_____
_____
_____

Case Study 3
Page 255
What Did Marlyne Do?
- ❑ Listened carefully and emphathetically to Thaddeus' problems and concerns with his crutches.
- ❑ Explained to Thaddeus that the crutches were adjusted to fit him properly at the office and that he may have caused some problems by readjusting them.
- ❑ Scheduled an appointment for Thaddeus to come in that day so the physician can examine him and his crutches can be checked for proper length.
- ❑ Went over crutch guidelines and crutch gaits with Thaddeus again when he came to the office for his appointment.
- ❑ Told Thaddeus that he should use a backpack to carry his books to keep his hands free to move on his crutches. Stressed that he should keep his backpack as light as possible and keep the weight evenly distributed on his back (i.e., use both straps).

What Did Marlyne Not *Do?*
- ❑ Did not tell Thaddeus to readjust the crutches himself.
- ❑ Did not tell Thaddeus that he should have paid more attention when he was being instructed in crutch guidelines.

What Would You Do/What Would You *Not* Do? Review Marlyne's response and place a checkmark next to the information you included in your response. List the additional information you included in your response.

_____
_____
_____
_____

APPLY YOUR KNOWLEDGE

Choose the best answer to each of the following questions.

1. Savannah Uriz recently played in a golf tournament; since then, she has been having low back pain. Dr. Walker recommended that she use a heating pad for 30 minutes every 2 hours for the next 3 days. Marlyne Cooper, CMA, is explaining the use of a heating pad to Savannah. Marlyne instructs Savannah to:
   A. Place a protective covering over the heating pad before using it.
   B. Place a wet towel between her back and the heating pad.
   C. Lie down flat with her back on the pad.
   D. Turn the setting higher if the pad no longer feels warm enough.

2. Brody Adams fell on the playground and has a large "goose egg" on his forehead. Dr. Walker directs Marlyne Cooper, CMA, to apply an ice bag. Marlyne uses small pieces of ice to fill the ice bag. The reason for this is:
   A. To prevent Brody's forehead from becoming too cold.
   B. So that the ice bag molds better to Brody's forehead.
   C. To prevent the goose egg from hatching.
   D. To prevent irritation to the affected skin.

3. Eunice Faye has osteoarthritis and for the past 3 days has been experiencing intense pain in the joints of the fingers of her right hand. Dr. Walker would be most likely to order which of the following ultrasound treatments for her condition?
   A. Prenatal ultrasound.
   B. Direct ultrasound.
   C. Underwater ultrasound.
   D. Hot wax ultrasound.

4. Michael Kasey broke his left wrist while playing football. He had a short arm fiberglass cast applied 3 hours after the accident. Marlyne Cooper, CMA, is instructing Michael on what to do to minimize swelling. Marlyne's explanation would include all of the following *except:*
   A. Elevate the cast above heart level for the first 24 to 48 hours.
   B. Cover the cast with a plastic bag.
   C. Apply an ice bag at the level of the injury.
   D. Gently move your fingers as often as possible.

5. Marlyne continues to instruct Michael on how to care for his cast. All of the following would be included in Marlyne's instructions *except:*
   A. Do not insert anything down into the cast.
   B. If the cast gets wet, dry it with a blow dryer on the high setting.
   C. Do not trim the cast or break off rough edges.
   D. Inspect the skin around the cast periodically.

6. Michael calls the office complaining of a problem with his cast. Which of the following would indicate that Michael should be seen immediately?
   A. His friends are unable to sign his cast with a ballpoint pen.
   B. He accidentally got his cast wet.
   C. There is a foul odor and drainage coming out of his cast.
   D. He decided he would rather have a purple cast instead of an orange one.

7. Katie Avery severely strained her left ankle. Dr. Walker asks Marlyne Cooper, CMA, to fit her for axillary crutches. If Katie's axillary crutches have been properly fitted:
   A. Her shoulders will be bent over the crutches.
   B. Two fingers can be inserted between the top of the crutch and her axilla.
   C. Her elbows will be flexed at a 45-degree angle.
   D. The axillary pads will fit snugly against her axillae.

8. Dr. Walker told Katie not to put weight on her left foot for the next 5 days. The most appropriate crutch gait for Katie to use would be the:
   A. Two-point gait.
   B. Three-point gait.
   C. Four-point gait.
   D. Swing-through gait.

9. Marlyne instructs Katie in the proper use of her crutches. Which of the following guidelines would be included in Marlyne's explanation?
   A. Support your body weight on your hands.
   B. Look straight ahead when walking.
   C. Keep the crutch tips dry.
   D. Report any tingling or numbness of the upper body.
   E. All of the above.

10. Marlyne fitted Katie's crutches correctly. When Katie gets home, she adjusts the crutches to a longer length. Katie is putting herself at risk for:
   A. Carpal tunnel syndrome.
   B. Sciatic nerve damage.
   C. Crutch palsy.
   D. Chickenpox.

❏ **The application of heat or cold** is used to treat pathologic conditions such as infection and trauma. Heat and cold are applied for short periods, usually ranging from 15 to 30 minutes. The type of heat or cold application depends on the purpose of the application, the location and condition of the affected area, and the age and general health of the patient.

❏ **The local effects of applying heat** to the body include dilation of the blood vessels in the area. Nutrients and oxygen are provided to the cells at a faster rate, and wastes are carried away faster. Erythema is redness of the skin caused by congestion of capillaries in the lower layers of the skin. Heat functions in relieving pain, congestion, muscle spasms, and inflammation.

❏ **The local application of cold** constricts the blood vessels. As a result, tissue metabolism decreases, less oxygen is used, and fewer wastes accumulate. The local application of cold is used to prevent edema and may be applied immediately after an individual has experienced direct trauma, such as a bruise, sprain, muscle strain, joint injury, or fracture.

❏ **Factors that affect the local application of heat and cold** include the age of the patient, the location of the application, impaired circulation and sensation, and individual tolerance to change in temperature.

❏ **Therapeutic ultrasound** uses high-frequency sound waves as a deep-heating agent for the soft tissues of the body. Ultrasound may be ordered to treat the following conditions: sprains, joint contractures, neuritis, arthritis, edema, synovitis, scar tissue, bursitis, fibrositis, strains, and dislocations. Ultrasound must not be used over the eyeball, over malignant tumors, directly over the spinal cord, over the heart or brain, over reproductive organs including a pregnant uterus, or over areas of impaired sensation or inadequate circulation.

❏ **A cast is a stiff cylindrical casing** that is used to immobilize a body part. Casts are applied most often when an individual sustains a fracture. Other uses of a cast are to support and stabilize weak or dislocated joints, to promote healing after a surgical correction, and to aid in the nonsurgical correction of deformities.

❏ **Casts are classified** according to the body part they cover. The types of cast most frequently applied are short arm cast, long arm cast, short leg cast, and long leg cast. The type of cast applied depends on the nature of the patient's injury or condition.

❏ **Splints and braces** are used to assist in the treatment of musculoskeletal injuries. A splint is a rigid removable device used to support and immobilize a displaced or fractured part of the body and to protect areas that are sprained or strained. A brace is designed to support a part of the body and hold it in its correct position to allow functioning of the body part while healing takes place.

❏ **Mechanical assistive devices** are used by individuals who require help to walk. Ambulatory aids include crutches, canes, and walkers. The device used depends on factors such as the type and severity of the disability, the amount of support required, and the patient's age and degree of muscular coordination.

❏ **Crutches are artificial supports** consisting of wood or tubular aluminum. They are used for patients who require assistance in walking as a result of disease, injury, or birth defects of the lower extremities. Crutches function by removing weight from the legs and transferring it to the arms.

❏ **The type of crutch gait** used depends on the amount of weight the patient is able to support with one or both legs, the patient's physical condition, and the patient's muscular coordination. Crutch gaits include the four-point gait, the two-point gait, the three-point gait, and the swing gaits.

❏ **A cane** is a lightweight, easily movable device used to provide balance and support. Canes are generally used by patients who have weakness on one side of the body.

❏ **A walker** is an ambulatory aid that is most often used by geriatric patients with weakness or balance problems.

pushed and rotated in a clockwise direction (Figure 8-4). In this way, a specimen from the ectocervix and the endocervix can be collected at the same time.

When the Pap specimen has been collected, the medical assistant is responsible for performing one of the following depending on the brand of liquid-based preparation being used:

1. Rinse the collection device in the vial of liquid preservative, and discard the collection device (performed with ThinPrep).
2. Remove the tip of the collection device, and deposit it in the vial of preservative. Discard the handle (performed with SurePath).

The preservative maintains the specimen and prevents it from drying out during transport to the laboratory. After being received by the laboratory, the vial is placed in an automated slide preparation processor. The automated processor performs several important functions. First, it separates the cells from debris present in the specimen, and then it disperses a representative cell sample onto a slide in a thin, uniform layer. The slide is next immersed in a fixative to maintain the normal appearance of the cells.

The ways in which the liquid-based method provides a better quality specimen than the direct smear method are as follows:

- With the direct smear method, only a small portion of the specimen is smeared on the slide; most of it is thrown away with the collection device. With the liquid-based method, the collection device is rinsed or the tip is deposited in a vial of liquid that preserves all or most of the specimen. Having more of the specimen available allows the laboratory to evaluate it better.
- When a Pap specimen is collected, it includes unnecessary debris, such as blood, mucus, and inflammatory cells. With the direct smear method, the debris is smeared on the slide along with the cells. This debris may obscure the cells in the

specimen, making it difficult to evaluate them. With the liquid-based method, the automated processor removes a large portion of the debris from the specimen and transfers the cells to a glass slide. This provides the cytotechnologist with a clear, unobstructed view of the epithelial cells.

- With the direct smear method, the cells have a tendency to clump together when they are smeared on the slide, making them more difficult to evaluate. With the liquid-based method, the automated processor disperses the cells onto the slide in a thin, even layer. In this way, the cells are spread out, making it easier for the cytotechnologist to evaluate them.

Cytology Request

A cytology request must accompany all Pap specimens. Figure 8-5 is an example of a cytology request form. The medical assistant is responsible for completing the request, which includes the following categories.

General Information

General information includes the physician's name, address, and phone number and the patient's name, address, identification number, date of birth, and date of last menstrual period (LMP). Insurance information also is required in this section for third-party billing.

Date and Time of Collection

The date and time of collection indicates to the laboratory the number of days that have passed since the collection, providing the laboratory with information regarding the freshness of the specimen.

Collection Method

Under the collection method category, the medical assistant must indicate whether the specimen is a direct smear (Pap smear) or a liquid-based preparation.

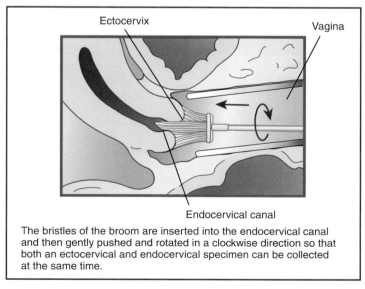

The bristles of the broom are inserted into the endocervical canal and then gently pushed and rotated in a clockwise direction so that both an ectocervical and endocervical specimen can be collected at the same time.

Figure 8-4. Collecting a Pap specimen using a broom.

GYN CYTOLOGY REQUISITION

THOMAS WOODSIDE, MD
501 MAIN ST
ST. LOUIS, MO 63146
(314) 555–0093

PATIENT INFO

Patient's Name (Last)	(First)	(MI)	Date of Birth	Collection Time	Collection Date	Patient's ID #
			MO	DAY	YR	: AM PM	MO	DAY	YR	

Patient's Address   Phone

City   State   ZIP

RESP. PARTY

Name of Responsible Party (if different from patient)

Address of Responsible Party   APT #

City   State   ZIP

INSURANCE

Patient's Relationship to Responsible Party   ☐ 1. Self   ☐ 2. Spouse   ☐ 3. Child   ☐ 4. Other

Insurance Comany Name	Plan	Carrier Code
Subscriber/Member #	Location	Group #
Insurance Address		Physician's Provider #
City	State	ZIP
Employer's Name or Number	Insured SSN	

Diagnosis/Signs/Symptoms in ICD-9 Format (Highest Specificity)

REQUIRED

ICD-9 codes are the internationally accepted method of describing the clinical picture of the patient. All diagnoses should be provided by the ordering physician or his or her authorized designee. The following is a partial list of of common diagnoses in ICD-9 format. Most third party payers require an ICD-9 code to indicate the medical necessity of the test(s) and or profile(s) ordered. For a complete list of all ICD-9 codes, please refer to a current ICD-9 manual.

V76.2 Routine Cervical Pap Smear	616.0 Cervicitis	626.8 Abnormal Bleeding
V15.89 High Risk Cervical Screening	616.10 Vaginitis	627.1 Postmenopausal Bleeding
V22.2 Pregnancy	617.0 Endometriosis, Uterus	627.3 Atrophic Vaginitis
079.4 Human Papillomavirus	622.1 Dysplasia, Cervix	795.0 Abnormal Cervical Pap Smear
180.0 Malignant Neoplasm, Cervix	623.0 Dysplasia, Vagina	

COLLECTION METHOD

Liquid-Based Prep
192055 ☐ ThinPrep Pap Test

192039 ☐ ThinPrep Pap Test w/reflex to HPV Hybrid Capture when ASC-US or SIL

192047 ☐ ThinPrep Pap Test w/reflex to high-risk only HPV Hybrid Capture when ASC-US

Pap Smear
009100 ☐ 1 Slide   009191 ☐ 2 Slides

Pap Smear and Maturation Index
009209 ☐ 1 Slide   190074 ☐ 2 Slides

SOURCE OF SPECIMEN

☐ Cervical
☐ Endocervical
☐ Vaginal

Date LMP

___ / ___ / ___
Mo   Day   Year

COLLECTION TECHNIQUE

☐ Spatula
☐ Brush
☐ Broom
☐ Other
_____

PATIENT HISTORY

☐ Pregnant
☐ Lactating
☐ Oral Contraceptives
☐ Postmenopausal
☐ Hormone Replacement Therapy

☐ PMP Bleeding
☐ Postpartum
☐ IUD
☐ Postcoital Bleeding
☐ DES Exposure
☐ Previous Abnormal Pap Test

☐ Other _____

PREVIOUS TREATMENT   Date/Results

☐ None
☐ Colposcopy and Bx   _____
☐ Cryosurgery   _____
☐ LEEP   _____
☐ Laser Vaporization   _____
☐ Conization   _____
☐ Hysterectomy   _____
☐ Radiation   _____
☐ Chemotherapy   _____

Figure 8-5. Cytology request form.

Source of the Specimen

The purpose of this category is to identify the origin of the specimen because it is impossible for the laboratory to obtain this information by looking at the specimen. The medical assistant checks one or more of the following boxes on the form: cervical, endocervical, or vaginal.

Collection Technique

The collection device or devices used to obtain the specimen must be indicated. The medical assistant checks one or more of the following boxes on the form: spatula, brush, or broom.

Patient History

Information on the present and past health status of the patient is specified under the patient history category. The medical assistant must check the following boxes that apply to the patient: pregnant, lactating, oral contraceptives, postmenopausal, hormone replacement therapy, postmenopausal bleeding, postpartum, IUD, postcoital bleeding, DES (diethylstilbestrol) exposure, and previous abnormal smear. This information assists the laboratory in evaluating the specimen.

Previous Treatment

Any previous treatment for a precancerous or cancerous condition of the cervix is indicated under this category. The medical assistant checks the appropriate box on the form if any of the following procedures have been performed on the patient: colposcopy and biopsy, cryosurgery, loop electrocautery excision procedure (LEEP), laser vaporization, conization, hysterectomy, radiation, and chemotherapy.

Evaluation of the Pap Specimen

Before a Pap slide can be evaluated, it must be stained by a laboratory technician. Staining is performed on slides prepared by the direct smear method and the liquid-based method. The purpose of staining is to allow better viewing of the morphology of the epithelial cells. The slide is studied under a microscope for evidence of abnormalities by a specially trained technician, known as a *cytotechnologist*. When an abnormality is detected, it is reviewed by a *cytopathologist* (a physician specializing in pathology), who makes a final evaluation. The findings are recorded on a cytology report and returned to the medical office.

A more recent development in the evaluation of Pap slides is the use of automated cytology computer-imaging devices. An abnormal slide may contain only a few abnormal cells among thousands of normal cells. Because of this, these abnormal cells may be missed during the evaluation by the cytotechnologist. A cytology computer-imaging device is able to examine every cell on the slide and select and display cells that appear "most abnormal." The cytotechnologist can evaluate these cells further under a microscope. In this way, the cytotechnologist is able to focus his

or her expertise and decision making on preselected areas of the slide.

Maturation Index

The maturation index must be performed on a sampling of cells taken from the upper third of the lateral vaginal wall. The *maturation index* refers to the percentage of parabasal, intermediate, and superficial cells present in the specimen. The maturation index provides the physician with an endocrine evaluation of the patient, which can assist in evaluating the cause of infertility, menopausal or postmenopausal bleeding, or amenorrhea and can help assess the results of treatment with hormones. If the physician orders a maturation index along with the Pap test, the medical assistant must indicate this on the cytology request by checking the box labeled *Maturation Index* (see Figure 8-5). Numerous factors affect the results of the maturation index; it is important to indicate on the cytology request the presence of abnormal bleeding; hormone treatment; or treatment with digitalis, corticosteroids, or thyroid medication.

Cytology Report

The Bethesda System (TBS) is the standard for reporting the results of a Pap test on the cytology report (Figure 8-6). The National Cancer Institute in Bethesda, Maryland, developed this system. It provides a detailed cytologic description, rather than a numerical result (as with the previous class I through V system). For this reason, TBS is a more effective means of communicating the results of the Pap test to the physician. TBS separates the cytology report into the following categories:

1. **Specimen Type.** This category identifies whether the specimen is a conventional cell sample (Pap smear) or a liquid-based cell sample (ThinPrep).
2. **Specimen Adequacy.** This category refers to the quality of the specimen collected by the physician. The specimen is described using one of the following classifications:
   - **Satisfactory for Evaluation.** This indicates that the specimen was of sufficient sampling and quality for a comprehensive assessment of the cells.
   - **Unsatisfactory for Evaluation.** This indicates that the overall sampling or quality of the specimen was inadequate. A reason is given for the inability to evaluate the Pap slide, such as too few cells were collected or the presence of blood or inflammation is obscuring the cells.
3. **General Categorization.** This category provides the medical office with a quick review of the report. The following classifications are used to categorize the specimen:
   - **Negative for Intraepithelial Lesion or Malignancy.** This indicates that the epithelial cells were normal and that there were no precancerous or cancerous findings. This classification also is assigned to a specimen that exhibits certain benign (noncancerous)

GYN CYTOLOGY REPORT

| RIVERVIEW MEDICAL LABORATORY
DEPARTMENT OF PATHOLOGY
2501 GRANT AVENUE
ST. LOUIS, MO 63146
(314) 555–3443 | **PATIENT:** Heather Jones
PATIENT NO: 45876
DOB: 10/20/65
SUBMITTING: T. Woodside, MD |

Date of Specimen: 7/01/08	**SPECIMEN TYPE**
Date Received: 7/02/08	[X] ThinPrep [ ] Conventional Pap Smear
Date Reported: 7/06/08	
Performed By: Richard McVay, Cytotechnologist	**Checked By:** Melissa Wagner, Pathologist

SPECIMEN ADEQUACY	GENERAL CATEGORIZATION
[X] **Satisfactory for Evaluation** [ ] **Unsatisfactory for Evaluation**	[ ] **Negative for Intraepithelial Lesion** **or Malignancy** (*see Interpretation/Result*) [X] **Epithelial Cell Abnormality** (*see Interpretation/Result*) [ ] **Other** (*see Interpretation/Result*)

INTERPRETATION/RESULT

A. BENIGN CELLULAR CHANGES

[ ] Infection:
- [ ] Trichomonas vaginalis
- [ ] Fungal organisms morphologically compatible w/ Candida species
- [ ] Cellular changes associated with herpes simplex virus
- [ ] Bacterial infection morphologically compatible with gardnerella
- [ ] Cytoplasmic inclusions suggestive of chlamydia

[ ] Reactive changes
- [ ] Without inflammation
- [ ] With inflammation
- [ ] Atrophy with inflammation (atrophic vaginitis)
- [ ] Radiation effect
- [ ] Repair
- [ ] Hyperkeratosis
- [ ] Parakeratosis

B. EPITHELIAL CELL ABNORMALITIES

[X] Squamous Cell
- [X] Atypical Squamous Cells of Undetermined Significance (ASC-US)
- [ ] Atypical Squamous Cells of Higher Risk (ASC-H)
- [ ] Low-Grade Squamous Intraepithelial Lesion (LSIL)
- [ ] High-Grade Squamous Intraepithelial Lesion (HSIL)
- [ ] Squamous Cell Carcinoma

[ ] Glandular Cell
- [ ] Atypical Glandular Cells of Undetermined Significance (AGUS)
- [ ] Adenocarcinoma

Figure 8-6. Cytology report form (The Bethesda System).

changes. Benign changes can be caused by vaginal infections, such as bacterial vaginosis, chlamydia, trichomoniasis, candidiasis, and herpes. Benign changes also can be caused by inflammation resulting from the normal cell repair process, radiation, and chemotherapy. Any benign findings of importance (e.g., vaginal infections) are described in detail in the Interpretation/Result section of the cytology report.

- **Epithelial Cell Abnormality.** This classification indicates abnormal cell changes. The abnormality is described in detail in the Interpretation/Result section of the report.
- **Other.** This classification is used to indicate that no abnormality was found in the cells, but the findings indicate some increased risk. The presence of normal-appearing endometrial cells in a postmenopausal

Table 8-1 Pap Test Results

Test Result	Interpretation
Negative for intraepithelial lesion or malignancy	Epithelial cells were normal, and there were no precancerous or cancerous findings
Atypical squamous cells of undetermined significance (ASC-US)	Cells are only slightly abnormal. Nature and cause of abnormality cannot be determined. These slightly altered cells usually return to normal on their own, resulting in negative results on subsequent Pap tests
Atypical squamous cells of higher risk (ASC-H)	Minor abnormal changes in cells with unknown causes, but at risk of progressing to high-grade lesion (HSIL). Further testing is required to determine whether this is a minor condition or one that may progress to HSIL
Low-grade squamous intraepithelial lesion (LSIL)	Abnormal cells that show definite minor changes, but are unlikely to progress to cancer (general term for this is *mild dysplasia*). LSIL may be caused by HPV infection, but of a type that is not likely to lead to cervical cancer
High-grade squamous intraepithelial lesion (HSIL)	Abnormal cell changes that have higher likelihood of progressing to cancer. Although not cancerous yet, abnormal cells may become cancerous if treatment is not obtained (general term for this is *moderate-to-severe dysplasia*). HSIL is often caused by HPV infection of a type associated with cervical cancer
Carcinoma	Usually means patient has cervical cancer. Most women with cervical cancer also test positive for HPV infection

HPV: human papillomavirus.

woman may indicate an abnormality of the endometrium. These findings are described in detail in the Interpretation/Result section of the report.

4. **Interpretation/Result.** This part of the report provides the physician with a detailed description of findings. This includes any significant benign changes (e.g., vaginal infections) and any abnormal changes in the epithelial cells. Table 8-1 lists and describes the findings most frequently reported.

5. **Automated Review.** This category indicates whether the specimen was evaluated using an automated computer-imaging device. The name of the device and the results are specified in this section.

6. **Ancillary Testing.** This category is used if an additional test method is used to evaluate the specimen. If abnormal cells are detected on the Pap slide, a human papillomavirus (HPV) test may be performed. The name of the test method and the results would be reported under this category.

Bimanual Pelvic Examination

After obtaining the smear for the Pap test, the physician withdraws the speculum and performs a bimanual pelvic examination. The physician inserts the index and middle fingers of a lubricated gloved hand into the vagina. The fingers of the other hand are placed on the woman's lower abdomen. Between the two hands, the physician can palpate the size, shape, and position of the uterus and ovaries and detect tenderness or lumps (Figure 8-7).

Rectal-Vaginal Examination

The last part of the pelvic examination is a rectal-vaginal examination. The physician inserts one gloved finger into the vagina and another gloved finger into the rectum to obtain information about the tone and alignment of the pelvic organs and the **adnexal** region (ovaries, fallopian

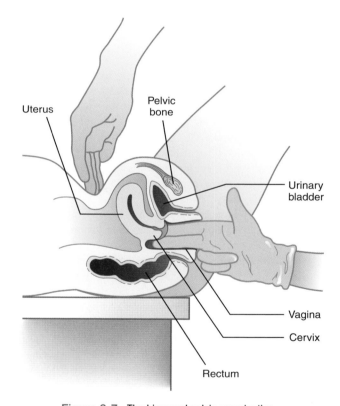

Figure 8-7. The bimanual pelvic examination.

tubes, and ligaments of the uterus). The presence of hemorrhoids, fistulas, and fissures also can be noted. During this examination, the physician may want to obtain some fecal material from the rectum to test for occult blood in the stool, which requires a guaiac slide test (e.g., Hemoccult). This is typically performed on women beginning at 40 years of age. The medical assistant is responsible for assisting with the collection and testing the specimen for occult blood. This procedure (fecal occult blood testing) is presented in detail in Chapter 13.

Text continued on p. 284

see DVD

PROCEDURE **8-1**   **Breast Self-Examination Instructions**

Outcome Instruct a patient in the procedure for performing a breast self-examination.

Equipment/Supplies

- Small pillow

1. **Procedural Step.** Greet the patient and introduce yourself. Identify the patient and inform the patient that you will be showing her how to perform a breast self-examination. Discuss with her the purpose of a breast self-examination and when to examine the breasts (see the box *Patient Teaching: Breast Self-Examination*).

2. **Procedural Step.** Explain to the patient that a complete breast self-examination should be performed in three ways—before a mirror, lying down, and in the shower. *Principle.* Using three methods results in a thorough examination, making it more likely that breast changes will be detected.

   Instruct the patient in the procedure for performing a breast self-examination as follows:

Before a Mirror

3. **Procedural Step.** Remove clothing from the waist up. Stand in front of a large mirror with your arms relaxed at your sides. Observe each breast for the following:
   a. Change in size or shape
   b. Swelling, puckering, or dimpling of the skin
   c. Change in skin texture
   d. Retraction of the nipple
   e. Changes in size or position of one nipple compared with the other
   Principle. Puckering and dimpling of the skin or retraction of the nipple may mean that a tumor is pulling the skin inward.

4. **Procedural Step.** Slowly raise your arms over your head, and repeat the same inspection listed in procedural step 3.
   Principle. When the arms are moved at the same time into the same positions, both breasts and nipples should react to the movement in the same way. A change in one breast (e.g., dimpling or puckering of the skin) and not the other should be reported to your physician.

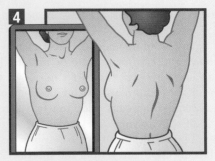

Raise your arms over your head.

5. **Procedural Step.** Rest your palms on your hips and press down firmly to flex your chest muscles. Repeat the inspection in procedural step 3.
   Principle. Flexing the chest muscles allows abnormalities to become more apparent.

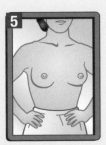

Press down firmly to flex the chest muscles.

6. **Procedural Step.** Gently squeeze the nipple of each breast with your fingertips and look for a discharge.

Lying Down

7. **Procedural Step.** To examine the right breast, lie on your back and place a small pillow (or folded towel) under your right shoulder. Place your right hand behind your head.
   Principle. The purpose of this step is to flatten the breast and distribute the breast tissue more evenly on the chest, making it easier to palpate the breast tissue.

8. **Procedural Step.** Extend your left hand with the fingers held flat. The pads of the middle three fingers of the left hand are used to perform the examination. The finger pads include the top third of each finger. Do not use the tips of the fingers. Use small rotating motions (about the size of a dime) and continuous firm pressure with the finger pads.

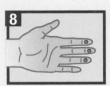

Use the pads of the middle three fingers.

Principle. The finger pads are more sensitive than the fingertips, making it easier to detect an abnormality.

9. Procedural Step. Use one of the following patterns to move around the breast: circular, vertical strip, or wedge. Choose the pattern that is easiest for you. When you have chosen a pattern, use the same pattern each time you examine your breasts.

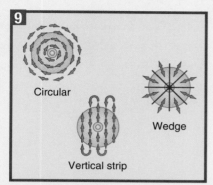

Use one of three patterns to examine the breasts.

Circular

a. Visualize the breast as a clock face.
b. Start at the outside top edge of the breast.
c. Proceed clockwise around the entire outer rim of the breast until your fingers return to the starting point.
d. Move in about 1 inch toward the nipple, and make the same circling motion again.
e. Move around the breast in smaller and smaller circles until you reach the nipple.

Vertical Strip

a. Mentally divide the breast into strips.
b. Start in the underarm area and slowly move your fingers downward until they are below the breast.
c. Move your fingers about 1 inch toward the middle, and slowly move back up.
d. Repeat until the entire breast has been examined.

Wedge

a. Mentally divide your breast into wedges similar to the pieces of a pie.
b. Starting at the outer edge of the breast, move your fingers toward the nipple and back to the edge of the breast.
c. Check your entire breast, covering one small wedge-shaped section at a time.

Principle. Using a specific pattern ensures that the entire breast is examined.

10. Procedural Step. Holding the middle three fingers of your hand together with the thumb extended, use your finger pads and the pattern you selected to examine the right breast thoroughly. Press firmly enough to feel the different breast tissues. The breast should be palpated for lumps, hard knots, and thickening. Breast tissue normally feels a little lumpy and uneven.

11. Procedural Step. Examine the entire chest area from your collarbone to the base of a properly fitted bra

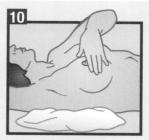

Examine the right breast.

and from the breastbone to the underarm. Pay special attention to the area between the breast and underarm, including the underarm itself. A ridge of firm tissue in the lower curve of the breast is normal. Continue the examination until every part of the breast has been examined, including the nipple.

Principle. An enlarged node in the armpit also can be a sign of breast cancer even if nothing can be felt in the breast.

12. Procedural Step. Repeat this procedure on the left breast. Place a small pillow (or folded towel) under the left shoulder, and place your left hand behind your head. Use the finger pads of the right hand to examine the left breast.

In the Shower

13. Procedural Step. Gently lather each breast.

Principle. Fingers glide easily over wet, soapy skin, making it easier to detect changes in the breast.

14. Procedural Step. Place your right hand behind your head. Extend your left hand with the fingers held flat. With the finger pads of the middle three fingers, use small rotating motions (about the size of a dime) and continuous firm pressure with the finger pads to examine the right breast. Use your preferred pattern (circular, vertical strip, or wedge) to palpate for lumps, hard knots, and thickening. Examine the area between the breast and underarm, including the underarm itself.

Principle. The upright position makes it easier to examine the upper and outer portions of the breast.

15. Procedural Step. Repeat the procedure on the left breast. Place the left arm behind the head, and use the right fingers to examine the left breast.

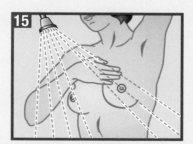

Examine the breasts in the shower.

Continued

PROCEDURE 8-1

PROCEDURE **8-1**   Breast Self-Examination Instructions—cont'd

16. **Procedural Step.** Instruct the patient to report lumps and other changes to the physician immediately. Reassure the patient that most breast lumps are not cancerous, but the only way to know for sure is to see the physician as soon as possible.

17. **Procedural Step.** Chart the procedure. Include the date and time and the type of instructions given to the patient. If you gave a printed instruction sheet or educational brochure to the patient, document this as well.

CHARTING EXAMPLE	
Date	
9/7/08	11:00 a.m. Instructions provided for a
	BSE. Pt given a BSE educational brochure.
	———————————— Y. Wu, RMA

PROCEDURE **8-2**   Assisting with a Gynecologic Examination

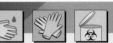

Outcome Assist with a gynecologic examination. The following procedure describes the medical assistant's role in assisting with a gynecologic examination consisting of breast and pelvic examinations, including a Pap test and a fecal occult blood test.

Equipment/Supplies

- Disposable gloves
- Examining gown and drape
- Disposable vaginal speculum
- Water-based lubricant
- Gauze pads

- Hemoccult slide and developing solution
- Tissues
- Cytology request form
- Biohazard specimen transport bag

Direct Smear Method

- Glass slides with frosted edge
- Cytology fixative
- Plastic spatula
- Endocervical brush
- Slide container

Liquid-Prep Method

- Vial with preservative (ThinPrep, SurePath)
- Plastic spatula and endocervical brush or cytology broom

1. **Procedural Step.** Sanitize your hands.
2. **Procedural Step.** Assemble the equipment. Complete as much of the cytology request form as possible. Some information on the form requires input from the patient, such as the last menstrual period (LMP),

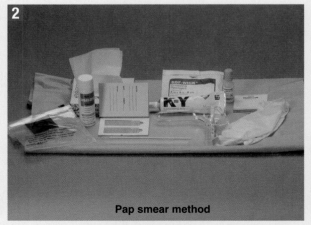

Pap smear method

Assemble equipment.

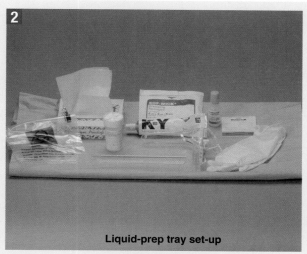

Liquid-prep tray set-up

Assemble equipment.

and must be completed later. Prepare the collection materials as follows:

Pap Smear Method. Using a lead pencil, identify the slides on the frosted edge with the patient's name, the date, and the source of the specimen using the following abbreviations: *V (vaginal), C (cervical),* and *E (endocervical).*

Liquid-Prep Method. Check the expiration date on the vial. Label the vial with the date and the patient's name and identification number. The identification number is located on the cytology request form.

Principle. If the vial is outdated, it should be discarded because it may lead to inaccurate test results.

3. **Procedural Step.** Greet the patient and introduce yourself. Identify the patient and explain the procedure.

4. **Procedural Step.** Escort the patient to the examining room and ask her to be seated. Seat yourself so that you are facing the patient. Ask the patient whether she has any problems or concerns, and record the information in the patient's chart. Ask the patient the necessary questions to complete the rest of the cytology request form.

5. **Procedural Step.** Measure the patient's vital signs, height, and weight, and chart the results.

6. **Procedural Step.** Instruct and prepare the patient for the examination as follows:
   a. Ask the patient whether she needs to empty the bladder before the examination. If a urine specimen is needed, instruct the patient in the proper collection of the specimen.
   b. Provide the patient with a patient gown. Instruct the patient to remove all clothing and to put on the patient gown with the opening in front. If the patient is wearing socks, tell her she can keep them on. Offer assistance if you sense the patient may have trouble undressing.

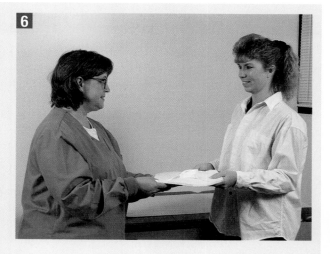

   c. Tell the patient to have a seat on the examining table after she has put on the examining gown.
   d. Inform the patient that the physician will be with her soon, and leave the room to give her privacy.

Principle. An empty bladder makes the examination easier and is more comfortable for the patient. Wearing socks helps keep the patient's feet warm during the examination.

7. **Procedural Step.** Make the medical record available for review by the physician. The medical office has a designated location where the record is placed, such as a small shelf mounted on the wall next to the outside of the examining room door or in a chart holder on the outside of the examining room door. Position the medical record so that patient-identifiable information is not visible.

Principle: Before going into the room, the physician will want to review the patient's measurements and urine test results documented by the medical assistant. HIPAA requires protection of a patient's health information.

8. **Procedural Step.** Check to make sure the patient is ready to be seen by the physician. Before entering a patient's room, always knock lightly on the door to let the patient know you are getting ready to enter the room. Inform the physician that the patient is ready. This may be done using a color-coded flagging system mounted on the wall next to the examining room.

9. **Procedural Step.** Assist the patient into a supine position, and properly drape her for the breast examination.

10. **Procedural Step.** Assist the patient into the lithotomy position for the pelvic examination.

11. **Procedural Step.** Prepare the vaginal speculum by removing it from the warming drawer and performing one of the following:

Pap Smear Method. Moisten the blades of the speculum with warm water.

Continued

PROCEDURE 8-2

PROCEDURE 8-2   Assisting with a Gynecologic Examination–cont'd

Liquid Prep Method. Thinly lubricate the blades of the speculum with a water-based lubricant.

Principle. Preparing the vaginal speculum facilitates its insertion into the vagina.

12. Procedural Step. Prepare the light for the physician as follows:

   a. *Overhead examination lamp:* Adjust and focus the light for the physician.

   b. *Speculum-illumination system:* Snap the light source device into the light holder on the vaginal speculum and turn it on. The lighting system produces a beam of light that shines through the blades of the speculum for visualization of the vagina and cervix.

   Principle. Visualization of the vagina and cervix requires direct light.

13. Procedural Step. Hand the vaginal speculum to the physician. Reassure the patient, and help her relax the abdominal muscles during the examination by telling her to breathe deeply, slowly, and evenly through the mouth.

   Principle. If the patient is relaxed, the examination proceeds more smoothly and is more comfortable for her.

14. Procedural Step. Apply gloves, and assist with the collection of the Pap specimen as follows:

   a. **Direct Smear Method**

   (1) Hold each slide so that the physician can smear the specimen on it.

   (2) Fix each slide immediately after collection by flooding it with 95% ethyl alcohol or by spraying it with a cytology fixative. The slide should be sprayed lightly with a continuous motion from a distance of 5 to 6 inches.

   (3) Allow the slides to air dry for 5 to 10 minutes, and place them in a protective slide container.

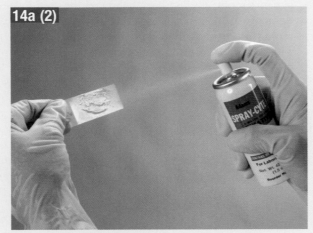

14a (2)

Spray lightly from a distance of 5 to 6 inches.

   b. **Liquid-Prep Method (ThinPrep)**
   Spatula and Brush Method

   (1) Remove the cap from the ThinPrep vial, and hold it so that the physician can insert the spatula into the vial.

   (2) Rinse the plastic spatula in the liquid preservative by vigorously swirling it around in the solution 10 times.

   (3) Discard the spatula in a biohazard waste container.

   (4) Hold the vial so that the physician can insert the endocervical brush into the vial.

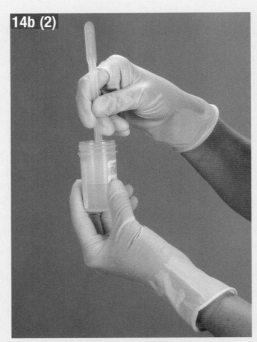

14b (2)

Vigorously swirl the spatula in the preservative.

   (5) Rinse the brush in the liquid preservative by vigorously rotating it in the solution 10 times while pushing the brush against the vial wall. Swirl the brush in the solution to further release cellular material.

   (6) Discard the brush in a biohazard waste container. Securely tighten the cap so that the torque line on the cap passes the torque line on the vial.

   Broom Method

   (1) Remove the cap from the ThinPrep vial, and hold it so that the physician can insert the broom into the vial.

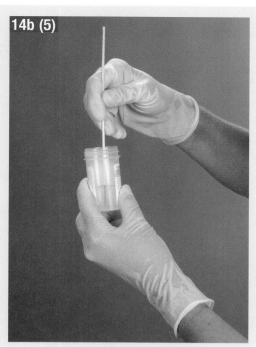

14b (5)

Rotate the brush in the preservative.

(2) Rinse the broom in the liquid preservative by pushing the broom vigorously into the bottom of the vial 10 times. This motion forces the broom bristles apart, releasing cervical cells into the solution. Swirl the broom vigorously in the liquid preservative to further release cellular material.

(3) Discard the broom in a biohazard waste container. Tighten the cap so that the torque line on the cap passes the torque line on the vial.

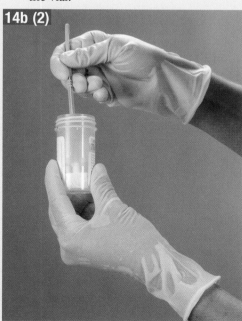

14b (2)

Push the broom vigorously into the bottom of the vial.

c. **Liquid-Prep Method (SurePath)**
  (1) Remove the cap from the SurePath vial, and hold it so that the physician can insert the collection device into the vial.
  (2) Break off or disconnect the tip of the collection device from the handle.
  (3) Discard the handle of the collection device in a waste container.
  (4) Repeat the above steps until the physician has collected all of the specimens needed for the Pap test.
  (5) Securely tighten the cap on the vial.

15. **Procedural Step.** Turn off the examining lamp or disconnect the light source from the vaginal speculum. Discard the disposable vaginal speculum in a biohazard waste container. Apply lubricant to a gauze square. Hold it out so that the physician can apply lubricant to his or her gloves to perform the bimanual and rectal-vaginal examinations. Assist with the collection of the fecal specimen for the fecal occult blood test.

Principle. Applying lubricant to a gauze square (rather than directly to the physician's gloved fingers) prevents the opening of the tube of lubricant from touching the physician's gloves and contaminating the contents of the tube.

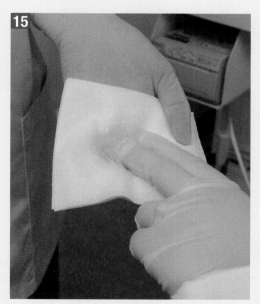

15

Hold the gauze with the lubricant for the physician.

16. **Procedural Step.** After the examination, assist the patient into a sitting position, and allow her the opportunity to rest for a moment. Offer the patient tissues to remove excess lubricant from the perineum. Assist the patient off the examining table.

Principle. Some patients (especially geriatric) become dizzy after being on the examining table and should be allowed to rest before sitting up.

PROCEDURE 8-2

Continued

PROCEDURE 8-2   Assisting with a Gynecologic Examination–cont'd

17. **Procedural Step.** Instruct the patient to get dressed. Tell the patient how and when she will be notified of Pap test results.

18. **Procedural Step.** Test the fecal occult blood specimen, and chart the results.

19. **Procedural Step.** Prepare the Pap specimen for transport to the laboratory. Place the specimen (slide container or vial) in a biohazard specimen transport bag, and seal the bag. Insert the cytology requisition into the outside pocket of the bag, and tuck the top of the requisition under the flap. Place the bag in the appropriate location for pickup by the laboratory.

20. **Procedural Step.** Chart the transport of the Pap specimen to an outside laboratory.

21. **Procedural Step.** Clean the examining room.

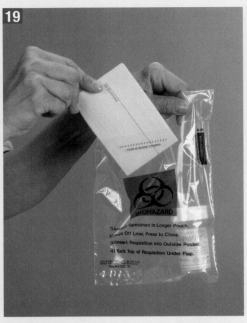

Insert the laboratory request into the outside pocket.

CHARTING EXAMPLE	
Date	
9/7/08	10:00 a.m. Hemoccult: negative.
	Instructions provided for BSE. ThinPrep
	Pap specimen to Medical Center Laboratory
	for cytology. ———————— Y. Wu, RMA

VAGINAL INFECTIONS

The vagina provides a warm, moist environment, which tends to encourage the growth of various organisms that can result in a vaginal infection, or *vaginitis.* If an unusual vaginal discharge is present, suggesting a vaginal infection, a specimen is obtained to identify the invading organism. A specimen of the discharge is collected at the medical office and is evaluated there or placed in a transport medium that is picked up by a laboratory courier and transported to an outside medical laboratory for evaluation. The patient should be instructed not to douche before coming to the medical office because the physician would be unable to observe the discharge or to obtain a specimen for microbiologic analysis.

The medical assistant is responsible for assembling the appropriate supplies for the collection and evaluation of the suspected invading organism. The medical assistant must label all specimens with the patient's name, the date, and the source of the specimen. If the specimen is to be transported to an outside medical laboratory for evaluation, a laboratory request form must be completed. The request form indicates the source of the specimen, the physician's clinical diagnosis, the microbiologic examination requested, and other pertinent information, such as medications the patient is taking.

The physician's clinical assessment of the patient's signs and symptoms, along with the results of the laboratory evaluation of the specimen, are used to diagnose the presence of a vaginal infection.

Medical assistants should protect themselves from infection with a pathogen while assisting with the collection and evaluation of the specimen by practicing good techniques of medical asepsis. Methods used to identify the invading organism and the supplies required for the collection and evaluation of organisms that cause common vaginal infections are presented next.

Trichomoniasis

Trichomonas vaginalis, the causative agent of trichomoniasis (trich), is a pear-shaped protozoan with four flagella, which allow for the motility of the organism (Figure 8-8). Trichomoniasis is usually, but not always, spread through sexual intercourse. Symptoms of this infection include a profuse, frothy vaginal discharge that is usually yellowish green and has an unpleasant odor; itching and irritation of the vulva and vagina; dyspareunia; and dysuria. The cervix may exhibit small red spots, a condition known as "strawberry cervix."

Trichomonas may be identified at the medical office by a wet preparation, which involves placing a small amount of the discharge on a microscope slide using a sterile swab, adding a drop of isotonic saline to it, and placing a coverslip over the mixture to protect it (Figure 8-9). The slide is examined under the microscope and observed for the presence of the lashing movements of the flagella and the motility of the organism.

If the physician prefers to have an outside laboratory evaluate the specimen, it must be placed in a tube containing a transport medium. The specimen must be transported

Wet Preparation

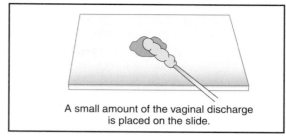

A small amount of the vaginal discharge is placed on the slide.

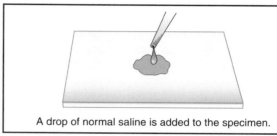

A drop of normal saline is added to the specimen.

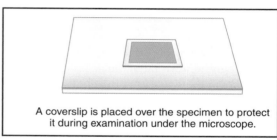

A coverslip is placed over the specimen to protect it during examination under the microscope.

Figure 8-9. Preparing a wet preparation for the identification of *Trichomonas vaginalis*.

as soon as possible (within 24 hours) to prevent it from dying, which would impede visualization of the motility of the organism.

Trichomoniasis is treated with the oral administration of metronidazole (Flagyl). The woman and her sexual partner must be treated at the same time to prevent reinfection because her partner may harbor the organism without displaying noticeable symptoms.

Candidiasis

Candida albicans is a yeastlike fungus normally found in the intestinal tract and is a frequent contaminant of the vagina; however, it usually does not produce symptoms indicating a vaginal infection. Conditions such as pregnancy, diabetes mellitus, and prolonged antibiotic therapy produce changes in the vagina that may precipitate a candidal infection of the vagina, commonly referred to as a "yeast infection." Symptoms of candidiasis include white patches on the mucous membrane of the vagina; a thick, odorless, cottage

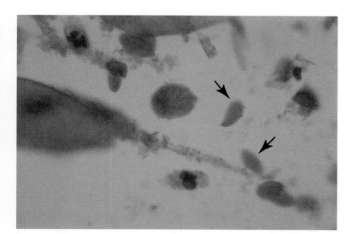

Figure 8-8. *Trichomonas vaginalis* under a microscope. (Modified from Mahon C, Manuselis G: *Textbook of diagnostic microbiology,* ed 2, Philadelphia, 2000, Saunders.)

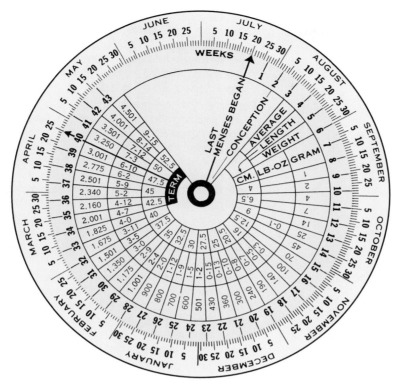

Figure 8-12. Gestation calculator. The last menstrual period is July 20, and the estimated date of delivery is April 25.

pelvic examinations) and a general physical examination of the other body systems, although the latter may be performed during a subsequent prenatal visit, depending on the medical office routine.

Women often have little or no medical supervision during their childbearing years; the physical examination is of particular importance in establishing a baseline for the woman's general state of health and in identifying high-risk prenatal patients. Conditions such as obesity, hypertension, severe varicosities, and uterine size inappropriate for the due date can be diagnosed by the physician, and necessary treatment or monitoring can be instituted to help prevent complications.

Preparation of the Patient

When the patient arrives at the medical office and the prenatal record form has been completed, the medical assistant is responsible for taking and recording the patient's vital signs, height, and weight to provide a database for subsequent prenatal visits. The patient is asked to disrobe completely and put on an examining gown with the opening in front. The medical assistant must give complete and thorough instructions so the patient knows exactly what is expected. The patient should be asked whether she needs to empty her bladder because an empty bladder facilitates the examination and is more comfortable for her. If the office policy is such that a specimen is needed for urine testing at the initial prenatal visit, the patient will be required to void.

Special precautions should be taken in assisting the prenatal patient. The medical assistant should support the patient as she gets onto and off the scale and examining table to ensure her safety and comfort. This is especially important as the pregnancy progresses and the patient becomes more awkward and off-balance.

The medical assistant is responsible for setting up the tray required for the examination. The setup includes the equipment and supplies required for the procedures to be performed. During the prenatal examination, the medical assistant is responsible for positioning the patient as required for each aspect of the examination and assisting the physician as necessary. Table 8-2 lists the procedures commonly included in the prenatal examination and the purpose, the implications, and (when applicable) the patient's position. Most of the procedures included in the initial prenatal examination are presented elsewhere in this book; the number of the chapter that contains the step-by-step procedure is included in Table 8-2.

Patient Education

At the conclusion of the initial prenatal examination and after the patient is dressed, the physician talks with her regarding instructions on diet, weight gain, rest, sleep, employment, exercise, travel, sexual intercourse, dental care, smoking, alcohol, and drugs. Many offices have a prenatal guidebook designed especially for this purpose that is given to each patient to use as a reference. Some offices also use a series of teaching films that the patient views during the return prenatal visit

Table 8-2 Components of the Initial Prenatal Examination

Procedure	Purpose and Implications
Vital Signs (see Chapter 4)	To provide baseline for subsequent prenatal visits. Blood pressure decreases slightly during first and second trimesters and returns to normal or slightly above normal during last trimester
Temperature Pulse Respiration Blood Pressure Weight (see Chapter 5)	Elevation in blood pressure during pregnancy in conjunction with other signs and symptoms indicates possible problems, such as pregnancy-induced hypertension or preeclampsia Patient position: sitting To provide baseline weight measurement for comparison with all future weight measurements at subsequent prenatal visits. Medical assistant charts patient's weight on flow sheet at each prenatal visit, and any deviations from expected progressions are evaluated by physician Measuring and recording maternal weight gain or loss are helpful in assessing fetal development and, to some extent, mother's nutrition and state of health. Sudden unexplained weight gain may indicate preeclampsia of pregnancy
Physical Examination (see Chapter 5)	To establish baseline for woman's general state of health to ensure patient is entering pregnancy in best possible physical condition. Physical examination includes examination of patient's eyes, ears, nose, and throat; chest, lungs, and heart; breasts; abdomen; reproductive organs; rectum; and extremities Of particular importance are breast, abdominal, and pelvic examinations
Breast Examination (Chapter 8)	To check for lumps, swelling, dimpling, puckering, and changes in skin texture To check for breast changes that occur during pregnancy, such as tenderness and fullness and darkening of nipple and areolae Patient position: supine
Abdominal Examination (Chapter 8)	To detect masses or lumps other than developing fetus. Abdomen is inspected for scars and striations, and initial measurement of fundal height is made to provide baseline for future fundal height measurements Patient position: supine

Pelvic Examination (Chapter 8)	To provide data to confirm pregnancy and to determine length of gestation
	To estimate gestational age of developing embryo (at 7 weeks, uterus is the size of an egg; at 10 weeks, it is the size of an orange; and at 12 weeks, it is the size of a grapefruit)
	To identify pelvic characteristics and any abnormalities that may result in complications during pregnancy or delivery. Pelvic examination generally includes the following:
	    Inspection of external genitalia
	    Speculum examination of vagina and cervix
	    Pap test
	    Specimen for chlamydia and gonorrhea tests
	    Vaginal specimen if infection is suspected
	    Bimanual examination
	Patient position: lithotomy

Rectal-Vaginal Examination (Chapter 8)	To assess strength and irregularity of posterior vaginal wall and posterior cervix Anus is inspected for hemorrhoids and fissures, and rectum is inspected for herniation and masses Patient position: lithotomy
Pelvic Measurements (Chapter 8)	To verify that size and shape of pelvis are within normal limits to allow full-term fetus to pass safely through pelvic inlet in normal vaginal route of delivery; if not, cesarean section will be required Some physicians delay taking pelvic measurements until later in pregnancy. At that time, the prenatal patient's perineal muscles are more relaxed, allowing pelvic measurements to be taken with less patient discomfort and more accuracy

while waiting to see the physician. The physician also prescribes a daily vitamin supplement to be taken during the prenatal period to ensure that the mother and fetus obtain an adequate supply of vitamins and minerals.

When the physician is finished talking with the patient, the medical assistant is responsible for scheduling the next prenatal visit and for ensuring that the patient understands the instructions for maintaining health and preventing disease during the pregnancy. The medical assistant should tell the patient to report the occurrence of any warning signs during the pregnancy (see the *Warning Signs during Pregnancy* box) and not to take any medications without first checking with the physician. The patient also should be encouraged to contact the medical office should any questions or problems arise.

Laboratory Tests

The physician orders many laboratory tests to assist in the assessment of the patient's state of health and to detect problems that may put the pregnancy at risk. Several tests, such as the Pap test and the chlamydia and gonorrhea tests, require the physician to collect the specimens at the medical office and have them transported by lab courier to an outside laboratory for evaluation. The specimen required for the prenatal blood tests must be obtained through a venipuncture to provide a sufficient quantity of blood for the number of tests ordered. The blood specimen is collected at the medical office or at an outside laboratory.

It is important to have these initial tests completed as soon as possible to provide the physician with the test results by the time of the next scheduled prenatal visit. Based on the results of the prenatal examination and the laboratory tests, the physician may order additional tests to assess the patient's condition. Certain tests and procedures are scheduled later in the pregnancy, such as the glucose challenge test (GCT) and the group B streptococcus (GBS) test. The prenatal laboratory tests that are usually performed on a pregnant woman are described next.

Urine Tests

Urinalysis

A complete urinalysis is performed, including physical, chemical, and microscopic analyses of the urine; a clean-catch midstream urine specimen is generally required for the test. If bacteria are found in the urine specimen, the physician usually requests a urine culture and sensitivity test to determine the possible presence of a urinary tract infection. A pregnancy test also may be performed on the urine specimen, if ordered by the physician.

Swab Tests

Pap Test

A Pap test is done for the detection of abnormalities of cell growth to diagnose precancerous or cancerous conditions of the cervix. This test also can be used for hormonal assessment (maturation index) and to assist in the detection of vaginal infections.

Chlamydia and Gonorrhea

Specimens are taken from the endocervical canal and sent to the laboratory to rule out chlamydia and gonorrhea. Chlamydia can be passed from an infected woman to her infant during childbirth, resulting in conjunctivitis and pneumonia in the newborn. If a gonorrheal infection is present at the time of delivery, the *N. gonorrhoeae* organism could infect the infant's eyes during passage through the birth canal. This results in *ophthalmia neonatorum,* which if not treated could lead to blindness. For this reason, most states require that pregnant women be tested for gonorrhea and that the eyes of newborns be treated with antibiotic or silver nitrate drops immediately after birth to kill any gonococcal bacteria that may be present. A patient who is diagnosed with chlamydia or gonorrhea requires immediate treatment with an appropriate antibiotic to prevent problems for herself and her child.

Trichomoniasis and Candidiasis

If an excessive irritating vaginal discharge is present, the physician obtains a specimen to rule out trichomoniasis and

---

Warning Signs during Pregnancy

Signs of Infection
- Fever
- Vaginal discharge
- Dysuria
- Increased frequency of urination
- Marked decrease in urinary output

Signs of Spontaneous Abortion
- Vaginal bleeding
- Persistent low back pain
- Abdominal pain and cramping

Signs of Preeclampsia
- Severe, persistent headache
- Dizziness
- Blurred vision
- Sudden swelling of hands, feet, or face
- Sudden rapid weight gain
- Abdominal pain

Signs of Placental or Fetal Problems
- Vaginal spotting or bleeding
- Abdominal pain and cramping
- Back pain
- Noticeable decrease in fetal activity
- No fetal movement

Signs of Preterm Labor
- Regular or frequent contractions (more than four to six per hour)
- Recurring low, dull backache
- Menstrual-like cramping
- Unusual pressure in the pelvis, low back, abdomen, or thighs

candidiasis. It is important to control candidiasis before delivery to prevent the development of thrush, a yeastlike infection of the infant's mucous membrane of the mouth or throat.

Group B Streptococcus

Group B streptococcus (GBS) is a common bacterium often found in the vagina and rectum of healthy women. Normally, one of four pregnant women carries GBS. GBS is not harmful to a pregnant woman, but it can cause life-threatening infections in the newborn. While passing through the birth canal, a newborn can become infected with the bacteria carried by the mother. When infected, the infant may develop an infection of the blood (septicemia), pneumonia, or meningitis.

To prevent GBS infection of the newborn, a pregnant woman is tested for the bacteria between 35 and 37 weeks' gestation. Using two swabs, the physician collects specimens from the vagina and the rectum. The specimen swabs are placed in a transport tube and sent to the laboratory to be cultured for GBS. If GBS is found, intravenous antibiotics are administered to the woman every 4 hours during labor until delivery. In most cases, this antibiotic administration prevents the newborn from becoming infected with GBS. In situations in which the newborn does become infected with GBS, antibiotics are administered immediately, and the infant is closely monitored.

Blood Tests

Complete Blood Count

The complete blood count (CBC) is a basic screening test used to assist in assessing the patient's state of health. It includes a hemoglobin, hematocrit, white blood cell count, red blood cell count, differential white blood cell count, platelet count, and red blood cell indices. Of particular importance with respect to the prenatal patient are the hemoglobin and hematocrit evaluations, which are described here.

Hemoglobin and Hematocrit

Low hemoglobin or hematocrit values are seen in cases of anemia. Prenatal patients have a tendency to develop anemia because there is an increased demand for and correlating increased production of red blood cells during

What Would You Do? What Would You *Not* Do?

Case Study 3

Johanna Kruger is 24 years old and pregnant with her first child. She is at the office for her first prenatal visit. She is quite upset. Her best friend just had her first baby and the baby died 24 hours later from a group B strep infection. Johanna is afraid that the same thing will happen to her baby. She wants to be tested for GBS as soon as possible. She has some antibiotics at home and is thinking of taking them. Johanna is worried because she has been experiencing some problems with her pregnancy. She is sick all day, her breasts hurt, and yesterday she had some spotting. Johanna is hesitant to tell all of this to the physician because he might think she worries too much. ■

pregnancy; the physician carefully reviews the results of these tests. If the hemoglobin or hematocrit value is low, further hematologic evaluation is usually required. If necessary, therapy is instituted, which usually consists of an iron supplement and nutritional counseling. The hemoglobin and hematocrit values are checked again at approximately 32 weeks of gestation as a precaution against anemia before delivery.

Rh Factor and ABO Blood Type

Tests are performed to anticipate ABO blood type and Rh factor incompatibilities. If the patient is Rh-negative, the father's blood type also must be evaluated. If the father's blood type is Rh-positive, the possibility of an Rh incompatibility exists. This situation warrants the performance of an Rh antibody titer test and repeat antibody titers throughout the pregnancy to determine whether the mother's antibody level is increasing. An increased Rh antibody level could be dangerous to the developing fetus. It can result in severe anemia, jaundice, brain damage, heart failure, and sometimes death of the fetus.

Glucose Challenge Test

A glucose challenge test is performed between 24 and 28 weeks of gestation to screen for gestational diabetes mellitus (GDM). This test works by assessing the body's response to a measured glucose solution. The patient does not need to fast for this test, and there is no preparation required other than arriving at the laboratory at the scheduled time. To perform the glucose challenge test, the patient is asked to drink 50 g of a glucose solution, and her glucose level is measured 1 hour later. A woman with a glucose level of less than 140 mg/dL does not have gestational diabetes mellitus and requires no further testing. If the glucose level is greater than 140 mg/dL, the test is abnormal. Not all women with elevated results have diabetes, however, and further testing using the 3-hour glucose tolerance test (GTT) must be performed before a final diagnosis can be made.

Serology Test for Syphilis

The microorganism that causes syphilis, *Treponema pallidum,* is able to cross the placental barrier and infect the fetus; this could result in intrauterine death or could cause the fetus to be born with congenital syphilis. Infants with congenital syphilis are often born with deformities and may become blind, deaf, paralyzed, or insane. The tests most commonly employed to screen for the presence of syphilis are the Venereal Disease Research Laboratory (VDRL) test and the rapid plasma regain (RPR) test. The test results are reported as nonreactive, weakly reactive, or reactive. Because these tests are screening tests, a weakly reactive or reactive test result warrants more specific testing to arrive at a diagnosis for syphilis. Examples of these tests are the fluorescent treponemal antibody absorption (FTA-ABS) test and the *Treponema pallidum* particle agglutination assay (TPPA) test.

A prenatal serology test for syphilis is mandated by most states and should be performed early in the pregnancy, before fetal damage occurs. A patient who has contracted syphilis requires treatment with an appropriate antibiotic.

Highlight on Gestational Diabetes Mellitus

Definition of Gestational Diabetes Mellitus

Gestational diabetes mellitus (GDM) is a condition in which a pregnant woman who has never had diabetes mellitus develops an elevated glucose level (hyperglycemia). Every year, approximately 2% to 5% of pregnant women in the United States are diagnosed with GDM. Because most women with GDM have no symptoms, the American Diabetes Association recommends that all pregnant women be screened for GDM during the second trimester of the pregnancy. The screening test used is the glucose challenge test, which is performed between 24 and 28 weeks of gestation.

Cause of Gestational Diabetes Mellitus

GDM develops from a physical interaction between the mother and the fetus. The placenta of the fetus produces hormones to preserve the pregnancy. These hormones are excreted into the mother's circulatory system in increasing amounts during the second trimester of pregnancy. These hormones counteract the effect of the mother's insulin, which results in a condition known as *insulin resistance.* In most cases, the mother's pancreas responds to insulin resistance by producing additional insulin to keep the blood glucose at a normal level. Some women are unable to produce enough extra insulin, however, which causes an elevation of their blood glucose level and results in GDM.

Problems for the Child

If GDM is not treated or if it is poorly controlled, problems can occur in the unborn child. The extra glucose crosses the placenta and enters the fetus' circulatory system. To decrease the elevated glucose level, the fetus' pancreas produces large amounts of insulin. The increased insulin converts the extra glucose into fat, resulting in the development of a large infant with a condition known as *macrosomia.* Infants with macrosomia may be too large to be born vaginally and may require a cesarean birth. Although the infant does not have diabetes, he or she is at risk for developing type 2 diabetes later in life. Other problems that can occur at birth include hypoglycemia, breathing difficulties, and jaundice.

Problems for the Mother

Problems that a mother with GDM develops include an increased incidence of preeclampsia, infection, postpartum bleeding, and injury to the birth canal if the infant is delivered vaginally. Another problem is the development of polyhydramnios (excess amount of amniotic fluid), which causes the uterus to stretch and take up more space in the abdominal cavity. This can result in breathing difficulties for the mother during the pregnancy. GDM almost always resolves after delivery. This is because when the placenta is removed, the hormones causing the problem also are removed. The mother's insulin can work normally without resistance. Some women go on to develop type 2 diabetes later in life, however.

Risk Factors for Gestational Diabetes Mellitus

Certain factors put some women at greater risk for developing GDM. These women are usually screened earlier and more often for GDM during the pregnancy. Risk factors for GDM include the following:

- Obesity
- Family history of diabetes mellitus
- Previous birth of an infant weighing more than 9 lb
- Previous birth of an infant who was stillborn or had a birth defect
- Previous GDM diagnosis
- Age older than 25 years old
- Polyhydramnios
- Belonging to an ethnic group known to have higher rates of GDM (Hispanic, African American, Native American, Asian, Pacific Islanders)

Treatment

If a woman is diagnosed with GDM, the treatment is focused on keeping her glucose at a safe level. This includes special meal plans, exercise, daily blood glucose testing, and insulin injections, if needed. If the blood glucose is controlled during pregnancy, most women with GDM are able to prevent maternal or fetal complications. ■

Rubella Antibody Titer

The rubella antibody titer assesses the level of antibody against rubella (German measles) in the patient's blood and is used to determine whether the woman is immune to rubella. If the mother contracts rubella during pregnancy, serious congenital abnormalities can occur in the fetus. Patients who lack immunity should be immunized against rubella within 6 weeks of delivery.

Rh Antibody Titer (on Rh-Negative Blood Specimens)

An Rh antibody titer detects the amount of circulating Rh antibodies against red blood cells. These antibodies can occur in a pregnant woman who is Rh-negative and is carrying an Rh-positive fetus; an Rh antibody titer is performed on all Rh-negative blood specimens. Repeat antibody titer levels also are performed during the pregnancy to determine whether the woman's antibody level is increasing. As previously indicated, an increased Rh antibody level could be dangerous to the developing fetus. As a preventive measure, Rh-negative women with the potential of having an Rh-positive infant and who test negative for Rh antibodies are given two injections of Rh immune globulin (RhoGAM). The Rh immune globulin prevents the formation of the Rh antibodies in the mother, which avoids Rh incompatibility complications during the next pregnancy. The first injection is given at 28 weeks of gestation, and the second injection is administered within 72 hours of delivery.

Hepatitis B and Human Immunodeficiency Virus

The Centers for Disease Control and Prevention recommends that pregnant women have a blood test, the HBsAg test, to screen for hepatitis B virus. Women who have positive HBsAg test results have an increased risk of spontaneous abortion or preterm labor. In addition, the mother may transmit hepatitis B to the infant, particularly during delivery or in the first few days of life. This risk can be greatly reduced by administering hepatitis B immune globulin (HBIG) and the hepatitis B vaccine within 12 hours of birth to the newborns of women who have tested positive for hepatitis B. It also is recommended that testing for human immunodeficiency virus (HIV), the virus that causes AIDS, be offered to all pregnant women, particularly women at risk for contracting HIV. Infants born to women who are HIV positive are at risk of developing the disease.

Return Prenatal Visits

Return prenatal visits provide the opportunity for a continuous assessment of the health of the mother and the fetus. During each visit, essential data are collected and recorded in the prenatal record, resulting in an updated record at each visit, as discussed in this section. If signs or symptoms of a pathologic condition are present, the physician performs selected aspects of the physical examination as necessary to diagnose and treat the condition. In addition, diagnostic and laboratory tests may be ordered to assist in diagnosis and treatment. The usual schedule of visits for prenatal care is listed below. A patient who exhibits complications is seen more frequently for closer monitoring.

- Every 4 weeks for the first 28 weeks
- Every 2 weeks until 36 weeks
- Weekly thereafter until delivery

The return prenatal visit also provides the opportunity for the physician and the medical assistant to lend support to the mother, to provide her with ongoing prenatal education to reduce apprehension and anxiety, and to ensure that the mother is well informed and prepared during her pregnancy, childbirth, and the postpartum period. The medical assistant plays an important role in prenatal education and should take the necessary time with each patient to provide appropriate information and to allow the patient to ask questions. Procedure 8-3 outlines the medical assistant's role in the return prenatal visit.

The patient is asked to obtain a urine specimen during each return prenatal visit. The medical assistant is responsible for testing the specimen for glucose and protein using a reagent strip and for recording results in the prenatal record. A positive reaction to glucose may indicate the development of gestational diabetes mellitus or a prediabetic condition, and a positive reaction to protein may indicate a urinary tract infection or preeclampsia. Further testing usually is needed to arrive at a final diagnosis and to institute treatment.

During the return visit, the physician performs one or more of the following procedures, depending on the stage of the pregnancy: (1) palpation of the woman's abdomen to measure fundal height, (2) measurement of the fetal heart rate, and (3) a vaginal examination. These procedures are discussed in detail next.

Fundal Height Measurement

The pregnant uterus rises gradually into the abdominal cavity, and the fundus is palpable between 8 and 13 weeks of gestation. The first fundal height measurement, which is usually performed during the first prenatal visit, is used as a guideline for all subsequent measurements. The physician measures the fundal height by placing one end of a flexible, nonstretchable centimeter tape measure on the superior aspect of the symphysis pubis and measuring to the crest or top of the uterine fundus (Figure 8-13). The measurement is recorded on a flow chart in the patient's prenatal record. By 20 weeks, the fundus reaches the lower border of the umbilicus, and between 36 and 37 weeks, it reaches the tip of the sternum. During the first and second trimesters, measuring the fundal height provides a rough estimate of the duration of the pregnancy (Figure 8-14). The fundal height measurement is considered accurate to within 4 weeks using McDonald's rule.

Calculation of the duration of the pregnancy using McDonald's rule is as follows:

Height of fundus (in centimeters) $\times$ 8/7 =
$$\text{duration of the pregnancy in weeks}$$

Example: 21 cm $\times$ 8/7 = 24 weeks

Height of fundus (in centimeters) $\times$ 2/7 =
$$\text{duration of the pregnancy in lunar months}$$

Example: 21 cm $\times$ 2/7 = 6 months

Because fetal weights vary considerably during the third trimester, it is difficult to use fundal height measurements as an estimate of the duration of the pregnancy in the last trimester.

In addition to assessing the duration of the pregnancy, the fundal height measurements permit variations from normal to become apparent and are used to assess whether fetal development is progressing normally. Growth that is too rapid or too slow must be evaluated further by the physician as a possible indication of high-risk conditions, such as multiple pregnancies, polyhydramnios, ovarian tumor, and intrauterine growth retardation, intrauterine death, or an error in estimating the fetal progress.

Fetal Heart Tones

The normal **fetal heart rate** is between 120 and 160 beats per minute with a regular rhythm. A very slow or rapid fetal heart rate usually indicates fetal distress. The term **fetal heart tones** refers to the heartbeat of the fetus as heard through the mother's abdominal wall. The fetal heart tones can be heard with a Doppler fetal pulse detector between 10 and 12 weeks

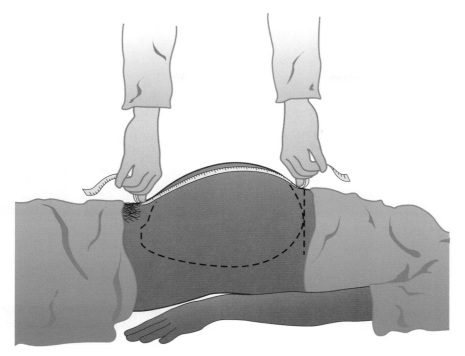

Figure 8-13. Measurement of fundal height. The physician places one end of a centimeter tape measure on the superior aspect of the symphysis pubis and measures to the top of the uterine fundus.

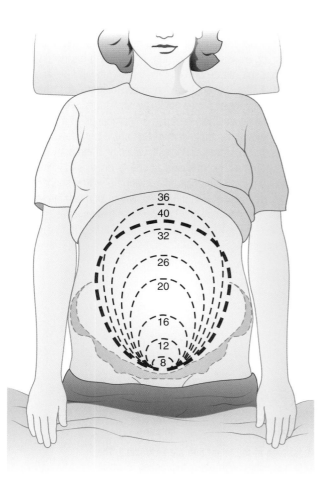

Figure 8-14. Fundal height showing gestational age in weeks.

of gestation. The Doppler fetal pulse detector converts ultrasonic waves into audible sounds of the fetal pulse.

The Doppler device consists of a main control unit and a probe (Figure 8-15A). The probe head contains a transducer and electronic components, which generate the sound waves. The probe head is delicate and must be handled carefully, making sure not to drop or knock the head to prevent damaging it.

Because air is a poor conductor of sound, an ultrasound coupling gel must first be spread on the mother's abdomen in the area to be examined. The gel is usually applied by the medical assistant, and its purpose is to increase conductivity of the sound waves between the abdomen and the transducer.

The physician places the head of the probe into the gel on the mother's abdomen and slowly moves it until the fetal heart tones are located. The Doppler device amplifies the fetal heart tones, and they are broadcast through a built-in loudspeaker in the main unit. A volume control provides adjustment of the sound level as required. (Fetal heart tones sound like the hoofbeats of a galloping horse, and when the probe is over the placenta, a windlike sound is heard.) The Doppler device also may have an LCD screen, which provides a digital display of the fetal pulse rate. Stereo headphones come with the Doppler device to allow private listening. The loudspeaker is muted when the headphones are connected (Figure 8-15B).

After the procedure, the medical assistant should remove excess gel from the mother's abdomen with a paper towel. The probe head is cleaned using a damp cloth or a paper

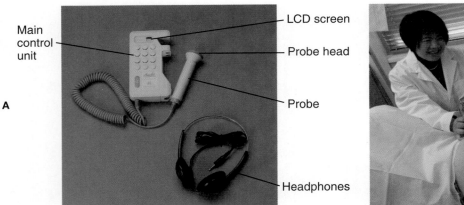

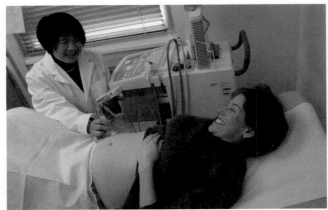

Figure 8-15. A, Parts of a Doppler device. **B,** The probe of the Doppler device is moved across the abdomen to detect the fetal pulse.

towel. The Doppler device should be properly stored in its carrying case to prevent it from becoming damaged.

Vaginal Examination

In the absence of vaginal bleeding, vaginal examinations may be performed at any time during the pregnancy; however, in a normal pregnancy, there is usually no need to perform a vaginal examination until the patient nears term. The vaginal examination is usually begun approximately 2 to 3 weeks from the EDD and is performed to confirm the presenting part and to determine the degree, if any, of cervical dilation and effacement. The purpose of dilation and effacement is to permit the passage of the infant from the uterus into the birth canal (Figure 8-16).

Special Tests and Procedures

The pregnancy can be evaluated with one or more of the following special tests and procedures: triple screen test, obstetric ultrasound scan, amniocentesis, and fetal heart rate monitoring. These are not considered routine procedures; however, they involve little or no risk to the mother or the fetus. Because some of these tests may be performed in the obstetric medical office, the medical assistant should have a general knowledge of these procedures.

What Would You Do? What Would You *Not* Do?

Case Study 4

Wynita Lopez is at the office with her husband. She is 32 years old and 18 weeks pregnant. It took Wynita a long time, almost 6 years, to get pregnant. She is excited and happy about being pregnant but, at the same time, sad and confused. Her test results on her triple screen test came back indicating the possibility that her baby has Down syndrome. A repeat test was done with the same results. Wynita just got finished having an ultrasound that showed a normal baby, but Wynita and her husband understand that the only way to know for sure is to have an amniocentesis. Wynita does not know what to do. She is afraid of having an amniocentesis because of the chance of miscarriage. She also knows her triple screen test could be a false-positive. Wynita is unsure what her decision would be if the baby did have Down syndrome. Her husband is visibly distressed and wants Wynita to make all the decisions, saying he will be supportive of whatever she decides. Right now she wants as much information as she can get about all of this before she makes a decision. She feels "safer" being at the medical office and does not want to go home just yet. ■

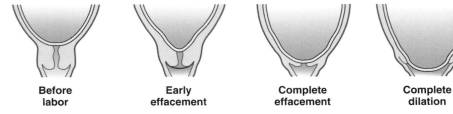

| **Before labor** | **Early effacement** | **Complete effacement** | **Complete dilation** |

Figure 8-16. Effacement and dilation occur to permit the passage of the infant into the birth canal. The cervical canal shortens from its normal length of 1 to 2 cm to a structure with paper-thin edges in which there is no canal at all. The cervix dilates from an opening a few millimeters wide to an opening large enough to allow the passage of the infant (approximately 10 cm).

Triple Screen Test

The triple screen test is a laboratory test available to pregnant women between 15 and 20 weeks of gestation. Its purpose is to screen for the presence of certain fetal abnormalities, which include neural tube defects, Down syndrome, trisomy 18, and ventral wall defect. Because the triple screen test has a high incidence of false-positive test results, it is not a mandatory prenatal test; however, the American College of Obstetricians and Gynecologists believes that this test should be offered to all pregnant women regardless of maternal age.

The triple screen test measures the level of the following three substances normally produced by the fetus and placenta and excreted into the mother's blood in the second trimester of pregnancy: alpha-fetoprotein (AFP), unconjugated estriol (uEST), and human chorionic gonadotropin (hCG).

AFP is a glycoprotein produced by the fetus. During pregnancy, some AFP crosses from the amniotic fluid to the mother's bloodstream. When the neural tube of the fetus is not properly formed, increased amounts of AFP appear in the maternal blood. Elevated AFP levels indicate the possibility of a neural tube defect in the fetus, such as spina bifida (incomplete closure of the spinal column) and anencephaly (incomplete closure of the brain).

A lower serum level of AFP and estriol, along with a higher level of hCG, is associated with an increased risk of having an infant with Down syndrome. A woman who is carrying a fetus with trisomy 18 may have lower blood levels of AFP, estriol, and hCG than women with unaffected fetuses.

The triple screen test is a screening test. Abnormal test results always require further testing, such as ultrasound or amniocentesis, to determine whether a fetal abnormality actually exists.

Obstetric Ultrasound Scan

An obstetric ultrasound scan is a diagnostic imaging technique, similar to sonar, used to view the fetus in utero. It allows continuous viewing of the fetus and shows fetal movement. The physician or an ultrasound technologist performs the procedure. The primary purpose of an ultrasound scan is to evaluate the health of the fetus and to determine gestational age. This is accomplished by viewing the image of the fetus and by taking various measurements of the image, such as the crown-rump length; biparietal diameter, which is a side-to-side measurement of the fetal head; femur length; and abdominal circumference.

Obstetric ultrasound scanning uses high-frequency sound waves that are directed into the uterus through a transducer. When the sound waves reach the uterus, they "bounce" back to the transducer, similar to an echo. These reflected sound waves are converted into an image, or *sonogram* (Figure 8-17), which is displayed on a monitor screen. The monitor is usually positioned so the mother can observe the image on the screen if she wishes. There are two methods for performing an ultrasound scan—the transabdominal method and the endovaginal method.

Transabdominal Ultrasound Scan

Transabdominal ultrasound is the scanning method performed most often. The patient must have a full bladder for this examination. This is accomplished by instructing the patient to consume 32 oz of fluid approximately 1 hour before the procedure. A full bladder acts as an "acoustic window" through which the sound waves can travel to provide a clear visualization of the uterus. In addition, a full bladder holds the uterus stable and pushes away any bowel that might interfere with the image. The patient lies on an examining table in a supine position and is draped with the abdomen exposed. A coupling agent, in the form of a liquid gel, is applied to the patient's abdomen to increase the transmission of the sound waves. An abdominal probe (containing a transducer) is placed into the gel, and the probe is moved slowly over the patient's abdomen; the image of the fetus is displayed on the screen of the monitor (see Figure 8-17).

Endovaginal Ultrasound Scan

In the early stages of the pregnancy (up to 12 weeks), endovaginal scanning is preferred over transabdominal scanning. The patient must have an empty bladder for this scan, which makes the examination more comfortable. The patient is placed in the lithotomy position, and a vaginal probe is placed in the patient's vagina. The image of the embryo is displayed on the screen of the monitor. An endovaginal ultrasound scan provides clearer visualization of the uterus in the beginning of the pregnancy because the probe is situated in the vagina, which places it closer to the uterus.

Although an obstetric ultrasound scan can be performed at any time during the pregnancy, it is often performed between 7 and 12 weeks of gestation and again between 18 and 20 weeks. A third scan is sometimes done around 34 weeks of gestation. Box 8-1 outlines this schedule and what can be assessed at these times.

Amniocentesis

Amniocentesis is a diagnostic procedure that can be performed between 15 and 18 weeks' gestation. Amniocentesis

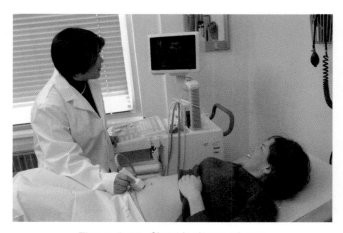

Figure 8-17. Obstetric ultrasound scan.

BOX 8-1 Purpose of Obstetric Ultrasound Scanning

Between 7 and 12 Weeks

- To confirm pregnancy by detecting fetal heart motion
- To determine gestational age by taking measurements of the embryo and embryonic sac
- To detect an ectopic pregnancy

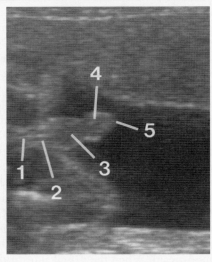

Erect fetal penis. *1,* urethra; *2,* corpus cavernosum; *3,* shaft; *4,* glans; *5,* foreskin. (From Callen P: *Ultrasonography in obstetrics and gynecology,* ed 4, Philadelphia, 2000, Saunders.)

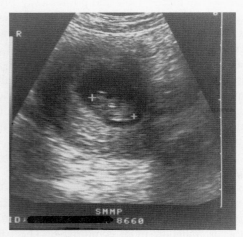

Embryo at approximately 9 weeks' gestation. (From Greer I, et al: *Mosby's color atlas and text of obstetrics and gynecology,* St. Louis, 2001, Mosby.)

Between 18 and 20 Weeks

- To determine fetal growth, size, and weight by taking measurements of the fetus
- To detect the presence of multiple fetuses
- To examine the brain, spinal cord, heart, lungs, gastrointestinal tract, reproductive organs, kidneys, bladder, bowel, and extremities of the fetus
- To detect congenital abnormalities
- To determine the location of the placenta
- To determine the cause of bleeding or spotting

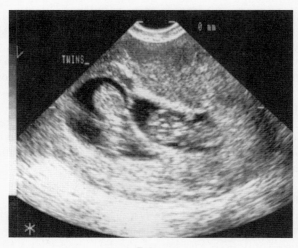

Twins.

aids in prenatal diagnosis of certain genetically transmitted errors of metabolism, congenital abnormalities, and chromosomal disorders such as Down syndrome. It also is used to detect fetal jeopardy or distress and, later in the pregnancy, to assess fetal lung maturity. Amniocentesis also can determine whether the infant is a boy or girl.

To perform the procedure, the physician inserts a long, thin needle through the mother's abdomen and into the amniotic sac surrounding the fetus (Figure 8-18). An obstetric ultrasound scan is always performed in conjunction with amniocentesis so that the physician can view the posi-

tion of the fetus, placenta, and amniotic fluid. This allows the physician to know the exact place to insert the needle. The physician withdraws a sample (about 1 tablespoon) of fluid, which contains fetal cells. The fluid is sent to a laboratory for study. It usually takes 1 to 3 weeks to evaluate the amniotic fluid and report the results.

Although the complication rate for an amniocentesis is extremely low, it is not risk-free. There is a slight risk of bleeding, leakage of fluid, and infection of the amniotic fluid. There also is a slight possibility of miscarriage. Because of these risks, amniocentesis is offered only to women whose

BOX 8-1 Purpose of Obstetric Ultrasound Scanning—cont'd

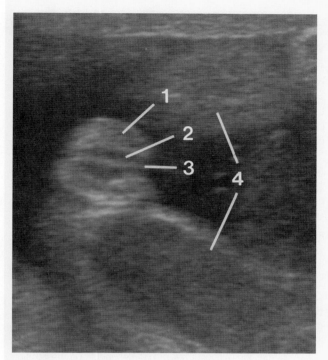

External female genitalia. *1,* major labium; *2,* minor labium; *3,* vaginal cleft; *4,* thighs. (From Callen P: *Ultrasonography in obstetrics and gynecology,* ed 4, Philadelphia, 2000, Saunders.)

At 34 Weeks

- To evaluate fetal growth, size, and weight by taking measurements of the fetus
- To verify location of the placenta
- To confirm fetal presentation in uncertain cases

Other Purposes

- To diagnose uterine and pelvic abnormalities during pregnancy
- To view the fetus, placenta, and amniotic fluid during tests such as amniocentesis and chorionic villus sampling
- To confirm intrauterine death

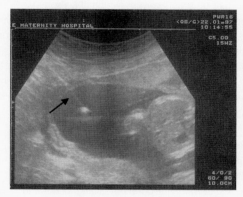

Amniocentesis being performed under ultrasound guidance. (From Greer I, et al: *Mosby's color atlas and text of obstetrics and gynecology,* St. Louis, 2001, Mosby.)

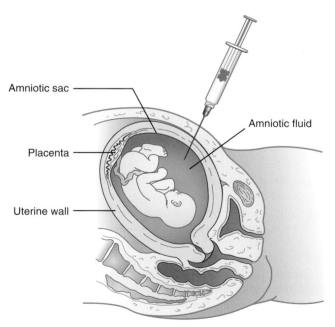

Figure 8-18. Amniocentesis.

pregnancies are at risk for fetal abnormalities. This includes women who are 35 years old or older, women who have a child with a genetic or neural tube defect, women who have abnormal triple screen test results, women who have or whose partner has a chromosomal abnormality, and women who are or whose partner is a carrier for a metabolic disease.

Fetal Heart Rate Monitoring

Fetal heart rate (FHR) monitoring is performed later in the pregnancy to obtain information on the physical condition of the fetus. Specific conditions that may warrant this procedure are fetal growth that is not progressing well, decreased amniotic fluid, decreased fetal activity, elevation of the mother's blood pressure, gestational diabetes, and an overdue infant.

To perform the procedure, an electronic microphone is strapped to the mother's abdomen to amplify the fetal heartbeat. A gel is usually applied under the microphone to make the sounds clearer. The fetal heartbeat is heard and displayed on a screen and printed on special paper.

PATIENT TEACHING **Obstetric Ultrasound Scan**

1. Emphasize the importance of preparing properly for the examination.
2. Provide the patient with educational materials on obstetric ultrasound.
3. Answer questions patients have about an obstetric ultrasound scan.

What is an ultrasound scan?

An ultrasound scan is performed to look at the fetus in the uterus with the use of sound waves. During the examination, a gel is spread over your abdomen, and a scanning device is moved lightly over the area. The baby's image is displayed on a monitor similar to a television screen. During the examination, pictures of your baby will be taken and you will be given a copy for your baby album. If you choose, you may bring a standard VHS tape for the ultrasonographer to record your baby on videotape. The ultrasound examination usually takes about 30 minutes.

Why is an ultrasound scan performed?

Ultrasound scanning is used to determine the age and position of the fetus, the location of the placenta, and the number of babies present, and overall to help the physician monitor and manage the pregnancy.

What preparation is needed?

To prepare for an obstetric (transabdominal) ultrasound scan, you will need to drink 32 oz of fluid 1 hour before the examination. Drink all the water within 15 to 20 minutes, and do not void until the examination has been completed. You should wear comfortable clothing. A two-piece outfit is recommended so that you do not have to undress completely.

Is an ultrasound scan safe?

There are no known side effects or risks to either mother or fetus during an ultrasound examination. Ultrasound does not use x-rays. No long-term risks have been detected. The procedure is painless, and the only discomfort is from a full bladder, which will make you want to go to the bathroom. When the examination is completed, you will have the opportunity to do so.

Can I learn the sex of my baby through an ultrasound scan?

Although an ultrasound scan is not performed only to determine the sex of the baby, it is sometimes possible (usually by 20 weeks) to tell whether the baby is a boy or girl, depending on the position of the baby in the uterus. Because not all parents want to know their baby's sex in advance, you will not automatically be told the baby's sex if it is determined, but you will be given the opportunity to make the choice of knowing or not knowing. ■

There are two kinds of fetal heart rate monitoring procedures—the nonstress test and the contraction stress test. The *nonstress test* (NST) monitors changes in the fetal heart rate in response to the fetus' spontaneous movements. The mother is instructed to press a button when she feels the fetus move. In a normal test, the fetus' heart rate increases when the fetus moves. To prepare for the nonstress test, the mother must be instructed to eat a light meal within 2 hours of the procedure to stimulate fetal movement.

If the results of the nonstress test are abnormal, a *contraction stress test* (CST) may be performed. This test is similar to the nonstress test except that mild contractions of the uterus are stimulated for a short period of time. The contraction stress test is used to evaluate the response of the fetus' heart rate to the contractions to determine whether the fetus would be able to withstand the stress of repeated contractions during labor. If the results of the test are ab-

normal, further evaluation is required to evaluate the well-being of the fetus and to determine how and when delivery of the fetus should be carried out.

Medical Assisting Responsibilities

The medical assistant has many important responsibilities in the return prenatal examination, which are outlined in Procedure 8-3. The medical assistant is responsible for assembling the equipment and supplies required for the examination, for obtaining information to update the prenatal record, for preparing the patient for the examination, and for assisting the physician during the examination. The physician depends on the medical assistant to have the urine test results and certain measurements, such as blood pressure and weight, completed and recorded in advance to allow him or her the opportunity to review these measurements before examining the patient.

Text continued on p. 309

PROCEDURE 8-3   Assisting with a Return Prenatal Examination

Outcome Assist with a return prenatal examination.

Equipment/Supplies

- Urine specimen container
- Centimeter tape measure
- Doppler fetal pulse detector
- Ultrasound coupling gel
- Paper towel

- Disposable vaginal speculum
- Disposable gloves
- Water-based lubricant
- Gauze pads
- Examining gown and drape

---

1. Procedural Step. Sanitize your hands.

2. Procedural Step. Set up the tray for the prenatal examination. The equipment and supplies depend on the procedures to be included in the examination, which may include one or more of the following:
   a. Fundal height measurement
   b. Measurement of fetal heart tones
   c. Examination of the legs, feet, and face for edema and development of varicosities
   d. Taking a specimen for the diagnosis of a vaginal infection
   e. Vaginal examination

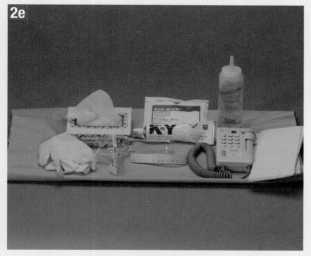

Set up the prenatal tray.

3. Procedural Step. Greet the patient and introduce yourself. Identify the patient and explain the procedure. Provide the patient with a urine specimen container, and ask her to obtain a urine specimen.
Principle. A urine specimen is needed to test for glucose and protein at each prenatal visit. In addition, an empty bladder makes the examination easier and is more comfortable for the patient.

4. Procedural Step. Escort the patient to the examining room, and ask her to be seated. Seat yourself so that you are facing the patient. Ask the patient whether she has experienced any problems since the last prenatal visit, and record information in the appropriate section in her prenatal record.
Principle. The physician investigates any unusual or abnormal signs or symptoms relayed by the patient.

5. Procedural Step. Measure the patient's blood pressure, and chart the results in the prenatal record. If the blood pressure is elevated, allow the patient to relax, and then measure the blood pressure again.
Principle. Taking the blood pressure again gives the opportunity to determine whether the elevation was due to emotional excitement.

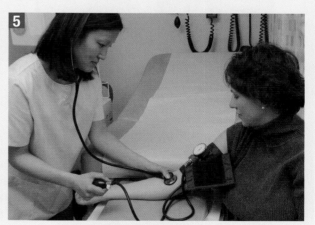

Measure the patient's blood pressure.

PROCEDURE 8-3

Continued

PROCEDURE 8-3　Assisting with a Return Prenatal Examination—cont'd

6. Procedural Step. Weigh the patient, and chart the results in the prenatal record.

Principle. Maternal weight gain or loss assists in assessing fetal development, as well as the mother's nutrition and state of health.

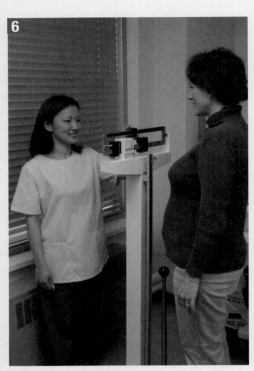

Weigh the patient.

7. Procedural Step. Instruct and prepare the patient for the examination. Have her remove or pull up her outer clothing to expose the abdominal area. If the physician will be performing a vaginal examination, the patient also must remove her panties; otherwise, she may leave them on. Tell the patient to have a seat on the examining table when she is finished getting ready for the exam. Inform the patient that the physician will be with her soon and leave the room to give her privacy.

8. Procedural Step. Using a reagent strip, test the urine specimen for glucose and protein, and chart the results. *Note:* The urine specimen may be tested at any time before the physician examines the patient; however, a convenient time to test the specimen is while the patient is disrobing.

Principle. The prenatal patient's urine must be tested at every visit to assist in the early detection and prevention of disease.

9. Procedural Step. Make the medical record available for review by the physician. The medical office has a designated location where the record is placed, such as a small shelf mounted on the wall next to the outside of the examining room door or in a chart holder on the outside of the examining room door. Position the medical record so that patient-identifiable information is not visible.

Principle: Before going into the room, the physician will want to review the patient's chart and information documented by the medical assistant. HIPAA requires protection of a patient's health information.

10. Procedural Step. Check to make sure the patient is ready to be seen by the physician. Before entering a patient's room, always knock lightly on the door to let the patient know you are getting ready to enter the room. Inform the physician. This may be done using a color-coded flagging system mounted on the wall next to the examining room.

11. Procedural Step. Assist the patient into a supine position, and properly drape her. Provide support and reassurance to the patient to help her relax during the examination.

Principle. The patient should be properly draped so that she is warm and comfortable.

12. Procedural Step. Assist the physician as required for the prenatal examination, as follows:

a. **Fundal Height Measurement:** Hand the physician the tape measure for the determination of the fundal measurement.

b. **Fetal Heart Tones:** Apply a liberal amount of coupling gel to the patient's abdomen. Turn on the Doppler fetal pulse detector and hand it to the physician. When the physician is finished, remove excess gel from the patient with a paper towel. Clean the probe head of the Doppler device with a damp cloth or a paper towel. Place the probe head back in its holder.

c. **Vaginal Specimen:** Assist the patient into the lithotomy position if a specimen is to be taken for the detection of a vaginal infection. Assist with the collection of the specimen as required.

d. **Vaginal Examination:** Assist the patient into the lithotomy position if a vaginal examination is to be performed.

13. Procedural Step. After the examination, assist the patient into a sitting position, and allow her the opportunity to rest for a moment. If a vaginal examination was performed, offer the patient tissues to remove excess lubricating jelly from the perineum. Assist her off the examining table to prevent falls. Instruct the patient to get dressed. Leave the room to provide the patient with privacy.

Principle. The patient may become dizzy after being on the examining table and should be allowed to rest

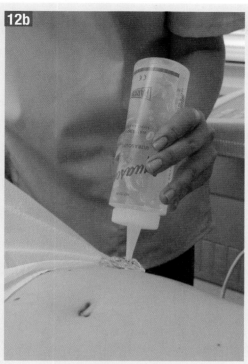

Apply a liberal amount of coupling gel.

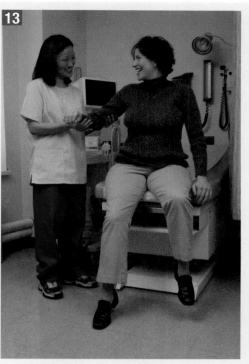

Assist the patient off the examining table.

before getting off the table. The medical assistant must provide for the safety of the prenatal patient while she is getting off the examining table.

14. **Procedural Step.** Provide prenatal patient teaching and further explanation of the physician's instructions as required to meet individual patient needs. Escort the patient to the reception area.

15. **Procedural Step.** Clean the examining room in preparation for the next patient, and, if necessary, prepare specimens for transport to an outside medical laboratory.

SIX WEEKS–POSTPARTUM VISIT

The **puerperium** includes the period of time in which the body systems are returning to their prepregnant or nearly prepregnant state, which usually is 4 to 6 weeks after delivery. During this time, numerous changes occur in the woman's body. The *involution of the uterus* (i.e., the process by which it returns to its normal size and state) occurs; this includes healing of any injuries sustained to the birth canal during delivery.

During the puerperium, the patient experiences a vaginal discharge shed from the lining of the uterus, known as **lochia.** Lochia consists of blood, tissue, white blood cells, mucus, and some bacteria. The color of the lochia is an indication of the progress of the healing of the uterus. For the first 3 days after delivery, the lochia consists almost entirely of blood and, because of its red color, is termed *lochia rubra.* By approximately 4 days postpartum, the amount of blood decreases, and the discharge becomes pink or brownish and is known as *lochia serosa.* By 10 days postpartum, the flow should decrease, and the lochia should become yellowish white; this is known as *lochia alba.* Lochia usually

continues in consistently decreasing amounts (from moderate to scant to occasional spotting) and becomes paler in color until the third week after delivery, when it usually disappears altogether. It would not be considered unusual for the discharge to last the entire 6 weeks, however.

The patient should be instructed to contact the medical office under the following circumstances: if the amount of discharge increases rather than decreases; if the discharge is absent within the first 2 weeks after delivery; if it changes to red after having been yellowish white, which indicates bleeding; or if it takes on a foul odor, which indicates infection. Menstruation usually begins approximately 2 months after delivery in a nonnursing mother and 3 to 6 months after delivery in a nursing mother.

During the puerperium, the patient should be encouraged to avoid fatigue, to avoid lifting heavy objects, and to consume a nutritious, well-balanced diet that helps maintain health and promote healing. The physician will want to see the patient at the medical office at the end of the 6-week period. The purpose of the 6 weeks–postpartum visit is to evaluate the general physical condition of the patient, to

Table 8-3 Six Weeks–Postpartum Examination

Procedure	Purpose

Vital Signs (see Chapter 4)
Temperature
    Pulse
    Respiration
    Blood pressure
	To ensure vital signs fall within normal limits and that blood pressure has returned to normal prepregnant level

Weight (see Chapter 5)	To determine whether patient's weight has returned to prepregnant measurement. If not, nutritional counseling may be indicated
Breast Examination (Chapter 8)	To ensure breasts are not sore or tender and no cysts or lumps are present In nonnursing mother, breasts are examined to determine whether they have returned to their prepregnant size In nursing mother, nipples are examined for cracks, redness, soreness, and fissures
Pelvic Examination (Chapter 8)	To ensure involution of uterus is complete and to determine whether cervix has healed To ensure episiotomy (if performed) and any injuries sustained by birth canal have healed To ensure no abnormal vaginal discharge is present
Rectal-Vaginal Examination (Chapter 8)	To ensure pelvic floor has regained its muscle tone To determine whether hemorrhoids are present
Evaluation of Patient's General Physical Condition (see Chapter 5)	To ensure body systems have returned to their prepregnant state

ensure there are no residual problems from childbearing, and to provide the patient with education regarding methods of contraception and infant care. During this visit the patient is queried about problems or abnormalities related to vaginal discharge, urinary or bowel function, and breastfeeding if she is nursing. This information is recorded in the patient's chart. The postpartum visit provides an excellent opportunity for the medical assistant to instruct the patient in the technique for performing a breast self-examination and to educate her in the importance of returning to the medical office annually for a Pap test.

During the postpartum examination, the physician evaluates the patient's general appearance, performs breast and pelvic examinations, and checks to determine whether the muscle tone has returned to the muscles of the abdominal wall. During the puerperium, atypical cells may be sloughed off into the cervical and vaginal mucus as part of the normal healing process. Because of this, the Pap test is not included in the postpartum visit. If the patient has problems with hemorrhoids or varicosities, the physician discusses any

further treatment required. If the patient does not have antibody protection to rubella, as has been evidenced through the prenatal laboratory tests, she receives rubella immunization at this time (if it was not administered in the hospital). In addition, hemoglobin and hematocrit determinations usually are performed on the postpartum patient to screen for anemia caused by blood loss during delivery and the puerperium.

The responsibilities of the medical assistant during the postpartum visit include measuring and recording the patient's vital signs and weight and preparing the patient for the examination. The patient is required to disrobe completely for this examination and to put on an examining gown with the opening in front. Table 8-3 lists the procedures commonly included in the 6 weeks–postpartum visit and the purpose of each.

 *Check out the **Companion CD** bound with the book to access additional interactive activities.*

MEDICAL PRACTICE *and the* LAW

Mature Minor

A difficult and complex issue facing policy makers today involves whether a minor should be able to obtain health care services without a parent's consent. A minor is an individual who has not reached the age of majority; in most states, minors reach majority

at 18 years old (at that time, individuals are legally able to make their own decisions regarding health care).

Over the past 3 decades, many states have passed legislation permitting minors to receive some health care services without parental consent. These include contraceptive services, testing and

MEDICAL PRACTICE and the LAW—cont'd

treatment for sexually transmitted diseases, prenatal care and delivery services, treatment for alcohol and drug abuse, and outpatient mental health care. States that have passed such legislation reason that some minors might avoid seeking the care that they need for certain conditions if they had to have parental consent. The one major exception to this is abortion. Most states have laws that require the involvement of at least one parent in a minor's decision to have an abortion.

In recent years, some states have given minors even greater authority to make health care decisions for themselves by adopting what is known as the *mature minor rule.* This allows an individual in the middle to late teens who exhibits the intelligence and maturity to understand the nature and consequences of a medi-

cal treatment to consent to such treatment without parental consent.

It is important for the medical assistant to become familiar with the laws in his or her state regarding a minor's right to consent to health care to help the medical assistant in making appropriate decisions with respect to minors. For example, if a state does not allow a minor to obtain prenatal care without parental consent, the medical assistant would not be permitted to make an appointment for a minor who is pregnant; rather, it would have to be scheduled by the minor's parent. Consent by minors to health care services will continue to be a complex issue; the medical assistant must keep up-to-date with changes in his or her state. ∎

What What You Do? What Would You *Not* Do? RESPONSES

Case Study 1
Page 268
What Did Yin-Ling Do?

❑ Reassured Mrs. Wooster that the physician is there to help her and stressed that he will be pleased that she has come to the office for an examination.

❑ Commended Mrs. Wooster on performing a breast self-examination at home and encouraged her to continue performing a BSE each month. Asked her whether she had any questions on how to perform a BSE.

❑ Told Mrs. Wooster that some breast changes are normal and others are not normal, and the only way to know for sure is to be examined by the physician.

❑ Told Mrs. Wooster that it is important to have a periodic gynecologic examination even if her periods are normal. Explained to her that some conditions can be present without symptoms. Took plenty of time with her so that she would feel comfortable coming back again in the future for a gynecologic examination. Gave Mrs. Wooster a patient information brochure on gynecologic examinations.

❑ Gave Mrs. Wooster a patient information brochure on mammograms, and explained the mammogram procedure to reduce her apprehension. Explained that the procedure is not painful, but there may be some minor discomfort. Provided her with some tips on reducing discomfort that may occur, such as avoiding caffeine several days before the procedure and having the office schedule the mammogram a week after her menstrual period.

What Did Yin-Ling Not Do?

❑ Did not criticize Mrs. Wooster for waiting so long to schedule a gynecologic examination.

❑ Did not tell Mrs. Wooster that there is no discomfort involved with a mammogram.

What Would You Do?/What Would You *Not* Do? Review Yin-Ling's response and place a checkmark next to the information you included in your response. List additional information you included in your response.

_____
_____
_____
_____

Case Study 2
Page 288
What Did Yin-Ling Do?

❑ Stressed to Dagny how important it is that she be seen by the physician. Explained that she could be infected with chlamydia and not know it because chlamydia often has no symptoms, especially in women.

❑ Explained to Dagny that state law allows her to be treated for a sexually transmitted disease without permission from her parents. Told her the law was created to encourage minors to seek treatment for sexually transmitted diseases.

❑ Commended Dagny on practicing safe sex. Relayed to her that if a condom is not used correctly, or if it tears, she might not be protected from getting a sexually transmitted disease. That is another reason she should be tested.

❑ Explained to Dagny what will occur during the examination and what the physician will be doing. Relayed techniques that Dagney could use to relax during the procedure.

What Did Yin-Ling Not Do?

❑ Did not tell Dagny everything would be all right and that she probably does not have chlamydia.

❑ Did not ask Dagny whether she knew how her boyfriend got chlamydia.

Continued

What What You Do? | What Would You *Not* Do? | RESPONSES—cont'd

❏ If Dagny still insisted on leaving, did not try to prevent her from doing so.

What Would You Do?/What Would You *Not* Do? Review Yin-Ling's response and place a checkmark next to the information you included in your response. List additional information you included in your response.

_____

_____

_____

_____

Case Study 3
Page 298
What Did Yin-Ling Do?

❏ Tried to calm Johanna by telling her that it is normal for her to be worried and concerned. Explained that the purpose of her prenatal visits are so that the physician can keep a close watch on her and detect any problems that might occur.

❏ Reassured Johanna that she does not need to be afraid to tell the physician any of her concerns because he is there to help her and her baby.

❏ Told Johanna that it is important not to take any medications during her pregnancy without first checking with the physician because some medications could be harmful to her baby.

❏ Told Johanna that her problems and concerns would be relayed to the physician and that he would want to talk to her about them. Explained that the physician also would talk with her about being tested for group B streptococcus.

What Did Yin-Ling Not *Do?*

❏ Did not tell Johanna that it was all right to take the antibiotics.

What Would You Do?/What Would You *Not* Do? Review Yin-Ling's response and place a checkmark next to the information you

included in your response. List additional information you included in your response.

_____

_____

_____

_____

Case Study 4
Page 302
What Did Yin-Ling Do?

❏ Escorted Mr. and Mrs. Lopez to a private room in the office. Tried to relax them and told them that whatever they choose to do will be the right decision for them. Reassured them that they could stay at the office for as long as they wanted.

❏ Gave Mrs. Lopez the information she requested that was available at the office and provided her with a list of resources approved by the physician that she could contact for further information.

❏ Asked Mr. and Mrs. Lopez whether they had any more questions they wanted to ask the physician.

What Did Yin-Ling Not *Do?*

❏ Did not give Mr. and Mrs. Lopez advice on what they should do.

What Would You Do?/What Would You *Not* Do? Review Yin-Ling's response and place a checkmark next to the information you included in your response. List additional information you included in your response.

_____

_____

_____

_____

🗣 APPLY YOUR KNOWLEDGE

Choose the best answer to each of the following questions.

Gynecology

1. Ashley Jacobs is 24 years old and has come to the office for her first gynecologic examination. While taking her medical history, Yin-Ling Wu, RMA, obtains the following information. Which of these puts Ashley at an increased risk for breast cancer?
   A. She is taking birth control pills.
   B. She started her periods at age 13.
   C. Her older sister has breast cancer.
   D. She has irregular periods and dysmenorrhea.

2. Yin-Ling helps Ashley into the lithotomy position for the pelvic examination. All of the following should be done when placing a patient in this position *except*:
   A. Positioning the stirrups so that they are level with the examining table.
   B. Pulling the stirrups out 1 foot from the table.
   C. Positioning the patient's buttocks 10 inches from the bottom edge of the table.
   D. Making sure the patient's knees are bent and relaxed.

3. Because Ashley is having a ThinPrep Pap test done, Yin-Ling prepares the disposable plastic vaginal speculum by:
   A. Lightly spraying it with a cytology fixative.
   B. Lubricating it with K-Y jelly.
   C. Polishing it with Windex.
   D. Moistening it with warm water.

4. Ashley asks Yin-Ling why a Pap test is being performed. Yin-Ling tells her:
   A. To diagnose vaginal infections.
   B. For the early detection of cervical cancer.
   C. To evaluate the cause of infertility.
   D. For the early detection of ovarian cancer.

5. After the gynecologic examination, Yin-Ling instructs Ashley on how to perform a breast self-examination. Yin-Ling explains to her that she should perform a BSE once a month:
   A. Any day during the month.
   B. Approximately 2 to 3 days after the start of her menstrual period.
   C. Approximately 2 to 3 days after her menstrual period ends.
   D. On the day she receives her electric bill.

6. Rachel Purdy comes to the office with the symptoms of a yeast infection. Yin-Ling Wu, RMA, is assembling the supplies that will be needed to prepare a vaginal specimen for the microscopic examination of candidiasis. She will need to have ready:
   A. A slide and normal saline.
   B. A live turkey.
   C. A collection and transport tube.
   D. A slide and a 10% KOH solution.

7. Mrs. Purdy has been diagnosed with candidiasis. Dr. Papanicolaou writes a prescription for Mrs. Purdy to treat her condition. A drug used to treat this vaginal infection is:
   A. Miconazole (Monistat).
   B. Azithromycin (Zithromax).
   C. Penicillin (Amoxil).
   D. Metronidazole (Flagyl).

Prenatal

1. Amanda Delaney, who is 33 years old, has come to the office for her first prenatal visit. Amanda asks Yin-Ling Wu, RMA, what is going to happen during the visit. Yin-Ling would relay all of the following *except*:
   A. Measurement of vital signs and weight.
   B. Breast and pelvic examination.
   C. Transabdominal ultrasound scan.
   D. Measurement of fundal height.

2. Yin-Ling obtains information from Amanda for the prenatal record. Amanda has been pregnant before and has a 6-year-old daughter. During the interview, Amanda relays the following information to Yin-Ling. Which statement does *not* provide information for the obstetric history?
   A. My daughter weighed 6 pounds and 8 ounces at birth.
   B. My daughter was born 3 weeks early.
   C. I was in labor for 8 hours with my daughter.
   D. I breastfed my daughter for 6 months.

3. After the prenatal examination, Amanda asks to talk with Yin-Ling in private. She tells Yin-Ling that she is upset that she is being tested for gonorrhea. She says that she has been happily married for 12 years and can't understand why the physician would think she has gonorrhea. Which of the following is the best response to help calm down Amanda?
   A. You may have contracted gonorrhea without knowing it, such as from a toilet seat in a public restroom.
   B. Gonorrhea can cause a serious eye infection in the newborn, which could lead to blindness.
   C. You may be happily married, but we don't know if the same is true for your husband.
   D. There is a state law that says we have to test all pregnant women for gonorrhea.

4. While proofreading the prenatal testing schedule just typed by the medical transcriber, Yin-Ling Wu, RMA, notices a mistake in the schedule. Which of the following should she ask the transcriber to correct?
   A. Transabdominal ultrasound: 18 to 20 weeks.
   B. Triple screen test: 15 to 20 weeks.
   C. GCT: 7 to 12 weeks.
   D. GBS test: 35 to 37 weeks.

5. Amanda Delaney has come to the office for a return prenatal visit. She is now 4 months pregnant. The responsibilities of Yin-Ling Wu, RMA, during this visit include all of the following *except*:
   A. Documenting any problems Amanda has experienced since the last visit.
   B. Testing Amanda's urine specimen for glucose and protein.
   C. Measuring Amanda's weight and blood pressure.
   D. Placing Amanda in the lithotomy position for a vaginal examination.

6. During Amanda's prenatal visit, Dr. Braxton listens for fetal heart tones using a Doppler device. He de-

Continued

APPLY YOUR KNOWLEDGE—cont'd

termines the fetal heart rate to be 145 beats per minute. What does this indicate?

  A. The heart rate is too fast; the fetus may be in distress.

  B. The heart rate is within normal limits.

  C. The heart rate is too slow; the fetus may not be receiving enough oxygen.

  D. The baby is going to have red hair.

7. Amanda is scheduled to have a transabdominal ultrasound scan performed at her next prenatal visit. Which of the following should Yin-Ling relay to Amanda regarding this examination?

  A. You need to drink 32 ounces of fluid 1 hour before the scan.

  B. You may have some spotting after the scan.

  C. You need to fast for 12 hours before the scan.

  D. You will find out whether the baby is a boy or girl.

8. Amanda delivers a healthy 8-lb, 3-oz boy on her due date. Toward the end of her pregnancy, Yin-Ling Wu, RMA, talked with Amanda regarding instructions on postpartum care. Which of the following instructions would Yin-Ling *not* have included in the discussion?

  A. Call the office if you have an increase in the amount of vaginal discharge.

  B. Make an appointment to come in 6 weeks after delivery.

  C. Do not use any type of birth control.

  D. Eat nutritiously and rest as much as possible.

CERTIFICATION REVIEW

❑ **Gynecology** is the branch of medicine that deals with diseases of female reproductive organs. A gynecologic examination includes breast and pelvic examinations. The purpose of the examination is to assess the health status of the female reproductive organs and to detect early signs of disease, leading to early diagnosis and treatment.

❑ **During the breast examination,** the physician inspects the breasts and nipples for swelling, dimpling, puckering, and change in skin texture. The nipples are checked for abnormalities, and the breasts and axial lymph nodes are palpated for lumps. Women should perform a breast self-examination at home each month starting at age 20, approximately 2 to 3 days after the menstrual period ends.

❑ **The purpose of the pelvic examination** is to assess the size, shape, and location of the reproductive organs and to detect the presence of disease. The pelvic examination consists of an inspection of the external genitalia, vagina, and cervix; collection of a specimen for a Pap test; bimanual pelvic examination; and rectal-vaginal examination.

❑ **The purpose of the Pap test** is early detection and treatment of cervical cancer. It also is used to detect abnormal cells that might develop into cancer if not treated. Abnormal cytologic findings on the Pap test indicate the need for further tests, such as colposcopy, cervical biopsy, and endocervical curettage.

❑ **The purpose of the bimanual pelvic examination** is to determine the size, shape, and position of the uterus and ovaries and detect tenderness or lumps. The purpose of the rectal-vaginal examination is to obtain information about the tone and alignment of the pelvic organs and the adnexal region and to collect a fecal specimen for occult blood testing. The presence of hemorrhoids, fistulas, and fissures also can be noted during this examination.

❑ **Trichomoniasis** is a vaginal infection caused by a protozoan and is most commonly spread through sexual intercourse. Symptoms include a profuse, frothy, yellowish-green vaginal discharge with an unpleasant odor; itching and irritation of the vulva and vagina; and dysuria. The cervix may exhibit small red spots; this is known as "strawberry cervix."

❑ **Candidiasis** is a vaginal infection caused by a yeastlike fungus. Conditions such as pregnancy, diabetes mellitus, and prolonged antibiotic therapy may precipitate a candidal infection, commonly referred to as a "yeast infection." Symptoms of candidiasis include white patches on the mucous membrane of the vagina, along with a thick, odorless, cottage cheese–like discharge that results in burning and intense itching.

❑ **Chlamydia** is caused by a bacterium and is the most frequently reported and fastest-spreading sexually transmitted disease in the United States. Most women with chlamydia have no symptoms. Women with symptoms have dysuria; itching and irritation of the genital area; an odorless, thick, yellowish-white vaginal discharge; dull abdominal pain; and bleeding between menstrual periods. If not treated, chlamydia can lead to pelvic inflammatory disease (PID), which can result in infertility.

❑ **Gonorrhea** is an infection of the genitourinary tract and is caused by a bacterium that is transmitted through sexual intercourse. Women who have contracted gonorrhea may be asymptomatic or may exhibit dysuria and a yellow vaginal discharge. As the disease progresses, it may spread to the lining of the uterus, resulting in PID.

❑ **Obstetrics** is the branch of medicine that deals with the supervision of women during pregnancy, childbirth, and the puerperium. *Prenatal* refers to the care of the pregnant woman before delivery of the infant to promote the health of the mother and fetus through the prevention of disease and early detection, diagnosis, and treatment of problems common to pregnancy.

❑ **The first prenatal examination** consists of the completion of a prenatal record form, an initial prenatal examination, prenatal patient education, and laboratory tests.

❑ **The prenatal record** provides information regarding the past and present health of the patient and serves as a database and flow sheet for subsequent prenatal visits. The past medical history focuses on conditions that could affect the health of the mother and fetus. The menstrual history provides information on the patient's menstrual cycle. The obstetric history provides information from the patient related to previous pregnancies. The present pregnancy history establishes a baseline for the present health status of the patient. The purpose of the interval prenatal history is to update the prenatal record at each return visit.

❑ **The expected date of delivery (EDD)** can be determined using Nägele's rule and a gestation calculator. Approximately 4% of patients deliver spontaneously on the EDD, and most patients deliver during the period from 7 days before to 7 days after the EDD.

❑ **The purpose of the initial prenatal examination** is to confirm the pregnancy and to establish a baseline for the woman's state of health. It includes a thorough gynecologic examination (breast and pelvic) and a general physical examination of the other body systems.

❑ **Numerous laboratory tests** are ordered to assist in the overall initial assessment of the patient's health and to detect problems that might put the pregnancy at risk. Prenatal laboratory tests that are performed include a complete urinalysis, Pap test, chlamydia and gonorrhea tests, tests for trichomoniasis and candidiasis (if warranted), group B streptococcus test (GBS) test, complete blood count (CBC), Rh factor and ABO blood type, glucose challenge test (GCT), serology test for syphilis, rubella antibody titer, Rh antibody titer, hepatitis B test, and HIV test.

❑ **Return prenatal visits** provide the opportunity for a continuous assessment of the health of the mother and fetus. During each return prenatal visit, the medical assistant is responsible for measuring the patient's blood pressure and weight and testing the patient's urine for glucose and protein. During the return visit, the physician performs one or more of the following procedures: palpation of the woman's abdomen to measure fundal height, measurement of the fetal heart rate, and a vaginal examination.

❑ **The triple screen test** is performed between 15 and 20 weeks of gestation to screen for certain fetal abnormalities. Abnormal test results may indicate the possibility of a neural tube defect, Down syndrome, trisomy 18, and ventral wall defect.

❑ **Obstetric ultrasound scanning** is used to view the fetus in utero. It is used most frequently to evaluate the health of the fetus and to determine gestational age. There are two methods for performing an ultrasound scan based on gestational age—endovaginal scan (up to 12 weeks' gestation) and transabdominal scan (after 12 weeks' gestation).

❑ **Amniocentesis** is performed to diagnose certain genetically transmitted errors of metabolism, congenital abnormalities, and chromosomal disorders such as Down syndrome. Fetal heart rate monitoring is performed to obtain information on the physical condition of the fetus.

❑ **The puerperium** includes the period of time in which the body systems are returning to the prepregnant or nearly prepregnant state, which usually is 4 to 6 weeks after delivery. The physician will want to see the patient at the medical office at the end of the 6-week period. The purpose of this postpartum visit is to evaluate the general physical condition of the patient, to ensure there are no residual problems from childbearing, and to provide the patient with education regarding methods of birth control and infant care.

⟳ TERMINOLOGY REVIEW

Abortion The termination of the pregnancy before the fetus reached the age of viability (20 weeks).

Adnexal Adjacent.

Amenorrhea The absence or cessation of the menstrual period. Amenorrhea occurs normally before puberty, during pregnancy, and after menopause.

Atypical Deviation from the normal.

Braxton Hicks contractions Intermittent and irregular painless uterine contractions that occur throughout pregnancy. They occur more frequently toward the end of pregnancy and are sometimes mistaken for true labor pains.

Cervix The lower narrow end of the uterus that opens into the vagina.

Colposcopy Examination of the cervix using a colposcope (a lighted instrument with a magnifying lens).

Cytology The science that deals with the study of cells, including their origin, structure, function, and pathology.

Dilation (of the cervix) The stretching of the external os from an opening a few millimeters wide to an opening large enough to allow the passage of an infant (approximately 10 cm).

Dysmenorrhea Pain associated with the menstrual period.

Dyspareunia Pain in the vagina or pelvis experienced by a woman during sexual intercourse.

Dysplasia The growth of abnormal cells. Dysplasia is a precancerous condition that may or may not develop into cancer.

Ectocervix The part of the cervix that projects into the vagina and is lined with stratified squamous epithelium.

EDD Expected date of delivery, or due date.

Effacement The thinning and shortening of the cervical canal from its normal length of 1 to 2 cm to a structure with paper-thin edges in which there is no canal at all. Effacement occurs late in pregnancy, during labor, or both. The purpose of effacement along with dilation is to permit the passage of the infant into the birth canal.

Embryo The child in utero from the time of conception to the beginning of the first trimester.

Endocervix The mucous membrane lining the cervical canal.

Engagement The entrance of the fetal head or the presenting part into the pelvic inlet.

Expected date of delivery (EDD) Projected birth date of the infant.

External os The opening of the cervical canal of the uterus into the vagina.

Fetal heart rate The number of times per minute the fetal heart beats.

Fetal heart tones The sounds of the heartbeat of the fetus heard through the mother's abdominal wall.

Fetus The child in utero from the third month after conception to birth; during the first 2 months of development, it is called an *embryo*.

Fundus The dome-shaped upper portion of the uterus between the fallopian tubes.

Gestation The period of intrauterine development from conception to birth; the period of pregnancy. The average pregnancy lasts about 280 days, or 40 weeks, from the date of conception to childbirth.

Gestational age The age of the fetus between conception and birth.

Gravidity The total number of pregnancies a woman has had regardless of duration, including a current pregnancy.

Gynecology The branch of medicine that deals with the diseases of reproductive organs of women.

Infant A child from birth to 12 months of age.

Internal os The internal opening of the cervical canal into the uterus.

Lochia A discharge from the uterus after delivery that consists of blood, tissue, white blood cells, and some bacteria.

Menopause The permanent cessation of menstruation, which usually occurs between the ages of 45 and 55.

Menorrhagia Excessive bleeding during a menstrual period, in the number of days or the amount of blood or both. Also called *dysfunctional uterine bleeding (DUB)*.

Metrorrhagia Bleeding between menstrual periods.

Multigravida A woman who has been pregnant more than once.

Multipara A woman who has completed two or more pregnancies to the age of fetal viability regardless of whether they ended in live infants or stillbirths.

Nullipara A woman who has not carried a pregnancy to the point of fetal viability (20 weeks of gestation).

Obstetrics The branch of medicine concerned with the care of the woman during pregnancy, childbirth, and the postpartal period.

Parity The condition of having borne offspring regardless of the outcome.

Perimenopause Before the onset of menopause, the phase during which the woman with regular periods changes to irregular cycles and increased periods of amenorrhea.

Perineum The external region between the vaginal orifice and the anus in a female and between the scrotum and the anus in a male.

Position The relation of the presenting part of the fetus to the maternal pelvis.

Postpartum Occurring after childbirth.

Preeclampsia A major complication of pregnancy, the cause of which is unknown, characterized by increasing hypertension, albuminuria, and edema. If this condition is neglected or not treated properly, it may develop into eclampsia, which could cause maternal convulsions and coma. Preeclampsia generally occurs between the 20th week of pregnancy and the end of the first week postpartum.

Prenatal Before birth.

Presentation Indication of the part of the fetus that is closest to the cervix and is delivered first. A cephalic presentation is a delivery in which the fetal head is presenting against the cervix. A breech presentation is a delivery in which the buttocks or feet are presented instead of the head.

Preterm birth Delivery occurring between 20 and 37 weeks of gestation regardless of whether the child was born alive or stillborn.

Primigravida A woman who is pregnant for the first time.

Primipara A woman who has carried a pregnancy to fetal viability (20 weeks of gestation) for the first time, regardless of whether the infant was stillborn or alive at birth.

Puerperium The period of time, usually 4 to 6 weeks after delivery, in which the uterus and the body systems are returning to normal.

Quickening The first movements of the fetus in utero as felt by the mother, which usually occurs between 16 and 20 weeks of gestation and is felt consistently thereafter.

Risk factor Anything that increases an individual's chance of developing a disease. Some risk factors (e.g., smoking) can be avoided, but others cannot (e.g., age and family history).

Term birth Delivery occurring after 37 weeks of gestation regardless of whether the infant was born alive or stillborn.

Toxemia A condition that can occur in pregnant women that includes preeclampsia and eclampsia. If preeclampsia goes undiagnosed or is not satisfactorily controlled, it could develop into eclampsia, characterized by convulsions and coma.

Trimester Three months, or one third, of the gestational period of pregnancy.

Vulva The region of the external female genital organs.

ON THE WEB

For Information on Sexually Transmitted Diseases:

National Institute of Allergy and Infectious Diseases: www.niaid.nih.gov

Centers for Disease Control Division of Sexually Transmitted Diseases (located under Disease Facts and Information): www.cdc.gov/std

Planned Parenthood: www.plannedparenthood.org

American Social Health Association: www.ashastd.org

Herpes Information: www.gotherpes.com

HPV Information: www.gothpv.com

For Information on Women's Health:

The National Women's Health Information Center: www.4women.gov

The Universe of Women's Health: www.obgyn.net

For Information on Contraceptives:

Planned Parenthood: www.plannedparenthood.org

Mayo Clinic Birth Control Options: www.mayoclinic.com/health/birth-control

Ultimate Birth Control Links: www.ultimatebirthcontrol.com

Reproductive Health Online: www.reproline.jhu.edu

For Information on Menopause:

North American Menopause Society: www.menopause.org

Menopause Online: www.menopause-online.com

For Information on Pregnancy and Childbirth:

Childbirth: www.childbirth.org

StorkNet's Pregnancy Guide: www.pregnancyguideonline.com

What to Expect: www.whattoexpect.com

The American College of Obstetricians and Gynecologists: www.acog.com

American Baby: www.americanbaby.com

Baby Zone: www.babyzone.com

Lamaze International: www.lamaze.org

LaLeche League: www.laleche.org

9

The Pediatric Examination

LEARNING OBJECTIVES

PROCEDURES

Pediatric Office Visits

1. List the components of the well-child visit.
2. State the usual schedule for well-child visits.
3. Explain the purpose of the sick-child visit.
4. List the procedures performed by the medical assistant during pediatric office visits.
5. Explain why it is important to develop a rapport with the pediatric patient.

Carry an infant using the following positions:
    Cradle
    Upright

Growth Measurements

1. State the importance of measuring the child's weight, height (or length), and head circumference during each office visit.
2. State the functions served by a growth chart.

Plot pediatric growth values on a growth chart.
Measure the weight and length of an infant.
Measure the head and chest circumference of an infant.

Pediatric Blood Pressure Measurement

1. State the importance of measuring a child's blood pressure.
2. List the three factors that determine whether a child has hypertension.

Measure the blood pressure of a child.

Collection of a Urine Specimen

1. List the reasons for collecting a urine specimen from a child.

Collect a urine specimen using a pediatric urine collector.

Pediatric Injections

1. State the range for the gauge and length of needles used for intramuscular and subcutaneous pediatric injections.
2. Explain the use of each of the following pediatric injection sites: dorsogluteal, vastus lateralis, and deltoid.

Locate the following pediatric intramuscular injection sites:
    Dorsogluteal
    Vastus lateralis
    Deltoid
Administer an intramuscular injection to an infant.
Administer a subcutaneous injection to an infant.

Immunizations

1. Describe the schedule for immunization of infants and children recommended by the American Academy of Pediatrics.
2. State the information that must be provided to parents as required by the National Childhood Vaccine Injury Act.
3. List the information that must be recorded in the medical record after administering an immunization.

Read and interpret a vaccine information statement.
Record information on a pediatric vaccine administration record.

Newborn Screening Test

1. Explain the purpose of a newborn screening test.
2. List the symptoms of phenylketonuria.
3. State what occurs if phenylketonuria is left untreated.

Collect a specimen for a newborn screening test.

NATIONAL COMPETENCIES

Clinical Competencies

Patient Care
Prepare and maintain examination and treatment areas.
Prepare patient for and assist with routine and specialty examinations.
Prepare patient for and assist with procedures, treatments, and minor office surgeries.
Maintain medication and immunization records.

General Competencies

Patient Instruction
Instruct individuals according to their needs.
Provide instruction for health maintenance and disease prevention.

KEY TERMS

adolescent
immunity (ih-MYOO-nih-tee)
immunization (IM-yoo-nih-ZAY-shun)
infant
length
pediatrician (PEE-dee-uh-TRIH-shun)
pediatrics (pee-dee-AT-riks)

preschool (PREE-skool) child
school-age child
toddler (TOD-ler)
toxoid (TOKS-oid)
vaccine (vak-SEEN)
vertex (VER-teks)

Introduction to the Pediatric Examination

Pediatrics is the branch of medicine that deals with the care and development of children and the diagnosis and treatment of diseases in children. A **pediatrician** is a physician who specializes in pediatrics. Many physicians in general practice accept pediatric patients. It is essential that the medical assistant develop the skills needed to assist the physician in the care and treatment of children.

PEDIATRIC OFFICE VISITS

There are two broad categories of pediatric patient office visits. The first is the *well-child visit* (also termed *health maintenance visit*), in which the physician progressively evaluates the growth and development of the child. A physical examination is performed during each well-child visit and is directed toward discovering any abnormal conditions commonly associated with the stage of development reached by the child. Table 9-1 provides an outline of normal development during infancy. The child also receives necessary immunizations during these visits.

Another important component of the well-child visit is *anticipatory guidance*. Anticipatory guidance is the process of providing parents with information to prepare them for anticipated developmental events and to assist them in promoting their children's well-being (Table 9-2). Topics that are commonly included are safety, nutrition, sleep, play, exercise, development, and discipline. Table 9-3 presents child safety guidelines by age group.

The interval between well-child visits depends on the medical office, but it frequently follows this schedule after

Text continued on p. 328

Table 9-1 Milestones of Gross and Fine Motor Development in Infancy

Average Age (Mo)	Gross Motor	Fine Motor
1	Turns head from side to side	Grasping reflex present
2	Holds head at 45-degree angle when prone	Holds rattle briefly
3	Begins rolling over	Grasps rattle or dangling objects
4	Slight head lag when pulled to sitting position	Brings objects to mouth
5	No head wobble when held in sitting position	Transfers objects from hand to hand
6	Sits without support	Manipulates and examines large objects with hands
7	Stands while holding on	Reaches for, grabs, and retains object
8	Pulls self to stand	Grasps objects with thumb and finger
9	Crawls backwards	Begins to show hand preference
10	Creeps on hands and knees	Hits cup with spoon
11	Walks using furniture for support	Picks up small objects with thumb and forefinger (pincer grasp)
12	Stands alone easily	Puts three or more objects into container
12-16	Walks alone easily	Turns two or three pages in large cardboard book

From Leahy JM, Kizilay PE: *Foundations of nursing practice,* Philadelphia, 1998, Saunders.

Table 9-2 Anticipatory Guidance

Issue	Rationale	Guidance
Infants		
Thumb sucking and pacifiers	Sucking is a major pleasure for infant Benefits such as decreased crying and increased relaxation have been identified by meeting infant's need for nonnutritive sucking Infants generally find their fingers or hands to suck on to meet this need without pacifier As need for nonnutritive sucking decreases, so does need for pacifier or thumb, unless their use is treated as reinforcement by parents to relieve infant distress	Explore parents' feelings regarding infant's need for pacifier If pacifiers are to be used, review safety considerations (e.g., preferably constructed in one piece, have flange with at least two ventilation holes and large enough to prevent aspiration; remove from infant when not in use; never secure to infant by tying with cord around neck) Thumb sucking is generally abandoned by the age when dental problems may become an issue (when permanent teeth erupt) If pacifier is used, try removing it around age 6 mo, when infant is not yet old enough to remember or miss it for long If pacifiers are used beyond the first year, unless you are meticulous about sterilizing them, they can be very unhygienic as child toddles around with them; this is a good reason to discontinue pacifier use
Teething	Teething seldom causes discomfort in infant <4 mo old At 5-6 mo, as first tooth emerges, drooling, chewing on hard objects, and some irritability may accompany minor inflammation of gums Most discomfort is felt by infant with eruption of first molars at age 12-15 mo	Believing that infant <4 mo old is irritable for long periods because of "teething" may cause parent to neglect illness Medical attention should be sought for any infant experiencing fever, diarrhea, vomiting, or loss of appetite; these are not symptoms of teething Avoid teething gels because they contain anesthetics that may cause untoward effects in infant if overused Provide something cold to bite on (e.g., frozen gel-filled teething ring)
Separation and stranger fear	Around 8 mo old, infants have sufficient capacity to recognize their primary caregivers and find comfort in their presence Because they have not yet developed the task of object permanence, infants experience great displeasure when their caregivers leave them alone or with unfamiliar substitute	Accustom infant to new persons, especially those who may baby-sit (more frequent the exposure, less likely the fear) Give infants opportunities to explore strangers at their own pace to allow "warm-up" of adjustment

From Leahy JM, Kizilay PE: *Foundations of nursing practice,* Philadelphia, 1998, Saunders.

Table 9-2 Anticipatory Guidance—cont'd		
Issue	**Rationale**	**Guidance**
Separation and stranger fear—cont'd	This behavior may continue into toddlerhood	Talk to infants when leaving them, and greet them when you return. This can aid development of object permanence and reassure them that you will always return Use transitional object (e.g., your scarf, toy) to reassure them of your continued presence
Spoiling and limit setting	When infants' needs are not promptly met, they become anxious, quick to fuss or cry, and slow to accept comfort; the less you meet infants' needs, the more demanding they become As infants become more mobile toward latter half of first year, parents need to set limits to provide for their safety; however, there is no substitute for vigilant parental monitoring	Prompt attention to crying infant often is greeted by infant's smile and comfort Delaying attention to crying infant leads to encounter with miserably distressed infant who does not settle down easily, has stomach full of air from excessive crying, and will most likely start crying again before long Set limits for older infants through consistent and age-appropriate methods Negative voice and stern eye-to-eye contact may be all that is needed Quiet period for infant in playpen may be warranted Parents who express concern about disciplining infant should recognize that the earlier it is started, the easier it is to maintain throughout childhood
Injury prevention	Unintentional injury is second-leading cause of death in infancy Common risks associated with this developmental stage include choking or suffocation, falls, motor vehicle crash injuries, burns	Parents and caregivers should know CPR, especially techniques for infants and children Parents should review home and environmental safety checklist
Crying and colic	Colicky infants cry for long periods (more than 3 hr daily) with legs drawn up Colic has no known cause, but has been associated with intolerance to cow's milk formula or ingestion of milk products by breastfeeding mothers and passive smoking As infants cry, they swallow more air, distend the abdomen, cry some more, and pass flatus, and the cycle continues Periods of crying up to 2 hr per day are a normal part of infant's temperament	Reassurance should be given to parents that crying is a release of energy for infant Parents should always initially respond to infant's cry to determine cause When no cause for crying episodes can be identified, time of onset should be noted; successful responses to infant are changing position, massaging abdomen, swaddling in blanket, taking for car ride, or placing infant in wind-up swing Continued long periods of crying should be reported to health care provider Avoid smoking near infant Provide small frequent feedings; burp during and after feeding; have infant sit upright for half an hour after feeding
Toddlers		
Toilet training	Ability to control elimination requires muscular maturation and cognitive maturity Toddler needs to understand instructions and purpose of this task, for which there is no tangible reward other than that of "pleasing" caregiver 84% of 3-yr-olds are dry throughout the day, and 66% are dry throughout the night	Most parents initiate toilet training at 20-24 mo Parents should be informed that "successful" toilet training at very early age is usually because parent is "trained" to recognize child's readiness and places child on potty at appropriate time Teach parents to record toddler's pattern and signals of elimination for several weeks before starting Have parents obtain sturdy potty chair, if possible, so that child can independently sit and get up, or sturdy step stool to access toilet with adult supervision Have parents dress child in loose clothing to aid access and prevent accidents Inform parents that when child signals that bowel movement or voiding may be on the way, they should casually suggest to child that he or she may want to sit on potty

Continued

Table 9-2 Anticipatory Guidance—cont'd

Issue	Rationale	Guidance
Toilet training—cont'd		Encourage parents not to force child to sit on potty or to show disappointment if attempts are unsuccessful Explain to parents that accidents happen and need to be taken in stride Nagging and punishing child for being uncooperative or for having "accidents" means certain failure; toddler becomes overwhelmed and confused about what is expected
Temper tantrums	Temper tantrums are common toward end of second year Tantrums are result of excessive frustration; when child becomes overwhelmed with emotion and feelings of tension, explosive outburst is means of release Tantrums often involve screaming, thrashing, and breath-holding spells	Parents should be taught that a temper tantrum is like an "emotional blown fuse," which is not something that toddler can control Parents need to recognize balance between frustration level that their child can tolerate and that is useful for learning and amount of frustration that causes fuse to blow During tantrum, parent should be instructed to protect child from harm, but not to overpower him or her because this physical restriction may heighten anger Reassure parents that breath-holding spells, although alarming to watch, do not result in physical harm. Body's natural reflex to breathe allows child to take in air before damage can occur
Stress, anxiety, and fear	Toddlers live on emotional seesaw, with most stress and tears arising from basic contradiction of wanting to be independent and to be protected and loved by their caregivers Toddlers need balance of autonomy and protection from separation anxiety Toddler feels anxious when his or her feelings become uncontrollable, leading to crying or temper tantrums	Inform parents to recognize cues from toddler that indicate impending problem (e.g., excessive clinginess, less adventurous behavior, increased shyness) Instruct parents to offer more affection, attention, and protection for several days until toddler regains a normal sense of independence and adventure
Bedtime struggles	50% of children 1-2 yr old engage in fussing or bedtime struggles lasting for more than 1 hr Sometimes these struggles are associated with family stress, such as illness or change in normal routines Most struggles are caused by continued infancy routines of "being put to sleep" by nursing, rocking, or coddling	Inform parents that this struggle is very common Inform parents that if they continue to coddle, rock, or nurse their toddlers to sleep at this age, it becomes harder to institute different bedtime routine Instruct parents to alter routine by providing about 20 min of sedentary activity, such as quiet conversation or storytelling Have parents keep night-light on if it makes child more comfortable Tell parents to finish their sedentary time with pleasant "goodnight," and if child begins to cry and continues for several minutes, they should go back in room, repeat "goodnight," and leave again; this performance should be repeated every few minutes for as long as it takes child to settle down Any sleep problem that persists over several months should be referred to child's health care provider
Unintentional injuries	Unintentional injury is leading cause of death and disability in toddlerhood Toddlers are especially vulnerable to unintentional injuries because of their activity level, developing motor skills, and inability to perceive dangerous situations Common risks associated with this developmental stage include drowning, burns or scalds, motor vehicle injuries, falls, poisoning	Parents and caregivers should know CPR Home and environmental safety checklist should be reviewed with parents and caregivers Reinforce with parents and caregivers importance of vigilant child monitoring and supervision during this highly vulnerable developmental stage

From Leahy JM, Kizilay PE: *Foundations of nursing practice,* Philadelphia, 1998, Saunders.

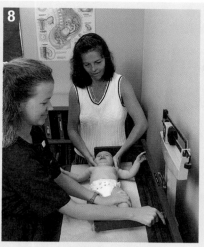

Properly position the infant.

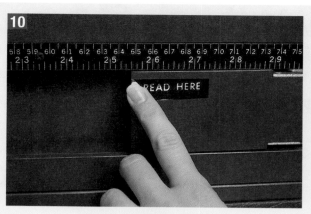

Read the length in inches.

10. **Procedural Step.** Read the infant's length in inches (to the nearest ⅛ inch) from the measure. Jot down this value or make a mental note of it. (*Note:* The result on this scale is 25½ inches.)

11. **Procedural Step.** Gently remove the infant from the table, and hand him or her to the parent. Return the headboard and footboard to their resting positions.

12. **Procedural Step.** Sanitize your hands, and chart the results.

CHARTING EXAMPLE

Date	
8/10/08	9:30 a.m. Wt. 15 lb 2 oz. Length 25 ½ in. ___
	_____ T. Powell, CMA

PROCEDURE 9-2 Measuring Head and Chest Circumference of an Infant

Outcome Measure the head and chest circumference of an infant.

Equipment/Supplies

- Flexible nonstretch tape measure

Measurement of Head Circumference

1. **Procedural Step.** Sanitize your hands, and assemble the equipment.

2. **Procedural Step.** Position the infant. The infant should be placed on his or her back on the examining table. An alternative position is to have the parent hold the infant.

3. **Procedural Step.** Position the tape measure around the infant's head at the greatest circumference. This is usually accomplished by placing the tape slightly above the eyebrows and pinna of the ears and around the occipital prominence at the back of the skull.

4. **Procedural Step.** Read the results in centimeters (or inches) to the nearest 0.5 cm (or ¼ inch). Jot down this value or make a mental note of it. Sanitize your hands, and chart the results.

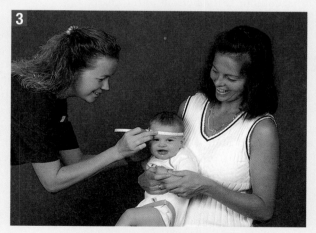

Position the tape measure around the infant's head.

CHARTING EXAMPLE

Date	
8/10/08	10:00 a.m. Head circumference: 42 ½ cm. ___
	_____ T. Powell, CMA

Continued

PROCEDURE 9-2   Measuring Head and Chest Circumference of an Infant—cont'd

Measurement of Chest Circumference

1. **Procedural Step.** Position the infant on his or her back on the examining table.
2. **Procedural Step.** Encircle the tape around the infant's chest at the nipple line. It should be snug, but not so tight that it leaves a mark.
3. **Procedural Step.** Read the results in centimeters (or inches) to the nearest 0.5 cm (or ¼ inch). Jot down this value or make a mental note of it. Sanitize your hands, and chart the results.

CHARTING EXAMPLE

Date	
8/15/08	10:00 a.m. Chest circumference: 42 cm. ___
	_____ T. Powell, CMA

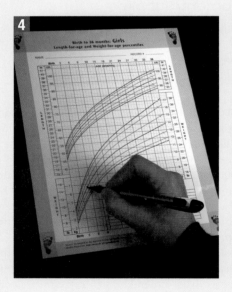

Encircle the tape around the infant's chest.

PROCEDURE 9-3   Calculating Growth Percentiles

Outcome Plot a pediatric growth value on a growth chart.

Equipment/Supplies

• Pediatric growth chart

1. **Procedural Step.** Select the proper growth chart.
2. **Procedural Step.** Locate the child's age in the horizontal column at the bottom of the chart.
3. **Procedural Step.** Locate the growth value in the vertical column under the appropriate category (weight, length or stature, and head circumference).
4. **Procedural Step.** Draw an imaginary vertical line from the child's age mark and an imaginary horizontal line from the child's growth mark. Find the site at which the two lines intersect on the graph, and place a dot on this site.
5. **Procedural Step.** To determine the percentile in which the child falls, follow the curved percentile line upward to read the value located on the right side of the chart. Interpolation is needed if the value does not fall exactly on a percentile line. (*Interpolation* means that you must estimate a percentile that falls between a larger and smaller known percentile.)
6. **Procedural Step.** Chart the results. Include the date and time and each growth percentile.
   Note: The weight (15 lb, 2 oz), length (25½ inches), and head circumference (42.5 cm) of the child in Procedures 9-1 and 9-2 have been plotted on a growth chart. This child is 5 months old. Locate these values on the appropriate growth chart to ensure you obtain the same percentiles.

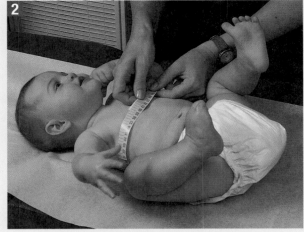

CHARTING EXAMPLE

Date	
10/22/08	10:30 a.m. Weight: 55%. Length: 70%. _____
	Head Circum: 67% _____ T. Powell, CMA

PROCEDURE 9-3   Calculating Growth Percentiles—cont'd

Birth to 36 months: Girls
Length-for-age and Weight-for-age percentiles

NAME _____

RECORD# _____

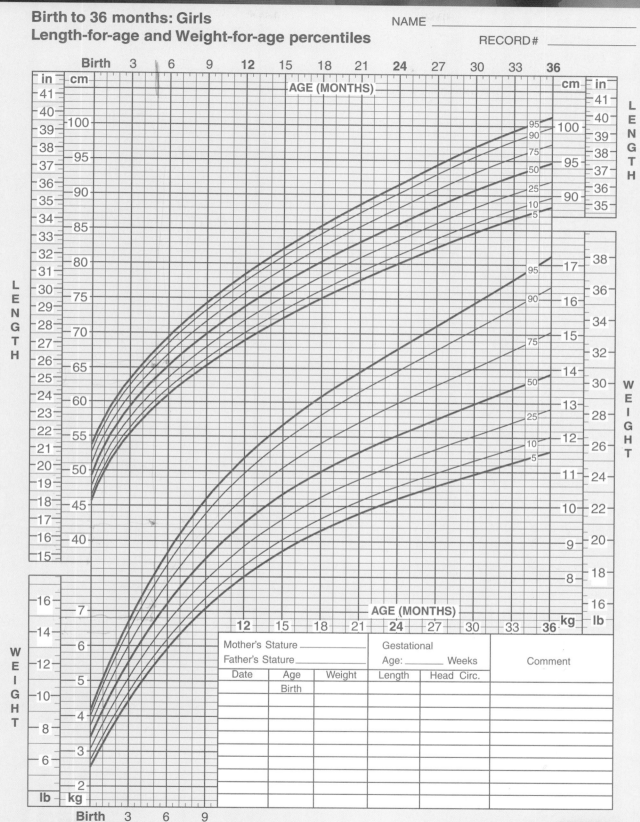

Mother's Stature _____
Father's Stature _____

Gestational
Age: _____ Weeks

Comment

Date	Age	Weight	Length	Head Circ.	
	Birth				

Published May 30, 2000 (modified 4/20/01).
SOURCE: Developed by the National Center for Health Statistics in collaboration with
the National Center for Chronic Disease Prevention and Health Promotion (2000).
http://www.cdc.gov/growthcharts

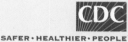

SAFER · HEALTHIER · PEOPLE™

PROCEDURE 9-3

Continued

PROCEDURE 9-3 Calculating Growth Percentiles—cont'd

Birth to 36 months: Girls
Head circumference-for-age and
Weight-for-length percentiles

NAME _____

RECORD# _____

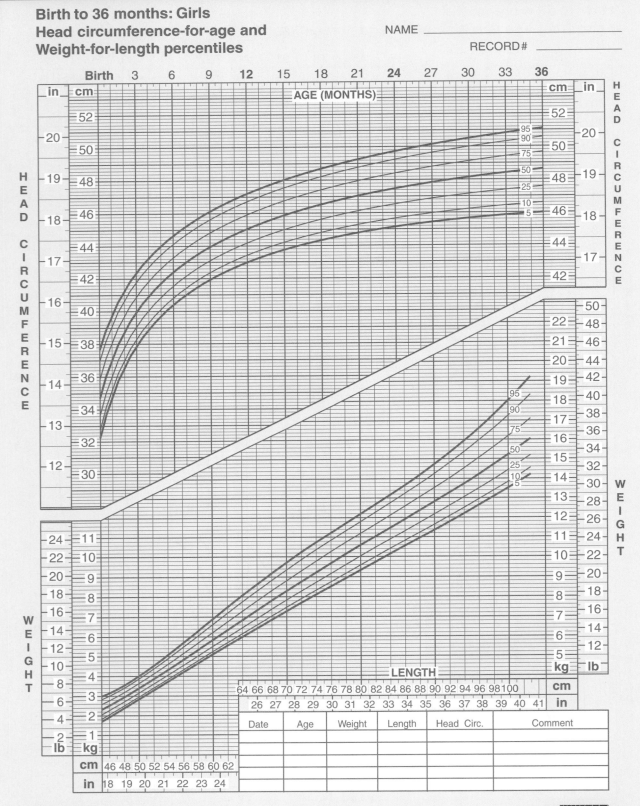

Published May 30, 2000 (modified 10/16/00).

SOURCE: Developed by the National Center for Health Statistics in collaboration with the National Center for Chronic Disease Prevention and Health Promotion (2000).

http://www.cdc.gov/growthcharts

SAFER • HEALTHIER • PEOPLE™

PROCEDURE 9-3   Calculating Growth Percentiles—cont'd

Birth to 36 months: Boys
Length-for-age and Weight-for-age percentiles

NAME _____

RECORD# _____

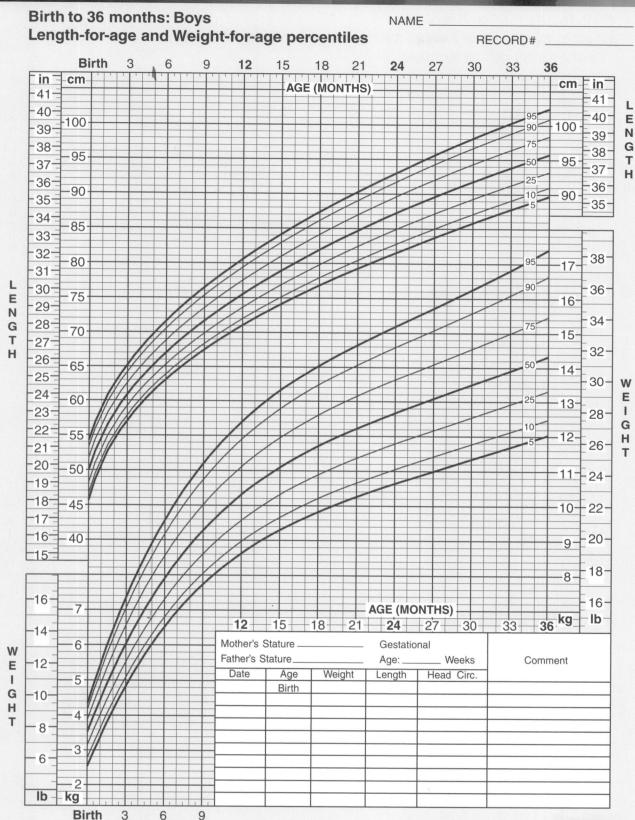

Mother's Stature _____   Gestational
Father's Stature _____   Age: _____ Weeks

Date	Age	Weight	Length	Head Circ.	Comment
	Birth				

Published May 30, 2000 (modified 4/20/01).
SOURCE: Developed by the National Center for Health Statistics in collaboration with
the National Center for Chronic Disease Prevention and Health Promotion (2000).
http://www.cdc.gov/growthcharts

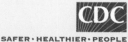

SAFER · HEALTHIER · PEOPLE™

Continued

PROCEDURE **9-3**   Calculating Growth Percentiles—cont'd

Birth to 36 months: Boys
Head circumference-for-age and
Weight-for-length percentiles

NAME _____

RECORD# _____

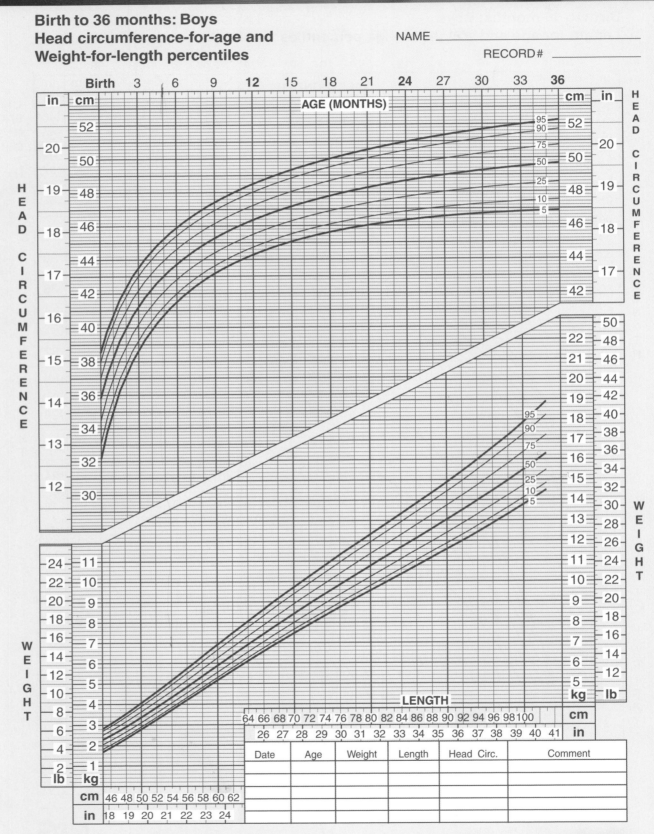

Published May 30, 2000 (modified 10/16/00).
SOURCE: Developed by the National Center for Health Statistics in collaboration with
the National Center for Chronic Disease Prevention and Health Promotion (2000).
http://www.cdc.gov/growthcharts

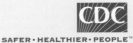

SAFER · HEALTHIER · PEOPLE™

PROCEDURE 9-3   Calculating Growth Percentiles—cont'd

2 to 20 years: Girls
Stature-for-age and Weight-for-age percentiles

NAME _____

RECORD# _____

Mother's Stature _____ Father's Stature _____

Date	Age	Weight	Stature	BMI*

*To Calculate BMI: Weight (kg) ÷ Stature (cm) ÷ Stature (cm) x 10,000
or Weight (lb) ÷ Stature (in) ÷ Stature (in) x 703

AGE (YEARS)

STATURE

WEIGHT

Published May 30, 2000 (modified 11/21/00).

SOURCE: Developed by the National Center for Health Statistics in collaboration with
the National Center for Chronic Disease Prevention and Health Promotion (2000).
http://www.cdc.gov/growthcharts

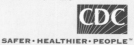

SAFER · HEALTHIER · PEOPLE™

PROCEDURE 9-3

Continued

PROCEDURE 9-3 Calculating Growth Percentiles—cont'd

2 to 20 years: Boys
Stature-for-age and Weight-for-age percentiles

NAME _____

RECORD# _____

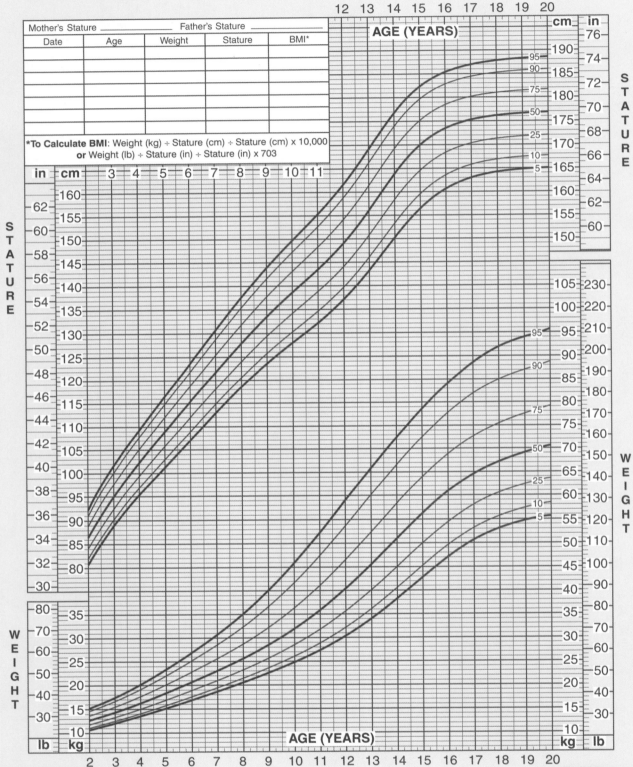

*To Calculate BMI: Weight (kg) ÷ Stature (cm) ÷ Stature (cm) x 10,000
or Weight (lb) ÷ Stature (in) ÷ Stature (in) x 703

Published May 30, 2000 (modified 11/21/00).
SOURCE: Developed by the National Center for Health Statistics in collaboration with
the National Center for Chronic Disease Prevention and Health Promotion (2000).
http://www.cdc.gov/growthcharts

SAFER • HEALTHIER • PEOPLE™

PEDIATRIC BLOOD PRESSURE MEASUREMENT

The American Academy of Pediatrics recommends that all children 3 years old and older have their blood pressure measured annually. Measuring pediatric blood pressure helps to identify children at risk for developing hypertension as adults. High blood pressure in children can be caused by kidney disease and, to a lesser degree, by heart disease. When the condition is treated, the blood pressure usually returns to normal. Overweight children usually have higher blood pressure than children of normal weight. Losing weight through a prescribed diet and regular physical activity often reduces blood pressure in these children.

Special Guidelines for Children

The procedure for measuring blood pressure in children is the same as that for adults and is presented in Chapter 4. Some special pediatric guidelines must be taken into consideration.

Correct Cuff Size

The most important criterion in obtaining an accurate pediatric blood pressure measurement is selecting the correct cuff size. If the cuff is too small, the reading may be falsely high. If the cuff is too large, the reading may be falsely low. Blood pressure cuffs come in a variety of sizes and are measured in centimeters (cm). The size of a cuff refers to its inner inflatable bladder, rather than its cloth cover. Table 9-5 lists the range of cuff sizes commercially available. The name of the cuff (e.g., child, adult) does not imply it is appropriate for

Table 9-5 Acceptable Bladder Dimensions for Arms of Different Sizes		
Cuff	Bladder Length (cm)	Arm Circumference Range at Midpoint (cm)
Newborn	6	Less than 6
Infant	15	6-15
Child	21	16-21
Small adult	24	22-26
Adult	30	27-34
Large adult	38	35-44
Adult thigh	42	45-52

that age. An 8-year-old overweight child may need an adult-sized cuff.

For an accurate blood pressure measurement, the bladder of the cuff should encircle 80% to 100% of the arm. The child's arm circumference should be assessed midpoint between the acromion process (shoulder) and the olecranon process (elbow). Figure 9-5 shows how to determine the correct pediatric cuff size.

Cooperation of the Child

Another important factor to consider when taking pediatric blood pressure is preparing the child for the procedure. It is important to gain the child's cooperation and to ensure that the child is relaxed. Apprehension can cause the blood pressure to be falsely high. To reduce a child's anxiety level, carefully explain the procedure to the child, and, if appro-

DETERMINATION OF PROPER CUFF SIZE

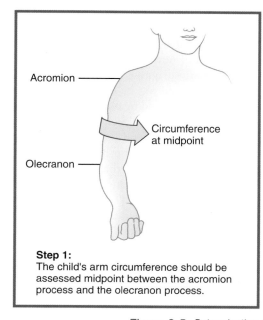

Step 1:
The child's arm circumference should be assessed midpoint between the acromion process and the olecranon process.

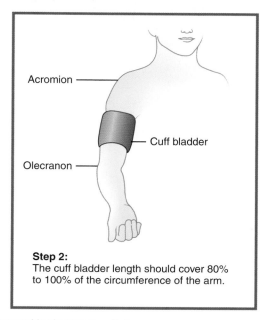

Step 2:
The cuff bladder length should cover 80% to 100% of the circumference of the arm.

Figure 9-5. Determination of proper blood pressure cuff size.

What Would You Do? What Would You *Not* Do?

Case Study 2

Wanda Tilley comes to the office with her 10-year-old daughter, Courtney. Courtney has a skin condition on her legs that needs to be evaluated by the physician. Courtney has been obese since she was 4 years old. Mrs. Tilley also is obese and is not too concerned about Courtney's weight. She says that Courtney must have inherited her "fat gene," and there's not much that can be done about it. Courtney's favorite activities are playing video games and reading. She would like to join the community swim team, but she's too embarrassed for anyone to see her in a bathing suit. Courtney says the other kids are always making fun of her at school. She says that they call her "two-ton Tilley" and "double-roll," and they don't want to sit with her at lunch. Courtney wants her mom to home-school her because she's getting to the point where she can't take it anymore. She doesn't want the doctor to examine her because he'll see how fat she is and say bad things about it. ■

priate, allow him or her to handle the equipment before measuring blood pressure. The blood pressure should be measured after the child has been sitting quietly for 3 to 5 minutes (Figure 9-6).

Blood Pressure Classifications

Blood pressure varies depending on the age of the child and his or her height and gender. The National High Blood Pressure Education Program (NHBPEP) prepared a set of tables that physicians use to determine whether a child's blood pressure is higher than the average among children of the same age and height. If a child has a blood pressure that is higher than 90% to 95% of most other children of the

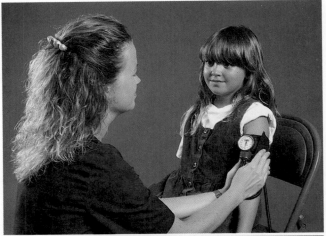

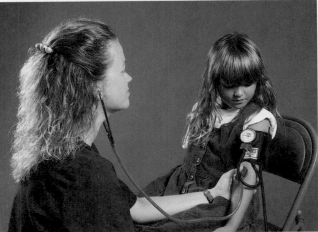

Figure 9-6. Traci measures the blood pressure of a pediatric patient.

same age, height, and gender, the child may have high blood pressure.

The NHBPEP tables (one for boys and one for girls) allow precise classification of blood pressure according to body size, which avoids misclassifying children at the extreme ends of normal growth. A very tall child would not be mistakenly diagnosed as having hypertension, and hypertension would not be missed in a very short child. The NHBPEP tables used by physicians to assist in the diagnosis of hypertension in children can be found at the National Heart, Lung, and Blood Institute website (www.nhlbi.nih.gov/health/prof/heart/hbp/hbp_ped.htm).

Blood pressure varies throughout the day in children as a result of normal fluctuations in physical activity and emotional stress. If a child's blood pressure is elevated, two more readings must be taken at different visits before the physician can make a diagnosis of hypertension.

COLLECTION OF A URINE SPECIMEN

A urinalysis may be performed on a pediatric patient for the following reasons: to screen for the presence of disease as part of a general physical examination, to assist in the diagnosis of

Memories *from* Externship

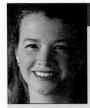

Traci Powell: I still remember how difficult it was at times as a student. I had been out of high school for more than a year, so I had to get back into the routine of studying. I worried about whether I would do well, whether I would be able to find a good job, and whether I would like medical assisting. Adding to these concerns was the financial burden of putting myself through school. I took advantage of grants and a student loan. Throughout the last 6 months of my education, I also worked full-time as an aide on the midnight shift at a nursing home while attending school full-time during the day. As if that were not enough, my first child was well on her way into this world as I was finishing up the last quarter of my degree. There were so many times that I was tired, frustrated, and broke, but I kept pushing myself to do my best because I knew this was going to be my lifetime career, and I wanted to excel in my profession. My determination paid off. Today I have a great medical assisting position that I love, with an institution that is one of the best employers in the area. ■

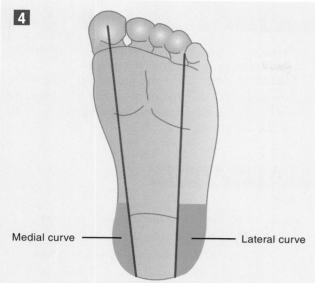

Medial curve ——————— Lateral curve

The shading indicates the appropriate
area for making the puncture.
Plantar surface of the heel.

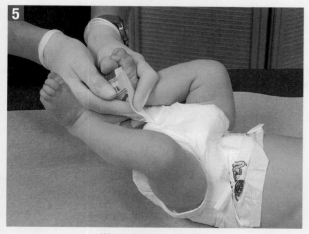

Warm the puncture site.

6. Procedural Step. Cleanse the puncture site with an antiseptic wipe, and allow it to air dry. Do not wipe the area with gauze to speed the drying process.

Principle. The site must be allowed to air dry to give the alcohol enough time to destroy microorganisms. If the site is wet, it will cause a stinging sensation when the puncture is made.

7. Procedural Step. Apply gloves. Grasp the infant's foot around the puncture site, and, without touching the cleansed site, make a puncture with the sterile lancet. The puncture should be made at a right angle to the lines of the skin. Dispose of the lancet in a biohazard sharps container.

Principle. Touching the site after cleansing would contaminate it, and the cleansing process would have to be repeated.

8. Procedural Step. Wipe away the first drop of blood with a gauze pad.

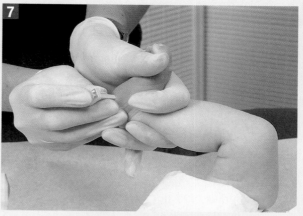

Grasp the infant's foot, and make the puncture.

Principle. The first drop of blood is diluted with alcohol and tissue fluid and is not a suitable specimen.

9. Procedural Step. Encourage a large drop of blood to form by exerting gentle pressure without excessively squeezing the area. Place one side of the filter paper next to the infant's heel. Touch the drop of blood to the center of the first circle on the test card, and completely fill the first circle with the blood specimen. The proper amount of specimen is obtained when the blood can be observed soaking completely through the filter paper from one side to the other.

Principle. Excessive squeezing would cause dilution of the blood sample with tissue fluid, leading to inaccurate test results.

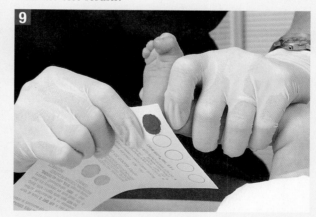

Completely fill the circle with the blood specimen.

10. Procedural Step. Repeat procedure step 9 until all the circles on the card are completely filled with blood. Be careful not to touch the blood specimens on the card with your gloved hand.

Principle. The circles must be completely filled to ensure enough of a blood sample to perform the test. Most repeat tests are required because of inadequate specimen collection. Touching the blood specimen could lead to inaccurate test results.

PROCEDURE 9-5

Continued

PROCEDURE 9-5   Newborn Screening Test—cont'd

11. **Procedural Step.** Hold a piece of gauze over the puncture site, and apply pressure to control the bleeding. Remain with the infant until the bleeding stops. If needed, apply an adhesive bandage.

12. **Procedural Step.** Remove the gloves, and sanitize your hands.

13. **Procedural Step.** Allow the test card to air dry in a horizontal position for at least 3 hours at room temperature on a nonabsorbent surface. Do not allow the wet blood specimen to come in contact with any other surface. Do not expose the test card to heat, moisture, or direct sunlight. Do not place the specimen in a biohazard specimen bag or any other type of plastic bag.

    Principle. Placing the test card in a plastic bag interferes with proper drying of the specimen.

14. **Procedural Step.** After the blood is completely dry, place the test card in its protective envelope, and mail it to an outside laboratory for testing within 48 hours.

    Principle. The test card should be mailed within 48 hours to ensure accurate test results.

15. **Procedural Step.** Chart the procedure. Include the date and time, the type of procedure, the puncture site location, and information regarding transfer to an outside laboratory.

CHARTING EXAMPLE

Date	
8/15/08	9:30 a.m. Blood specimen collected from medial heel. Sent to Newborn Screening Lab on 8/15/08 for newborn screening test.
	———————————— T. Powell, CMA

CD *Check out the **Companion CD** bound with the book to access additional interactive activities.*

MEDICAL PRACTICE *and the* LAW

Children are not small adults. They must be treated as individuals, according to their developmental level. Pediatric patients (except for emancipated minors) cannot give written or verbal consents. Make sure a parent or legal guardian is available for consent. A babysitter or grandparent cannot give consent for treatment without written permission from a parent or legal guardian. Similarly, patient information can be given only to a parent or legal guardian.

If your office sees pediatric patients, you have a responsibility to be aware of developmental needs and milestones of children at various ages. This is necessary for accurate developmental assessment. ∎

What Would You Do? What Would You *Not* Do? RESPONSES

Case Study 1
Page 327
What Did Traci Do?

❏ Listened patiently to Mrs. Chang and allowed her to vent her frustrations.

❏ Reassured Mrs. Chang that her milk is very nutritious for Christopher. Gave her a brochure on breastfeeding that included information on what to do for sore nipples and engorgement.

❏ Gave Mrs. Chang the names and phone numbers of community resources for nursing mothers.

❏ Told Mrs. Chang that Christopher's weight and length do not fall in the underweight category on his growth chart. Showed her Christopher's growth chart so that she could see that Christopher is progressing normally.

What Did Traci Not Do?

❏ Did not tell Mrs. Chang to cheer up because the colic would eventually go away on its own.

❏ Did not give a personal opinion on whether Mrs. Chang should breastfeed or bottle-feed her infant.

What Would You Do?/What Would You *Not* Do? Review Traci's response and place a checkmark next to the information you included in your response. List additional information included in your response.

_____
_____
_____
_____

Case Study 2
Page 342
What Did Traci Do?

❏ Explained to Mrs. Tilly that childhood obesity has doubled in the past 20 years and has become a serious health concern.

❏ Told Mrs. Tilly that she could have a big impact on Courtney's life by preparing healthy meals and eating them with her and by becoming involved in activities with Courtney, such as taking walks.

❏ Spent some time talking with Courtney about her interests and complimented Courtney on her achievements.

❏ Encouraged Courtney to join the swim team. Told her that lots of people do not like to be seen in a bathing suit and encouraged her not to let that stand in her way of doing something she wants to do.

❏ Reassured Courtney that the doctor wants to help her and that he would never say anything bad about her weight.

What Did Traci Not Do?

❏ Did not agree with Mrs. Tilly that there is nothing that can be done about Courtney's weight problem.

❏ Did not tell Courtney that she needs to lose weight or she might develop serious health problems such as diabetes.

What Would You Do?/What Would You *Not* Do? Review Traci's response and place a checkmark next to the information you included in your response. List additional information included in your response.

_____
_____
_____
_____

Case Study 3
Page 346
What Did Traci Do?

❏ Explained to Stacy that it is rare, but sometimes a child develops polio from getting the oral polio vaccine. Told her that this does not occur with the injectable polio vaccine.

❏ Explained to Stacy that chickenpox is usually a mild disease, but it can be serious, especially in young infants and adults.

❏ Explained to Stacy that most side effects from vaccines are mild, and the complications from the diseases far outweigh the possible side effects.

❏ Told Stacy that these diseases have been reduced to very low levels in the United States, but they still occur in other countries. Explained that infected travelers can bring these diseases to the United States and infect individuals who are not immunized.

❏ Reminded Stacy that these immunizations are required for Matthew to start kindergarten.

❏ Talked with Matthew on his level about why he needs to be immunized.

❏ Told Matthew that they would play a game so that it wouldn't hurt as much. Taught him to hold up his finger and pretend that it was a birthday candle; when the injection was given, told him to keep blowing out the candle until he was told to stop.

❏ Told Matthew that he could choose a prize from the treasure chest after he had his immunizations.

What Did Traci Not Do?

❏ Did not ignore or minimize Stacy's concerns.

❏ Did not tell Stacy that the answers to all her questions are in the vaccine information sheets that she was just given.

❏ Did not tell Stacy it would be all right to skip Matthew's immunizations.

❏ Did not refer to the immunizations as "shots" when talking with Matthew.

❏ Did not tell Matthew that it would not hurt when he gets his immunizations.

What Would You Do?/What Would You *Not* Do? Review Traci's response and place a checkmark next to the information you included in your response. List additional information included in your response.

_____
_____
_____
_____

APPLY YOUR KNOWLEDGE

Choose the best answer to each of the following questions.

1. Trisha Jordan, a surgical nurse, brings her 6-month-old daughter, Amy, to the office for a well-child visit. To prepare the examination room for her visit, Traci Powell, CMA, would have available all of the following *except*:
   A. A pediatric balance scale.
   B. A growth chart for Girls: Birth to 36 Months.
   C. A blood pressure cuff and stethoscope.
   D. A centimeter tape measure.

2. All of the following immunizations will be given to 6-month-old Amy at this visit *except*:
   A. DTaP
   B. MMR
   C. Hib
   D. IPV

3. Traci Powell, CMA, measures Amy's weight and length and calculates her growth values. Amy is in the 75th percentile for weight and the 25th percentile for length. Traci notices that Amy has been in approximately these same percentiles since birth. Which of the following would Dr. Immunity most likely relay to Mrs. Jordan regarding Amy's growth?
   A. Amy needs to have some growth evaluation tests.
   B. You have a short fat baby.
   C. Amy is growing normally.
   D. You need to stop breastfeeding.

4. Traci asks Mrs. Jordan some questions regarding Amy's stage of development. Which of the following should Amy be able to do now that she is 6 months old?
   A. Sit without support.
   B. Ride a bike.
   C. Stand alone.
   D. Pick up small objects.

5. John Whitmore, a stay-at-home dad, brings his 6-year-old daughter, Samantha, to the office for her kindergarten physical. Samantha is to receive an MMR immunization at this visit. Mr. Whitmore wants to know what vaccines are in an MMR. Traci Powell, CMA, tells him that MMR includes:
   A. Meningitis, mumps, and rubella.
   B. Measles, mumps, and rubella.
   C. Measles, mumps, and roseola.
   D. Measles, mononucleosis, and rat-bite fever.

6. Samantha also is scheduled for a DTaP immunization during this visit. Mr. Jordan wants to know whether this immunization has side effects. Which of the following should Traci Powell, CMA, relay to Mr. Jordan?
   A. Amy may be fussy and tired 1 to 3 days after the injection.
   B. The vaccine may cause a slight fever 1 to 3 days after the injection.
   C. There may be some swelling and redness at the injection site.
   D. All of the above.

7. Samantha is very upset about having to get "shots." A developmentally appropriate approach that Traci could use to reduce Samantha's anxiety level might be:
   A. Tell Samantha that she is a "big girl" and should not cry.
   B. Have Samantha count from ten to one backwards while the injections are being administered.
   C. Have Samantha's father give her the injections.
   D. Have Samantha read the VIS for these vaccines so that she will understand why she needs them.

8. Samantha is crying after receiving her immunizations. Traci would respond to her behavior by:
   A. Telling Samantha that she is disappointed because she thought Samantha would be braver about this.
   B. Leaving the room and letting Samantha's father handle the situation.
   C. Giving Samantha a hug and letting her pick a prize from the treasure chest.
   D. Having the physician do a tap dance for Samantha to cheer her up.

9. After administering the DTaP injection, Traci is required by the NCVIA to record all of the following in Samantha's chart *except*:
   A. The expiration date of the vaccine.
   B. The lot number of the vaccine.
   C. The manufacturer of the vaccine.
   D. The date the injection was administered.

10. Cecilia Morales, a radiologic technician, comes in with her newborn son, Sandro, who is 1 week old. Sandro had a PKU test done in the hospital but now must have another one done at the medical office. Mrs. Morales wants to know why the PKU test has to be repeated. Traci Powell, CMA, is aware that Mrs. Morales is breastfeeding and includes all of the following statements in her explanation *except*:

A. Breastfed infants can be tested earlier for PKU than formula-fed infants.
B. The PKU test is not accurate until the infant is consuming milk.
C. The first few days after delivery a nursing mother produces colostrum, which is not "true" milk.
D. Colostrum causes invalid PKU test results.

CERTIFICATION REVIEW

❑ **Pediatrics** is the branch of medicine that deals with the care and development of children and the diagnosis and treatment of diseases in children. A pediatrician is a physician who specializes in pediatrics.

❑ **There are two categories of pediatric office visits:** the well-child visit and the sick-child visit. The purpose of the well-child visit is to receive necessary immunizations and to observe for abnormal conditions associated with the child's stage of development. The purpose of the sick-child visit is to diagnose the condition of a child who is exhibiting the signs and symptoms of disease.

❑ **To evaluate the progress of a child,** the weight, height (or length), and head circumference are measured during each visit and plotted on a growth chart. The child's weight is used to determine nutritional needs and the proper dosage of a medication to administer to the child. Growth charts provide a means for assessing the child's rate of growth; the physician investigates any significant change or rapid increase or decrease in the child's growth pattern.

❑ **Blood pressure** should be measured in children 3 years old and older to identify children at risk for developing hypertension as adults. To obtain an accurate pediatric blood pressure measurement, the correct cuff size must be used. Blood pressure varies depending on the age of the child and his or her height and gender.

❑ **A urine specimen** may be required from a pediatric patient as part of a general physical examination to assist in the diagnosis of a pathologic condition or to evaluate the effectiveness of therapy. Collecting a urine specimen from an infant or young child who cannot urinate voluntarily requires the use of a pediatric urine collector.

❑ **Administering an injection to a child** uses the same basic technique as that used to administer an injection to an adult. The vastus lateralis muscle is the recommended intramuscular injection site for infants and young children. It is large enough to accommodate the injected medication. The dorsogluteal site should not be used until the child has been walking for at least 1 year.

❑ **Immunity** is the resistance of the body to the effects of harmful agents, such as pathogenic microorganisms and their toxins. Immunizations build the body's defenses and protect an individual from attack by certain infectious diseases.

❑ **The National Childhood Vaccine Injury Act** requires that parents be provided with information about the benefits and risks of childhood immunizations through vaccine information sheets (VIS) developed by the Centers for Disease Control and Prevention.

❑ **Phenylketonuria (PKU)** is a congenital hereditary disease. If left untreated, PKU can result in mental retardation and other abnormalities. Most states require that infants undergo PKU screening because early diagnosis and treatment can lead to a better prognosis. In addition to the PKU test, other tests are performed on the blood specimen to screen for congenital hypothyroidism, galactosemia, and homocystinuria.

TERMINOLOGY REVIEW

Adolescent An individual 12 to 18 years old.

Immunity The resistance of the body to the effects of a harmful agent, such as a pathogenic microorganism and its toxins.

Immunization (active, artificial) The process of becoming immune or of rendering an individual immune through the use of a vaccine or toxoid.

Infant A child from birth to 12 months old.

Length (recumbent) The measurement from the vertex of the head to the heel of the foot in a supine position.

Pediatrician A physician who specializes in the care and development of children and the diagnosis and treatment of children's diseases.

Pediatrics The branch of medicine that deals with the care and development of children and the diagnosis and treatment of children's diseases.

Preschool child A child 3 to 6 years old.

School-age child A child 6 to 12 years old.

Toddler A child 1 to 3 years old.

Toxoid A toxin (a poisonous substance produced by a bacterium) that has been treated by heat or chemicals to destroy its harmful properties. It is administered to an individual to prevent an infectious disease by stimulating the production of antibodies in that individual.

Vaccine A suspension of attenuated (weakened) or killed microorganisms administered to an individual to prevent an infectious disease by stimulating the production of antibodies in that individual.

Vertex The top of the head.

ON THE WEB

For Information on Child Health:

KidsHealth: www.kidshealth.com

Healthy Kids: www.healthykids.com

ParentCenter: parentcenter.babycenter.com

Pediatric on Call: www.pediatriconcall.com

Kids Source Online: www.kidsource.com

American Academy of Pediatrics: www.aap.org

For Information on Childhood Conditions:

Attention-Deficit Hyperactivity Disorder: www.add-adhd.org

Attention Deficit Disorder Association: www.add.org

Cerebral Palsy: www.about-cerebral-palsy.org

American Academy for Cerebral Palsy and Developmental Medicine: www.aacpdm.org

Child Abuse: www.preventchildabuse.org

American Professional Society on the Abuse of Children: apsac.fmhi.usf.edu

Cystic Fibrosis: www.cysticfibrosis.com

Cystic Fibrosis Foundation: www.cff.org

Dental Health: Colgate World of Care: www.colgate.com

American Denistry Association: www.ada.org

The Tooth Fairy Online: www.asis.com/toothfairy

Diabetes: American Diabetes Association: www.diabetes.org

Children with Diabetes: www.childrenwithdiabetes.com

Down Syndrome: www.downsyndrome.com

National Down Syndrome Society: www.ndss.org

Spina Bifida Association of America: www.sbaa.org

National SIDS/Infant Death Resource Center: www.sidscenter.org

Influenza Information: www.cdc.gov/flu

SIDS Alliance: www.sidsalliance.org

For Information on Immunizations:

Centers for Disease Control and Prevention: Vaccine Information Statements: www.cdc.gov/nip

American Academy of Pediatrics Childhood Immunization Support Program: www.cispimmunize.org

American Academy of Family Physicians: Recommendations for Immunizations: www.aafp.org

The Children's Hospital of Philadelphia Vaccine Education Center: www.chop.edu

Every Child by Two: www.ecbt.org

National Network for Immunization Information: www.immunizationinfo.org

10

Minor Office Surgery

LEARNING OBJECTIVES

Surgical Asepsis

1. Identify procedures that require the use of surgical asepsis.
2. Describe the medical assistant's responsibilities during a minor surgical procedure.
3. List the guidelines to follow to maintain surgical asepsis during a sterile procedure.
4. Identify and explain the use and care of instruments commonly used for minor office surgery.

Wound Healing

1. Explain the difference between a closed and an open wound, and give examples.
2. List and explain the three phases of the healing process.
3. List and describe the different types of wound drainage.
4. List the functions of a dressing.

Sutures

1. Explain the method used to measure the diameter of suturing material.
2. Describe the two types of sutures (absorbable and nonabsorbable), and give examples of their uses.
3. Categorize suturing needles according to type of point and shape.

Medical Office Surgical Procedures

1. Explain the purpose of and procedure for each of the following minor surgical operations: sebaceous cyst removal, incision and drainage of a localized infection, needle biopsy, ingrown toenail removal, colposcopy, cervical punch biopsy, and cryosurgery.
2. Explain the principles underlying each step in the minor office surgery procedures.

PROCEDURES

Apply and remove sterile gloves.
Open a sterile package.
Add an article to a sterile field.
Pour a sterile solution.

Change a sterile dressing.

Remove sutures.
Remove surgical staples.
Apply and remove adhesive skin closures.
Set up a tray for each of the following surgical procedures:
    Suture insertion
    Sebaceous cyst removal
    Incision and drainage of a localized infection
    Needle biopsy
    Ingrown toenail removal
    Colposcopy
    Cervical punch biopsy
    Cryosurgery

Assist the physician with minor office surgery.

LEARNING OBJECTIVES

Bandaging

1. State the functions of a bandage, and list the guidelines for applying a bandage.
2. Identify the common types of bandages used in the medical office.
3. Explain the use of a tubular gauze bandage.

PROCEDURES

Apply each of the following bandage turns:
    Circular
    Spiral
    Spiral-reverse
    Figure-eight
    Recurrent
Apply a tubular gauze bandage.

CHAPTER OUTLINE

Introduction to Minor Office Surgery
Surgical Asepsis
Instruments Used in Minor Office Surgery
    Scalpels
    Scissors
    Forceps
    Miscellaneous Instruments
    Gynecologic Instruments
    Care of Surgical Instruments
Commercially Prepared Sterile Packages
Wounds
    Wound Healing
Sterile Dressing Change
Sutures
    Types of Sutures
    Suture Size and Packaging
    Suture Needles
    Insertion of Sutures
    Suture Removal
    Surgical Skin Staples
    Adhesive Skin Closures

Assisting with Minor Office Surgery
    Tray Setup
    Skin Preparation
    Local Anesthetic
    Assisting the Physician
Medical Office Surgical Procedures
    Sebaceous Cyst Removal
    Surgical Incision and Drainage of Localized Infections
    Needle Biopsy
    Ingrown Toenail Removal
    Colposcopy
    Cervical Punch Biopsy
    Cryosurgery
Bandaging
    Guidelines for Application
    Types of Bandages
    Bandage Turns
    Tubular Gauze Bandages

NATIONAL COMPETENCIES

Clinical Competencies
Patient Care
Prepare patient and assist with procedures, treatments, and minor office surgeries.

General Competencies
Legal Concepts
Identify and respond to issues of confidentiality.
Perform within legal and ethical boundaries.

Patient Instruction
Provide instruction for health maintenance and disease prevention.

KEY TERMS

abrasion (ah-BRAY-shun)
abscess (AB-sess)
absorbable suture (ab-SOR-ba-bul SOO-chur)
approximation (ah-PROKS-ih-MAY-shun)
bandage
biopsy (BYE-op-see)
capillary action (KAP-ill-air-ee AK-shun)
colposcope (KOL-poe-skope)

colposcopy (kol-POS-koe-pee)
contaminate (kon-TAM-in-ate)
contusion (kon-TOO-shun)
cryosurgery (KRY-oh-SURJ-er-ee)
exudate (EKS-oo-date)
fibroblast (FYE-broh-blast)
forceps (FORE-seps)
furuncle (FYOOR-un-kul)

hemostasis (hee-moe-STAY-sis)
incision (in-SIH-shun)
infection (in-FEK-shun)
infiltration (in-fill-TRAY-shun)
inflammation (in-flah-MAY-shun)
laceration (Lass-ur-AY-shun)
ligate (LIH-gate)
local anesthetic (LOE-kul an-es-STET-ik)
Mayo (MAY-oe) tray
needle biopsy (NEE-dul BYE-op-see)
nonabsorbable suture (non-ab-SOR-ba-bul SOO-chur)
postoperative (post-OP-er-uh-tiv)

preoperative (pree-OP-er-uh-tiv)
puncture (PUNK-shur)
scalpel (SKAL-pul)
scissors
sebaceous cyst (suh-BAY-shus SIST)
serum (SEER-um)
sterile (STARE-ul)
surgical asepsis (SUR-jih-kul ay-SEP-sis)
sutures (SOO-churz)
swaged (SWAYJD) needle
wound

Introduction to Minor Office Surgery

Various types of minor surgical operations are performed in the medical office, such as insertion of sutures, sebaceous cyst removal, mole removal, incision and drainage of infections, needle biopsies, cervical biopsies, and ingrown toenail removal. The physician explains the nature of the surgical procedure and any risks to the patient and offers to answer questions. The medical assistant is responsible for explaining the patient preparation required for the procedure and for obtaining the patient's signature on a written consent to treatment form, which grants the physician permission to perform the surgery (Figure 10-1).

Additional responsibilities of the medical assistant include preparing the treatment room, preparing the patient, preparing the minor surgery tray, assisting the physician during the procedure, administering postoperative care to the patient, and cleaning the treatment room after the procedure.

The treatment room must be spotlessly clean, and the medical assistant should ensure that the physician has adequate lighting for the procedure. The patient is positioned and draped according to the procedure to be performed. The skin is prepared as specified by the physician. Hair around the operative site is a contaminant and may need to be removed by shaving. The skin is cleansed, and an appropriate antiseptic is applied to the area to reduce the number of microorganisms present.

The medical assistant prepares the minor surgery tray using **sterile** technique. The specific instruments and supplies included in each setup vary, depending on the type of surgery to be performed and the physician's preference. The medical assistant must become familiar with the instruments and supplies required for each surgical procedure performed in the medical office.

During the minor surgery, the medical assistant is present to assist the physician as needed and to lend support to the patient. The medical assistant should become completely familiar with the assisting techniques (e.g., swabbing blood from the operative site) required for each surgical procedure performed in the medical office and learn to anticipate the physician's needs to help the procedure go quickly and smoothly.

After the minor surgery, the medical assistant should remain with the patient as a safety precaution to prevent accidental falls and other injuries and to make sure the patient understands the postoperative instructions. The medical assistant removes and properly cares for all used instruments and supplies and cleans the treatment room in preparation for the next patient.

SURGICAL ASEPSIS

Surgical asepsis, also known as *sterile technique,* refers to practices that keep objects and areas sterile, or free from all living microorganisms and spores. Surgical asepsis protects the patient from pathogenic microorganisms that may enter the body and cause disease. It is always employed under the following circumstances: when caring for broken skin, such as open wounds and suture punctures; when a skin surface is being penetrated, as by a surgical incision for a mole removal or the administration of an injection (the needle must remain sterile); and when a body cavity is entered that is normally sterile, such as during the insertion of a urinary catheter. Sterility of instruments and supplies is achieved through the use of disposable sterile items or by sterilizing reusable articles.

A sterile object that touches any unsterile object is automatically considered contaminated and must not be used. If the medical assistant is in doubt or has a question concerning the sterility of an article, he or she should consider it contaminated and replace it with a sterile article.

Sterility of the hands cannot be attained. Sanitizing the hands renders them medically aseptic and must be

---

(attach label or complete blanks)

First name: _____   Last name: _____

Date of Birth: _____ Month _____ Day _____ Year

Account Number: _____

Procedure Consent Form

I, _____ , hereby consent to have

Dr. _____ perform _____ .

I have been fully informed of the following by my physician:

1. The nature of my condition.
2. The nature and purpose of the procedure.
3. An explanation of risks involved with the procedure.
4. Alternative treatments or procedures available.
5. The likely results of the procedure.
6. The risks involved with declining or delaying the procedure.

My physician has offered to answer all questions concerning the proposed procedure.

I am aware that the practice of medicine and surgery is not an exact science, and I acknowledge that no guarantees have been made to me about the results of the procedure.

Patient _____   Date _____
                   (or guardian and relationship)

Witnessed _____   Date _____

Figure 10-1. Consent to treatment form.

Guidelines for Surgical Asepsis

1. Take precautions to prevent sterile packages from becoming wet. Wet packages draw microorganisms into the package owing to the capillary action of the liquid, resulting in contamination of the sterile package. If a sterile package that has been prepared at the medical office becomes wet, it must be rewrapped and resterilized; if a disposable sterile package becomes wet, it must be discarded.
2. A 1-inch border around the sterile field is considered contaminated or unsterile because this area may have become contaminated while the sterile field was being set up.
3. Always face the sterile field. If you must turn your back to it or leave the room, a sterile towel must be placed over the sterile field.
4. Hold all sterile articles above waist level. Anything out of sight might become contaminated. The sterile articles also should be held in front of you and should not touch your uniform.
5. To avoid contamination, place all sterile items in the center, not around the edges, of the sterile field.
6. Be careful not to spill water or solutions on the sterile field. The area beneath the field is contaminated, and microorganisms are drawn up onto the field by the capillary action of the liquid, resulting in contamination of the field.
7. Do not talk, cough, or sneeze over a sterile field. Water vapor from the nose, mouth, and lungs is carried outward by the air and contaminates the sterile field.
8. Do not reach over a sterile field. Dust or lint from your clothing may fall onto it, or your unsterile clothing may accidentally touch it.
9. Do not pass soiled dressings over the sterile field.
10. Always acknowledge if you have contaminated the sterile field so that proper steps can be taken to regain sterility.

Explain the following to the patient regarding wounds:
- The type of wound that the patient has: incision, laceration, puncture, or abrasion.
- The purpose of suturing the wound: to close the skin and protect against further contamination, to facilitate healing, and to leave a smaller scar.
- If a tetanus toxoid has been administered, explain the purpose of this immunization: to protect against tetanus (lockjaw).
- Teach the patient how to care for the wound, as follows:
  - Keep the dressing clean and dry. If it becomes wet, contact the medical office to schedule a sterile dressing change.
  - Apply an ice bag for swelling (if prescribed by the physician).

- Report immediately any signs that the wound is infected. These signs include:
  a. Fever
  b. Persistent or increased pain, swelling, or drainage
  c. Red streaks radiating away from the wound
  d. Increased redness or warmth
- Notify the office if the sutures become loose or break.
- Return as instructed by the physician for the removal of sutures.
- Teach the patient how to apply an ice bag (if prescribed by the physician).
- Give the patient written instructions on wound care to refer to at home.

destroy invading microorganisms and to restore the structure and function of the damaged tissues, as is described next.

Phases of Wound Healing

Wound healing occurs in three phases, which are described here and illustrated in Figure 10-5.

Phase 1

Phase 1, also called the *inflammatory phase,* begins as soon as the body is injured. This phase lasts approximately 3 to 4 days. During this phase, a fibrin network forms, resulting in a blood clot that "plugs" up the opening of the wound and stops the flow of blood. The blood clot eventually becomes the scab. The inflammatory process also occurs during this phase. **Inflammation** is the protective response of the body to trauma, such as cuts and abrasions, and to the entrance of foreign matter, such as microorganisms. During inflammation, the blood supply to the wound increases, which brings white blood cells and nutrients to the site to assist in the healing process. The four local signs of inflammation are redness, swelling, pain, and warmth. The purpose of inflammation is to destroy invading microorganisms and to remove damaged tissue debris from the area so that proper healing can occur.

Phase 2

Phase 2 is also called the *granulation phase* and typically lasts 4 to 20 days. During this phase, **fibroblasts** migrate to the wound and begin to synthesize collagen. Collagen is a white protein that provides strength to the wound. As the amount of collagen increases, the wound becomes stronger, and the chance that the wound will open decreases. There also is a growth of new capillaries during this phase to provide the damaged tissue with an abundant supply of blood. As the capillary network develops, the tissue becomes a translucent red color. This tissue is known as *granulation tissue.* Granulation tissue consists primarily of collagen and is fragile and shiny and bleeds easily.

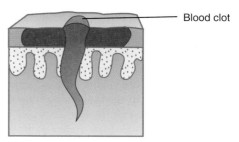

Phase 1: Inflammatory Phase

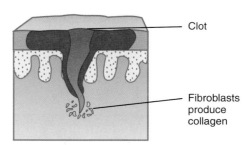

Phase 2: Granulation Phase

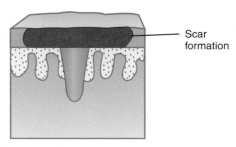

Phase 3: Maturation Phase

Figure 10-5. Phases of wound healing.

Phase 3

Phase 3, also known as the *maturation phase,* begins as soon as granulation tissue forms and can last for 2 years. During this phase, collagen continues to be synthesized, and the granulation tissue eventually hardens to white scar tissue. Scar tissue is not true skin and does not contain nerves or have a blood supply.

The medical assistant should always inspect the wound when providing wound care. The wound should be observed for signs of inflammation and the amount of healing that has occurred. This information should be charted in the patient's record.

Wound Drainage

The medical term for drainage is **exudate.** An exudate is material, such as fluid and cells, that has escaped from blood vessels during the inflammatory process. The exudate is deposited in tissue or on tissue surfaces and is often present in a wound. When providing wound care, the medical assistant should always inspect the wound for drainage and chart this information in the patient's record. There are three major types of exudates: serous, sanguineous, and purulent.

- **Serous exudate.** A serous exudate consists chiefly of **serum,** which is the clear portion of the blood. Serous drainage is clear and watery. An example of a serous exudate is the fluid in a blister from a burn.
- **Sanguineous exudate.** A sanguineous exudate is red and consists of red blood cells. This type of drainage results when capillaries are damaged, allowing the escape of red blood cells, and is frequently seen in open wounds. A bright-red sanguineous exudate indicates fresh bleeding, and a dark exudate indicates older bleeding.
- **Purulent exudate.** A purulent exudate contains pus, which consists of leukocytes, dead liquefied tissue debris, and dead and living bacteria. Purulent drainage is usually thick and has an unpleasant odor. It is white in color, but may acquire tinges of pink, green, or yellow depending on the type of infecting organism. The process of pus formation is *suppuration.*

In addition to the exudates just described, mixed types of exudates are often observed in a wound. A *serosanguineous exudate* consists of clear and blood-tinged drainage and is commonly seen in surgical incisions. A *purosanguineous exudate* consists of pus and blood and is often seen in a new wound that is infected.

STERILE DRESSING CHANGE

Surgical asepsis must be maintained when one is caring for and applying a dry sterile dressing (abbreviated as *DVD*) to an open wound. The medical assistant must take care to prevent infection in clean wounds and to decrease infection in wounds already infected. The function of a sterile dressing is to protect the wound from contamination and trauma, to absorb drainage, and to restrict motion, which may interfere with proper wound healing. The size, type, and amount of dressing material used during a sterile dressing change depend on the size and location of the wound and the amount of drainage.

Sterile folded *gauze pads* are used in the medical office for a sterile dressing change. This type of dressing absorbs drainage, but the gauze has a tendency to stick to the wound when the drainage dries. Gauze pads come in a variety of sizes, including 4×4, 3×3, and 2×2; the 4×4 size is used most frequently.

Nonadherent pads also are used as a sterile dressing; they have one surface impregnated with agents that prevent the dressing from sticking to the wound. One brand of this type of material is Telfa pads. The nonadherent side, which is shiny, is placed next to the wound. Telfa dressings are often used to cover burned skin. Procedure 10-4 presents the procedure for changing a sterile dressing.

Text continued on p. 380

PROCEDURE 1O-4   Changing a Sterile Dressing

Outcome   Change a sterile dressing.

Equipment/Supplies

- Mayo stand
- Biohazard waste container

Side Table

- Clean disposable gloves
- Antiseptic swabs
- Sterile gloves
- Plastic waste bag
- Hypoallergenic adhesive tape
- Scissors

Sterile Field

- Sterile dressing
- Sterile thumb forceps

1. **Procedural Step.** Wash your hands with an antimicrobial soap.
2. **Procedural Step.** Assemble the equipment. Set up the nonsterile items on a side table or counter. Position the waterproof waste bag in a location convenient for disposal of contaminated items.
3. **Procedural Step.** Greet the patient and introduce yourself. Identify the patient and explain the procedure. Instruct the patient not to move during the procedure. Adjust the light so that it is focused on the dressing.
4. **Procedural Step.** Apply clean gloves. Loosen the tape on the dressing, and pull it toward the wound. Care-

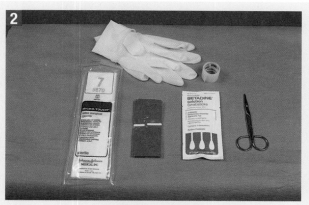

Prepare the side table.

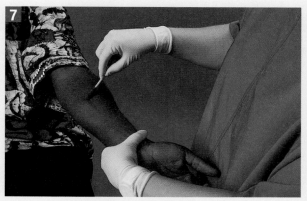

Apply an antiseptic to the wound.

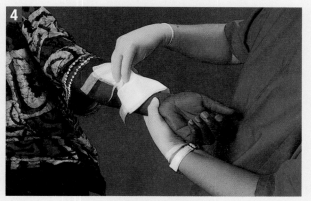

Remove the soiled dressing.

fully and gently remove the soiled dressing by pulling it upward. Do not touch the inside of the dressing that was next to the open wound. If the dressing is stuck to the wound, it can be loosened by moistening it with a normal saline solution. Place the soiled dressing in the waste bag without allowing the dressing to touch the outside of the bag.

Principle. Gentle dressing removal avoids unnecessary stress on the wound. Touching the inside of the dressing can transfer an infected discharge to your gloves.

5. **Procedural Step.** Inspect the wound, and observe for the following: amount of healing; presence of inflammation; and presence of drainage, including the amount (scant, moderate, or profuse) and type of drainage.

Principle. Drainage is classified as serous (containing serum), sanguineous (red and composed of blood), serosanguineous (containing serum and blood), or purulent (containing pus and appearing white with tinges of yellow, pink, or green, depending on the type of infecting microorganism). Purulent drainage is usually thick and has an unpleasant odor.

6. **Procedural Step.** Open the pouch containing the sterile antiseptic swabs, and place it in a convenient location or hold it in your nondominant hand.

7. **Procedural Step.** Using the antiseptic swabs, apply the antiseptic to the wound. Apply the antiseptic

from the top to the bottom of the wound, working from the center to the outside of the wound. Use a new swab for each motion. Discard each contaminated swab in the waste bag after use.

Principle. The purpose of the antiseptic is to decrease the number of microorganisms in the wound.

8. **Procedural Step.** Remove the clean disposable gloves, and discard them in the waste bag without contaminating yourself. Sanitize your hands and prepare the sterile field using surgical asepsis. Items are either placed onto a sterile field or contained in a prepackaged set-up. Instruct the patient not to talk, laugh, sneeze, or cough over the sterile field.

Principle. Microorganisms are carried in water vapor from the mouth, nose, and lungs, and can be transferred onto the sterile field.

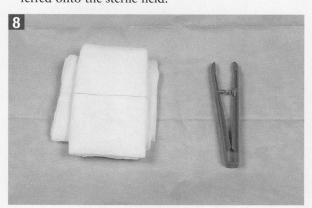

Prepare the sterile field.

9. **Procedural Step.** Open a package of sterile gloves, and apply them.

10. **Procedural Step.** Pick up the sterile dressing with your gloved hand or sterile forceps. Place the sterile dressing over the wound by lightly dropping it in place. Do not move the dressing once you have dropped it into place. Discard the gloves or forceps in the waste bag.

Principle. Dropping the dressing over the wound and not moving it prevents the transfer of microorganisms from the skin to the center of the wound.

Continued

PROCEDURE 10-4

PROCEDURE 10-4   Changing a Sterile Dressing—cont'd

11. **Procedural Step.** Apply hypoallergenic adhesive tape to hold the dressing in place. The tape must be long enough to adhere to the skin, but not so long that it loosens when the patient moves. The strips of tape should be evenly spaced, with strips at each end of the dressing.

12. **Procedural Step.** Instruct the patient in wound care as follows:
 a. Provide the patient with written wound care instructions (see the patient teaching box on wound care in this chapter).
 b. Explain the wound care instructions, and ask the patient whether he or she has any questions. Tell the patient to keep the wound clean and dry and to contact the office if signs of infection occur such as excessive swelling, pain, or discharge.
 c. Ask the patient to sign the instruction sheet on the appropriate line.
 d. Witness the patient's signature by signing your name in the appropriate space on the form. Include today's date.

 e. Before the patient leaves the medical office, make a copy of the instruction sheet. Give a signed copy of the wound care instructions to the patient, and file the original in the patient's medical record.
 Principle. The filed copy protects the physician legally in the event that the patient fails to follow the instructions and causes further harm or damage to the wound.

13. **Procedural Step.** Return the equipment. Tightly secure the bag containing the soiled dressing and contaminated articles, and dispose of it in a biohazard waste container.
 Principle. Contaminated items must be disposed of properly to prevent the spread of infection.

14. **Procedural Step.** Sanitize your hands.

15. **Procedural Step.** Chart the procedure. Include the date and time, location of the dressing, condition of the wound, type and amount of drainage, care of the wound, and any problems the patient experienced with the wound. Also chart the instructions given to the patient on wound care.

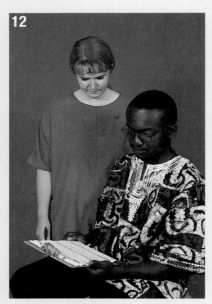

Instruct the patient in wound care.

CHARTING EXAMPLE

Date	
9/20/08	10:30 a.m. Dressing changed (L) ant forearm.
	Scant amt of serous drainage noted. Sl
	redness around incision line. Sutures intact
	and suture line in good approximation. Incision
	cleaned c̄ Betadine and DSD applied. No
	complaints of pain or discomfort. Explained
	wound care. Written instructions provided.
	Signed copy filed in chart. To return in 2 days
	for suture removal. ———— T. Browning, CMA

SUTURES

The insertion and removal of **sutures** are commonly performed in the medical office. Sutures may be required to close a surgical incision or to repair an accidental wound. They **approximate,** or bring together, the edges of the wound with surgical stitches and hold them in place until proper healing can occur. Sutures also protect the wound from further contamination and minimize the amount of

scar formation. A **local anesthetic** is necessary to numb the area before the sutures are inserted.

Types of Sutures

Sutures are available in two types: absorbable and nonabsorbable. **Absorbable sutures** consist of surgical gut or synthetic materials, such as polyglycolic acid (Dexon), polyglactin 910 (Vicryl), polydioxanone (PS II), polyglyconate

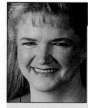

Trudy Browing: I remember observing my first minor office surgery during my externship. It was a sebaceous cyst removal. The cyst was located on the calf of the patient's left leg. I helped in setting up the surgical tray and prepared and draped the site. I tried to explain to the patient what was going on to prepare her for the procedure. I think the patient was calmer than I was. The physician entered the room with a medical assistant on hand. Although I was in the room primarily to observe, I helped the physician with his surgical gloves and in numbing the site. I watched the physician make the incision and cut out and remove a large cyst.

Everything was going smoothly until the physician started to suture the wound. I felt like someone had turned the heat up really high; the room seemed to get really hot. I started to feel dizzy. I smiled at the physician and excused myself. He just smiled back at me, and I left the room. I went outside the room and caught my breath. I regained my composure and reentered the room. The physician was still suturing the wound. As I watched him run the needle through the skin and pull the suture tight, it really got to me. I smiled and told the physician that I would wait outside until they were done. After the physician left the room, I went back to help clean up. I felt so stupid. Later that day, the physician looked at me and said: "Got a little warm in there, didn't it?" He just laughed and said that what I did was normal and not to worry about it. He made me feel better about myself. After that incident, I went in alone and helped him with cyst removals, and it didn't bother me at all. ■

(Maxon), and poliglecaprone (Monocryl) (Figure 10-6A). Surgical gut is made from sheep or cow intestine. This type of suturing material is gradually digested by tissue enzymes and absorbed by the body's tissues 5 to 20 days after insertion, depending on the kind of surgical gut employed. Plain surgical gut has a rapid absorption time, whereas chromic surgical gut is treated to slow down its rate of absorption in the tissues. Absorbable sutures frequently are used to suture subcutaneous tissue, fascia, intestines, bladder, and peritoneum and to **ligate,** or tie off, vessels. Because the suturing

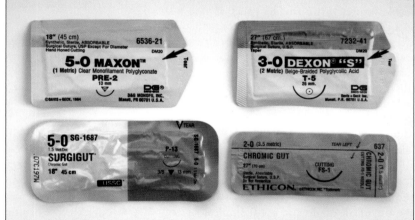

A, Absorbable sutures.

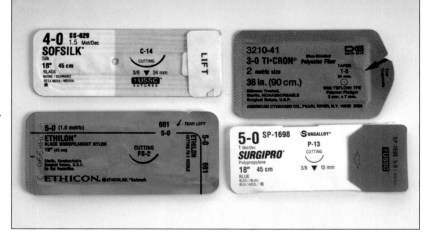

B, Nonabsorbable sutures.

Figure 10-6 Swaged suture packets.

of this type of tissue is generally done during surgery performed by the physician in the hospital with the patient under a general anesthetic, the medical office may not stock absorbable suture material.

Nonabsorbable sutures (Figure 10-6B) are not absorbed by the body and either remain permanently in the body tissues and become encapsulated by fibrous tissue or are removed (e.g., skin sutures). Nonabsorbable sutures are used to suture skin; this type of suture is used frequently in the medical office. Nonabsorbable sutures are made from materials that are not affected by tissue enzymes. These materials include silk, cotton, nylon (Ethilon), braided polyester (Ti-Cron), polypropylene (Prolene), stainless steel, and surgical skin staples.

Suture Size and Packaging

Sutures are measured by their gauge, which refers to the diameter of the suturing material. The size ranges from numbers below 0 (pronounced "aught") to numbers above 0. The diameter of the suture material increases with each number above 0 and decreases with each number below 0. If the size of a particular suture material ranges from 6-0 to 4, the available sizes include 6-0, 5-0, 4-0, 3-0, 2-0, 0, 1, 2, 3, and 4. Size 6-0 are very fine sutures, and size 4 are very heavy sutures. Size 2-0 (00) sutures have a smaller diameter than size 0 sutures.

Nonabsorbable sutures with a smaller gauge (5-0 to 6-0) are used for suturing incisions in delicate tissue, such as the face and neck, whereas nonabsorbable heavy sutures are used for firmer tissue, such as the chest and abdomen. Finer sutures also leave less scar formation and are used when cosmetic results are desired.

Sutures come in individual packages that consist of an outer peel-apart package and a sterile inner packet. They are labeled according to the type of suture material (e.g., surgical silk), the size (e.g., 4-0), and the length of the suturing material (e.g., 18 inches). The type and size of material used are based on the nature and location of the tissue being sutured and the physician's preference. To repair a laceration of the arm, the physician might use a 4-0 surgical silk suture. The physician informs the medical assistant of the type and size of sutures needed.

Suture Needles

Needles used for suturing are categorized according to their type of point and their shape. A needle with a sharp point is a *cutting needle,* and one with a round point is a *noncutting needle.* Cutting needles (Figure 10-7A) are used for firm tissues such as skin; the sharp point helps push the needle through the tissue. Noncutting or blunt needles are used to penetrate tissues that offer a small amount of resistance, such as the fascia, intestine, liver, spleen, kidney, subcutaneous tissue, and muscle.

A suture needle is either curved or straight (see Figure 10-7A). *Curved needles* permit the physician to dip in and out of the tissue. A needle holder must be used with a curved needle. A *straight needle* is used when the tissue can

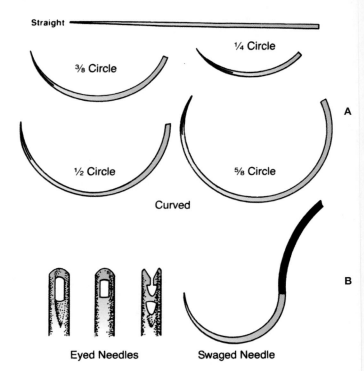

Figure 10-7. Common suture needles. **A,** Needles with a cutting point. **B,** Eyed needles and a swaged needle. (**A** modified from *Perspectives on sutures,* courtesy Davis & Geck, Danbury, Conn; **B,** modified from Nealon TF Jr: *Fundamental skills in surgery,* ed 4, Philadelphia, 1994, Saunders.)

be displaced sufficiently to permit the needle to be pushed and pulled through the tissue. Straight needles do not require the use of a needle holder.

Some needles have an eye through which the suture material is inserted, and some needles are **swaged** (Figure 10-7B). *Swaged* means that the suture and needle are one continuous unit; the needle is permanently attached to the end of the suture. Swaged needles are used frequently because they offer several advantages over eyed needles. One advantage is that the suture material does not slip off the needle, as might occur with suture material threaded through the eye of a needle. Another advantage is that tissue trauma is reduced because a swaged needle has only a single strand of suture that must be pulled through the tissue compared with a double strand in an eyed needle. The swaged needle can be pulled through the tissue with less resulting trauma. Swaged suture packets are labeled to specify the gauge, type, and length of suture material and the type of needle point (cutting or noncutting) and the needle shape (curved or straight) (see Figure 10-6).

Insertion of Sutures

The medical assistant may be responsible for preparing the suture tray and for assisting the physician during the insertion of the sutures. The physician designates the size and type of suture material and needle required. Because sutures, needles, and suture-needle combinations (swaged needles) are contained in peel-apart packages, they can be added to the sterile field by flipping them onto the sterile

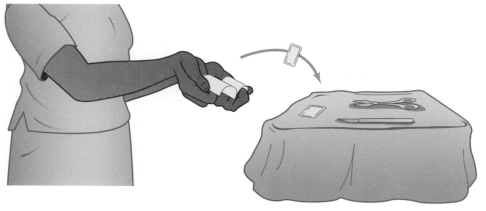

Flipping sutures onto the sterile field.

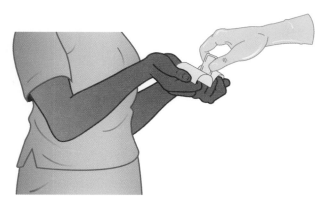

The physician removing the sutures with a sterile gloved hand.

Figure 10-8. Adding sutures to a sterile field.

field or by placing them there with a sterile gloved hand (Figure 10-8).

Suture Insertion Setup
The items required for a suture insertion setup are listed next.

Items Placed to the Side of the Sterile Field
- Clean disposable gloves
- Antiseptic solution
- Surgical scrub brush
- Antiseptic swabs

- Sterile gloves
- Local anesthetic
- Antiseptic wipe to cleanse the vial
- Tetanus toxoid with needle and syringe

Items Included on the Sterile Field
- Fenestrated drape
- Syringe and needle for drawing up the local anesthetic
- Hemostatic forceps
- Thumb forceps

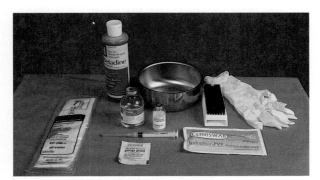

Suture insertion side table.

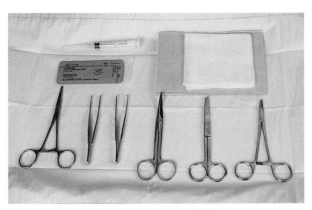

Suture insertion sterile field.

- Tissue forceps
- Dissecting scissors
- Operating scissors
- Needle holder
- Suture
- Sterile 4 × 4 gauze

Suture Removal

When the wound has healed such that it no longer needs the support of nonabsorbable suture material, the sutures must be removed. The length of time the sutures remain in place depends on their location and the amount of healing that must occur. Some areas of the body, such as the head and neck, have a good blood supply; the sutures do not need to remain there as long as they do in other areas because this area heals more rapidly.

Sutures must always be left in place long enough for proper healing to occur. The physician determines the length of time, but in general, skin sutures inserted in the face and neck are removed in 3 to 5 days, and sutures inserted in other areas, such as the skin of the chest, arms, legs, hands, and feet, are removed in 7 to 10 days.

Surgical Skin Staples

Surgical skin staples are often used to close wounds. Stapling is the fastest method of closure of long skin incisions. In addition, trauma to the tissue is reduced because the tissue does not have to be handled much when inserting the staples. Surgical staples are stainless steel and are inserted into the skin using a special skin stapler. Skin staplers are available as reusable or disposable devices. The skin stapler holds a cartridge that contains a prescribed number and size of staples (Figure 10-9).

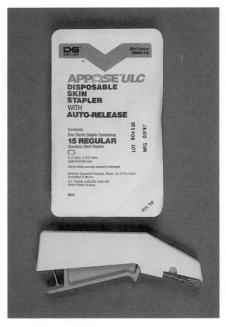

Figure 10-9. Disposable skin stapler.

The physician inserts the staples by gently approximating the tissues with tissue forceps. The skin stapler is held over the site, and the staple is inserted into the skin. Skin stapling produces excellent cosmetic results, and the staples are easy to remove with a specially designed staple remover.

The medical assistant is frequently responsible for removing sutures and staples. This procedure should be done only after the physician has given a written or verbal order to the medical assistant. Procedure 10-5 presents the method used to remove sutures and skin staples.

Text continued on p. 387

What Would You Do? What Would You *Not* Do?

Case Study 1

Kerry Ventura brings her 6-year-old son Cory to the medical office. Cory got a new bike for his birthday and just learned how to ride it without training wheels. While going around a corner, he lost his balance and fell and cut his left knee. The incision is about 1½ inches long. Cory is going to need sutures to approximate the wound. Mrs. Ventura is very upset and blames herself. She says that she should have been watching him more closely. Mrs. Ventura wants to know why Steri-Strips can't be used to close the incision. She says that it would be a lot less painful for Cory than having stitches. When asked to sign the consent to treatment form for Cory, Mrs. Ventura says she does not want to sign the form until her husband has a chance to read it. She says that right now he is in Japan for 2 weeks on a business trip. ∎

PROCEDURE 10-5   Removing Sutures and Staples

Outcome Remove sutures and staples.

Equipment/Supplies

- Antiseptic swabs
- Clean disposable gloves
- Sterile 4 × 4 gauze

For Suture Removal

- Suture removal kit, which includes:
  - Suture scissors
  - Thumb forceps
  - Sterile 4 × 4 gauze

For Staple Removal

- Staple removal kit, which includes:
  - Staple remover
  - Sterile 4 × 4 gauze

1. Procedural Step. Wash your hands with an antimicrobial soap. Assemble the equipment.
Principle. Washing the hands with an antimicrobial soap removes microorganisms from the hands and also

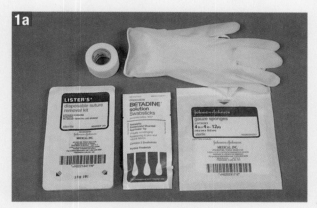

Suture removal setup.

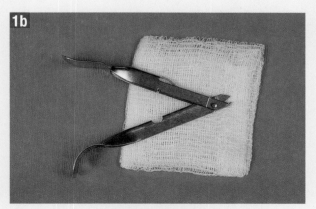

Staple removal setup.

- Surgical tape
- Mayo stand
- Biohazard waste container

deposits an antimicrobial film on your hands to discourage the growth of bacteria.

2. Procedural Step. Greet the patient and introduce yourself. Identify the patient and explain the procedure.

3. Procedural Step. Position the patient as required to provide good access to the site. Adjust the light so that it is focused on the wound. Verify that the sutures (or staples) are intact and that the incision line is approximated and not gaping. Check that the incision line is not infected. If the incision line is not approximated or if redness, swelling, or a discharge is present, do not remove the sutures; notify the physician.
Principle. The sutures (or staples) should not be removed unless the incision line is approximated and free from infection.

4. Procedural Step. Open the suture or staple removal kit, keeping the contents of the kit sterile. Most kits are opened by peeling back a top cover, which exposes a plastic tray that holds the necessary instruments and supplies.

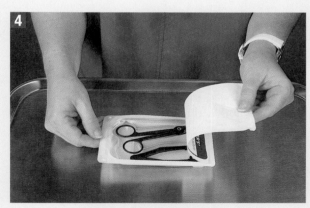

Open the suture removal kit.

5. Procedural Step. Apply clean gloves. Cleanse the incision line with an antiseptic swab to destroy microorganisms and to remove any dried exudate encrusted around the sutures or staples. Clean the wound from the top to the bottom, working from the center to the outside of the wound. Use a new swab for each cleansing motion. Allow the skin to dry.
Principle. Dried exudate must be removed to allow unimpeded removal of the sutures or staples.

Continued

PROCEDURE 10-5

6. Procedural Step. Remove the sutures or staples. Tell the patient that he or she will feel a pulling or tugging sensation as each suture (or staple) is removed, but that it will not be painful. Count the number of sutures or staples removed. Check the patient's chart to make sure the same number are removed as were inserted by the physician.

To remove sutures:

a. Using the sterile thumb forceps provided in the kit, pick up the knot of the first suture.

b. Place the curved tip of the suture scissors under the suture. Using the sterile suture scissors, cut the suture below the knot on the side of the suture closest to the skin. Cut the suture as close to the skin as possible.

c. Using a smooth, continuous motion, gently pull the suture out of the skin. Remove the suture without allowing any portion that was previously outside to be pulled back through the tissue lying beneath the incision line. Place the suture on the 4 × 4 gauze included in the suture kit.

d. Continue in this manner until all the sutures have been removed.

Principle. To prevent infection, the suture must be removed without pulling any portion that has been outside the skin back through the tissue lying beneath the incision line.

To remove staples:

a. Gently place the bottom jaws of the staple remover under the staple to be removed.

b. Firmly squeeze the staple handles until they are fully closed.

c. Carefully lift the staple remover upward to remove the staple from the incision line. Place the staple on the 4 × 4 gauze included in the staple kit.

d. Continue in this manner until all the staples have been removed.

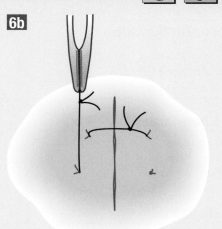

Gently pull the suture out. (From Nealon TF Jr: *Fundamental skills in surgery,* ed 4, Philadelphia, 1994, Saunders.)

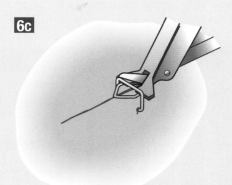

Place the bottom jaws of the staple remover under the staple.

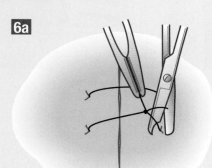

Cut the suture below the knot on the side closest to the skin. (From Nealon TF Jr: *Fundamental skills in surgery,* ed 4, Philadelphia, 1994, Saunders.)

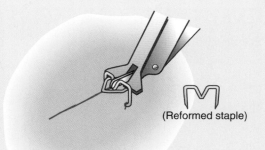

(Reformed staple)

Firmly squeeze the staple handles until they are fully closed. (Courtesy Ethicon, Somerville, NJ.)

7. **Procedural Step.** Cleanse the site with an antiseptic swab. Some physicians want the medical assistant to apply adhesive skin closures after removing the sutures or staples to provide additional support to the wound as it continues to heal.

8. **Procedural Step.** Apply a dry sterile dressing if indicated by the physician.

9. **Procedural Step.** Dispose of the sutures (or staples) and the gauze in a biohazard waste container.

10. **Procedural Step.** Remove the gloves, and sanitize your hands.

11. **Procedural Step.** Chart the procedure. Include the date and time, the status of the sutures (or staples) and incision line, the number of sutures (or staples) removed, the location of the site, care of the wound (i.e., application of an antiseptic or dressing), and the patient's reaction. Chart any instructions given to the patient.

CHARTING EXAMPLE	
Date	
9/20/08	10:30 a.m. Sutures intact and incision line in good approximation. No signs of infection. Sutures x6 removed from Ⓡ ant forearm. Incision line cleaned c̄ Betadine and DSD applied. Instructions provided on dressing care. —————————— T. Browning, CMA

PROCEDURE 10-5

Adhesive Skin Closures

Adhesive skin closures may be used for wound repair to approximate the edges of a laceration or incision. Skin closures consist of sterile, hypoallergenic tape that is commercially available in a variety of widths and lengths and is strong enough to approximate a wound until healing occurs. Brand names for adhesive skin closures are Steri-Strip (3M Corporation) and Proxi-Strip (Johnson & Johnson) (Figure 10-10).

Adhesive skin closures may be used when not much tension exists on the skin edges. The strips of tape are applied transversely across the line of incision to approximate the skin edges. The advantages of adhesive skin closures are that they eliminate the need for sutures and a local anesthetic, they are easy to apply and remove, they have a lower incidence of wound infection compared with sutures, and they result in less scarring than sutures. The disadvantage of this method is that there is less precision in bringing the wound edges together compared with suturing the wound. In addition, adhesive skin closures cannot be used on certain areas of the body where the adhesive has difficulty adhering to the skin. This includes areas that harbor moisture (e.g., palms of the hands, soles of the feet, axilla) and hairy areas of the body (e.g., scalp, a man's chest).

The medical assistant frequently is responsible for applying adhesive skin closures. Procedure 10-6 outlines this pro-

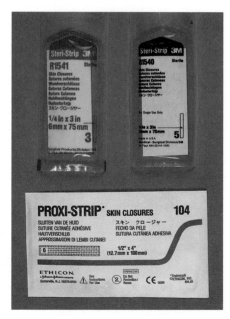

Figure 10-10. Adhesive skin closures in different sizes.

cedure. Approximately 5 to 10 days after application, the skin closures usually loosen and fall off on their own. If they require removal by the medical assistant, the method presented at the end of Procedure 10-6 should be followed.

Text continued on p. 391

PROCEDURE 10-6   Applying and Removing Adhesive Skin Closures

Outcome Apply and remove adhesive skin closures.

Equipment/Supplies

- Clean disposable gloves
- Sterile gloves
- Antiseptic solution
- Surgical scrub brush
- Antiseptic swabs

- Tincture of benzoin
- Sterile cotton-tipped applicator
- Adhesive skin closure strips
- Sterile 4 × 4 gauze pads
- Surgical tape

Application of Adhesive Skin Closures

1. Procedural Step. Wash your hands with an antimicrobial soap and assemble the equipment.

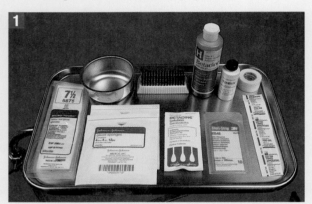

Assemble the equipment.

2. Procedural Step. Greet the patient and introduce yourself.

3. Procedural Step. Identify the patient and explain the procedure.

4. Procedural Step. Position the patient as required for application of the strips. Adjust the light so that it is focused on the wound. Apply clean gloves. Inspect the wound for signs of redness, swelling, and drainage. (*Note:* Chart this information in the patient's record after completing the procedure.)

5. Procedural Step. Gently scrub the wound using an antiseptic solution (e.g., Betadine solution) and a ster-

ile gauze pad or a surgical scrub brush. Clean at least 3 inches around the wound, removing all debris, skin oil, and exudates. Allow the skin to dry or pat dry with gauze squares. (*Note:* Change gloves as needed to maintain cleanliness.)

6. Procedural Step. Apply an antiseptic to the site using antiseptic swabs such as Betadine swabs. Apply the antiseptic from the top to the bottom of the wound, working from the center to the outside of the wound. Use a new swab for each motion. Allow the skin to dry completely.

Principle. The antiseptic decreases the number of microorganisms in the wound. The skin must be completely dry to ensure adhesion of the skin closures to the skin.

7. Procedural Step. If dictated by the medical office policy, apply a thin coat of tincture of benzoin to the skin parallel to each side of the wound with a sterile cotton-tipped applicator. Do not allow the tincture of benzoin to touch the wound. Allow the skin to dry. Remove the gloves, and wash your hands with an antimicrobial soap.

Principle. Tincture of benzoin facilitates adhesion of the strips to the skin.

8. Procedural Step. Open the plastic peel-apart package of strips using sterile technique as follows:

a. Grasp each flap of the package between the thumbs and bent index fingers. Pull the package apart.

b. Peel back the package until it is completely open.

c. Lay the opened package flat on a clean dry surface. The inside of the package serves as the sterile field.

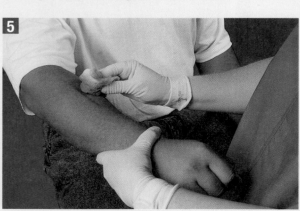

Clean the wound.

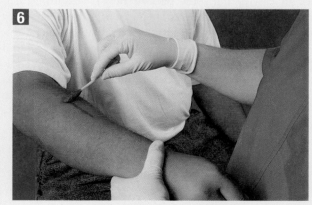

Apply an antiseptic to the wound.

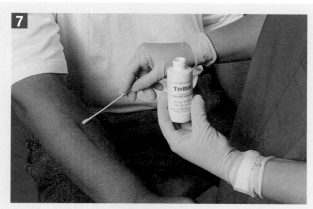

Apply tincture of benzoin.

9. Procedural Step. Apply sterile gloves. Fold the card of strips along its perforated tab, and tear off the tab, which exposes the ends of the strips, making them easier to grasp. Peel a strip of tape off the card at a 45-degree angle to the card.

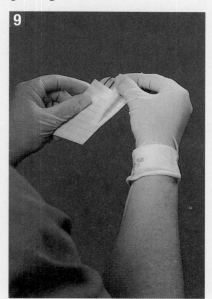

Peel a strip of tape off the card.

10. Procedural Step. Check that the skin surface is dry. Position the first strip over the center of the wound as follows:
   a. Secure one end of the strip of tape to the skin on one side of the wound by pressing down firmly on the tape.
   b. Stretch the strip transversely across the line of the incision until the edges of the wound are approximated exactly. If necessary, use your gloved hand to assist in bringing the edges of the wound together.
   c. Secure the strip on the skin on the other side of the wound by pressing down firmly on the tape.

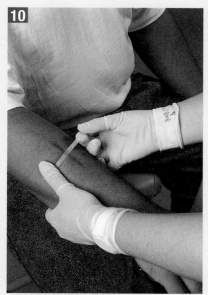

Position the first strip over the center of the wound.

Principle. Approximating the wound exactly facilitates good healing and minimizes scar formation.

11. Procedural Step. Apply the second strip perpendicular to the wound on one side of the center strip. The space between the strips should be approximately ⅛ inch. Apply a third strip on the other side of the center strip at a ⅛-inch interval. Continue applying the strips at ⅛-inch intervals until the edges of the wound are approximated. If at any time the skin surfaces become moist with perspiration, blood, or serum, wipe the area dry with a sterile gauze pad before applying the next strip.

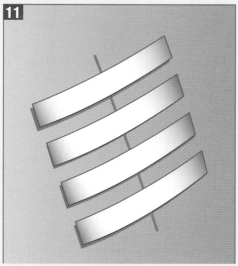

Apply the strips until the edges of the wound are approximated.

Continued

PROCEDURE 10-6

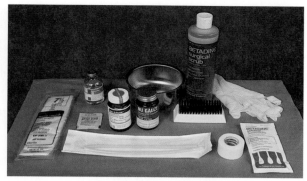

Incision and drainage side table.

Items Included on the Sterile Field
- Fenestrated drape
- Needle or syringe for drawing up the local anesthetic
- Scalpel and blade
- Dissecting scissors
- Hemostatic forceps
- Tissue forceps
- Thumb forceps
- Operating scissors
- Sterile 4 × 4 gauze

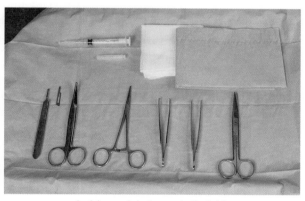

Incision and drainage sterile field.

Procedure
Localized infections, such as abscesses, furuncles, and infected sebaceous cysts, that do not rupture and drain naturally may need to be incised and drained by the physician as follows:
1. A local anesthetic is generally used for the procedure.
2. A scalpel is used to make the incision. Either a rubber Penrose drain or a gauze wick is inserted into the wound to keep the edges of the tissues apart, which facilitates drainage of the exudate. The exudate contains pathogenic microorganisms; the medical assistant should be careful to avoid contact with the exudate while assisting with the minor surgery.
3. A sterile dressing of several thicknesses is applied over the operative site to absorb the drainage.

Postoperative Instructions
The physician may prescribe the application of warm compresses to be applied by the patient at home. Applying heat to the operative site helps to promote healing. If the physician orders this treatment, the medical assistant should instruct the patient in this procedure properly according to the information outlined in Chapter 7 (see Procedure 7-3).

Needle Biopsy

A **biopsy** is the removal and examination of tissue from the living body. The tissue usually is examined under a microscope. Biopsies are most often performed to determine whether a tumor is malignant or benign; however, a biopsy also may be used as a diagnostic aid for other conditions, such as infections. A **needle biopsy** is a type of biopsy in which tissue from deep within the body is obtained by the insertion of a biopsy needle through the skin. A biopsy needle consists of an outer needle for making the puncture and a forked inner needle for obtaining the tissue specimen (Figure 10-18A). The inner needle detaches tissue from a part of the body and brings it to the surface through its lumen (Figure 10-18B). The advantage of a needle biopsy is that a sample of tissue can be obtained that might otherwise require a major surgical operation.

Needle Biopsy Setup
The items required for a needle biopsy are listed.

Items Placed to the Side of the Sterile Field
- Clean disposable gloves
- Antiseptic solution
- Surgical scrub brush
- Antiseptic swabs
- Sterile gloves
- Local anesthetic
- Antiseptic wipe to cleanse the vial
- Specimen container with preservative and label
- Laboratory request form
- Surgical tape

Items Included on the Sterile Field
- Fenestrated drape
- Needle and syringe for drawing up the local anesthetic
- Biopsy needle
- Sterile 4 × 4 gauze

Procedure
1. The procedure is performed under a local anesthetic, and because an incision is not required, the patient does not have to undergo the discomfort and inconvenience of an operative recovery.
2. The tissue specimen is placed in a container with a preservative and sent to the laboratory for examination by a pathologist.
3. A small dressing, placed over the needle puncture site, is usually sufficient to protect the operative site and promote healing.

Figure 10-18. Biopsy needle. **A,** A biopsy needle consists of an outer needle for making the puncture and a forked inner needle for obtaining the specimen. **B,** The inner needle detaches tissue from a part of the body and brings it to the surface through its lumen. (Modified from Nealon TF Jr: *Fundamental skills in surgery,* ed 4, Philadelphia, 1994, Saunders.)

4. After the procedure, the patient should be observed for any evidence of complications related to the procedure.

Ingrown Toenail Removal

An ingrown toenail occurs when the edge of the toenail grows deeply into the nail groove and penetrates the surrounding skin, resulting in pain and discomfort to the patient (Figure 10-19A). Ingrown toenails are caused by external pressure, such as from tight shoes, or from trauma, improper nail trimming, or infection. The protruding nail acts as a foreign body, usually resulting in secondary infec-

tion and inflammation. In mild cases, this condition is treated by inserting a small piece of cotton packing under the toenail to raise the nail edge away from the tissue of the nail groove (Figure 10-19B). In severe and recurring cases, part of the nail must be surgically removed, which relieves pain by decreasing the nail pressure on the soft tissues.

Ingrown Toenail Removal Setup

The items required for the removal of an ingrown toenail are listed.

Items Placed to the Side of the Sterile Field
- Clean disposable gloves
- Antiseptic solution
- Surgical scrub brush
- Antiseptic swabs
- Sterile gloves
- Local anesthetic
- Antiseptic wipe to cleanse the vial
- Surgical tape

Items Included on the Sterile Field
- Fenestrated drape
- Needle and syringe for drawing up the local anesthetic
- Surgical toenail scissors
- Hemostatic forceps
- Operating scissors
- Sterile 4 × 4 gauze

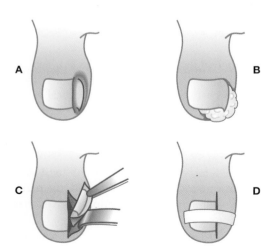

Figure 10-19. Ingrown toenail. **A,** The edge of the toenail grows deeply into the nail groove. **B,** In mild cases, treatment consists of inserting a small piece of cotton packing under the toenail. **C,** In severe and recurring cases, a wedge of the nail is surgically removed. **D,** A strip of surgical tape is applied over the area. (From Nealon TF Jr: *Fundamental skills in surgery,* ed 4, Philadelphia, 1994, Saunders.)

Procedure

An ingrown toenail is removed as follows:
1. Before the surgical procedure is performed, the affected foot must be soaked in tepid water containing an antibac-

terial skin solution for 10 to 15 minutes to soften the nail plate and decrease the possibility of bacterial infection.

2. The patient is placed in a reclining position with the foot adequately supported, and the toe is shaved to remove hair, which would act as a contaminant.

3. An antiseptic is applied to the affected toe, which is numbed using a local anesthetic.

4. Using surgical toenail scissors, the physician surgically removes a wedge of the nail (Figure 10-19C).

5. A sterile gauze dressing or a strip of surgical tape is applied over the area to protect the operative site and to promote healing (Figure 10-19D).

Colposcopy

Colposcopy is the visual examination of the vagina and cervix by means of a lighted instrument with a binocular magnifying lens, known as a **colposcope** (Figure 10-20). The purpose of colposcopy is to examine the vagina and cervix to determine areas of abnormal tissue growth. Colposcopy is performed following abnormal Pap test results, to evaluate a vaginal or cervical lesion observed during a pelvic examination, or after treatment for cancer of the cervix. To prepare for the procedure, the patient should be instructed not to insert anything (eg., tampons, vaginal medications, spermicides) into the vagina for 24 to 48 hours before the procedure. The lens of the colposcope is positioned approximately 12 inches (30 cm) from the opening of the vagina. The lens magnifies

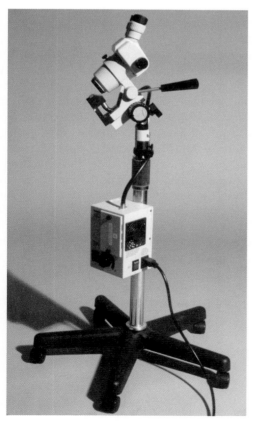

Figure 10-20. A colposcope. (From Apgar BS, Brotzman GL, Spitzer M: *Colposcopy: principles and practice—an integrated textbook and atlas*, Philadelphia, 2002, Saunders.)

tissue, facilitating the inspection of cervical cells and the obtaining of a biopsy specimen. For a routine colposcopic examination, a magnification ranging from 6× to 15× is generally used. The colposcope may be placed on an adjustable stand or attached to the side of the examining table and swung out before use.

Colposcopy Setup
The items required for colposcopy are listed.

Items Placed to the Side of the Sterile Field
- Colposcope
- Sterile gloves
- Normal saline
- Acetic acid (3%)
- Lugol's iodine solution

Items Included on the Sterile Field
- Vaginal speculum
- Long, sterile, cotton-tipped applicators
- Uterine tenaculum
- Uterine dressing forceps

Procedure
Colposcopy is performed as follows:

1. The patient is assisted into a lithotomy position and prepared as for a pelvic examination.

2. The physician inserts a vaginal speculum into the vagina.

3. A long, cotton-tipped applicator moistened with saline is used to wipe the cervix to remove the mucous film that normally covers it. The saline also provides better visualization of the cervical epithelium because dry cervical epithelium is not transparent and does not allow satisfactory viewing of the vascular pattern of the cervix.

4. The colposcope is focused on the cervix, and the physician inspects the saline-moistened cervix.

5. The cervix is swabbed with acetic acid, using a long, cotton-tipped applicator. The acetic acid dissolves cervical mucus and other secretions; the acetic acid provides the best contrast between normal and abnormal tissue, allowing easier visualization of dysplastic and neoplastic epithelium.

6. The cervical epithelium also may be stained with Lugol's iodine solution using a long, cotton-tipped applicator. This provides another means to identify unhealthy epithelium. The healthy epithelium of the cervix contains glycogen, which is able to absorb the iodine, causing the epithelium to stain a dark brown color. Conversely, abnormal epithelium, such as would constitute a malignancy, does not contain glycogen and is unable to absorb the iodine.

7. If an abnormal area is observed, the physician obtains a cervical biopsy specimen using punch biopsy forceps, which is described next.

Cervical Punch Biopsy

A cervical biopsy is performed in combination with colposcopy to remove a cervical tissue specimen for examination by

Case Study 3

Sadira Wisal has been referred to the office for a colposcopy by her family physician. Her last Pap test came back as abnormal, and a repeat Pap test 3 months later also was abnormal. While having her vital signs taken, Sadira bursts into tears. She tearfully explains that she's afraid that she has cancer, and that no one at her regular physician's office told her what to expect from this procedure. Sadira does not understand why she has to have this procedure done, and she does not know what the physician will be doing during the procedure. She says that she feels stupid, but she does not even know what a cervix is. Sadira also worries that the procedure will affect her ability to have children. ■

a pathologist. The purpose of the biopsy is to determine whether the specimen is benign or malignant. Cervical biopsies are often performed following abnormal Pap test results. The procedure usually is performed 1 week after the end of the menstrual period, when the cervix is the least vascular. To prepare for the procedure, the patient should be told not to douche; use tampons, vaginal medications, or spermicides; or have intercourse for 2 days before the examination.

Cervical Punch Biopsy Setup

The items required for a cervical punch biopsy are listed.

Items Placed to the Side of the Sterile Field
- Colposcope
- Sterile gloves
- Lugol's iodine solution
- Monsel's solution
- Specimen container with preservative and label
- Laboratory request form
- Sanitary pad

Items Included on the Sterile Field
- Vaginal speculum
- Long, sterile, cotton-tipped applicators
- Cervical punch biopsy forceps
- Uterine dressing forceps
- Uterine tenaculum
- Sterile 4 × 4 gauze

Procedure

A cervical biopsy is performed as follows:

1. The patient is positioned and draped in a lithotomy position. An anesthetic is not needed; because the cervix has few pain receptors, the patient experiences little discomfort from the procedure. Some patients experience mild cramping and pinching when the specimen is being removed from the cervix.
2. The physician inserts a vaginal speculum into the vagina for proper visualization of the cervix.
3. To assist in obtaining the specimen, the physician may stain the cervix with Lugol's solution.

4. The colposcope is focused on the cervix, and the physician inspects the cervix.
5. Using cervical biopsy punch forceps, the physician obtains several tissue specimens (Figure 10-21A) from the abnormal cervical epithelium (Figure 10-21B).
6. The specimen is placed in a container with a preservative and is sent to the laboratory for examination by a pathologist.
7. If bleeding occurs, the physician controls it with gauze packing, a hemostatic solution (e.g., Monsel's solution), or electrocautery.
8. The patient is given a sanitary pad at the office after the procedure to absorb any discharge.

Postoperative Instructions

Postoperative instructions include the following:

1. The patient should be informed that a minimum amount of bleeding may follow the procedure.
2. The patient should be instructed to contact the physician if bleeding is heavier than normal menstrual bleeding.
3. A foul-smelling, gray-green vaginal discharge may occur several days after the procedure and continue for 3 weeks. The patient should be informed that this discharge results from normal healing of cervical tissue and gradually diminishes as the healing progresses.
4. An appointment is scheduled approximately one week following the procedure to make sure that healing is taking place and to discuss the biopsy results.

Cryosurgery
Cervical

Cervical **cryosurgery,** also known as *cryotherapy,* is often used to treat chronic cervicitis and cervical erosion through the use of freezing temperatures. The procedure can be performed without an anesthetic, although occasionally a mild analgesic is necessary immediately afterward. The cryosurgery unit consists of a long metal probe attached to a cooling-agent tank (Figure 10-22). The principal cooling agents are liquid nitrogen, nitrous oxide, and carbon dioxide gas; of these, liquid nitrogen is used most often. The probe is placed in contact with the infected area, and the cooling agent flows through the probe, freezing the cervical tissue to 40°C to 80°C. This causes the cells to die and slough off so that the cervical covering can eventually be replaced with new, healthy epithelial tissue. The regeneration of cervical tissue occurs within approximately 4 to 6 weeks after the procedure.

Cryosurgery Setup

The items required for cryosurgery are listed.

Items Placed to the Side of the Sterile Field
- Cryosurgery unit
- Sanitary pads

Items Included on the Sterile Field
- Vaginal speculum
- Acid-saline solution
- Long, cotton-tipped applicators

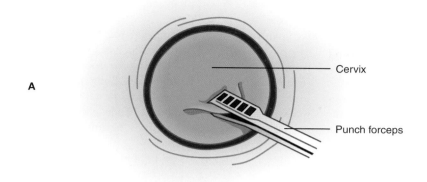

A

— Cervix

— Punch forceps

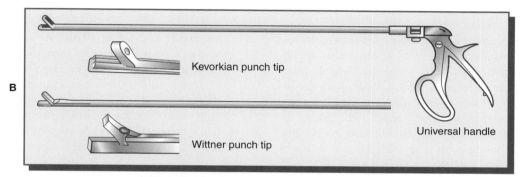

B

Kevorkian punch tip

Wittner punch tip

Universal handle

Figure 10-21. Cervical punch biopsy. **A,** Obtaining a tissue specimen from the cervix using cervical biopsy punch forceps. **B,** Cervical biopsy punch forceps. (Courtesy Elmed, Addison, Ill.)

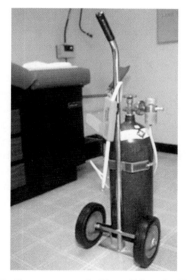

Figure 10-22. Cryosurgery unit. (From Zakus S: *Clinical skills for medical assistants,* ed 4, Philadelphia, 2001, Saunders.)

Procedure

Cryosurgery is performed as follows:
1. The patient is draped and assisted into the lithotomy position.
2. The physician inserts a vaginal speculum for proper visualization of the cervix.

3. The cervix is swabbed with an acid-saline solution to remove mucus and other contaminants.
4. The metal probe is placed in contact with the affected area, and the cryosurgery unit is turned on.
5. The cooling agent is permitted to flow over the cervical area for approximately 3 minutes. During the procedure, the patient may experience some pain resembling menstrual cramping, which usually lasts about 30 minutes.
6. When the procedure has been completed, the medical assistant should assist the patient as necessary and observe her for signs of discomfort or vertigo.
7. The patient is given a sanitary pad at the office after the procedure to absorb any discharge.

Postoperative Instructions

Postoperative instructions include the following:
1. The patient should be informed of the type of discharge that normally occurs after the cryosurgery. On the first postoperative day, the patient will develop a heavy, clear, watery vaginal discharge, which usually reaches its maximum by the sixth day.
2. The patient should be told to use sanitary pads, rather than tampons, at home. In addition, a vaginal cream may be prescribed to promote healing and the formation of new epithelial tissue.
3. The patient should be told that continuation of the discharge for approximately 4 weeks is normal, but that

the development of a foul odor should be reported to the physician.

4. The patient should be informed that the next menstrual period will be heavier than normal and may involve some cramping.

5. The patient usually is instructed to abstain from intercourse for 4 weeks after the procedure and to douche with a solution of dilute vinegar and water.

6. The patient must schedule a return visit 6 weeks after the procedure to ensure that proper healing has occurred.

Skin Lesions

In the medical office, cryosurgery also may be used to remove benign skin lesions, such as common warts. Only a small amount of cooling agent is required for skin lesions, so the cryosurgery unit is considerably smaller than the one described for cervical cryosurgery. Most physicians use liquid nitrogen contained in a small, pressurized, stainless steel canister with an attached probe. The physician applies the liquid nitrogen to the skin lesion until it turns white, which indicates that freezing of the tissue has occurred. During the procedure, the patient feels a slight burning or stinging sensation as the cooling agent is applied. After cryosurgery, a blister develops and dries to a scab in 1 week to 10 days and eventually sloughs off. The patient should be told to keep the area clean and dry until the scab has sloughed off. In some cases, the treatment may not result in complete destruction of the lesion; two or more treatments may be required to remove the lesion.

BANDAGING

A **bandage** is a strip of woven material used to wrap or cover a part of the body. The function of the bandage may be to apply pressure to control bleeding, to protect a wound from contamination, to hold a dressing in place, or to protect, support, or immobilize an injured part of the body.

Guidelines for Application

The bandage should be applied so that it feels comfortable to the patient, and it must be fastened securely with metal clips or adhesive tape. Guidelines for applying a bandage are as follows:

1. Observe the principles of medical asepsis during the application of a bandage.
2. Ensure that the area to which a bandage is applied is clean and dry.
3. Do not apply a bandage directly over an open wound. To prevent contamination of the wound, apply first a sterile dressing and then the bandage. The bandage should extend at least 2 inches (5 cm) beyond the edge of the dressing,
4. To prevent irritation, do not allow the skin surfaces of two body parts (e.g., two fingers) to touch. In addition, the patient's perspiration provides a moist environment

that encourages the growth of microorganisms. A piece of gauze should be inserted between the two body parts.

5. Ensure that joints and prominent parts of bones are padded to prevent the bandage from rubbing the skin and causing irritation.
6. Bandage the body part in its normal position with joints slightly flexed to avoid muscle strain.
7. Apply the bandage from the distal to the proximal part of the body to aid the venous return of blood to the heart.
8. As you apply the bandage, ask the patient whether it feels comfortable. The bandage should fit snugly enough that it does not fall off, but not so tightly that it impedes circulation.
9. If possible, leave the fingers and toes exposed when bandaging an extremity. This provides the opportunity to check them for signs of impairment in circulation. Signs indicating that the bandage is too tight include coldness, pallor, numbness, cyanosis of the nailbeds, swelling, pain, and tingling sensations. If any of these signs occurs, loosen the bandage immediately.
10. If a bandage roll is dropped during the procedure, obtain a new bandage and begin again.

Types of Bandages

Three basic types of bandages are used in the medical office. A *roller bandage* is a long strip of soft material wound on itself to form a roll. It ranges from ½ to 6 inches (1.3 to 15.2 cm) wide and from 2 to 5 yards (1.83 to 4.57 m) long. The width used depends on the part being bandaged. Roller bandages usually are made of sterilized gauze. Gauze is porous and lightweight, molds easily to a body part, and is relatively inexpensive and easily disposed of. Because it is made of loosely woven cotton, however, it may slip and fray easily. *Kling gauze* is a special type of gauze that stretches; this allows it to cling, and, as a result, it molds and conforms better to the body part than does regular gauze.

Elastic bandages are made of woven cotton that contains elastic fibers. One brand name of elastic bandages is the Ace bandage. Although elastic bandages are expensive, they can be washed and used again. The medical assistant must be extremely careful when applying an elastic bandage because it is easy to apply it too tightly and impede circulation. Elastic adhesive bandages also may be used; these have an adhesive backing to provide a secure fit.

Bandage Turns

Five basic bandage turns are used, alone or in combination. The type of turn used depends on which body part is to be bandaged, and whether the bandage is used for support or immobilization or for holding a dressing in place.

The *circular turn* is applied to a part of uniform width, such as toes, fingers, or the head. Each turn completely overlaps the previous turn. Two circular turns are used to anchor a bandage at the beginning and end of a spiral, spiral-reverse, figure-eight, or recurrent turn (Figure 10-23).

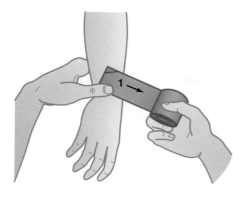

1. Place the end of the roller bandage on a slant.

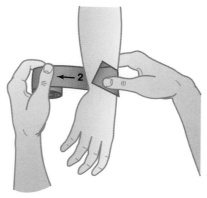

2. Encircle the part while allowing the corner of the bandage to extend.

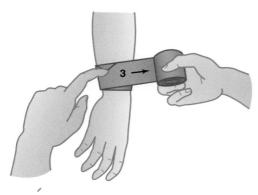

3. Turn down the corner of the bandage.

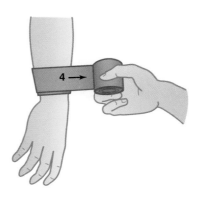

4. Make another circular turn around the part.

Figure 10-23. Procedure for anchoring a bandage.

The *spiral turn* is applied to a part of uniform circumference, such as the fingers, arms, legs, chest, or abdomen. Each spiral turn is carried upward at a slight angle and should overlap the previous turn by one half to two thirds the width of the bandage (Figure 10-24).

The *spiral-reverse turn* is useful for bandaging a part that varies in width, such as the forearm or lower leg. Reversing each spiral turn allows for a smoother fit and prevents gaping caused by the variation in the contour of the limb. The thumb is used to make the reverse halfway through each spiral turn. The bandage is directed downward and folded on itself while it is kept parallel to the lower edge of the previous turn. Each turn should overlap the previous one by two thirds of the width of the bandage. The reverse turn is used as often as necessary to provide a uniform fit (Figure 10-25).

The *figure-eight turn* generally is used to hold a dressing in place or to support and immobilize an injured joint, such as the ankle, knee, elbow, or wrist. The figure-eight turn consists of slanting turns that alternately ascend and descend around the part and cross over one another in the middle, resembling the figure 8. Each turn overlaps the previous one by two thirds of the width of the bandage (Figure 10-26).

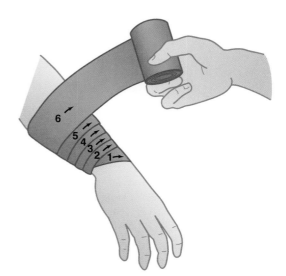

Figure 10-24. Procedure for making the spiral turn.

The *recurrent turn* is a series of back-and-forth turns used to bandage the tips of fingers or toes, the stump of an amputated extremity, or the head. The bandage is anchored by using two circular turns and is passed back and forth over the tip of the part to be bandaged, first on one side and

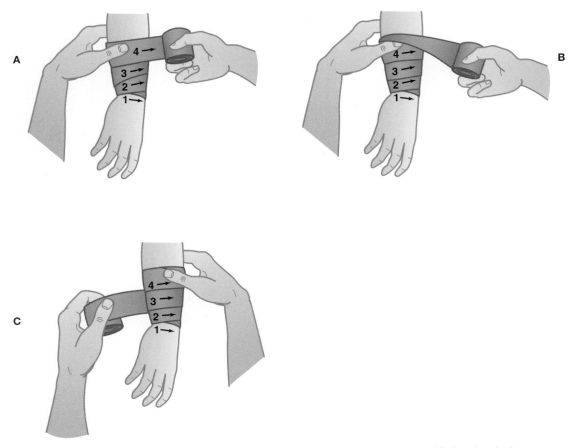

Figure 10-25. Procedure for making the spiral-reverse turn. **A,** Encircle the part while keeping the bandage at a slant. **B,** Reverse the spiral turn using the thumb or index finger, and direct the bandage downward and fold it on itself. **C,** Keep the bandage parallel to the lower edge of the previous turn.

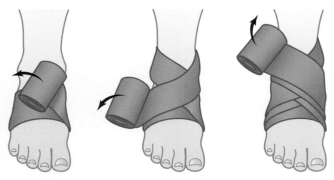

Figure 10-26. Procedure for applying an elastic bandage around the ankle using a figure-eight turn. (From Leake MJ: *A manual of simple nursing procedures,* Philadelphia, 1971, Saunders.)

then on the other side of the first center turn. Each turn should overlap the previous turn by two thirds of the width of the bandage (Figure 10-27).

Tubular Gauze Bandages

A tubular gauze bandage consists of seamless elasticized gauze fabric dispensed in a roll. It is used to cover round body parts, such as fingers, toes, arms, and legs, and fits like

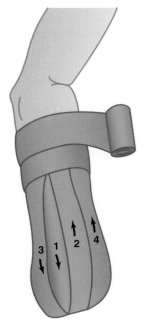

Figure 10-27. Procedure for using the recurrent turn to bandage the end of a stump.

a sleeve. This type of bandage is easier to apply than a roller bandage, and it adheres more securely to the body part. Tubular gauze is not sterile and should not be applied over open wounds; however, it can be applied over a sterile dressing to hold it in place. The gauze is available in varying widths; selection of the width is based on the body part to be bandaged. Table 10-1 lists tubular gauze widths and the body parts each size can be used to bandage.

The gauze is applied by means of a plastic or metal frame-like applicator, which comes in different sizes. The applicator must be larger than the part to be bandaged to allow the gauze to slide easily over the body part. To assist in selecting the proper gauze width, each applicator is marked with a size that corresponds to the size on the tubular gauze bandage box. Procedure 10-8 outlines the method to apply a tubular gauze bandage to a finger.

Table 10-1 Tubular Gauze Bandage Widths and Recommended Application Sites	
Width (inches)	**Recommended Application Sites**
⅝	Fingers and toes of infants Small fingers and toes of adults
1	Hands and feet of infants Fingers and toes of adults Over bulky dressings
1½	Arms and legs of infants Arms and feet of children Small hands, arms, and feet of adults
2⅝	Legs, thighs, and heads of children Arms and lower legs of adults Small thighs and small heads of adults
3⅝	Legs, thighs, lower legs, shoulders, arms, and heads of adults Trunks of infants
5	Large heads and small trunks of adults
7	Trunks of adults

PROCEDURE 10-8   Applying a Tubular Gauze Bandage

Outcome Apply a tubular gauze bandage.

Equipment/Supplies

- Applicator
- Roll of tubular gauze
- Adhesive tape
- Bandage scissors

1. **Procedural Step.** Sanitize your hands. Greet the patient and introduce yourself. Identify the patient and explain the procedure.

2. **Procedural Step.** Assemble the equipment. The applicator selected should be larger than the part to be bandaged. The proper gauze width must be used to ensure a secure fit.

   Principle. The applicator should be larger than the body part to allow the gauze to slide easily over the body part.

3. **Procedural Step.** Place the gauze bandage on the applicator as follows:
   a. Pull a sufficient length of gauze from the dispensing box roll.
   b. Spread apart the open end of the gauze, using your fingers.
   c. Slide the gauze over one end of the applicator. Continue loading the applicator by gathering enough gauze on the applicator to complete the bandage.
   d. Cut the roll of gauze near the opening of the box.

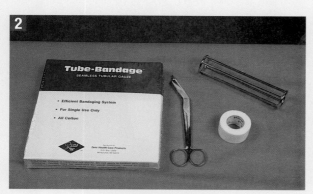

Assemble the equipment.

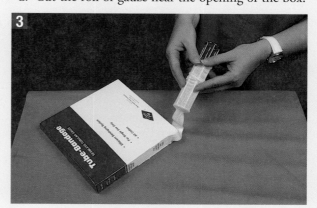

Slide the gauze over one end of the applicator.

Continued

PROCEDURE 1O-8   Applying a Tubular Gauze Bandage—cont'd

4. Procedural Step. Place the applicator over the proximal end of the patient's finger.

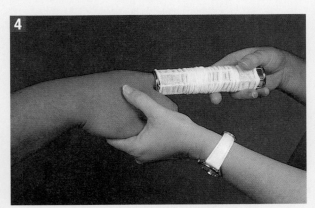

Place the applicator over the patient's finger.

5. Procedural Step. Move the applicator from the proximal end to the distal end of the patient's finger, while leaving the bandage on the length of the finger. The bandage should be held in place at the base of the patient's fingers with your fingers.
Principle. The bandage should be held in place to prevent it from sliding, which would not ensure complete coverage of the affected part.

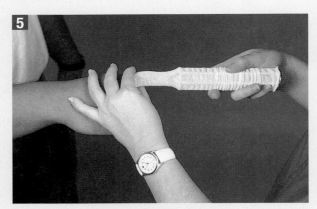

Move the applicator from the proximal to the distal end of the patient's finger.

6. Procedural Step. Pull the applicator 1 to 2 inches past the end of the patient's finger. Continue to hold the bandage in place with your fingers.
Principle. The bandage must extend beyond the length of the patient's finger to secure it at the distal end.

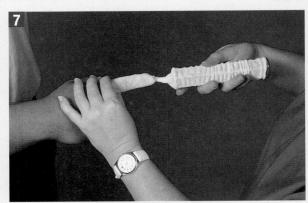

Rotate the applicator one full turn.

7. Procedural Step. Rotate the applicator one full turn to anchor the bandage.
Principle. Anchoring the bandage holds it securely in place.

8. Procedural Step. Move the applicator forward again toward the proximal end of the patient's finger.
Principle. Moving the applicator forward applies a second layer of bandaging material to the patient's finger.

9. Procedural Step. Move the applicator forward approximately 1 inch past the original starting point of the bandage, and anchor it using another rotating motion.
Principle. Anchoring the bandage holds it securely in place.

10. Procedural Step. Repeat this procedure for the number of layers desired. Finish the last layer at the proximal end. Cut unused gauze from the applicator, and remove the applicator.

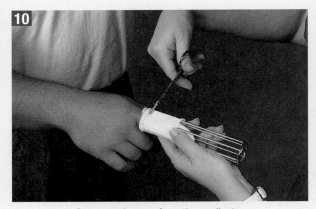

Cut unused gauze from the applicator.

11. **Procedural Step.** Apply adhesive tape at the base of the finger to secure the bandage.

12. **Procedural Step.** Sanitize your hands, and record the procedure. Include the date and time and location of the bandage application and any instructions given to the patient.

CHARTING EXAMPLE	
Date	
9/30/08	10:00 a.m. Tubular gauze bandage applied
	to Ⓡ index finger. Explained bandage care.
	———————— T. Browning, CMA

*Check out the **Companion CD** bound with the book to access additional interactive activities.*

MEDICAL PRACTICE and the LAW

Surgical procedures are invasive and painful, and they have the potential for harmful complications and subsequent lawsuits. Before having a surgical procedure performed, the patient must sign a consent to treatment form. It is the medical assistant's responsibility to witness the patient's signature, but it is the physician's responsibility to inform the patient of the procedure to be performed and its risks, alternative procedures, and benefits. The physician may delegate some or all of these tasks to the medical assistant, but *do not* accept this responsibility. Patients cannot sign for themselves if they are minors or if they are impaired by drugs or disease, such as Alzheimer's disease. In these cases, consent must be obtained from the legal guardian or next of kin. Before asking a patient to sign a consent to treatment form, ask whether he or she has any questions. If so, make sure the information is given before the consent is signed. Make sure you know what procedures require informed consent in your office.

During the procedure, your duty is to assist the physician and maintain surgical asepsis. If this is broken, you must inform the physician and remedy the situation. There is no such thing as "almost sterile."

After the surgical procedure, the medical assistant must give the patient home care instructions. Home care must be performed exactly to ensure proper healing. Instructions should be given verbally, demonstrated, and given in writing. Written instructions must be in the correct language and at the patient's reading level. Pictures included with the written instructions can clarify difficult points. Many offices purchase preprinted instructions for common surgical procedures. Make sure the signs of infection are listed on these sheets, along with instructions to call the physician if they occur, or if any other problems or questions arise. ∎

What Would You Do? What Would You *Not* Do? RESPONSES

Case Study 1
Page 384

What Did Trudy Do?

❑ Tried to calm and reassure Mrs. Ventura. Told her that children at this age are prone to accidents and that she should not blame herself.

❑ Told Mrs. Ventura that Cory's wound could not be held together effectively with Steri-Strips. Explained that sutures would help the wound heal better.

❑ Told Mrs. Ventura that the doctor could not perform the procedure unless she signs the consent form. Explained that Cory's wound should be sutured as soon as possible to prevent infection and to minimize scarring.

❑ Asked Mrs. Ventura whether she would like to talk with the doctor again about any questions she has about the procedure before signing the form.

What Did Trudy Not Do?

❑ Did not prepare Cory for the suture insertion procedure until Mrs. Ventura signed the consent to treatment form.

What Would You Do?/What Would You *Not* Do? Review Trudy's response and place a checkmark next to the information you included in your response. List additional information you included in your response.

_____

_____

_____

_____

What Would You Do? What Would You *Not* Do?   RESPONSES—cont'd

Case Study 2
Page 393
What Did Trudy Do?
- ❑ Explained to Abbey that the antiseptic contains iodine, which appears orange when it is applied to the skin. Assured her that the iodine would not stain her skin permanently and that it would wear off in a few days.
- ❑ Calmly and discreetly opened a new pair of sterile gloves so that the physician could reapply sterile gloves. Reminded Abbey not to move during the procedure.
- ❑ Told Abbey that all tissues removed from patients are routinely sent to the laboratory for a biopsy. Reassured her that the doctor has told her everything he knows about her condition.
- ❑ Made it clear to Abbey that her neighbor is not permitted to remove her sutures. Stressed to her that the doctor needs to check her incision before the sutures are removed to ensure that proper healing has occurred.

What Did Trudy Not *Do?*
- ❑ Did not scold Abbey for contaminating the physician's sterile gloved hand.

What Would You Do?/What Would You *Not* Do? Review Trudy's response and place a checkmark next to the information you included in your response. List additional information you included in your response.

_____
_____
_____
_____
_____

Case Study 3
Page 404
What Did Trudy Do?
- ❑ Listened empathetically to Sadira, and tried to calm and reassure her.
- ❑ Spent some time going over the colposcopy procedure and what to expect.
- ❑ Answered as many of Sadira's questions as possible. Reassured her that a lot of people do not know what a cervix is and that she was asking some very good questions.
- ❑ Asked the physician to spend some time talking with Sadira before the procedure to answer the questions that Trudy was not qualified to answer.
- ❑ Ensured that Sadira understood all of the information about the procedure before asking her to sign a consent to treatment form.

What Did Trudy Not *Do?*
- ❑ Did not tell Sadira that her family physician and staff should have spent some time explaining the procedure to her so that she did not have to worry so much.
- ❑ Did not tell Sadira that she does not have cancer.

What Would You Do?/What Would You *Not* Do? Review Trudy's response and place a checkmark next to the information you included in your response. List additional information you included in your response.

_____
_____
_____
_____

 APPLY YOUR KNOWLEDGE

Choose the best answer to each of the following questions.

1. Dr. Xylocaine will be suturing a large laceration on Seth James's left thigh. Trudy Browning, CMA, is assisting the physician. Trudy explains to Mr. James that he should not talk during the procedure. He asks her, "Why?" Trudy explains:
   A. It is easier for the physician to concentrate when it is quiet.
   B. The local anesthetic will work faster.
   C. The wound will not heal properly.
   D. Microorganisms from his mouth can contaminate the sterile field.

2. After opening and setting up the sterile suture insertion tray for Mr. James's laceration, Trudy notices that she forgot to bring in sutures. Trudy should:
   A. Leave the room and obtain the sutures as quickly as possible.
   B. Send Mr. James out to get the sutures.
   C. Cover the tray with a sterile towel and leave to get the sutures.
   D. Leave to get the sutures and then set up a new sterile suture tray after returning.

3. Dr. Xylocaine has started suturing Mr. James's laceration. He asks Trudy for more sterile gauze. Of the following methods, Trudy would best maintain surgical asepsis by:
   A. Using her bare hands to place the gauze on the sterile field.
   B. Opening the sterile package and allowing Dr. Xylocaine to remove the gauze with his gloved hand.
   C. Applying clean gloves and adding the sterile gauze to the tray.
   D. Handing a sterile gauze package to Dr. Xylocaine.

4. Dr. Xylocaine tells Mr. James to return to the office in 10 days to have his sutures removed. Trudy realizes that by that time Mr. James would be in which of the following phases of the healing process?
   A. Phase 1, or the inflammatory phase.
   B. Phase 2, or the granulation phase.
   C. Phase 3, or the maturation phase.
   D. Phase 4, or the final phase.

5. Mr. James returns to the office to have his sutures removed. On inspection of Mr. James's sutures, Trudy notices that he has a small gaping area at the bottom of his laceration with greenish-yellow, foul-smelling drainage. She would document this as:
   A. Laceration well approximated with serous drainage.
   B. Laceration unapproximated at distal end with serosanguineous drainage.
   C. Laceration gaping with sanguineous drainage.
   D. Purulent drainage noted from unapproximated area at distal end of laceration.

6. Dr. Xylocaine tells Trudy not to remove the sutures and to apply Steri-Strips to the gaping area of Mr. James's laceration. To prepare the area for the application, Trudy would:
   A. Cleanse the laceration with normal saline, and allow it to dry.
   B. Cleanse the laceration with phenol, and apply tincture of benzoin directly on the laceration.
   C. Cleanse the laceration with Betadine, and apply tincture of benzoin on each side of the laceration.
   D. Wipe the laceration clean with sterile gauze, and apply the Steri-Strips.

7. Eric Link is 16 years old and has come to the office with his mother to have surgery on his ingrown toenail. Before starting the procedure, Trudy Browning, CMA, must:
   A. Inform Eric of the risks of the procedure and have him sign a consent to treatment form.
   B. Obtain verbal consent from Eric's mother for the surgery.
   C. Make sure that Eric is not allergic to bee stings.
   D. Verify that Eric's mother has discussed the procedure with Dr. Xylocaine and has signed a consent to treatment form.

8. Before the surgical procedure is started, which of the following would be appropriate to do preoperatively for Eric's ingrown toenail?
   A. Soak his foot in tepid water and an antiseptic solution.
   B. Scrub his foot and toe with a surgical scrub sponge moistened with 90% ethyl alcohol.
   C. Ask him to wiggle his big toe.
   D. Trim as much of the toenail away as possible.

9. Dr. Xylocaine will use Betadine to cleanse the area of the toe before making an incision. He asks Trudy to pour some Betadine into the basin on the sterile field. Which of the following would represent an *error* in technique when pouring the Betadine into the sterile basin?
   A. Placing the bottle cap on a flat surface with the open end facing down.
   B. Palming the label of the Betadine bottle.
   C. Making sure the Betadine is not expired.
   D. Pouring the solution from a height of 6 inches.

10. After Eric's surgery, Trudy is teaching him signs that might indicate he has an infection at his surgical site. These would include all of the following *except:*
   A. Bruising.
   B. Warmth.
   C. Edema.
   D. Redness.

Table 11-1 Classification of Drugs Based on Action

Drug Category	Primary Use and Major Therapeutic Effects	Commonly Prescribed Drugs	
		Generic	Brand
Analgesics (Opioid)	**Used** to manage moderate to severe pain	codeine/APAP	▶Tylenol w/Codeine (III)
	Work by altering perception of and response to painful stimuli	fentanyl	Actiq
	Vicodin	hydrocodone/APAP	▶Vicodin (III)
	VICODIN	hydrocodone/ASA	Lortab (III)
	500/5 mg	meperidine	Demerol (II)
	Darvocet-N	oxycodone	▶Oxycontin (II)
	DARVOCET N 50	oxycodone/APAP	▶Percocet (II)
	50/325 mg	oxycodone/ASA	Percodan (II)
	DARVOCET-N 100	propoxyphene	Darvon (IV)
	100/650 mg	propoxyphene N/APAP	▶Darvocet-N (IV)
		tramadol	▶Ultram
Analgesics/ Antipyretics	**Used** to manage mild to moderate pain and to reduce fever	acetaminophen	Tylenol*
		aspirin	Bayer*
	Work by relieving pain and reducing fever		Ecotrin*
	Naprosyn	**NSAID**	
	NAPROSYN 250	diclofenac	Voltaren
	250 mg	ibuprofen	Advil*
			Motrin*
	375 mg 500 mg	meloxicam	Mobic
		naproxen	Aleve*
			Anaprox
			Naprosyn
Anesthetics (Local)	**Used** to produce local anesthesia through loss of feeling to a body part	lidocaine	Xylocaine
	Work by preventing initiation and conduction of normal nerve impulses in body part	dibucaine	Nupercainal ointment*
Antacids	**Used** to treat heartburn, hyperacidity, indigestion, and gastroesophageal reflux disease, and to promote healing of ulcers	aluminum hydroxide/ magnesium hydroxide	Maalox* Mylanta*
	Work by neutralizing gastric acid to relieve gastric pain and irritation	calcium carbonate	Tums*
		sodium bicarbonate/ASA	Alka-Seltzer*
Anti-Alzheimer's Agents	**Used** to treat mild to moderate dementia associated with Alzheimer's disease	donepezil	Aricept
	Work by elevating acetylcholine concentration in cerebral cortex		
Antianemics	**Iron Supplements**		
	Used to prevent or cure iron-deficiency anemia	ferrous sulfate	Feosol*
	Work by increasing amount of iron in body	iron dextran	DexFerrum
	Vitamin B$_{12}$ Injections		InFed
	Used to treat pernicious anemia	cyanocobalamin	Cobex
	Work by increasing amount of vitamin B$_{12}$ in body		Cyanoject
	Folic Acid Supplements	folic acid	▶Folvite
	Used to promote normal fetal development		
	Work by stimulating production of red blood cells, white blood cells, and platelets		

*Available OTC (over-the-counter).
▶Top-200 most prescribed drugs.
(II): schedule II drug, (III): schedule III drug, (IV): schedule IV drug.

Continued

Table 11-1 Classification of Drugs Based on Action—cont'd

Drug Category	Primary Use and Major Therapeutic Effects	Commelly Prescribed Drugs	
		Generic	Brand
Antianginals	*Used* to relieve or prevent angina attacks *Work* by increasing blood supply to myocardial tissue **Imdur** 60 mg **Nitrostat** 0.3 mg 0.4 mg 0.6 mg	**Nitrates** isosorbide dinitrate isosorbide mononitrate nitroglycerin **Beta Blockers** atenolol propranolol **Calcium Channel Blockers** amlodipine bepridil diltiazem nifedipine verapamil	Sorbitrate Imdur Nitro-Bid Nitro-Dur Nitrostat Tenormin Inderal Norvasc Vascor ▶Cardizem Dilacor XR Adalat Procardia-XL Calan Isoptin Verelan
Antianxiety Agents	*Used* to treat anxiety *Work* at many levels in central nervous system to produce anxiolytic (anxiety-relieving) effect **Xanax** 0.25 mg 0.5 mg 1 mg 2 mg	alprazolam buspirone chlordiazepoxide diazepam lorazepam	▶Xanax (IV) BuSpar Librium (IV) Valium (IV) ▶Ativan (IV)
Anticholinergics	*Used* to decrease preoperatively oral and respiratory secretions *Work* by blocking effects of acetylcholine in autonomic nervous system	atropine	Atro-Pen
Anticoagulants	*Used* to prevent and treat venous thrombosis, pulmonary embolism, and myocardial infarction by preventing clot extension and formation *Work* by delaying or preventing blood coagulation **Coumadin** 1 mg 2 mg	warfarin heparin	▶Coumadin
Anticonvulsants	*Used* to prevent or relieve seizures *Work* by decreasing incidence and severity of seizures **Neurontin** 100 mg 300 mg 400 mg	carbamazepine clonazepam divalproex gabapentin lamotrigine phenytoin topiramate valproic acid	Tegretol ▶Klonopin (IV) ▶Depakote ▶Neurontin ▶Lamictal ▶Dilantin Topamax Depakene

*Available OTC (over-the-counter).
▶Top-200 most prescribed drugs.
(II): schedule II drug, (III): schedule III drug, (IV): schedule IV drug.

Table 11-1 Classification of Drugs Based on Action—cont'd

Drug Category	Primary Use and Major Therapeutic Effects	Commonly Prescribed Drugs	
		Generic	Brand
Antidepressants	*Used* to prevent, cure, or alleviate depression, and to treat anxiety disorders (panic attacks) and obsessive-convulsive disorder *Work* by inhibiting reuptake of neurotransmitters in central nervous system **Prozac** 10 mg 20 mg **Wellbutrin-SR** 100 mg 150 mg	**Selective Serotonin Reuptake Inhibitors (SSRIs)** citalopram escitalopram oxalate fluoxetine paroxetine sertraline **Miscellaneous** amitriptyline bupropion mirtazapine nefazodone trazodone venlafaxine	►Celexa ►Lexapro ►Prozac ►Paxil ►Zoloft ►Elavil ►Wellbutrin-SR ►Remeron Serzone ►Desyrel ►Effexor XR
Antidiabetics	**Oral Hypoglycemics** *Used* to manage non–insulin-dependent type 2 diabetes mellitus *Work* by stimulating release of insulin from pancreas and increasing sensitivity to insulin **Insulins** *Used* to manage diabetes mellitus *Work* by reducing blood glucose levels **Amaryl** 2 mg 4 mg **Glucotrol XL** 5 mg 10 mg	glimepiride glipizide glyburide metformin pioglitazone rosiglitazone regular insulin NPH insulin NPH/regular insulin insulin glargine insulin lispro	►Amaryl ►Glucotrol XL ►DiaBeta ►Micronase ►Glucophage ►Actos ►Avandia Humulin R* Novolin R* ►Humulin N* Novolin N* ►Humulin 70/30* Novolin 70/30* Lantus Humalog
Antidiarrheals	*Used* to control and relieve diarrhea *Work* by inhibiting peristalsis, reducing fecal volume, and preventing loss of fluids and electrolytes **Lomotil** 2.5/0.025 mg	bismuth subsalicylate diphenoxylate/atropine kaolin/pectin loperamide	Pepto-Bismol* Lomotil (V) Kaopectate* Imodium*
Antidysrhythmics	*Used* to control or prevent cardiac dysrhythmias *Work* by decreasing myocardial excitability and slowing conduction velocity **Inderal** 10 mg 20 mg 40 mg 60 mg 80 mg	procainamide propranolol	Pronestyl Inderal

Continued

Table 11-1 Classification of Drugs Based on Action—cont'd

Drug Category	Primary Use and Major Therapeutic Effects	Commonly Prescribed Drugs	
		Generic	Brand
Antiemetics	*Used* to prevent or relieve nausea and vomiting *Work* by depressing chemoreceptor trigger zone in central nervous system to inhibit nausea and vomiting	dronabinol ondansetron prochlorperazine promethazine meclizine	Marinol (III) Zofran Compazine ▶Phenergan Bonine*
Antiflatulents	*Used* to relieve discomfort of excess gas and bloating in gastrointestinal tract *Work* by causing coalescence of gas bubbles in intestinal tract	simethicone	Gas-X* Mylanta Gas*
Antifungals	*Used* to treat fungal infections *Work* by killing or inhibiting growth of susceptible fungi **Diflucan** 50 mg 100 mg 200 mg	amphotericin B clotrimazole fluconazole ketoconazole miconazole nystatin terconazole	Fungizone Gyne-Lotrimin* ▶Diflucan Nizoral Monistat* Mycostatin* Terazol
Antigout Agents	*Used* to prevent attacks of gout *Work* by inhibiting production of uric acid **Zyloprim** 100 mg 300 mg	allopurinol colchicine	▶Zyloprim Colchicine tablets
Antihelmintics	*Used* to treat worm infections (pinworms, roundworms, hookworms) *Work* by destroying worms	mebendazole	Vermox
Antihistamines	*Used* to relieve symptoms associated with allergies (increased sneezing; rhinorrhea; itchy eyes, nose, and throat) *Work* by blocking effects of histamine at histamine receptor sites **Allegra** 60 mg 180 mg	brompheniramine cetirizine chlorpheniramine desloratadine diphenhydramine fexofenadine hydroxyzine loratadine promethazine	Dimetaine* ▶Zyrtec Chlor-Trimetron* Teldrin* ▶Clarinex Benadryl* ▶Allegra ▶Atarax Vistaril ▶Claritin* Phenergan
Antihypertensives	*Used* to manage hypertension *Work* by causing systemic vasodilation to reduce blood pressure **Accupril** 5 mg 10 mg 20 mg 40 mg	**Angiotensin-Converting Enzyme (ACE) Inhibitors** benazepril captopril enalapril	 Lotensin Capoten ▶Vasotec

*Available OTC (over-the-counter).
▶Top-200 most prescribed drugs.
(II): schedule II drug, (III): schedule III drug, (IV): schedule IV drug.

Table 11-1 Classification of Drugs Based on Action—cont'd

Drug Category	Primary Use and Major Therapeutic Effects	Commonly Prescribed Drugs	
		Generic	Brand
Antihypertensives—cont'd	**Cozaar** 25 mg 50 mg **Toprol XL** 50 mg 100 mg 200 mg **Cardizem** 30 mg 60 mg 90 mg 120 mg	lisinopril quinapril ramipril	►Prinivil ►Accupril ►Altace
		Peripherally Acting Adrenergic Blockers clonidine doxazosin prazosin	►Catapres ►Cardura Minipress
		Angiotensin II Receptor Antagonists candesartan irbesartan losartan olmesartan medoxomil valsartan	Atacand ►Avapro ►Cozaar ►Benicar ►Diovan
		Beta Blockers atenolol bisoprolol fumerate carvedilol metoprolol propranolol timolol	►Tenormin ►Zebeta ►Coreg Lopressor ►Toprol XL ►Inderal Blocadren
		Calcium Channel Blockers amlodipine diltiazem felodipine	►Norvasc ►Cardizem Plendil
		Vasodilators hydralazine	Apresoline
		Miscellaneous amlodipine/benazepril bisoprolol/hydrochloro- thiazide losartan/hydrochloro- thiazide nadolol/bendroflume- thiazide	►Lotrel Ziac ►Hyzaar Corzide
Antiimpotence Agents	*Used* to treat erectile dysfunction *Work* by promoting increased blood flow to penis **Viagra** 25 mg 50 mg 100 mg	sildenafil	►Viagra

Continued

Table 11-1 Classification of Drugs Based on Action—cont'd

Drug Category	Primary Use and Major Therapeutic Effects	Commonly Prescribed Drugs	
		Generic	Brand
Antiinfectives	*Used* to treat infections *Work* by killing or inhibiting growth of bacteria	**Penicillins** amoxicillin amoxicillin/clavulanate benzathine penicillin penicillin V procaine penicillin	►Amoxil Trimox ►Augmentin Bicillin Veetids Wycillin
	Amoxil 125 mg 250 mg 250 mg 500 mg	**Macrolides** azithromycin clarithromycin erythromycin	►Zithromax ►Biaxin Ery-Tab Pediazole
	Zithromax 250 mg 250 mg	**Cephalosporins** cefaclor cefdinir cefprozil ceftriaxone cephalexin	Ceclor ►Omnicef ►Cefzil Rocephin ►Keflex
	Keflex 250 mg 500 mg	**Fluoroquinolones** ciprofloxacin levofloxacin ofloxacin	►Cipro ►Levaquin Floxin
	Cipro 250 mg 500 mg 750 mg	**Tetracyclines** doxycycline minocycline tetracycline	►Doryx Vibramycin ►Arestin Achromycin Sumycin
	Macrobid 100 mg	**Aminoglycosides** gentamicin kanamycin neomycin tobramycin	Garamycin Kantrex Neobiotic Tobrax
		Sulfonamides sulfamethoxazole trimethoprim/sulfa- methoxazole	Gantanol Bactrim
		Miscellaneous chloramphenicol mupirocin nitrofurantoin vancomycin	Chloromycetin ►Bactroban ►Macrobid Macrodantin Vancocin
Antiinflammatory Agents	*Used* to relieve signs and symptoms of osteoarthritis and rheumatoid arthritis in adults	aspirin	Bayer* Ecotrin*

*Available OTC (over-the-counter).
►Top-200 most prescribed drugs.
(II): schedule II drug, (III): schedule III drug, (IV): schedule IV drug.

Table 11-1 Classification of Drugs Based on Action—cont'd

Drug Category	Primary Use and Major Therapeutic Effects	Commonly Prescribed Drugs	
		Generic	Brand
Antiinflammatory Agents—cont'd	*Work* by decreasing pain and inflammation **Celebrex** 100 mg / 200 mg	celecoxib etodolac ibuprofen indomethacin nabumetone naproxen valdecoxib	►Celebrex Lodine Advil* Motrin* Indocin ►Relafen Aleve* Anaprox Naprosyn ►Bextra
Antimanics	*Used* to treat bipolar affective disorders *Work* by altering cation transport in nerves and muscles **Eskalith** 300 mg **Eskalith CR** 450 mg	lithium	Eskalith Eskalith CR
Antimigraines	*Used* in acute treatment of migraine attacks *Work* by causing vasoconstriction in large intracranial arteries	sumatriptan	►Imitrex
Antineoplastics	*Used* to treat tumors *Work* by preventing development, growth, or proliferation of malignant cells	cyclophosphamide methotrexate	Cytoxan Mexate Folex
Anti-Parkinson's Agents	*Used* to treat symptoms of Parkinson's disease *Work* by restoring balance between acetylcholine and dopamine in central nervous system **Sinemet** 10/100 mg / 25/100 mg / 50/200 mg / 25/250 mg	carbidopa/levodopa	Sinemet
Antiprotozoals	*Used* to treat protozoal infections *Work* by destroying protozoa **Flagyl** 250 mg / 500 mg / 375 mg	metronidazole	Flagyl

Continued

Table 11-1 Classification of Drugs Based on Action—cont'd

Drug Category	Primary Use and Major Therapeutic Effects	Commonly Prescribed Drugs	
		Generic	Brand
Antipsychotics	*Used* to treat psychotic disorders *Work* by blocking dopamine and serotonin receptors in central nervous system **Risperdal** 1 mg 2 mg 3 mg 4 mg	haloperidol olanzapine risperidone quetiapine	Haldol ▶Zyprexa Risperdal ▶Seroquel
Antiretrovirals	*Used* to manage HIV infections and to reduce maternal-fetal transmission of HIV *Work* by inhibiting replication of retroviruses **Retrovir** 100 mg	zidovudine	Retrovir
Antispasmodics	*Used* to control hypermotility in irritable bowel syndrome, spastic colitis, spastic bladder, and pylorospasm *Work* by preventing or relieving spasms of gastrointestinal or genitourinary tracts	dicyclomine hyoscyamine	Bentyl Levsin
Antituberculars	*Used* to treat tuberculosis *Work* by killing or inhibiting growth of mycobacteria	isoniazid pyrazinamide rifampin	Isotamine (INH) PMS- Pyrazinamide Rifadin
Antitussives	*Used* in prevention or relief of coughs caused by minor viral upper respiratory infections or inhaled irritants *Work* by suppressing cough reflex by direct effect on cough center in central nervous system	benzonatate chlorpheniramine/ hydrocodone dextromethorphan guaifenesin/codeine	Tessalon Tussionex (III) Robitussin DM* Robitussin A-C (V)
Antiulcers	*Used* to manage ulcers, gastroesophageal reflux disease, heartburn, indigestion, and gastric hyperacidity *Work* by preventing accumulation of acid in stomach **Prevacid** 15 mg 30 mg	**Gastric Pump Inhibitors** esomeprazole lansoprazole omeprazole pantoprazole rabeprazole **H₂-Receptor Antagonists** cimetidine famotidine ranitidine	 Nexium ▶Prevacid Prilosec* ▶Protonix ▶Aciphex Tagamet* Pepcid AC* ▶Zantac*
Antivirals	*Used* to manage herpes infections *Work* by inhibiting viral replication **Valtrex** 500 mg 1 g	acyclovir valacyclovir	▶Zovirax Valtrex

*Available OTC (over-the-counter).
▶Top-200 most prescribed drugs.
(II): schedule II drug, (III): schedule III drug, (IV): schedule IV drug.

Table 11-1 Classification of Drugs Based on Action—cont'd

		Commonly Prescribed Drugs	
Drug Category	Primary Use and Major Therapeutic Effects	Generic	Brand
Bone Resorption Inhibitors	*Used* to treat and prevent osteoporosis *Work* by inhibiting resorption of bone **Fosamax** 5 mg 10 mg 40 mg	alendronate raloxifene risedronate	▶Fosamax ▶Evista ▶Actonel
Bronchodilators	*Used* to manage reversible airway obstruction caused by asthma or chronic obstructive pulmonary disease *Work* by relaxing smooth muscle of respiratory tract resulting in bronchodilation **Singulair** 4 mg 5 mg 10 mg	albuterol fluticasone/salmeterol ipratropium/albuterol montelukast salmeterol theophylline zafirlukast	▶Proventil ▶Advair Diskus ▶Combivent ▶Singulair Serevent Bronkodyl Accolate
Cardiac Glycosides	*Used* to treat congestive heart failure and cardiac arrhythmias *Work* by increasing strength and force of myocardial contractions and slowing heart rate **Lanoxicaps** 0.1 mg	digitoxin digoxin	Crystodigin ▶Digitek Lanoxicaps ▶Lanoxin
Central Nervous System Stimulants	*Used* to treat narcolepsy and manage attention-deficit/hyperactivity disorder *Work* by increasing level of catecholamines in central nervous system **Adderal (II)** 5 mg 10 mg 20 mg 30 mg	atomoxetine dextroamphetamine dextroamphetamine saccharate and sulfate methylphenidate	▶Strattera Dexedrine (II) ▶Adderall (II) Ritalin (II) ▶Concerta (II)
Contraceptives (Hormonal)	*Used* to prevent pregnancy and to regulate menstrual cycle *Work* by inhibiting ovulation **Ortho-Novum** 7/7/7 1/35	**Oral Contraceptives** ethinyl estradiol/ desogestrel	Apri

Continued

- **Subscription.** The subscription gives directions to the pharmacist. At present, it is generally used to designate the number of doses to be dispensed. To prevent a prescription from being altered illegally, it is recommended that numbers and letters be used to indicate the quantity to be dispensed (e.g., #30 [thirty]).
- **Signatura.** The signatura (abbreviated *Sig.*) is a Latin term that means "write" or "label" and indicates the information to be included on the medication label. It consists of directions to the patient for taking the medication. The name of the medication also is included on the label so that the patient can identify the medication.
- **Refill.** This part of the prescription indicates the number of times the prescription may be refilled.
- **Physician's signature.** A prescription cannot be filled unless it is signed by the physician.
- **DEA number.** The number assigned to the physician by the Drug Enforcement Administration must appear on the prescription for a controlled drug. See Table 11-4 for examples of controlled drugs.

Generic Prescribing

Generic prescribing means that the physician writes the prescription using the generic rather than the brand name of the drug. Because many pharmaceutical manufacturers may produce the same generic drug and sell it under different brand names, price competition often results. If the physician prescribes a drug using its generic name, the pharmacist is permitted to fill it with the drug that offers the best savings to the patient. In addition, most states allow the pharmacist the option of filling the prescription with a chemically equivalent generic drug, even if the drug has been prescribed by brand name. If the physician wants the prescription be filled with a specific brand of drug, instructions must be indicated on the prescription form, such as "Dispense as Written (DAW)," or words of a similar meaning (see Figure 11-2).

Completing a Prescription Form

The physician is responsible for having accurate and pertinent information on the prescription form. If delegated by

---

PATIENT TEACHING **Prescription Medications**

To avoid adverse reactions, teach patients the proper guidelines for taking prescription medication. These guidelines are as follows:

Know the names of all your prescription and nonprescription medications. Nonprescription drugs are known as *over-the-counter* (OTC) drugs; they are drugs that can be purchased without a prescription. Vitamin supplements and herbal products are considered OTC drugs.

Know why you are taking each medication. It is important to know the desired therapeutic outcome and the common side effects of each medication and guidelines ("do's and dont's") to follow when taking the medication.

Take your medication exactly as prescribed, at the right times and in the right amounts. The medication may not work properly if it is not taken as directed. If the dose is too small, the drug may not produce its intended therapeutic effect; exceeding the recommended dosage could result in a toxic effect.

Inform the physician if new symptoms or adverse effects develop when you are taking the medication. The physician may need to change your dosage or prescribe a different medication. There are usually alternative medications that the physician can prescribe to treat your condition.

Take the medication for the prescribed duration of time, even after you begin to feel better. If you do not complete the entire course of drug therapy, your condition may recur. Not taking all of a prescribed antibiotic may cause an infection to return, and it may be worse than the first infection.

Tell the physician if you decide not to take your medication. Otherwise, the physician may think your medication is not working. Not taking a medication prescribed by the physician could be serious because it may allow your condition to worsen.

Do not take additional medications, including OTC medications, without checking with the physician. All drugs, including OTC medications, are designed to have an effect on the body. Some combinations of drugs cause serious reactions. In some cases, one drug cancels the effects of another and prevents it from working.

Never take a medication that was prescribed for someone else. Physicians prescribe medication based on an individual's age, weight, sex, and condition. Taking a medication prescribed for someone else can have serious results.

Keep all medications in their original containers to avoid taking the wrong medication by mistake. Store your medications in their original containers from the pharmacy. Basic information about your medication is on the original container. Medications that are not clearly marked may be taken inadvertently by the wrong person.

Store your medications in a safe place, away from the reach of children. Ask for child-resistant safety closures, and ensure that the caps of the bottles are closed tightly. Accidental drug poisoning in children is a common and preventable problem. Also, do not take your medication in front of young children because they may want to mimic your behavior.

Store medications in a cool, dry place or as stated on the label. Do not store capsules or tablets in the bathroom or kitchen because heat or moisture may cause the medication to break down.

Discard unused portions of prescription medications and outdated OTC medications. Medications should be discarded by flushing them down the toilet. Medications that are past their expiration date may produce adverse effects in the body.

the physician, a prescription form can be completed by the medical assistant and signed by the physician. The physician must review the prescription thoroughly before signing it to ensure all of the information is correct. If the medical assistant is delegated this responsibility, he or she must carefully follow the important guidelines presented in the box *Guidelines for Completing a Prescription Form.*

MEDICATION RECORD

The medical office may use a preprinted form to record the medications (Rx and OTC) that a patient is taking; vitamin supplements and herbal products the patient is taking also should be recorded on the form. A medication record form (Figure 11-3) includes detailed information about each medication so that the physician can tell at a glance what medications and how much the patient is taking. The medication record is part of the patient's medical record. The medical assistant may be responsible for documenting medication information on this form. Care must be taken to ensure the information is correct and clearly written.

A medication record form typically includes the following information:
- Patient's name and date of birth
- Any drug allergies

What Would You Do? What Would You *Not* Do?

Case Study 2

Linda Cardwell calls the medical office. Her daughter Rachel, 9 years old, was seen in the office 10 days ago. Rachel was diagnosed with strep throat, and the physician ordered Amoxil 250 mg tid × 7 days. Mrs. Cardwell says that after 3 days of taking the medication, Rachel was much better, so she stopped giving her the Amoxil because it was causing her to have diarrhea. Mrs. Cardwell says that her 12-year-old son started feeling achy all over and she gave him the Amoxil for 2 days, and it seemed to help. She also says that her husband started complaining of sinus problems, so she also gave him the Amoxil for 2 days. Mrs. Cardwell says that now Rachel's throat is hurting again, and she has a fever. She wants to know whether Rachel has developed another case of strep throat. Mrs. Cardwell says she does not know what to do because she does not have any Amoxil left to give Rachel. ■

- Date the medication was prescribed (Rx) or date the patient started taking the medication (OTC)
- Name and dose of the medication
- Frequency of administration of the medication
- Route of administration

MEDICATION RECORD

Patient _John Walsh_
Birthdate _6/10/49_

ALLERGY
Ø

DATE	MEDICATION AND DOSAGE	FREQUENCY	RX	OTC	REFILLS		STOP
2/18/06	Cipro 250mg	÷ q 12 h po x 10 days	X				2/28/06
6/10/06	Prevacid 15mg	÷ qd po	X				7/10/06
6/10/06	Lipitor 10mg	÷ qd po	X		1/6/04		
6/10/06	Prozac 20mg	÷ qd po	X		1/6/04		
12/3/06	Tobrex Ophthalmic Solution	÷ gtt q3h OD	X				12/10/06
2/5/07	Echinacea	÷ qd po		X			
3/15/07	Nitrostat 0.4mg	÷ prn pain SL Rep q 5 min prn pain, not to exceed 3 tabs	X				
3/15/07	Inderal 40mg	÷ bid po	X				
3/15/07	St Joseph ASA Enteric Coated 81 mg	÷ qd po		X			

Figure 11-3. Example of a medication record.

- Prescription or OTC medication category
- Refills (Rx medication only)
- Date the patient stopped taking the medication

FACTORS AFFECTING DRUG ACTION
Therapeutic Effect

Each drug has an intended therapeutic effect—the reason the patient takes the medication. Certain factors affect the therapeutic action of drugs in the body, causing patients to respond differently to the same drug. Because of this, the drug therapy may need to be adjusted to meet these variations, which include the following.

Age

Children and the elderly tend to respond more strongly to drugs than do young and middle-aged adults. The physician may calculate smaller doses for very young and old patients.

Route of Administration

Medications administered by different routes are absorbed at different rates. Drugs administered orally are absorbed slowly because they must be digested first. Parenterally administered drugs are absorbed more quickly than orally administered drugs because they are injected directly into the body.

Size

A patient's body size has an effect on drug action. A thin individual may require a smaller quantity of a drug, and an obese individual may require more.

Time of Administration

A drug administered through the oral route is absorbed more rapidly when the stomach is empty than when it contains food. A drug may not produce the desired effect or may be absorbed too slowly if it is taken when food is present. Some drugs irritate the stomach's lining, however, and must be taken with food. The drug package insert or a drug reference should always be consulted to determine when a drug should be taken.

Tolerance

A patient taking a certain drug over a period of time may develop a tolerance to it. This means that the same dose of a drug no longer produces the desired effect after prolonged administration. The physician should be notified to determine whether a change of drug or dosage is needed.

Undesirable Effects of Drugs

A drug may cause undesirable effects, which may occur immediately or be delayed hours or even days after administration of the medication.

Adverse Reactions

Most drugs produce unintended and undesirable effects known as **adverse reactions.** Adverse reactions are second-

Memories *from* Externship

Theresa Cline: I can clearly remember the first time I gave an injection at my externship site. I was worried that I would forget how to give an injection and look bad in front of my externship supervisor and the patient. What made things worse is that the patient was a woman with very thin arms. I was giving her a flu shot, and I was so scared that the needle would hit her bone even though I was only using a 1-inch needle. When I walked into the room, my supervisor told the woman that I was a student and asked her if it was all right if I gave her the flu injection. The woman laughed and said, "Well, I guess so." That made me feel even more nervous. The patient then asked if it was my first shot. I told her "yes" and she said, "Just don't hurt me." When it came time to give the injection, everything that I had ever learned about injections came back to me. I gave the injection, and the woman told me I did a good job and that she didn't even feel it. That made me feel so good! My supervisor said, "If you can give a shot to her, you can give a shot to anyone." Every injection after that was a "piece of cake." I've learned just to take a deep breath before each difficult situation encountered in the office, and everything will work out. ∎

ary effects that occur along with the therapeutic effect of the drug. Some adverse reactions, referred to as *side effects,* are harmless and often tolerated by the patient to obtain the therapeutic effect of the drug. Most patients are willing to tolerate the dry mouth and drowsiness that may accompany an antihistamine to obtain its therapeutic effect. Other adverse reactions, such as a decrease in blood pressure or an allergic reaction, can be harmful to the patient and warrant discontinuing the medication.

Drug Interactions

When certain medications are used at the same time, drug interactions may produce undesirable effects. The medical assistant should inquire about other medications the patient is taking and record this information in the patient's chart for review by the physician.

Allergic Drug Reaction

The patient may exhibit an allergic reaction to a drug. The reaction is usually mild and takes the form of a rash, rhinitis, or pruritus. Occasionally, a patient has a severe allergic reaction that occurs suddenly and immediately. This is known as an **anaphylactic reaction.**

An anaphylactic reaction is the least common but the most serious type of allergic reaction. Symptoms begin with sneezing, urticaria (hives), itching, *angioedema, erythema,* and disorientation. Erythema is the reddening of the skin caused by dilation of superficial blood vessels in the skin. Angioedema is a localized urticaria of the deeper tissues of the body. If not treated, the symptoms of anaphylaxis quickly increase in severity and progress to dyspnea, cyanosis, and shock. Blood pressure decreases, and the pulse becomes weak and thready. Convulsions, loss of consciousness, and death may occur if treatment is not initiated promptly.

To prevent an anaphylactic reaction to a drug or to reduce its danger, the medical assistant should stay with the patient after administration of the medication. The medical assistant should be especially alert for signs of an anaphylactic reaction after administering allergy skin tests or a penicillin or allergy injection. If a reaction occurs, the physician should be notified immediately so that he or she can begin treatment immediately. Treatment generally consists of one or more injections of epinephrine, depending on the severity of the reaction. Epinephrine goes to work immediately to reverse the life-threatening symptoms of anaphylaxis. When the patient is stabilized, he or she is usually given an injection of an antihistamine. The antihistamine takes longer to begin working but helps alleviate urticaria, itching, angioedema, and erythema. The medical assistant must ensure that an ample supply of epinephrine is on hand at all times. Many offices maintain emergency crash carts for this purpose.

Idiosyncratic Reaction

An idiosyncratic reaction is an abnormal or peculiar response to a drug that is unexplained and unpredictable. Elderly patients are most prone to idiosyncratic reactions to drugs and should be monitored closely when they are taking a new medication.

GUIDELINES FOR PREPARATION AND ADMINISTRATION OF MEDICATION

To prevent medication errors, the medical assistant should follow these guidelines when preparing and administering any drug:

1. Work in a quiet, well-lit atmosphere that is free of distractions.
2. Always ask if you have a question about the medication order.
3. Know the drug to be given.
4. Select the proper drug. Check the label of the medication three times—as it is taken from its storage location, before preparing the medication, and after preparing the medication. Do not use a drug if the label is missing or is difficult to read.
5. Do not use a drug if the color has changed, if a precipitate has formed, or if it has an unusual odor.
6. Check the expiration date before preparing the drug for administration.
7. Prepare the proper dose of the drug. The term **dose** refers to the quantity of a drug to be administered at one time. Each medication has a dose range, or range of quantities of the drug that can produce therapeutic effects. It is important to administer the exact dose of the drug. A dose that is too small would not produce a therapeutic effect, and a dose that is too large could be harmful or even fatal to the patient.
8. Correctly identify the patient so that the drug is administered to the intended patient. When administer-

ing medication, the patient should be identified by his or her full name and date of birth.
9. Before administering the medication, check the patient's records or question the patient to ensure that he or she is not allergic to the medication.
10. If you are giving an injection, determine the appropriate route and site at which to administer the injection; the route and site are dictated by the type of injection being given. An allergy injection is given through the SC route, and an antibiotic injection is given through the IM route. The site must be free from abrasions, lesions, bruises, and edema.
11. Use the proper technique to administer the medication.
12. Stay with the patient after administering the medication.
13. Document information properly in the patient's chart immediately after administering the drug. Make sure the recording is clear and legible to avoid confusion by others who read it. Include the date and time, the name of the medication, the lot number (if required), the dose given, the route of administration, the site of administration, and any unusual observations or patient reactions. Sign the recording with your name and credentials. If you administer a medication that contains a fraction of a unit, place a 0 before the decimal point (e.g., 0.5 mg, not .5 mg) so that the dosage is not misread as 5 mg. A decimal point and a zero should never be placed after a whole number. The decimal point may be overlooked and misread, resulting in a 10-fold overdose error (e.g., 20 mg, not 20.0 mg).
14. Always follow the seven "rights" of preparing and administering medication in the medical office:
    Right drug
    Right dose
    Right time
    Right patient
    Right route
    Right technique
    Right documentation

ORAL ADMINISTRATION

The oral route is the most convenient and the most used method of administering medication. **Oral administration** means that the drug is given by mouth in either a solid form (e.g., a tablet or capsule) or a liquid form (e.g., a suspension or a syrup). Absorption of most oral medication occurs in the small intestine, although some may be absorbed in the mouth and stomach.

Many patients find it easier to swallow a tablet or capsule with a glass of water. Water should not be offered after the patient has received a cough syrup, however, because the water would dilute the medication's beneficial effects. Unless the patient has a malabsorption problem or is unable to swallow, the oral route is considered the safest and most desirable route for administering medication. Procedure 11-1 outlines the procedure for the administration of oral medications.

Text continued on p. 452

PROCEDURE **11-1** Administering Oral Medication

Outcome Administer oral solid and liquid medications.

Equipment/Supplies

- Medication ordered by the physician
- Medicine cup
- Medication tray

1. **Procedural Step.** Sanitize your hands.
2. **Procedural Step.** Assemble the equipment.
3. **Procedural Step.** Work in a quiet, well-lit atmosphere.
   Principle. Good lighting aids the medical assistant in reading the medication label.
4. **Procedural Step.** Select the correct medication from the shelf. Compare the medication with the physician's instructions. Check the drug label three times—while removing the medication from storage, while preparing the medication, and after preparing the medication. Check the expiration date.
   Principle. If the medication is outdated, consult the physician because it may produce undesirable effects for which the medical assistant could be held responsible. To prevent a drug error, the medication should be carefully compared with the physician's instructions.

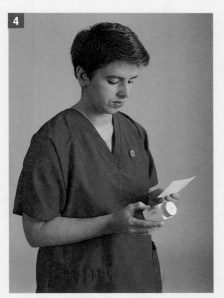

Compare the medication with the physician's instructions.

5. **Procedural Step.** Calculate the correct dose to be given, if necessary.
6. **Procedural Step.** Remove the bottle cap, touching the outside of the lid only.
   Principle. Touching the inside of the lid contaminates it.
7. **Procedural Step.** Check the drug label again, and pour the medication.

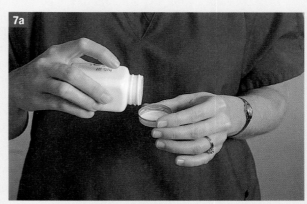

Pour the correct number of capsules or tablets into the bottle cap.

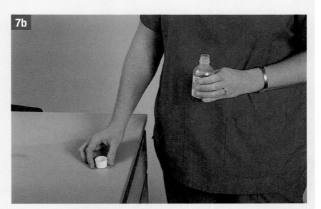

Place the lid of the bottle on a flat surface with the open end facing up.

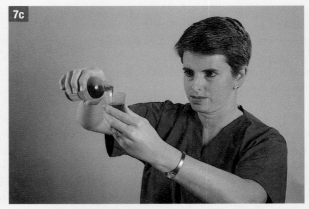

Hold the cup at eye level, and pour the medication.

Continued

PROCEDURE 11-1   Administering Oral Medication—cont'd

Solid Medications. Pour the correct number of capsules or tablets into the bottle cap. Transfer the medication to a medicine cup, being careful not to touch the inside of the cup.

Principle. Pouring the medication into the lid prevents contamination of the medication and lid.

Liquid Medications. Place the lid of the bottle on a flat surface with the open end facing up. Palm the surface of the label. With the opposite hand, place the thumbnail at the proper calibration on the medicine cup, and hold the cup at eye level. Pour the medication, and read the dose at the lowest level of the meniscus. (The meniscus is the curved surface of the liquid in a container. When a liquid is poured into a medicine cup, capillary action causes the liquid in contact with the cup to be drawn upward, resulting in a curved surface in the middle.)

Principle. Placing the bottle cap with the open end up prevents contamination of the inside of the cap. Palming the medication label prevents the medication from dripping on the label and obscuring it.

8. **Procedural Step.** Replace the bottle cap, and check the drug label a third time to ensure it is the correct medication. Return the medication to its storage location.

9. **Procedural Step.** Greet the patient and introduce yourself. Identify the patient by full name and date of birth and explain the procedure. Explain the purpose of administering the medication.

Principle. It is crucial that no error be made in patient identity.

10. **Procedural Step.** Hand the medicine cup containing the medication to the patient, along with a glass of water. (If the medication is a cough syrup, do not offer water.)

Principle. Water helps the patient swallow the medication.

11. **Procedural Step.** Remain with the patient until the medication is swallowed. If the patient experiences any unusual reaction, notify the physician.

12. **Procedural Step.** Sanitize your hands.

13. **Procedural Step.** Chart the procedure. Include the date and time, the name of the medication, the dosage given, the route of administration, and any significant observations or patient reactions. The Latin abbreviation *po,* which means "by mouth," can be used to indicate the route of administration.

CHARTING EXAMPLE	
Date	
2/12/08	9:30 a.m. Acetaminophen, 650 mg, po.
	——————————————— T. Cline, CMA

PARENTERAL ADMINISTRATION

The parenteral route of drug administration has several advantages. Medications given subcutaneously, intramuscularly, and intravenously are absorbed more rapidly and completely than medications given orally. In some cases, the parenteral route is the only way a drug can be given. If the patient is unconscious or has a gastric disturbance, such as nausea or vomiting, the parenteral route would be used. If state laws permit, the medical assistant is usually responsible for administering SC, IM, and intradermal injections. IV medications are sometimes administered in the medical office and are discussed in more detail later in the section on IV therapy.

The parenteral route also has disadvantages, such as pain and the possibility of infection as a result of breaking the skin. The medical assistant can minimize pain by inserting and withdrawing the needle quickly and smoothly and by withdrawing the needle at the same angle as for insertion. If injections are given repeatedly (e.g., allergy injections), the sites should be rotated to prevent the overuse of one site, which may cause irritation and tissue damage. Rotating sites also allows better absorption of the drug.

When recording the administration of a medication in the patient's chart, the medical assistant must include the site of the injection (e.g., right upper arm, left dorsogluteal). This assists in proper site rotation for patients who receive repeated injections. In addition, the information provides a reference point should a problem arise with the injection site.

Medical asepsis must be used when parenteral medications are administered. In addition, the needle and the inside of the syringe must remain sterile. These practices reduce the danger of microorganisms entering the patient's body during the administration of medication. The medical assistant must follow the OSHA standard when administering medication as a means of protecting himself or herself from bloodborne pathogens (see Chapter 2). Procedure 11-2 describes how to prepare an injection.

Parts of a Needle and Syringe

Needle

The needle consists of several parts (Figure 11-4). The *hub* of the needle fits onto the top of the syringe. The *shaft* is inserted into the body tissue. The opening in the shaft of

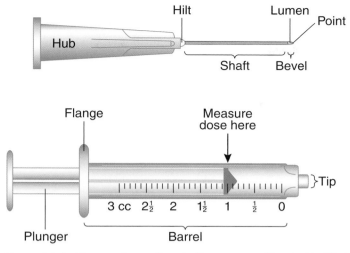

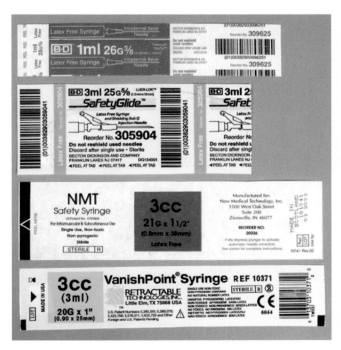

Figure 11-4. Diagram of a needle and a 3-cc syringe, with parts identified.

the needle, known as the *lumen,* is continuous with the needle hub. Medication flows from the syringe and through the lumen of the needle. The *point* of the needle is located at the end of the needle shaft. The point is sharp so that it can penetrate body tissues easily. The top of the needle is slanted and is called the *bevel.* The bevel is designed to make a narrow, slitlike opening in the skin. This narrow opening closes quickly when the needle is removed to prevent leakage of medication, and it heals quickly.

Each needle has a certain **gauge;** needle gauges for administering medication range between 18 G and 27 G. The gauge of a needle is determined by the diameter of the lumen: As the size of the gauge increases, the diameter of the lumen decreases. A needle with a gauge of 23 has a smaller lumen diameter than a needle with a gauge of 21. Thick or oily preparations must be given with a large lumen because they are too thick to pass through a smaller one. A needle with a larger lumen makes a larger needle track in the tissues. To reduce pain and tissue damage, a needle with the smallest gauge appropriate for the solution and route of administration is always chosen.

The length of the needle ranges between ⅜ and 3 inches; the length used is based on the type of injection being given and the size of the patient. To administer an IM injection to an obese adult requires a longer needle to reach the muscle tissue than would be required for a normal-size adult. To administer an IM injection to a thin patient requires a shorter needle to avoid inserting a needle too deeply and possibly penetrating the bone. The needle used to give an IM injection must be longer than one used for an SC injection so that it penetrates deeply enough to reach the muscle tissue.

Syringe

The syringe is used for inserting fluids into the body. It is made of plastic and must be disposed of after one use. The syringe with an attached needle is packaged in a cellophane wrapper or a rigid plastic container. Information regarding the syringe's capacity and the needle's length and gauge is printed on the wrapper of the syringe and needle (Figure 11-5). Syringes and needles also are available in separate packages. In this case, the medical assistant must attach a needle to the syringe before drawing medication into the syringe.

The parts of a syringe are the barrel, flange, and plunger (see Figure 11-4). The *barrel* of the syringe holds the medication and contains calibrated markings to measure the

Figure 11-5. Examples of syringe and needle packages labeled according to contents.

proper amount of medication. Most syringes are calibrated in cubic centimeters (cc), the unit of measurement used most often to administer parenteral medication. The medical assistant should become familiar with reading the graduated scales on syringes. At the end of the barrel is a rim known as the *flange,* which helps in injecting the medication. The flange also prevents the syringe from rolling when it is placed on a flat surface. The *plunger* is a movable cylinder that slides back and forth in the barrel. It is used to draw medication into the syringe when preparing an injection and to push medication out of the syringe when administering an injection.

Various types of syringes are available to administer injections. The choice is based on the type of injection being given (e.g., tuberculin skin test, allergy injection, antibiotic injection) and the amount of medication being administered. The types of syringes used most often in the medical office include hypodermic, insulin, and tuberculin (Figure 11-6).

Hypodermic syringes are available in 2-, 2.5-, 3-, and 5-cc sizes and are calibrated in cubic centimeters. They are commonly used to administer IM injections.

The *insulin syringe* is designed especially for the administration of an insulin injection, and the barrel is calibrated in units. The most common type is the U-100 syringe, which is calibrated into 100 units in increments of 2.

Tuberculin syringes are employed to administer a small dose of medication, such as when administering a tuberculin test. The tuberculin syringe has a capacity of 1 cc, and the calibrations are divided into tenths (0.10) and hundredths (0.01) of a cubic centimeter.

Syringes also are available with capacities of 10, 20, 30, 50, and 60 cc; however, they are not used for administering medication, but rather for medical treatments, such as irrigating wounds and draining fluid from cysts.

Safety Engineered Syringes

The Occupational Safety and Health Administration (OSHA) stipulates requirements to reduce needlestick and other sharps injuries among health care workers. As discussed in Chapter 2, employers are required to evaluate and implement commercially available safer medical devices that reduce occupational exposure to the lowest extent feasible.

Safer medical devices include safety engineered syringes. *Safety engineered syringes* incorporate a built-in safety feature to reduce the risk of a needlestick injury. Figure 11-7 illustrates types of safety engineered syringes and the methods for using them.

Preparation of Parenteral Medication

Medication used for injections is available in various types of dispensing units—vials, ampules, and prefilled syringes and cartridges.

Vials

A **vial** is a closed glass container with a rubber stopper; a soft metal or plastic cap protects the rubber stopper and must be removed the first time the medication is used. An injectable medication may be available in a single-dose vial, a multiple-dose vial, or both (Figure 11-8).

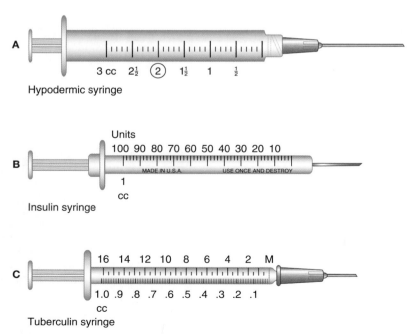

Figure 11-6. Various syringes used to administer injections. **A,** Hypodermic. **B,** Insulin (U-100). **C,** Tuberculin.

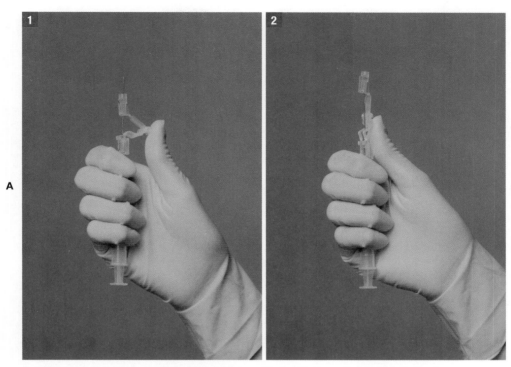

A. Safety Engineered Syringes Hinged Shield Syringe (Becton-Dickinson Safety Glide Syringe)
1. After administering the injection, push the lever of the hinged-shield forward.
2. Continue pushing until the needle tip is fully covered by the shield, then discard the syringe in a biohazard sharps container.

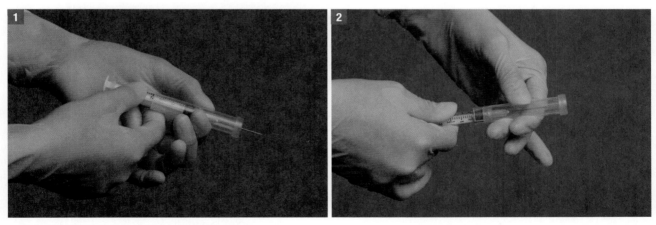

B. Sliding Shield Syringe (Monoject Safety Syringe)
1. After administering the injection, extend the sliding shield forward fully until a click is heard.
2. Lock the shield by twisting it in either direction until a click is heard. Discard the syringe in a biohazard sharps container.

Figure 11-7. Safety engineered syringes.

Continued

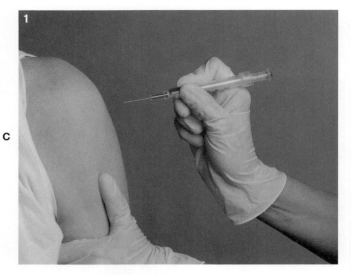

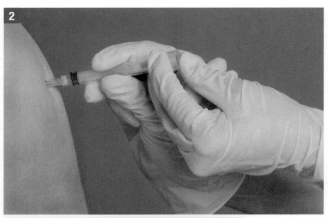

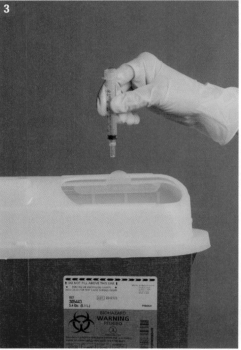

C

C. Retractable Needle (Vanish Point Syringe)

1. Administer the injection following the proper technique.
2. After administering the medication, continue depressing the plunger with the thumb. Use firm pressure past the point of initial resistance. This action delivers the full dose of medication to the patient and activates the needle retraction device, causing the needle to retract automatically from the patient's skin and into the barrel of the syringe.
3. Discard the syringe in a biohazard sharps container.

Figure 11-7, cont'd. Safety engineered syringes.

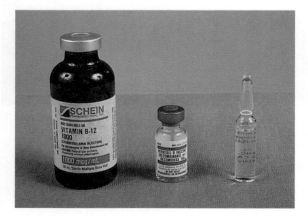

Figure 11-8. The multiple-dose vial *(left)* and the single-dose vial *(middle)* consist of a closed glass container with a rubber stopper. The ampule *(right)* consists of a small, sealed glass container that holds a single dose of medication.

Before the medication can be withdrawn, some vials require mixing (e.g., reconstituting a powdered drug or mixing a vial that separates on standing). Vials that require mixing should be rolled between the hands rather than shaken because shaking would cause the medication to foam, creating air bubbles that may enter the syringe when the medication is withdrawn.

To remove medication from a vial, an amount of air exactly equal to the amount of liquid to be removed is injected into the vial. The air should be inserted above the fluid level to avoid creating bubbles in the medication. If air is not injected first, a partial vacuum is created, and it is difficult to remove the medication. During the withdrawal of medication, the needle opening should be inserted below the fluid level to prevent the entrance of air bubbles. Air bubbles can be removed by tapping the barrel of the syringe with the fingertips. If the bubbles are allowed to remain, they take up space that the medication should occupy, which would prevent the patient from receiving the full dose of medication.

Ampules

An **ampule** is a small, sealed glass container that holds a single dose of medication (see Figure 11-8). An ampule has a constriction in the stem, known as the *neck*, which helps in opening it. Before opening, the medical assistant must ensure that there is no medication in the stem by tapping it lightly. A colored ring around the neck indicates where the ampule is prescored for easy opening. The ampule is opened by holding it firmly with gauze and breaking off the stem with a strong steady pressure.

A hazard with medication in ampules is the possibility of small glass particles getting into the ampule as the stem is broken off. When the medication is withdrawn into the syringe, the glass particles also might be withdrawn. To prevent this problem, a needle with a filter should be used that filters out small glass particles (Figure 11-9).

The needle opening is inserted into the base of the ampule below the fluid level to withdraw medication. To prevent contamination, the needle should not be permitted to touch the outside of the ampule. Air should never be injected into the ampule because it could force out some of the medication.

Prefilled Syringes and Cartridges

Some drugs come in *prefilled disposable syringes,* or cartridges. Using this type of dispensing unit does not require drawing up the medication. The name of the drug, the dose, and the expiration date are printed on the syringe or cartridge (Figure 11-10). An example is the Tubex Injector, which consists of a reusable device that holds a Tubex sterile cartridge-needle unit. The procedure for administering an injection using the Tubex Injector is presented in Figure 11-11.

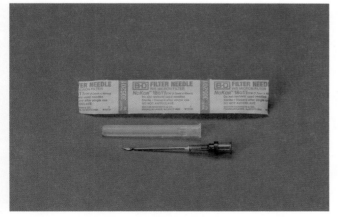

Figure 11-9. Filter needle used to withdraw medication from an ampule.

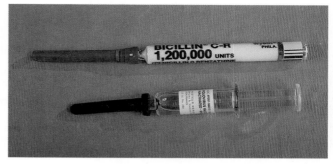

Figure 11-10. *Top,* A prefilled disposable cartridge of medication. Disposable cartridges must be inserted into a specially designed syringe for administration of the injection. *Bottom,* A prefilled disposable syringe.

Storage

The medical assistant should always read the drug package insert to determine the proper method for storing each parenteral medication because improper storage may alter the effectiveness of the medication.

Reconstitution of Powdered Drugs

Some parenteral medications are stable for only a short time in liquid form; these medications are prepared and stored in powdered form and require the addition of a liquid before administration. The process of adding a liquid to a powdered drug is known as *reconstitution.* The liquid used to reconstitute a powdered drug is known as the *diluent* and usually consists of sterile water or normal saline. The powdered drug is contained in a single-dose or multiple-dose vial and is accompanied by specific instructions for reconstitution. An example of a parenteral medication that requires reconstitution is the measles, mumps, and rubella (MMR) immunization (Figure 11-12). The procedure for reconstituting powdered drugs is outlined in Procedure 11-3.

Subcutaneous Injections

A **subcutaneous injection** is made into the subcutaneous tissue, which consists of adipose (fat) tissue and is located just under the skin (Figure 11-13). Subcutaneous tissue is located all over the body; however, certain sites are more commonly used because they are located where bones and blood vessels are not near the surface of the skin. These sites include the upper lateral part of the arms, the anterior thigh, the upper back, and the abdomen (Figure 11-14). Absorption of medication from a SC injection occurs mainly through capillaries, resulting in a slower absorption rate than with IM injections. To ensure proper absorption, tissue that is grossly adipose, hardened, inflamed, or edematous should not be used as an injection site.

The needle length varies from ½ to ⅝ inch, and the gauge ranges from 23 G to 25 G. Elderly and dehydrated patients tend to have less SC tissue, and obese patients have more. The length of the needle should be adjusted accordingly to ensure the medication is administered into the subcutaneous tissue and not into muscle tissue.

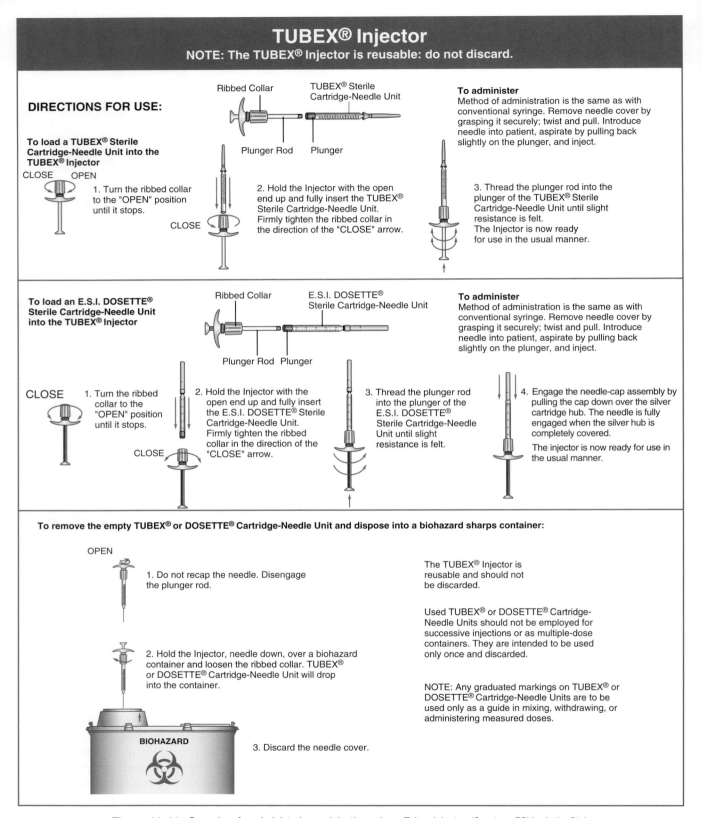

Figure 11-11. Procedure for administering an injection using a Tubex Injector. (Courtesy ESI Lederle, Division of American Home Products Corporation, St. Davids, Penn.)

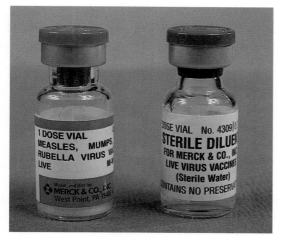

Figure 11-12. The measles, mumps, and rubella (MMR) vaccine is a parenteral medication that requires reconstitution before administration. The vial on the left contains the medication in powdered form, and the vial on the right contains the sterile diluent.

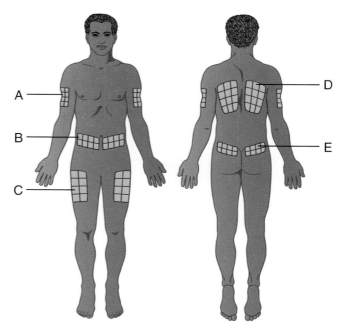

Figure 11-14. Common sites for subcutaneous injections. **A,** Upper outer arm. **B,** Lower abdomen. **C,** Upper outer thigh. **D,** Upper back. **E,** Flank region.

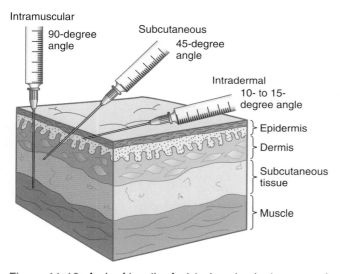

Figure 11-13. Angle of insertion for intradermal, subcutaneous, and intramuscular injections.

Subcutaneous tissue is sensitive to irritating solutions and large volumes of medications; therefore drugs given subcutaneously must be isotonic, nonirritating, nonviscous, and water-soluble. The amount of medication injected through the SC route should not exceed 1 cc. More than this amount results in pressure on sensory nerve endings, causing discomfort and pain.

Medications commonly administered through the SC route include epinephrine, insulin, and allergy injections. Patients who receive allergy injections must wait in the medical office for 15 to 20 minutes after the injection to be observed for an allergic reaction. Procedure 11-4 outlines the administration of a subcutaneous injection.

Intramuscular Injections

Intramuscular injections are made into the muscular layer of the body, which lies below the skin and subcutaneous layers (see Figure 11-13). The amount of medication that can be injected into muscle tissue is more than the amount that can be injected into subcutaneous tissue. An amount up to 3 cc can be injected into the gluteal or vastus lateralis muscles, although older and very thin adults are able to tolerate only 2 cc or less in these sites.

Absorption is more rapid by this route than by the SC route because there are more blood vessels in muscle tissue. Medication that is irritating to subcutaneous tissue is often given intramuscularly because there are fewer nerve endings in deep muscle tissue. Most parenteral medications administered in the medical office are given through the IM route; examples include immunizations, antibiotics, injectable contraceptives, vitamin B_{12}, and corticosteroids.

The length of the needle for an adult must be long enough to reach muscle tissue and varies from 1 to 3 inches. A 1½-inch needle is typically used for an average-sized adult, whereas a 1-inch needle is often used for a thin adult or child and a needle of 2 to 3 inches may be needed for an obese adult. The gauge of the needle used ranges from 18 G to 23 G, depending on the viscosity of the medication. Procedure 11-5 outlines the technique for the administration of an IM injection.

Intramuscular Injection Sites
The sites chosen for IM injections are away from large nerves and blood vessels. The medical assistant should practice locating these sites to become familiar with them. The

area should always be fully exposed to permit clear visualization of the injection site.

Dorsogluteal Site

The dorsogluteal site is often used to administer IM injections in the medical office. In adults and children older than 3 years of age, the gluteal muscles are well developed and can absorb a large amount of medication. The patient should lie on the abdomen with the toes pointed inward, which aids in relaxation of the gluteal muscles. The medication is injected into the upper outer quadrant of the gluteal area, in the area located above and outside a diagonal line drawn from the greater trochanter to the posterior superior iliac spine. These landmarks should be identified through palpation. The medical assistant must be *extremely* careful to maintain the proper boundary lines to avoid injection into the sciatic nerve or superior gluteal artery (Figure 11-15).

Deltoid Site

The deltoid area is easily accessible and can be used when the patient is sitting or lying down. This site is small be-

cause major nerves and blood vessels surround it, and large amounts of medication (no more than 1 cc) and repeated injections should not be given in this area. The medication is injected into the deltoid muscle.

The medical assistant should ensure that the entire arm is exposed by having the patient's sleeve completely pulled up or by removing the sleeve from the arm if it cannot be pulled up. A tight sleeve constricts the arm and causes unnecessary bleeding from the puncture site.

The deltoid site is located by palpating the lower edge of the acromion process, which forms the base of a triangle in line with the midpoint of the lateral side of the arm, opposite the axilla (see Figure 11-15). This site also may be located by placing four fingers horizontally across the deltoid muscle with the top finger along the acromion process. The injection site is located three finger widths below the acromion process.

Vastus Lateralis Site

The vastus lateralis is used because it is not near major nerves and blood vessels and is a relatively thick muscle (see

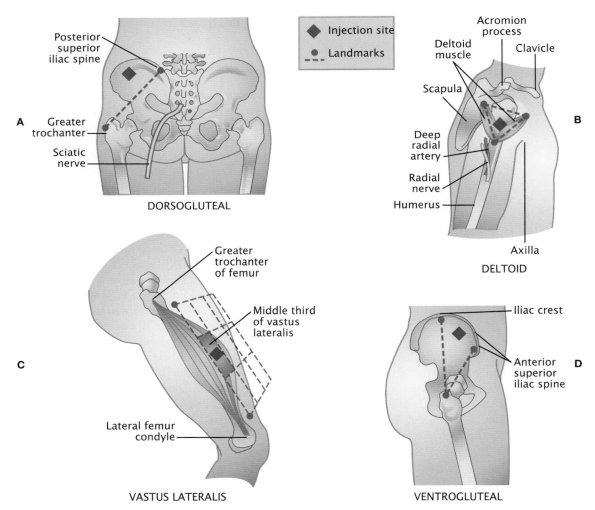

Figure 11-15. Sites of intramuscular injections. **A,** Dorsogluteal muscle. **B,** Deltoid muscle. **C,** Vastus lateralis. **D,** Ventrogluteal muscle. (From Leahy JM, Kizilay PE: *Foundations of nursing practice: a nursing process approach,* Philadelphia, 1988, Saunders.)

Figure 11-15). This site is particularly desirable for infants and children younger than 3 years old whose gluteal muscles are not yet well developed. The area is bounded by the midanterior thigh on the front of the leg and the midlateral thigh on the side. The proximal boundary is a hand's breadth below the greater trochanter, and the distal boundary is a hand's breadth above the knee. It is easier to give an injection in the vastus lateralis if the patient is lying down, but a sitting position also can be used.

Ventrogluteal Site

The ventrogluteal site is growing in acceptability as an IM injection site because the subcutaneous layer is relatively small and the muscle layer is thick. The site is located away from major nerves and blood vessels. Through palpation, the greater trochanter of the femur, the anterior superior iliac spine, and the iliac crest can be located. If the injection is being made into the patient's left side, the palm of the right hand is placed on the greater trochanter, and the index finger is placed on the anterior superior iliac spine. The middle finger is spread posteriorly as far as possible away from the index finger, to touch the iliac crest. The hand position is reversed if the injection is being made into the patient's right side. The triangle formed by the fingers is the area into which the injection is given. An injection into the ventrogluteal site can be administered when the patient is lying prone or on one side (see Figure 11-15).

Z-Track Method

Medications that are irritating to subcutaneous and skin tissue or that discolor the skin must be given intramuscularly using the Z-track method; one medication that is administered by this method is iron dextran (Imferon). The dorsogluteal, ventrogluteal, and vastus lateralis sites all can be used as areas to administer a Z-track injection.

The Z-track method is similar to the IM injection procedure except that the skin and subcutaneous tissue at the injection site are pulled to the side before the needle is inserted. This causes a zigzag path through the tissues when the needle is removed and the skin is released. The zigzag path prevents the medication from reaching the subcutaneous layer or skin surface by sealing off the needle track (Figure 11-16). The procedure for administering medication using the Z-track method is outlined in Procedure 11-6.

Text continued on p. 471

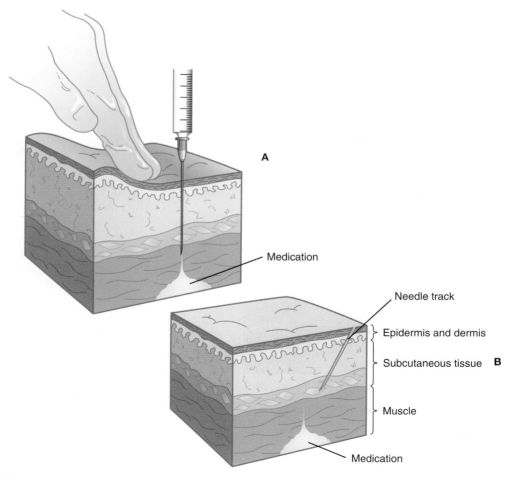

Figure 11-16. Z-track intramuscular injection method. **A,** The skin and subcutaneous tissue are pulled to the side before the needle is inserted. **B,** This causes a zigzag path through the tissue when the skin is released, which seals off the needle track.

Outcome Prepare an injection from an ampule and a vial.

Equipment/Supplies

- Medication ordered by the physician
- Appropriate needle and syringe
- Antiseptic wipe
- Medication tray

1. **Procedural Step.** Sanitize your hands.
2. **Procedural Step.** Assemble the equipment.
3. **Procedural Step.** Work in a quiet and well-lit atmosphere.
   Principle. Good lighting aids the medical assistant in reading the medication label.
4. **Procedural Step.** Select the proper medication. Compare the medication with the physician's instructions. Check the drug label three times—while removing the medication from storage, before withdrawing the medication into the syringe, and after preparing the medication. Check the expiration date.
   Principle. The medication should be carefully identified to prevent the administration of the wrong medication. Outdated medication should not be used because it could produce undesirable effects.

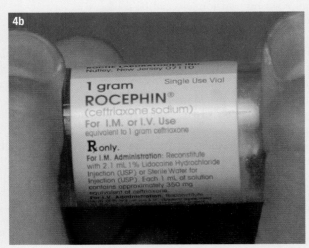

Check the drug label three times.

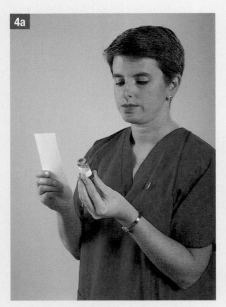

Compare the medication with the physician's instructions.

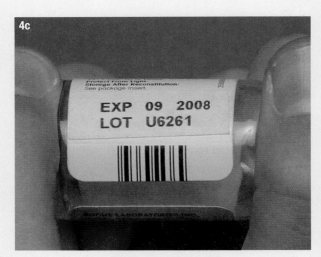

Check the expiration date.

5. **Procedural Step.** Calculate the correct dose to be given, if necessary. If you have any questions regarding the administration of the medication, check the package insert accompanying the drug.

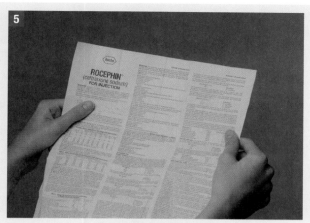

Check the package insert.

6. Procedural Step. Open the syringe and needle package. If necessary, assemble the needle and syringe.
Principle. Disposable needles and syringes may come already assembled together in a package or in separate packages that require assembly of the needle and syringe.

7. Procedural Step. Check to ensure that the needle is attached firmly to the syringe by loosening the guard on the needle, grasping the needle at the hub, and tightening it. Break the seal on the syringe by moving the plunger back and forth several times.

8. Procedural Step. Check the drug label again to ensure it is the correct medication. If required, mix the medication by rolling the vial between your hands to obtain a uniform suspension of the medication.

9. Procedural Step. Withdraw the medication following these steps.

Withdrawing Medication from a Vial

a. Procedural Step. Remove the soft metal or plastic cap protecting the rubber stopper of the vial. Open the antiseptic; wipe and cleanse the rubber stopper.
Principle. Cleansing the top of the vial removes dust and bacteria.

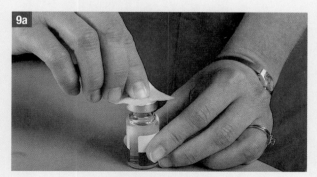

Cleanse the rubber stopper.

b. Procedural Step. Place the vial in an upright position on a flat surface. Remove the needle guard. Pull

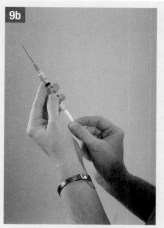

Draw air into the syringe.

back on the plunger to draw an amount of air into the syringe equal to the amount of medication to be withdrawn from the vial.
Principle. Air must be injected into the vial first to prevent the formation of a partial vacuum in the vial, which would make it difficult to remove medication.

c. Procedural Step. Using moderate pressure, insert the needle through the center of the rubber stopper at a 90-degree angle, until it reaches the empty space between the stopper and fluid level. Be careful not to bend the needle. Push down on the plunger to inject the air into the vial, keeping the needle opening above the fluid level. (*Note:* If you are using a retractable safety syringe, do not push too hard on the plunger to avoid activating the retracting mechanism prematurely.)

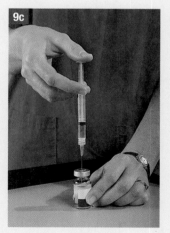

Inject air into the vial.

Principle. The air must be inserted above the fluid level to avoid creating air bubbles in the medication.

Continued

PROCEDURE 11-2

d. Procedural Step. Invert the vial while holding onto the syringe and plunger. Hold the syringe at eye level, and withdraw the proper amount of medication. Keep the needle opening below the fluid level.

Principle. The needle opening must be below the fluid level to prevent the entrance of air bubbles into the syringe.

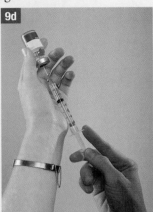

Withdraw the proper amount of medication.

e. Procedural Step. Remove any air bubbles in the syringe by holding the syringe in a vertical position and tapping the barrel with the fingertips until they disappear.

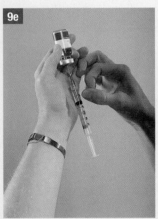

Tap the barrel with the fingertips to remove air bubbles.

Principle. Air bubbles take up space the medication should occupy, preventing the patient from getting the proper dose of medication.

f. Procedural Step. Remove any air remaining at the top of the syringe by slowly pushing the plunger forward and allowing the air to flow back into the

vial. Carefully remove the needle from the rubber stopper, and replace the needle guard.

Principle. The needle must remain sterile. The needle guard prevents the needle from becoming contaminated.

g. Procedural Step. Check the drug label for the third time, and return the medication to its proper storage location.

Withdrawing Medication from an Ampule

a. Procedural Step. Remove the needle (and needle guard) from the syringe, and attach a filter needle (and needle guard).

b. Procedural Step. Open the antiseptic wipe, and cleanse the neck of the ampule.

Principle. Cleansing the neck of the ampule removes dust and bacteria.

c. Procedural Step. Tap the stem of the ampule lightly to remove any medication in the neck of the ampule.

d. Procedural Step. Check the medication label a second time and place a piece of gauze around the neck of the ampule. Hold the base of the ampule between the first two fingers and the thumb of one hand. Hold the neck of the vial between the first two fingers and the thumb of the other hand. Apply a strong steady pressure with the thumbs, and break off the stem by snapping it quickly and firmly away from the body. Discard the stem and gauze in a biohazard sharps container.

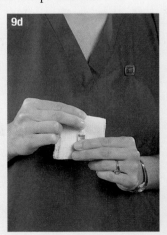

Snap off the stem away from the body.

e. Procedural Step. Place the ampule on a flat surface. Remove the needle guard. Insert the filter needle opening below the fluid level.

Principle. The filter needle prevents glass particles from being withdrawn into the syringe.

f. **Procedural Step.** Withdraw the proper amount of medication by pulling back on the plunger. Keep the needle opening below the fluid level to prevent the entrance of air bubbles into the syringe. Tilt the ampule as needed to keep the needle opening immersed in the fluid.

Principle. Air bubbles take up space the medication should occupy, resulting in an inaccurate measurement of medication.

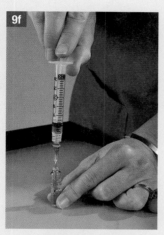

Withdraw the medication.

Note: There is another method that can be used to remove medication from an ampule. Choose the method that is easiest for you. To perform this method, invert the ampule, making sure to keep the needle opening below the fluid level. Withdraw the proper amount of medication by pulling back on the plunger. Move the needle downwards as necessary to keep the needle opening immersed in the fluid.

g. **Procedural Step.** Remove the needle from the ampule, and replace the needle guard. Check the drug label for the third time, and dispose of the glass ampule in a biohazard sharps container.

h. **Procedural Step.** Remove the filter needle (and guard) from the syringe, and discard it in a biohazard sharps container. Reapply the needle (and guard) for administering the medication.

i. **Procedural Step.** If air bubbles are in the syringe, remove the needle guard, hold the syringe in a vertical position, and tap the barrel with the fingertips until the bubbles disappear. Remove the air at the top of the syringe by slowly pushing the plunger forward. If the syringe contains excess fluid, hold the syringe vertically over a sink with the needle tip up and slanted toward the sink. Slowly eject the excess fluid into the sink. Replace the needle guard.

PROCEDURE **11-3**   Reconstituting Powdered Drugs

Outcome Reconstitute a powdered drug for parenteral administration.

Equipment/Supplies

- Medication ordered by the physician
- Appropriate needle and syringe
- Antiseptic wipe
- Medication tray

1. **Procedural Step.** Follow steps 1 through 8 of Procedure 11-2.

2. **Procedural Step.** From the vial of the powdered drug, withdraw an amount of air equal to the amount of liquid to be injected into the vial.

   Principle. Removing air from the powdered drug vial allows room for injection of the diluent.

3. **Procedural Step.** Inject the air removed from the powdered drug vial into the vial of diluent.

   Principle. Air must be injected into the vial to prevent formation of a partial vacuum in the vial, which would make it difficult to remove the diluent.

4. **Procedural Step.** Invert the diluent vial, and withdraw the proper amount of liquid into the syringe. Remove air bubbles from the syringe, and carefully remove the needle from the vial.

5. **Procedural Step.** Insert the needle into the powdered drug vial, and inject the diluent into the vial. Remove the needle from the vial, and replace the needle guard.

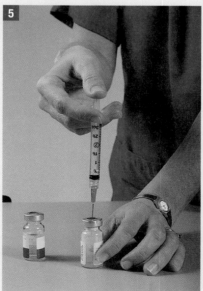

Inject the diluent into the vial.

Continued

PROCEDURE 11-3

PROCEDURE 11-3   Reconstituting Powdered Drugs—cont'd

6. **Procedural Step.** Roll the vial between the hands to mix the powdered drug and liquid (unless indicated otherwise by the drug package insert).
Principle. Shaking the vial may cause air bubbles to form.

7. **Procedural Step.** Label multiple-dose vials with the date of preparation and your initials.

8. **Procedural Step.** Follow step 9 (a through g) of Procedure 11-2.

9. **Procedural Step.** Store multiple-dose vials as indicated by the manufacturer's instructions. Because reconstituted drugs are stable for a short time, carefully check the date of preparation on the multiple-dose vial before administering it again.

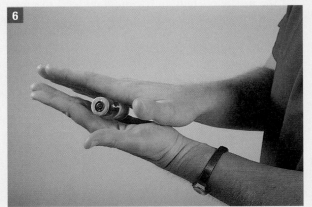

Roll the vial between the hands.

PROCEDURE 11-4   Administering a Subcutaneous Injection

Outcome Administer a subcutaneous injection.

Equipment/Supplies

- Medication ordered by the physician
- Appropriate needle and syringe
- Antiseptic wipe
- Sterile 2 × 2 gauze pad
- Disposable gloves
- Biohazard sharps container

1. **Procedural Step.** Sanitize your hands, and prepare the injection.

2. **Procedural Step.** Greet the patient and introduce yourself. Identify the patient by full name and date of birth. Explain the procedure and purpose of the injection.
Principle. It is crucial that no error be made in patient identity. An apprehensive patient may need reassurance.

3. **Procedural Step.** Select an appropriate injection site. The upper arm, thigh, back, and abdomen are recommended sites for a subcutaneous injection. See Figure 11-14.
Principle. The entire area should be exposed to ensure a safe and comfortable injection.

4. **Procedural Step.** Prepare the injection site. Cleanse the area with an antiseptic wipe. Using a circular motion, start with the injection site, and move outward. Do not touch the site after cleansing it.
Principle. Using a circular motion carries contaminants away from the injection site. Touching the site after cleansing contaminates it, and the cleansing process needs to be repeated.

5. **Procedural Step.** Allow the area to dry completely.

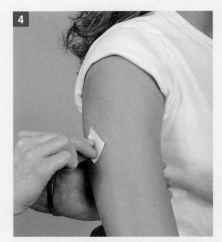

Cleanse the area with an antiseptic wipe.

Principle. If the area is not permitted to dry, the antiseptic may enter the tissues when the skin is pierced, resulting in irritation and patient discomfort.

6. **Procedural Step.** Apply gloves, and remove the needle guard. Position your nondominant hand on the area

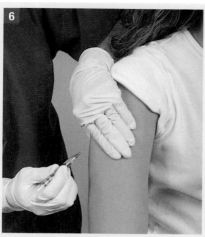

Grasp the area surrounding the injection site.

surrounding the injection site. The skin may be held taut, or the area surrounding the injection site may be grasped and held in a cushion fashion.

Principle. Gloves provide a barrier against blood-borne pathogens. In normal adults, the needle enters the subcutaneous tissue when the skin is held taut. Grasping the area around the injection site is recommended for a thin or dehydrated patient. This ensures that the subcutaneous tissue, and not muscle tissue, is entered.

7. Procedural Step. Hold the barrel of the syringe between your thumb and index finger. Insert the needle quickly and smoothly at a 45-degree or 90-degree angle, depending on the length of the needle. With a ½-inch needle, a 90-degree angle should be used; with a ⅝-inch needle, a 45-degree angle should be used. Insert the needle to the hub.

Principle. Inserting the needle quickly and smoothly minimizes tissue trauma and pain. Needle length de-

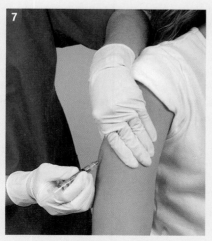

Insert the needle at a 45-degree angle.

termines the angle of insertion to ensure placement of the medication in subcutaneous tissue.

8. Procedural Step. Remove your hand from the skin. *Principle.* Medication injected into compressed tissue causes pressure against nerve fibers and is uncomfortable for the patient.

9. Procedural Step. Hold the syringe steady and pull back gently on the plunger to determine whether the needle is in a blood vessel, in which case blood would appear in the syringe. If blood appears, withdraw the needle, prepare a new injection, and begin again.

Principle. Moving the syringe after the needle has entered the tissue causes patient discomfort. Drugs intended for subcutaneous administration but injected into a blood vessel are absorbed too quickly, and undesirable results may occur.

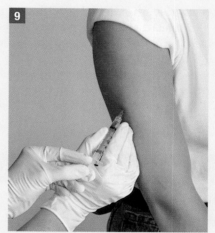

Pull back gently to determine whether the needle is in a blood vessel.

10. Procedural Step. Inject the medication slowly and steadily by depressing the plunger. If you are using a retractable safety syringe, activate it at this time following the steps outlined in Figure 11-7, and continue to step 12.

Principle. Rapid injection creates pressure and destroys tissue, which are uncomfortable for the patient.

11. Procedural Step. Place the antiseptic wipe or a gauze pad gently over the injection site, and quickly remove the needle, keeping it at the same angle as for insertion.

Principle. Withdrawing the needle quickly and at the same angle as for insertion reduces patient discomfort. The antiseptic wipe or gauze pad placed over the injection site helps prevent tissue movement as the needle is withdrawn, reducing patient discomfort. Using a gauze pad prevents a stinging sensation from the alcohol.

Continued

PROCEDURE 11-4   Administering a Subcutaneous Injection—cont'd

12. **Procedural Step.** Apply gentle pressure to the injection site with the antiseptic wipe or gauze pad. If you are using a safety syringe with a shield, activate the safety feature at this time following the steps outlined in Figure 11-7.
    Principle. Gentle pressure helps distribute the medication so that it is completely absorbed. Avoid vigorous massaging because it could damage underlying tissue.

13. **Procedural Step.** Properly dispose of the needle and syringe in a biohazard sharps container.
    Principle. Proper disposal is required by the OSHA standard to prevent accidental needlestick injuries.

14. **Procedural Step.** Remove gloves, and sanitize your hands.

15. **Procedural Step.** Chart the procedure. Include the date and time, the name of the medication, the lot number (if required), the dosage given, the route of administration, the injection site used, and any significant observations or patient reactions.
    Principle. The lot number indicates the batch in which the medication was made. Should a problem arise with that batch, the drug can be recalled, and individuals who received it can be identified.

16. **Procedural Step.** Stay with the patient to ensure that he or she is not experiencing any unusual reactions. *Note:* If an allergy injection has been given, the patient should remain at the medical office for at least 15 minutes to ensure that an allergic reaction does not occur.) Check the patient's arm after the waiting period and observe for induration and redness. If the patient experiences such a reaction, notify the physician immediately.

CHARTING EXAMPLE

Date	
2/17/08	3:30 p.m. Ragweed allergy inj, 0.20 cc, SC ®️
	upper arm. Arm checked 15 min. after admin.
	No reaction noted. ———————— T. Cline, CMA

 PROCEDURE 11-5   Administering an Intramuscular Injection

Outcome Administer an intramuscular injection.

Equipment/Supplies

- Medication ordered by the physician
- Appropriate needle and syringe
- Antiseptic wipe
- Sterile 2 × 2 gauze pad
- Disposable gloves
- Biohazard sharps container

1. **Procedural Step.** Sanitize your hands, and prepare the injection.

2. **Procedural Step.** Greet the patient and introduce yourself. Identify the patient by full name and date of birth and explain the procedure.
   Principle. Make sure that you administer the medication to the right patient. Explain the purpose of the injection. Assistance may be needed for restraining infants and children.

3. **Procedural Step.** Select an appropriate IM injection site. See Figure 11-15 for the recommended IM injection sites. Remove the patient's clothing as necessary to ensure the entire area is exposed.
   Principle. Major nerves and blood vessels may lie in close proximity to the intramuscular injection sites. The medical assistant should develop skill and accuracy in locating the proper sites.

4. **Procedural Step.** Prepare the injection site. Cleanse the area with an antiseptic wipe. Using a circular motion, start with the injection site, and move outward. Do not touch the site after cleansing it.
   Principle. Using a circular motion carries contaminants away from the injection site. Touching the site after cleansing contaminates it, and the cleansing process needs to be repeated.

5. **Procedural Step.** Allow the area to dry completely.
   Principle. If the area is not permitted to dry, the antiseptic may enter the tissues when the skin is pierced, resulting in irritation and patient discomfort.

6. **Procedural Step.** Apply gloves, and remove the needle guard. Using the thumb and first two fingers of the nondominant hand, stretch the skin taut over the injection site.

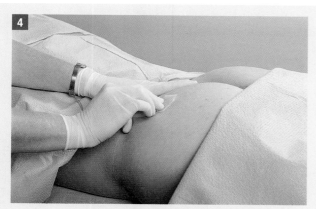

Cleanse the site with an antiseptic wipe.

Principle. Gloves provide a barrier against blood-borne pathogens. Stretching the skin taut permits easier insertion of the needle and helps ensure that the needle enters muscle tissue.

7. **Procedural Step.** Hold the barrel of the syringe like a dart, and insert the needle quickly and smoothly at a

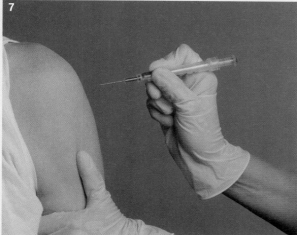

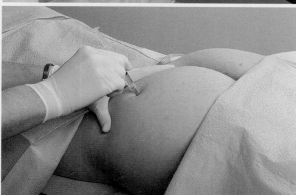

Insert the needle at a 90-degree angle.

90-degree angle to the patient's skin with a firm motion. Insert the needle to the hub.

Principle. The needle is inserted at a 90-degree angle to ensure that it reaches muscle tissue. Inserting the needle quickly and smoothly minimizes tissue trauma and pain.

8. **Procedural Step.** Hold the syringe steady, and pull back gently on the plunger to determine whether the needle is in a blood vessel. If blood appears, withdraw the needle, prepare a new injection, and begin again.

Principle. Moving the syringe after the needle has penetrated the tissue causes patient discomfort. If drugs intended for intramuscular administration are injected into a blood vessel, the result is faster absorption of the medication. This may produce undesirable results.

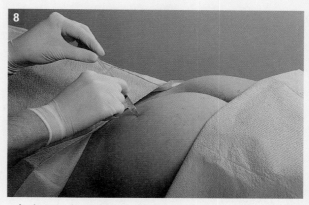

Aspirate to determine whether the needle is in a blood vessel.

9. **Procedural Step.** Inject the medication slowly and steadily by depressing the plunger. If you are using a retractable safety syringe, activate it at this time following the steps outlined in Figure 11-7, and continue to step 11.

Principle. Rapid injection creates pressure and destroys tissue, causing discomfort for the patient.

10. **Procedural Step.** Place the antiseptic wipe or gauze pad gently over the injection site, and remove the needle quickly, keeping it at the same angle as for insertion.

Principle. Withdrawing the needle quickly and at the same angle as for insertion reduces patient discomfort. Placing the antiseptic wipe or gauze pad over the injection site helps prevent tissue movement as the needle is withdrawn, also reducing patient discomfort. Using a gauze pad prevents a stinging sensation from the alcohol.

Continued

PROCEDURE 11-5

CHARTING EXAMPLE

Date	
2/15/08	10:00 a.m. Tubersol Mantoux test 5 TU,
	0.10 ml, ID. Connaught Laboratories,
	Lot #: C0832AA. Admin Ⓡ ant forearm.
	Pt to return on 2/17/08 to have results
	read. ———————————— T. Cline, CMA

Reading Mantoux Test Results
Equipment/Supplies

- Millimeter ruler
- Disposable gloves
- Tuberculin test record card

1. **Procedural Step.** Greet the patient and introduce yourself. Identify the patient by full name and date of birth and explain the procedure.
2. **Procedural Step.** Work in a quiet, well-lit atmosphere. Check the patient's chart to determine which arm was used to administer the test.
3. **Procedural Step.** Sanitize your hands, and apply gloves.
4. **Procedural Step.** Ask the patient to flex the arm at the elbow.
5. **Procedural Step.** Locate the application site. The result should be read horizontally to the long axis of the forearm, meaning "across" the forearm.
6. **Procedural Step.** Gently rub your finger over the test site, and lightly palpate for the presence of induration. If induration is present, the area should be lightly rubbed from the area of normal skin (without induration) to the indurated area to assess the size of the area of induration.
Principle. Induration is the only criterion used in determining a positive reaction. If erythema is present without induration, the results are interpreted as negative.

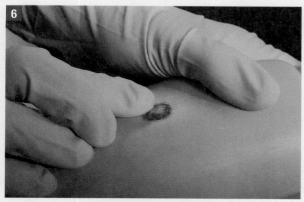

Lightly palpate for induration.

7. **Procedural Step.** Measure the diameter of the induration with a flexible millimeter ruler (supplied by the

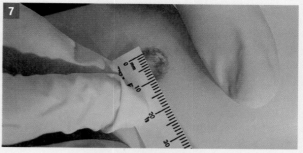

Measure the induration.

manufacturer). The results of the Mantoux test are interpreted as follows:
Positive Reaction: Vesiculation or induration 10 mm or more.
Doubtful Reaction: Induration 5 to 9 mm.
Negative Reaction: Induration less than 5 mm.
8. **Procedural Step.** Remove gloves, and sanitize your hands.
9. **Procedural Step.** Chart the results. Include the date and time, the name of the test (Mantoux), and the test results (recorded in millimeters). If no induration is present, 0 mm should be recorded.
10. **Procedural Step.** Complete a tuberculin test record card, and give it to the patient.
Principle. The record card provides the patient with a permanent record of the test results.

TUBERCULOSIS TEST RECORD

Name		Date Admin: 2/15/08	
Carrie Fee		Date Read: 2/17/08	
MANTOUX TEST	**RESULT**		
	Negative	Doubtful	Positive
Tubersol, 5 TU	___ mm	9 mm	___ mm

Logan Family Practice
401 St. George St.
St. Augustine, FL 32084
(904) 555-3933

Performed by ____ *T. Cline, CMA* ____

CHARTING EXAMPLE

Date	
2/17/08	3:00 p.m. Tubersol Mantoux test: 9mm.
	Pt provided c̄ TB record card. Scheduled
	for TB retesting on 2/28/08. ———————
	———————————— T. Cline, CMA

PROCEDURE 11-7

INTRAVENOUS THERAPY

Intravenous (IV) therapy is the administration of a liquid agent directly into a patient's vein, where it is distributed throughout the body by way of the circulatory system (Figure 11-22). The veins most commonly used for IV therapy are the peripheral veins of the arm and hand. The liquid agent may consist of basic fluids, medication, nutrients, blood, or blood products. When fluids, medications, or nutrients are administered through the IV route, the technique is called an **infusion.** When whole blood or blood products are administered through the IV route, the procedure is called a **transfusion.**

Most IV therapy occurs in a hospital setting on an inpatient and outpatient basis. IV therapy also is administered in outpatient ambulatory settings, such as medical offices and clinics, urgent care centers, ambulatory infusion clinics, and the patient's home (Figure 11-23).

Advantages of Outpatient Intravenous Therapy

Administration of IV therapy in an outpatient setting is growing in acceptance by patients and the medical community. Outpatient IV therapy is more convenient for the patient and reduces medical costs through earlier discharge from the hospital or by avoiding hospitalization altogether.

Earlier Hospital Discharge

When a hospitalized patient is receiving IV therapy and requires continued therapy, it is not always necessary or cost-effective to keep the patient in the hospital. If the patient is medically stable, he or she may no longer need the careful observation and daily nursing care provided by a hospital. By receiving IV therapy in an outpatient setting, the patient can be discharged earlier. Most patients, particularly children, are more comfortable in their home environment, which often contributes to faster healing. An example of this is a hospitalized patient with an infection who still needs IV antibiotic therapy, but no longer needs to be hospitalized, and receives the therapy at an infusion clinic.

Avoidance of Hospitalization

Outpatient IV therapy provides an alternative to patients with an acute or chronic illness that requires IV therapy.

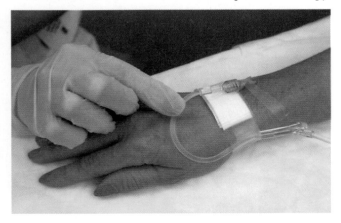

Figure 11-22. IV therapy. (From Potter PA, Perry AG: *Basic nursing: essentials for practice,* ed 5, St. Louis, 2002, Mosby.)

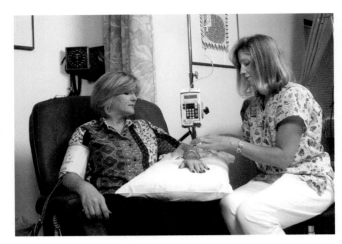

Figure 11-23. Patient receiving IV therapy in an outpatient setting. (Photo by Margaret Hartshorn: Courtesy of the Arizona Arthritis Center [www.arthritis.arizona.edu].)

Patients who do not require hospitalization for their condition are able to obtain their IV therapy in an outpatient setting. This allows patients the option of being able to continue their daily routine without major interruptions and provides them with more independence and control over their condition. An example of this is a patient with rheumatoid arthritis who needs IV infliximab (Remicade) therapy and receives that therapy at the rheumatology medical office.

Medical Office–Based Intravenous Therapy

Some medical offices provide outpatient IV therapy. Outpatient IV therapy may be provided in an oncology office for the administration of IV chemotherapy. With the advent of newer rheumatology medications that must be given intravenously, some rheumatology offices have started to provide this service. There are distinct advantages to medical office–based IV therapy. It allows the physician to provide closer monitoring of a patient's response to the IV therapy and any adverse reactions exhibited by the patient. These benefits have prompted more physicians to consider office-based IV therapy.

Based on the potential future growth of IV therapy in the medical office and the current growth of other IV outpatient settings, such as infusion clinics and the patient's home, there is a need for medical assistants to acquire some basic knowledge in IV therapy. The medical assistant is often responsible for scheduling IV therapy and providing the patient with IV therapy instructions, such as the length of time required for the therapy. In addition, patients may have questions that the medical assistant may need to answer (or refer to the proper individual for answering) regarding their outpatient IV therapy. The entry-level medical assistant should be familiar with the basic theory of outpatient IV therapy, which is presented here.

Advanced IV theory and initiating, maintaining, and discontinuing IV therapy are not entry-level medical assisting competencies and are not addressed in this text. Certain requirements must be met before the medical assistant can perform IV therapy in the medical office. The medical assistant first should check the laws of his or her state to determine whether it is legally permissible for the medical assistant to perform this procedure. The medical assistant must acquire the proper training (theory and skills) by completing a recognized IV therapy training program including supervised clinical practice. Although the IV procedure can appear simple when performed by an expert, it is a difficult skill that requires considerable practice to perfect.

Indications for Outpatient Intravenous Therapy

Outpatient IV therapy has been shown to be a safe and effective alternative to inpatient IV therapy for the treatment of certain conditions. Before prescribing outpatient IV therapy, the physician assesses the need for the therapy by determining whether the following criteria are met: The patient's condition warrants the use of IV therapy, no alternative routes are feasible or appropriate to deliver the therapy, and the patient does not need to be hospitalized to receive the IV therapy. After determining the need for outpatient IV therapy, the physician prescribes the appropriate medication or fluid and treatment plan, orders laboratory tests to monitor the patient's progress, and assesses the patient after the IV therapy.

Scheduling the IV Therapy

If the patient receives the IV therapy at an outpatient site other than the medical office (e.g., an infusion clinic), the medical assistant may be responsible for scheduling the necessary services and providing the patient with IV therapy instructions, such as the length of time required for the therapy, any dietary restrictions, whether to wear loose-fitting comfortable clothing, and whether someone needs to transport the patient to and from the appointment.

Medical Office Guidelines

Medical offices that provide IV therapy onsite usually set up a special room to deliver the therapy, which often includes a lounge chair to provide for patient comfort during the therapy. With office-based IV therapy, the entry-level medical assistant is responsible for scheduling the IV therapy and providing the patient with the IV therapy instructions listed previously. The medical office employs an IV practitioner, such as a nurse or specially trained medical assistant, to initiate, maintain, and discontinue the IV therapy. This practitioner must be completely familiar with all aspects of the IV therapy, including indications and uses, actions, dose and rate of infusion, incompatibilities, contraindications and precautions, antidote, and adverse effects. During the IV therapy, the practitioner must monitor carefully the patient's response to the therapy and be alert for adverse or allergic reactions. After the therapy is completed, the IV practitioner provides the patient with follow-up instructions, such as normal side effects that may occur when the patient returns home and any adverse reactions that need to be reported to the medical office.

Administration of IV Therapy

IV therapy may be administered in an outpatient setting for a variety of reasons. These include the following, which are discussed in more detail in the next section:

- Administration of IV medication
- Replacement of fluids and electrolytes
- Administration of nutritional supplements
- Administration of blood products
- Emergency administration of IV medication and fluids

Administration of Intravenous Medication

IV medication administration is the process of delivering medication directly into a patient's vein. The IV route provides a rapid and effective method for administering medication to a patient. It also provides more accurate dosing than other routes because the medication enters the body directly from the circulatory system. This allows the medication to bypass barriers to drug absorption, such as the digestive tract (from oral administration) or muscle tissue (from IM administration), which makes it easier to control the actual amount of drug delivered to the body.

Medication may have to be administered through the IV route, as opposed to other, less invasive, routes such as oral administration, for many reasons, including the following:

- A rapid systemic response to the medication is desired.
- Therapeutic blood levels of the medication need to be maintained.
- The medication is destroyed by stomach acids, digestive enzymes, or both.
- The medication cannot be absorbed into the body through the gastrointestinal tract.
- The medication is toxic and could damage the lining of the gastrointestinal tract.
- The medication is painful or irritating when given by other parenteral routes (IM or SC injection).

Intravenous Administration Methods

IV medication can be administered by three methods: direct IV injection, intermittent IV administration, and continuous IV administration.

Direct Intravenous Injection

The direct IV injection method (known as an *IV push*) involves the administration of the medication as a single dose into the vein over a short time, usually less than 10 minutes. It is usually administered through a vascular access device that is already in place. Medication administered through this method produces immediate and predictable results and is a good way to administer lifesaving medications in an emergency.

Intermittent Intravenous Administration

Intermittent IV administration is employed frequently in outpatient settings. It involves the administration of a medication over a specific amount of time (termed the *rate of infusion*) and at specified intervals. Before administering, the medication first must be diluted in a moderate amount of an IV fluid (25 to 250 ml). The amount and type of IV fluid are indicated in the drug insert accompanying the medication. The intermittent IV administration of ceftriaxone (Rocephin) (an antibiotic) requires that it first be reconstituted and then diluted in 50 to 100 ml of an IV fluid, such as sterile water or 0.9% sodium chloride.

The rate of infusion for administering an IV medication intermittently depends on the medication being administered and typically ranges from 15 minutes to several hours. This information also is specified in the drug insert accompanying the medication. The recommended rate for the intermittent infusion of ceftriaxone is 15 to 30 minutes. The recommended rate of infusion for IV infliximab is at least 2 hours.

The interval of time between doses is determined by the physician and depends on the medication being administered and the patient's condition. The physician may prescribe the following outpatient treatment plan for a patient with Lyme disease: IV ceftriaxone intermittently once a day for 14 days. In this instance, the interval of time between doses is 24 hours, or 1 day.

Continuous Intravenous Administration

Continuous IV administration, also known as an *IV drip,* is most often used in a hospital or home setting. It involves the infusion of medication over a continuous period of time (4 to 24 hours). Continuous IV administration is used to maintain a constant therapeutic blood level of the medication. The medication is diluted in a large quantity (250 to 1000 ml) of an IV fluid (Figure 11-24), such as 0.9% sodium chloride (normal saline) or 5% dextrose in water (D5W). Because of the time required for continuous administration, this method of administration is not generally used to administer IV medications in the medical office.

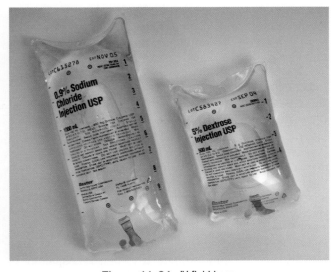

Figure 11-24. IV fluid bags.

Intravenous Medications Administered in an Outpatient Setting

Medications that are most commonly administered intravenously in an outpatient setting are listed next, along with the conditions each is used to treat.

Antibiotics

The physician may prescribe IV antibiotic therapy to treat a serious infection to prevent the infection from spreading and to avoid the development of serious complications. The IV route allows the antibiotic to achieve high blood concentrations quickly, permitting it to go to work on the infection immediately.

Examples of infections for which the physician may prescribe IV antibiotic therapy in an outpatient setting include osteomyelitis, cellulitis endocarditis, bacterial meningitis, Lyme disease, bacterial pneumonia, bacterial septicemia, pyelonephritis, pelvic inflammatory disease, AIDS-related infections, severe urinary tract infections, and nonhealing wound infections.

Chemotherapy

Chemotherapy is broadly defined as the use of chemicals to treat disease. More specifically, chemotherapy refers to the use of antineoplastic medications to treat different types of cancer. In most cases, chemotherapy works by interfering with the ability of the cancer cells to grow or reproduce. The IV route is commonly used to administer chemotherapy because most antineoplastic medications are toxic and irritating and must be delivered to the body through a vein. These types of medications cause pain and trauma to the tissues if administered by other parenteral routes (i.e., IM or SC).

IV chemotherapy may take only a few minutes to administer or several hours and may be given on a daily, weekly, or monthly basis. The frequency and length of the chemotherapy treatment depend on the type of cancer being treated, the medications that are being administered, and the patient's overall health and ability to tolerate the medications. IV chemotherapy is often administered in an outpatient setting, such as a medical oncology office or an infusion clinic.

Monoclonal Antibodies

One use of monoclonal antibodies is to treat inflammatory diseases; infliximab (Remicade) is a monoclonal antibody. Individuals with certain inflammatory disease have too much of a normally occurring protein (tumor necrosis factor [TNF]) in their bodies. TNF causes inflammation in the body, but in too large amounts, it attacks healthy tissues. Infliximab works by binding with TNF and blocking its action, reducing the inflammatory response of the body. In doing so, however, infliximab also lowers the ability of the body to fight infection.

IV infliximab therapy is often administered in an outpatient setting for treatment of the following conditions: Crohn's disease, rheumatoid arthritis, ulcerative colitis, ankylosing spondylitis, and psoriatic arthritis. Infliximab works to reduce the symptoms of the patient's condition and to initiate and maintain remission of the disorder. Infliximab has some undesirable side effects and is very expensive. Because of this, it is administered only when patients with these conditions have had an inadequate response to conventional therapy.

Analgesics

When a patient is not able to manage pain using oral pain medication, the physician may prescribe a narcotic pain medication administered through the IV route. Conditions for which the physician may prescribe IV analgesic therapy in an outpatient setting include migraine headaches, cancer-related pain, and the pain associated with AIDS conditions.

Some patients receive IV narcotic analgesics at home through the use of an ambulatory IV pump (Figure 11-25) that is controlled by the patient. This type of IV analgesic therapy is known as *patient-controlled analgesia* (PCA). When the patient experiences pain, he or she presses a button attached to the PCA pump. The PCA pump is programmed to deliver a predetermined dose of the narcotic analgesic intravenously to the patient to relieve the pain. The pump is preset to prevent overmedication, and it includes a locking device for security of the medication.

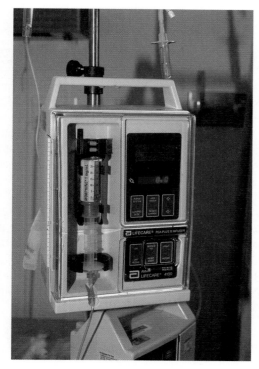

Figure 11-25. Patient-controlled anesthesia pump. (From Elkin MK, Perry AG, Potter PA: *Nursing interventions and clinical skills*, ed. 3, St. Louis, 2004, Mosby.)

Replacement of Fluids and Electrolytes

To remain healthy, the body must maintain an adequate fluid and electrolyte balance. This balance can be altered by a variety of conditions. Conditions that may cause a depletion of fluids and electrolytes include vomiting and diarrhea, excessive perspiration (from fever or hot weather), and starvation. If an individual experiences an excessive loss of fluids or electrolytes, they must be replaced as soon as possible to prevent dehydration. Infants and children are especially vulnerable to dehydration.

The best way to replace fluids and electrolytes is through oral consumption; however, this may not always be possible, such as when the patient is experiencing excessive vomiting. In these instances, IV fluid therapy may be prescribed. The physician determines the specific IV fluid and amount of fluid to treat the patient's condition using the following information:

- Patient's diagnosis (e.g., prolonged diarrhea)
- Other coexisting medical conditions
- Length of the current illness
- Patient's body size and weight
- Physician's findings from the physical examination
- Laboratory test results

Examples of IV fluids commonly used to replace fluids and electrolytes include 0.9% sodium chloride and Ringer's solution. IV fluids are administered by continuous administration in the following outpatient settings: urgent care centers, infusion clinics, and the patient's home. Because of the length of time required for continuous administration, the medical office does not typically administer IV fluids and electrolytes except in an emergency situation (see later).

Administration of Nutritional Supplements

IV therapy can be used to administer nutritional supplements to patients in an outpatient setting who are unable to eat or have conditions causing poor absorption of nutrients from the gastrointestinal tract. IV nutritional therapy provides the nutrients necessary for basic health maintenance and to promote healing. The IV route is used only when the patient has a condition that prevents other routes of administration, such as the oral or enteral routes. **Enteral nutrition** is the delivery of nutrients through a tube inserted into the gastrointestinal tract.

Examples of specific conditions that may require the IV administration of nutritional supplements include ulcerative colitis, Crohn's disease, short bowel syndrome, celiac disease, pancreatitis, esophageal cancer, AIDS-related malnutrition, and malnutrition related to an eating disorder. Parenteral IV nutrition is often administered in the following outpatient settings: infusion clinics and the patient's home.

Administration of Blood Products

Blood products can be administered to a patient in an outpatient setting. The most frequently administered blood products are discussed next.

Introduction to Electrocardiography

The **electrocardiograph** is an instrument used to record the electrical activity of the heart. The **electrocardiogram (ECG)** is the graphic representation of this activity. The ECG exhibits the amount of electrical activity produced by the heart and the time required for the impulse to travel through the heart.

Electrocardiography is used for the following purposes:

- To detect an abnormal cardiac rhythm (**dysrhythmia**)
- To help diagnose damage to the heart caused by a myocardial infarction
- To assess the effect on the heart of digitalis or other cardiac drugs
- To determine the presence of electrolyte disturbances
- To assess the progress of rheumatic fever
- To determine the presence of hypertrophy of the heart chambers
- Performed before surgery to assess cardiac risk during surgery

An ECG cannot detect all cardiovascular disorders. In addition, it cannot always detect impending heart disease. The ECG is generally used in combination with other diagnostic and laboratory tests to assess cardiac functioning.

The medical assistant is frequently responsible for recording ECGs in the medical office. Because of this, knowledge and skill must be acquired in the following aspects of electrocardiography: preparation of the patient, operation of the electrocardiograph, identification and elimination of artifacts, labeling the completed ECG, and care and maintenance of the electrocardiograph.

Electrocardiographs are available in single-channel and three-channel recording formats. Because most medical offices use a three-channel ECG, the information in this chapter focuses on the three-channel electrocardiograph (Figure 12-1).

STRUCTURE OF THE HEART

The human heart consists of four chambers: The right and left atria are the upper chambers, and the right and left ventricles are the lower chambers (Figure 12-2). Blood enters the right atrium from two large veins, the superior vena cava and the inferior vena cava, which bring it back from its circulation through the body. The blood entering the right atrium is deoxygenated, meaning it contains very little oxygen and is high in carbon dioxide.

From the right atrium, the blood enters the right ventricle. It is pumped from here to the lungs via the pulmonary artery. It picks up oxygen in the lungs in exchange for carbon dioxide and returns to the left atrium of the heart via the pulmonary veins. From the left atrium, the blood enters the left ventricle. This is the most powerful chamber of the heart and serves to pump blood to the entire body. Blood exits from the left ventricle via the aorta, which distributes it to all parts of the body to nourish the tissues with oxygen and nutrients.

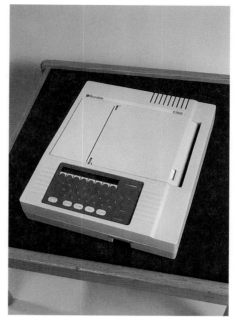

Figure 12-1. A three-channel electrocardiograph.

CONDUCTION SYSTEM OF THE HEART

The *sinoatrial (SA) node* is located in the upper portion of the right atrium, just below the opening of the superior vena cava. It consists of a knot of modified myocardial cells that have the ability to send out an electrical impulse without an external nerve stimulus. In this way, the SA node initiates and regulates the heartbeat.

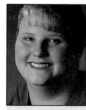

Putting It All into Practice

My Name is Janet Canterbury, and I work in the medical laboratory of an internal medicine office. I also run electrocardiograms, hook up and read Holter monitors, and perform pulmonary function tests and assist with cardiac stress testing.

One of my most rewarding experiences was when a young woman came into the office with severe chest pains. I immediately helped her back to an examining room. I ran an electrocardiogram as ordered by the physician. After the physician read the electrocardiogram, he indicated the results did not look good and that the patient would have to be transported to the hospital. I went into the patient's room to comfort her. She asked me if she was going to have to go to the hospital. I replied, "Possibly." She immediately said, "No!" Then I began to explain to her how important it was to have more tests to make sure she would be allright. She finally agreed to go. After being taken to the hospital by an ambulance, she was later transferred to another hospital for a heart catheterization. A few weeks passed, and she came into the office. She hugged me and thanked me for possibly saving her life. It felt so good that I could help make a difference in a patient's life. ∎

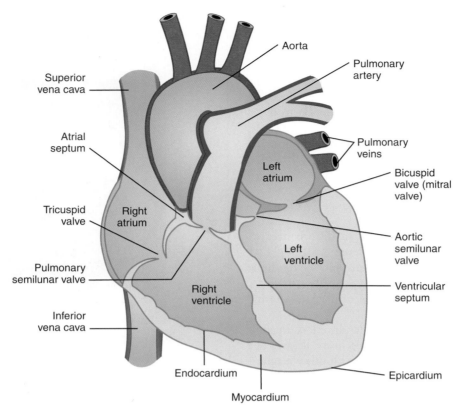

Figure 12-2. Diagram of the heart.

Each electrical impulse discharged by the SA node is distributed to the right and left atria and causes them to contract. This contraction forces blood through the open cuspid valves and into the ventricles. The impulse is picked up by the *atrioventricular (AV) node,* another knot of modified myocardial cells located at the base of the right atrium. The AV node delays the impulse momentarily to give the ventricles a chance to fill with blood from the atria. The AV node then transmits the electrical impulse to the *bundle of His.* The bundle of His divides into right and left branches known as the *bundle branches,* which relay the impulse to the *Purkinje fibers.* The Purkinje fibers distribute the impulse evenly to the right and left ventricles, causing them to contract; this forces blood out of the ventricles and into the pulmonary artery and aorta. The entire heart relaxes momentarily. The SA node initiates a new impulse, and the cycle repeats (Figure 12-3).

CARDIAC CYCLE

The **cardiac cycle** represents one complete heartbeat. It consists of the contraction of the atria, the contraction of the ventricles, and the relaxation of the entire heart (as described previously). The electrocardiograph records the electrical activity that causes these events in the cardiac cycle. The **ECG cycle** is the graphic representation of the cardiac cycle (Figure 12-4).

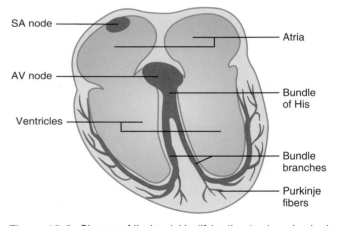

Figure 12-3. Diagram of the heart, identifying the structures involved with the conduction of an electrical impulse through the heart.

Waves

The normal ECG cycle consists of a P wave; the Q, R, and S waves (known as the *QRS complex*); and a T wave. The ECG cycle is recorded from left to right, beginning with the P wave.

P wave   The P wave represents the electrical activity associated with the contraction of the atria, or *atrial depolarization.*

QRS complex   The QRS complex represents the electrical activity associated with the contraction of the ventricles,

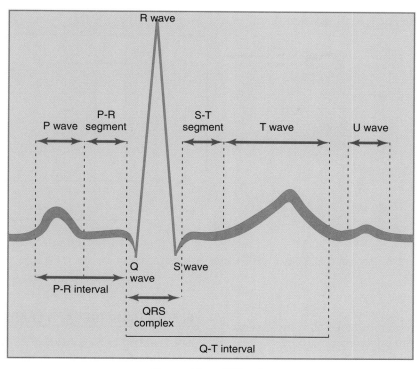

Figure 12-4. ECG cycle.

or *ventricular depolarization,* and consists of the Q wave, the R wave, and the S wave.

T wave   The T wave represents the electrical recovery of the ventricles, or *ventricular repolarization.* The muscle cells are recovering in preparation for another impulse.

U wave   Occasionally, a U wave follows a T wave. It is a small wave that is associated in some as yet undefined way with repolarization.

Baseline, Segments, and Intervals

The flat, horizontal line that separates the various waves is known as the **baseline.** The waves deflect either upward (positive deflection) or downward (negative deflection) from the baseline. The baseline is divided into segments and intervals for the purpose of interpretation and analysis of the ECG by the physician. A **segment** is the portion of the ECG between two waves, and an **interval** is the length of a wave or the length of a wave with a segment.

Segments:

P-R segment   The P-R segment represents the time interval from the end of the atrial depolarization to the beginning of the ventricular depolarization. It is the time needed for the impulse to be delayed at the AV node and then travel through the bundle of His and Purkinje fibers to the ventricles.

S-T segment   The S-T segment represents the time interval from the end of the ventricular depolarization to the beginning of repolarization of the ventricles.

Intervals:

P-R interval   The P-R interval represents the time interval from the beginning of the atrial depolarization to the beginning of the ventricular depolarization.

Q-T interval   The Q-T interval is the time interval from the beginning of the ventricular depolarization to the end of repolarization of the ventricles.

Baseline   The baseline after the T wave (or U wave, if present) represents the period when the entire heart returns to its resting, or polarized, state.

ELECTROCARDIOGRAPH PAPER

Electrocardiograph paper is divided into two sets of squares for accurate and convenient measurement of the waves, intervals, and segments (Figure 12-5). Each small square is 1 mm high and 1 mm wide. Each large square (made up of 25 small squares) is 5 mm high and 5 mm wide. By measuring the various waves, intervals, and segments of the graph cycle, the physician is able to determine whether the electrical activity of the heart falls within normal limits.

Electrocardiograph paper consists of a black or blue base with a white plastic coating. A black or red graph is printed on top of the plastic coating. A heated stylus moves over the heat-sensitive paper and melts away the plastic coating, resulting in the recording of the ECG cycles. In addition to being heat-sensitive, the paper is pressure-sensitive and should be handled carefully to avoid making impressions that would interfere with the proper reading of the ECG.

STANDARDIZATION OF THE ELECTROCARDIOGRAPH

The electrocardiograph machine must be standardized when recording an ECG. This is a quality control measure that ensures an accurate and reliable recording. It means

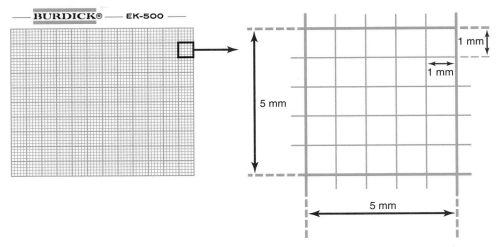

Figure 12-5. Diagram of ECG paper with a section enlarged to indicate the size of the large and small squares.

that an ECG run on one electrocardiograph compares inaccuracy with a recording run on another machine.

By international agreement, 1 millivolt (mV) of electricity should cause the stylus to move 10 mm high in **amplitude** (10 small squares). A three-channel electrocardiograph automatically records standardization marks on the tracing. During the recording, the machine allows 1 mV to enter the electrocardiograph machine, which should result in an upward deflection of 10 mm. The marking on the ECG paper is known as the *standardization mark* (Figure 12-6). The width of the mark made by the machine is approximately 2 mm (two small squares). If the standardization mark is more or less than 10 mm in amplitude, it can be adjusted. The manufacturer's operating manual must be consulted for proper adjustment information. An electrocardiograph must never be adjusted without use of the operating manual.

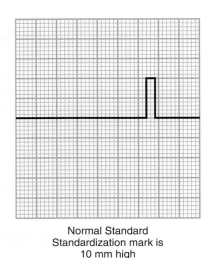

Normal Standard
Standardization mark is
10 mm high

Figure 12-6. Standardization mark.

ELECTROCARDIOGRAPH LEADS

The standard ECG consists of 12 leads. Each lead provides an electrical "photograph" of the heart's activity from a different angle. Together, the 12 leads, or "photographs," facilitate a thorough interpretation of the heart's activity.

The electrical impulses given off by the heart are picked up by **electrodes** and conducted into the machine through lead wires. Electrodes are composed of a substance that is a good conductor of electricity. The impulses given off by the heart are very small. To produce a readable ECG, they must be made larger, or amplified, by a device known as an *amplifier,* located within the electrocardiograph. The amplified voltages are changed into mechanical motion by the *galvanometer* and recorded on the electrocardiograph paper by a heated stylus (Figure 12-7).

There are four limb electrodes: the right arm electrode (RA), the left arm electrode (LA), the right leg electrode (RL), and the left leg electrode (LL). The right leg electrode is known as the *ground.* It is not used for the actual recording, but serves as an electrical reference point. The chest leads are abbreviated V or C and use six chest electrodes.

Disposable electrodes are typically used with a three-channel electrocardiograph. A disposable electrode consists of a self-adhesive tab that contains an electrolyte. An **electrolyte** is a substance that facilitates the transmission of the heart's electrical impulse. The electrode is applied to the skin and held in place with its adhesive backing; it is thrown away after use.

Bipolar Leads

The first three leads of the 12-lead ECG are the bipolar leads; they are leads I, II, and III. The bipolar leads use two of the limb electrodes to record the heart's electrical activity. Lead I records the heart's voltage difference between the right arm and the left arm, lead II records the difference between the right arm and the left leg, and lead III records the difference between the left arm and the left leg (Figure 12-8).

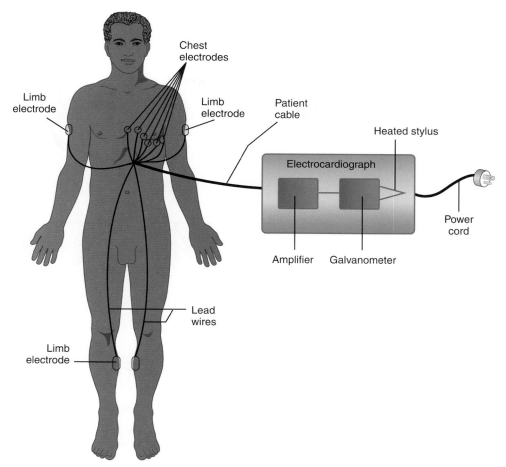

Figure 12-7. Diagram of the basic components of the electrocardiograph. The limb electrodes are attached to the fleshy parts of the limbs, and the lead wires are arranged to follow body contour. The patient cable is not dangling, and the power cord points away from the electrocardiograph.

Lead II shows the heart's rhythm more clearly than the other leads. Because of this, the physician often requests a *rhythm strip,* which is a longer recording (approximately 12 inches) of lead II.

Augmented Leads

The next three leads are the augmented leads: aVR (augmented voltage—right arm), aVL (augmented voltage—left arm), and aVF (augmented voltage—left leg or foot). Lead aVR records the heart's voltage difference between the right arm electrode and a central point between the left arm and left leg. Lead aVL records the heart's voltage difference between the left arm electrode and a central point between the right arm and left leg. Lead aVF records the heart's voltage difference between the left leg electrode and a central point between the right and left arms. Leads I, II, III, aVR, aVL, and aVF record the voltage from side to side and from the top to the bottom of the heart (see Figure 12-8).

What Would You Do? | What Would You *Not* Do?

Case Study 1

Camilla Rossi is 22 years old and works at a waffle house during the day and goes to business school at night. She comes to the office because she has been experiencing some heart problems. Over the past month, she has had three episodes of tachycardia, palpitations, trouble breathing, and profuse sweating. She is really scared that she has heart disease. Her beloved grandfather just died from a heart attack, and she is afraid she will die next.

The physician orders an ECG, but Camilla is reluctant to have the procedure. She is embarrassed about having to take her top off, and she is worried that she will get shocked by all the wires coming out of the machine. She says that she does not have health insurance, and she does not know how she would pay for such a fancy test. She wants to know whether there is a cheaper way to find out what is wrong with her. ∎

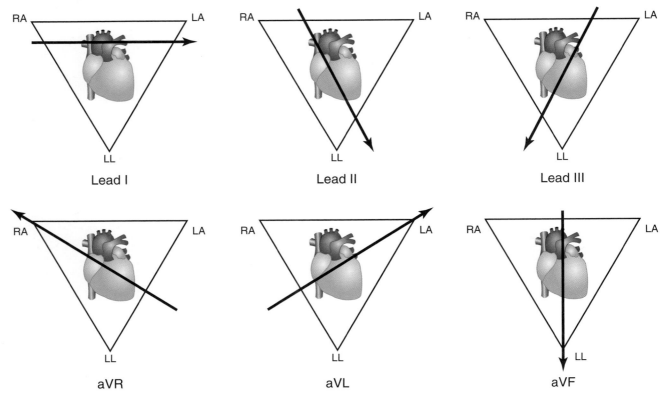

Figure 12-8. Diagram of the heart's voltage for leads I, II, III, aVR, aVL, and aVF.

Highlight on Stress Testing

Description
Exercise tolerance testing, also called *stress testing,* is a diagnostic procedure used to evaluate the cardiovascular system. It is usually performed in a hospital under the direction of a cardiologist and an exercise tolerance technician so that emergency equipment and trained personnel are available to deal with unusual situations that might arise.

Purpose
The purpose of exercise tolerance testing is as follows:
1. To diagnose ischemic heart disease that cannot be detected by a standard resting electrocardiogram. Ischemic heart disease is heart disease that occurs as a result of inadequate blood supply to the myocardium, as in a myocardial infarction and angina pectoris.
2. To assist in evaluating the cause of cardiac symptoms, such as chest discomfort and dysrhythmias.
3. To assess the effectiveness of cardiac drug therapy.
4. To follow the course of rehabilitation after a myocardial infarction or a cardiac surgical procedure, such as a coronary bypass operation or a coronary stent placement.
5. To determine an individual's fitness for a strenuous exercise program, such as jogging.

How the Test Works
Exercise tolerance testing involves the continuous electrocardiographic monitoring of an individual during physical exercise. The patient's blood pressure, heart rate, and physical symptoms also are monitored during the test. The tolerance testing is accomplished by having the patient use a treadmill. The intensity of the physical exertion is increased gradually until the patient's target heart rate is reached, unless the signs and symptoms of cardiac ischemia appear, in which case the test is stopped. These symptoms include claudication (severe leg pain), severe dyspnea, chest discomfort or pain, pallor, and dizziness.

Interpretation of Results
The patient's response to the exercise tolerance testing is used to determine normal or abnormal results. A normal response is a gradual increase in the patient's blood pressure as the physical exertion increases, whereas an abnormal response is a sudden increase or decrease of the patient's blood pressure. The electrocardiogram of a normal individual exhibits a shortened P-R interval and a compressed QRS complex. An abnormal tracing indicative of myocardial ischemia results in a depressed S-T segment and an inverted T wave. An abnormal exercise tolerance test usually warrants further testing, such as a coronary angiogram. ■

Chest Leads

The last six leads are the chest, or precordial, leads: V_1, V_2, V_3, V_4, V_5, and V_6. These leads record the heart's voltage from front to back. The voltage is recorded from a central point "inside" the heart to a point on the chest wall where the electrode is placed. These points correspond to the chest leads. Figure 12-9 shows the proper location of the six chest leads. To ensure an accurate and reliable recording, the medical assistant must be able to locate them accurately. When first learning to locate the chest leads, it helps to mark their location on the patient's chest with a felt-tipped pen.

Normally, the ECG is recorded with the paper moving at a speed of 25 mm/sec. Occasionally, the ECG cycles are close together, making the recording difficult to read. The medical assistant can change the paper speed to 50 mm/sec to spread out the cycles. To alert the physician to the change, the medical assistant must make a notation of it on the recording.

MAINTENANCE OF THE ELECTROCARDIOGRAPH

Electrocardiographs require very little maintenance. The casing of the electrocardiograph should be cleaned frequently with a soft cloth, slightly dampened with a mild detergent, to remove dust and dirt. Commercial solvents and abrasives should not be used because they can damage the finish of the casing. The patient cables, lead wires, and power cord should be cleaned periodically with a cloth

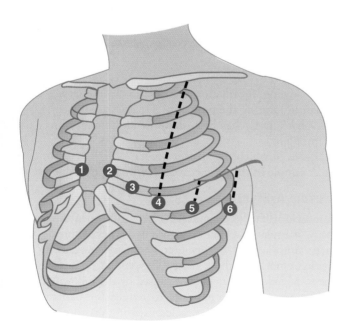

Figure 12-9. Recommended positions for ECG chest leads:
1. V_1, fourth intercostal space at right margin of sternum
2. V_2, fourth intercostal space at left margin of sternum
3. V_3, midway between positions 2 and 4
4. V_4, fifth intercostal space at junction of left midclavicular line
5. V_5, at horizontal level of position 4 at left anterior axillary line
6. V_6, at horizontal level of position 4 at left midaxillary line

moistened with a disinfectant cleaner. The cables should never be immersed in the cleaning solution because this could damage them.

ELECTROCARDIOGRAPHIC CAPABILITIES

Electrocardiographs have a variety of capabilities that permit specific recording options.

Three-Channel Recording Capability

An electrocardiograph with a three-channel recording capability can record electrical activity through three leads simultaneously. This is in contrast to a single-channel electrocardiograph, which records only one lead at a time. The advantage of a three-channel electrocardiograph is that an ECG can be produced in less time than would be required if each lead were recorded separately.

The leads that are recorded simultaneously are leads I, II, and III; followed by aVR, aVL, and aVF; followed by V_1, V_2, and V_3; followed by V_4, V_5, and V_6. Recording three leads at one time requires three-channel recording paper, which is designed in a standard $8\frac{1}{2} \times 11$-inch format. This size of the printout fits easily into the patient's chart. Most three-channel electrocardiographs have a *copy capability* that quickly produces an accurate tracing of the last ECG recorded. Figure 12-10 is an example of a three-channel ECG recording that also includes a rhythm strip. Procedure 12-1 describes how to run a 12-lead three-channel ECG.

Teletransmission

An electrocardiograph with teletransmission capabilities can transmit a recording performed at the medical office over the telephone line to an ECG data interpretation site. The recording is interpreted by a cardiologist (often along with a computer analysis) at the ECG site, and a printout of the recording along with the interpretation is electronically transmitted to the sending office the same day. Patient information (e.g., age, sex, height, weight, medications) must be relayed to the ECG site to assist in the interpretation. This information is entered into the electrocardiograph by the medical assistant (using a keyboard) and transmitted automatically with the ECG recording.

Interpretive Electrocardiograph

An electrocardiograph with interpretive capabilities has a built-in computer program that analyzes the recording as it is being run. Interpretive electrocardiographs provide immediate information on the heart's activity, leading to earlier diagnosis and treatment. Patient data are used in the interpretation of the ECG and must be entered into the electrocardiograph using a keyboard before running the recording. The data generally required are the patient's age, sex, height, weight, and medications. The computer analysis of the ECG is printed at the top of the recording, along with the reason for each interpretation (Figure 12-11). The results are reviewed and interpreted further by the physician before a diagnosis is made and treatment is initiated.

Name JANE DOE
ID 12346
34YR Female

13:57 11/22/03
Vent   Durations   Axes
Rate PR QRS QT/QTC   P--QRS--T
 71   188 68 400/423   42 31 71

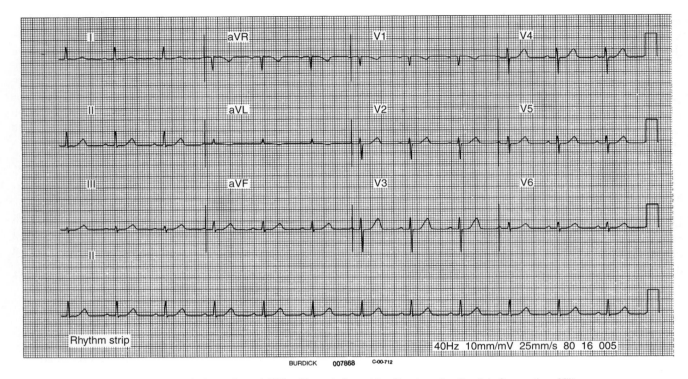

Figure 12-10. A three-channel ECG with a rhythm strip. (Courtesy the Burdick Corporation, Milton, Wisc.)

ARTIFACTS

The medical assistant is responsible for producing a clear and concise ECG recording that can be read and interpreted easily by the physician. Structures sometimes appear in the recording that are not natural and interfere with the normal appearance of the ECG cycles. They are known as **artifacts** and represent additional electrical activity that is picked up by the electrocardiograph. The medical assistant should be able to identify artifacts and correct them. There are several types of artifacts; the most common are muscle, wandering baseline, and alternating current (AC) (Figure 12-12).

In some circumstances, as when individuals have trouble holding still or in buildings with older electrical systems, normal methods to eliminate muscle and AC artifacts may be unsuccessful. Electrocardiographs have an artifact filter that can reduce artifacts when all else fails. Because the *artifact filter* also affects the diagnostic accuracy of the ECG, it should be used as little as possible.

If the medical assistant is unable to correct an artifact, the physician should be consulted. It is possible that the machine is broken. If an electrocardiograph service technician has to be contacted, the medical assistant should have the following information available to aid the service technician in locating the problem:

1. What already has been done to locate and correct the problem
2. Leads in which the artifact occurs
3. A sample of the artifact recorded by the machine

Muscle Artifact

A muscle artifact (see Figure 12-12A) can be identified by its fuzzy, irregular baseline. There are two types of muscle artifacts: those caused by involuntary muscle movement (somatic tremor) and those caused by voluntary muscle movement. Muscle artifacts may be caused by the following:

1. **An apprehensive patient.** To reduce the patient's apprehension and relax muscles, explain the procedure and reassure the patient that having an ECG recorded is a painless procedure.
2. **Patient discomfort.** Ensure that the table is wide enough to support the patient's arms and legs adequately. The patient can be made more comfortable by placing a pillow under his or her head. Check that the room temperature is comfortable for the patient. A temperature

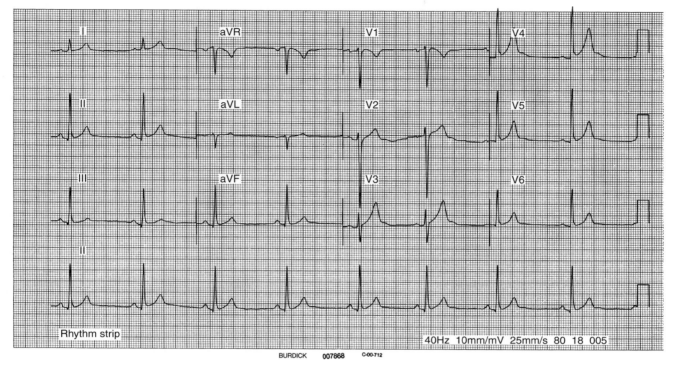

Name JOHN DOE   SINUS BRADYCARDIA
ID 12345   POSSIBLE LEFT VENTRICULAR HYPERTROPHY [VOLTAGE CRITERIA PLUS LAE OR QRS WIDENING]
36YR Male   ABNORMAL ECG

14:04 11/22/03
Vent   Durations   Axes
Rate PR QRS QT/QTC   P--QRS--T
 48 176 100 428/396   77 75 51

Figure 12-11. An ECG recording with a rhythm strip that has been analyzed by an interpretive electrocardiograph. The computer analysis is printed at the top of the recording, along with the reason for each interpretation. (Courtesy the Burdick Corporation, Milton, Wisc.)

that is warm enough for the medical assistant may be too cold for the patient who has removed clothing. This could result in shivering, which also would produce a muscle artifact on the ECG.

3. **Patient movement.** The patient must be instructed to lie still and not talk during the recording.

4. **A physical condition.** Several nervous system disorders, such as Parkinson's disease, prevent relaxation, and the patient trembles continually. The medical assistant must be understanding and try to record while the tremor is at a minimum.

Wandering Baseline Artifact

A wandering baseline artifact (see Figure 12-12B) can be caused by the following:

1. **Loose electrodes.** The medical assistant should ensure that the disposable adhesive electrodes are attached firmly to the patient's skin. If an electrode pulls loose, it can be reattached with hypoallergenic tape or replaced with a new electrode. The alligator clips should be attached firmly to the electrodes. To prevent pulling or

twisting of the patient cable, it should be well supported on the table or the patient's abdomen and not be allowed to dangle.

2. **Body creams, oils, or lotions** on the skin in the area where the electrode is applied. The medical assistant should remove these by rubbing with alcohol, using friction.

Alternating Current Artifact

AC artifacts (see Figure 12-12C) are caused by electrical interference. Alternating electric current can "leak" or spread out from the power used by electrical appliances in the room in which the ECG is being run. This current may be picked up by the patient and carried into the electrocardiograph, where it would show up on the ECG recording as an AC artifact. An AC artifact appears as small, straight, spiked lines that are consistent. AC artifacts can be caused by the following:

1. **Lead wires not following body contour.** Dangling lead wires can pick up AC. Arrange the wires to follow body contour and to lie flat.

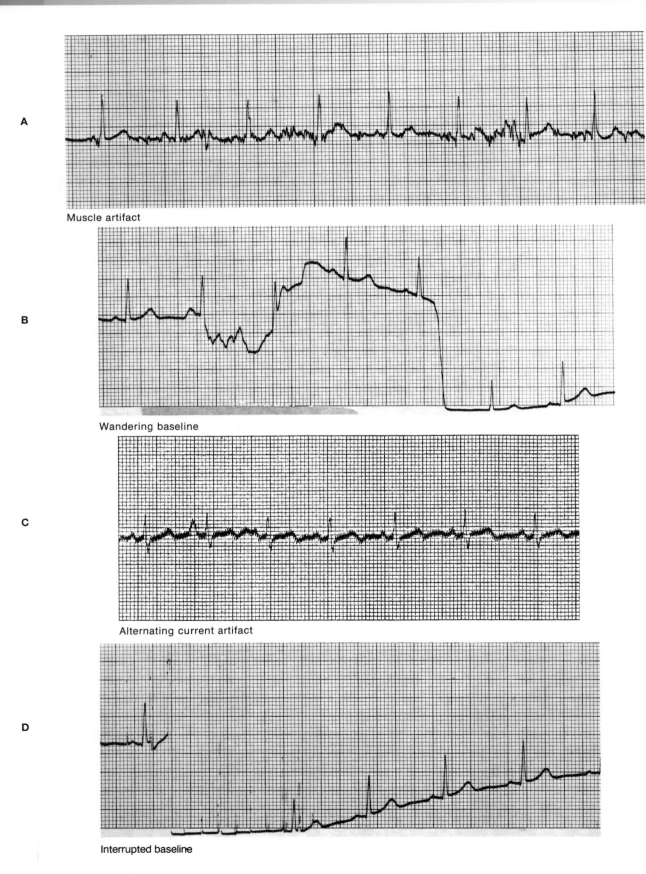

A

Muscle artifact

B

Wandering baseline

C

Alternating current artifact

D

Interrupted baseline

Figure 12-12. **A-D,** Examples of ECG artifacts. (Courtesy the Burdick Corporation, Milton, Wisc.)

2. **Other electrical equipment in the room.** Lamps, autoclaves, electrically powered examining tables, or other electrical equipment that is plugged in may be leaking AC. Unplug all nearby electrical equipment.
3. **Wiring in the walls, ceilings, or floors.** Try moving the patient table away from the walls.
4. **Improper grounding of the electrocardiograph.** The machine is automatically grounded when it is plugged in. Ensure that the plug is securely in the wall outlet. The right leg electrode is not used for recording the leads, but it picks up AC that has "leaked" onto the patient and carries it into the electrocardiograph. The AC is carried away by the machine's grounding system.

Interrupted Baseline Artifact

Occasionally, an interrupted baseline (see Figure 12-12D) occurs that may be caused by the metal tip of a lead wire becoming detached or by a broken patient cable. If the latter is the case, a new patient cable should be ordered from the manufacturer.

Text continued on p. 507

PROCEDURE **12-1**   Running a 12-Lead, Three-Channel Electrocardiogram

Outcome Record a 12-lead electrocardiogram.

Equipment/Supplies

- Three-channel electrocardiograph
- Disposable electrodes
- ECG paper

1. **Procedural Step.** Work in a quiet, relaxing atmosphere away from sources of electrical interference.
2. **Procedural Step.** Sanitize your hands, and assemble the equipment. Greet the patient and introduce yourself. Identify the patient by full name and date of birth.
3. **Procedural Step.** Help the patient relax by explaining the procedure. Tell the patient that having an ECG recording is painless. Explain that he or she must lie still and not talk while the ECG is being recorded so that an accurate ECG can be obtained.
   Principle. Explaining the procedure helps reassure apprehensive patients. The patient should be mentally and physically relaxed for an accurate ECG recording; an apprehensive or moving patient produces muscle artifacts.
4. **Procedural Step.** Prepare the patient. Ask him or her to remove clothing from the waist up. The lower legs also must be uncovered. Assist the patient into a supine position on the table. The table should support the arms and legs adequately so that they do not dangle. Properly drape the patient to prevent exposure and to provide warmth. A pillow can be used to support the patient's head.
   Principle. The chest, upper arms, and lower legs must be uncovered to allow proper placement of the electrodes. The patient should be kept warm, and the arms and legs should not be allowed to dangle; otherwise, muscle artifacts could result.
5. **Procedural Step.** Position the electrocardiograph so that the power cord points away from the patient and does not pass under the table. It is usually easier for the medical assistant to work on the left side of the patient.

Principle. Proper positioning of the electrocardiograph reduces AC artifacts.

6. **Procedural Step.** Prepare the patient's skin for application of the disposable electrodes. If the patient has oily skin or has used lotion, wipe the area to which the electrode will be applied with alcohol, and allow it to dry. If the patient's chest is hairy, dry shave it at each electrode site before applying the electrode.
   Principle. The patient's skin must be dry and free of oil and body hair so that the adhesive backing of the electrodes sticks to the patient's skin and stays on during the procedure.
7. **Procedural Step.** Apply limb electrodes. Firmly apply the adhesive backing of the electrodes to the fleshy part of each of the four limbs (upper arms and lower legs). The tabs of the arm electrodes should point downward, and the tabs of the leg electrodes should point upward. The adhesive backing of the electrode allows it to adhere firmly to the patient's skin.

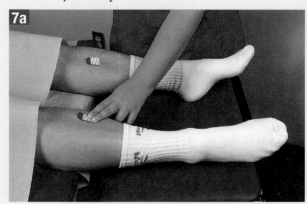

Apply the leg electrodes.

Continued

PROCEDURE 12-1   Running a 12-Lead, Three-Channel Electrocardiogram—cont'd

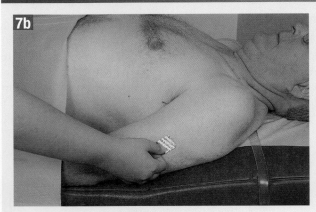

Apply the arm electrodes.

Principle. The tab of the electrodes should be positioned toward the cable to provide a more stable connection when the lead wire is attached to the electrode and to prevent the lead wires from pulling and causing artifacts.

8. Procedural Step. Apply the chest electrodes. Properly locate each chest position, and apply the electrode with the tab pointing downward. Continue until all six of the chest electrodes have been applied.

Principle. Positioning the tabs of the electrodes downward prevents the lead wires from pulling and causing artifacts.

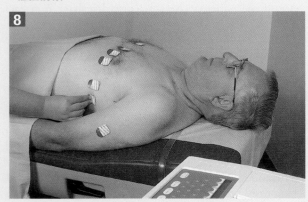

Apply the chest electrodes.

9. Procedural Step. Connect the lead wires to the electrodes. This is accomplished by inserting an alligator clip onto the metal tip of each electrode. The alligator clip is attached to the tab of each electrode. The ends of the lead wires are usually color-coded and identified with abbreviations to help the medical assistant connect the proper lead to each electrode. Arrange the lead wires to follow body contour.

Principle. Arranging the lead wires to follow body contour reduces the possibility of AC artifacts.

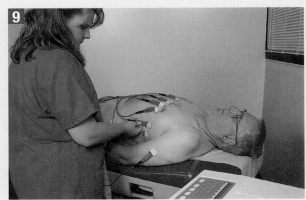

Connect the lead wires to the electrodes.

10. Procedural Step. Plug the patient cable into the machine. The cable should be supported on the table or on the patient's abdomen to prevent pulling or twisting.

11. Procedural Step. Turn on the electrocardiograph. Enter patient data using the soft-touch keypad. Always use your fingertips to enter the data. Pencils or other sharp objects can damage the keyboard. As the data are entered, they are displayed on the LCD screen. The patient data to be entered generally include the patient's name, a patient identification number, age, sex, height, weight, and medications.

Principle. The patient data and the date and time of the recording are printed at the top of the recording. If the electrocardiograph is equipped with interpretive capabilities, this information also is used in the computer-assisted interpretation of the ECG.

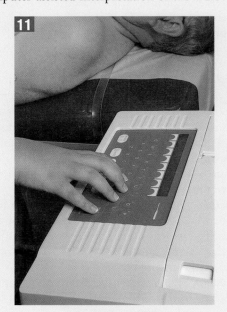

Enter patient data.

12. Procedural Step. Remind the patient to lie still and not to talk. Press the AUTO (automatic) button, and run the recording. The machine automatically inserts a standardization mark at the beginning of the recording, followed by the recording of the 12-lead ECG in a three-channel format.

13. Procedural Step. After the ECG has been recorded:
a. Check the printout to ensure the standardization mark is 10 mm high. If it is more or less than 10 mm, adjust the standardization mark according to the manufacturer's instructions, and run another ECG.

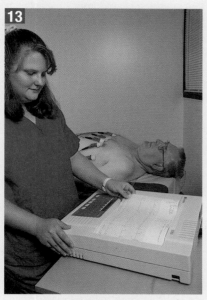
Check the standardization mark.

b. Check the direction of the R wave in Lead 1. If your patient's limb leads are attached correctly, the R wave on Lead 1 should have a positive deflection. If it has a negative deflection, the limb leads are not attached correctly. Reattach the limb leads properly and run another recording.
c. Observe the recording for artifacts. If an artifact is present, determine the cause of the artifact, correct the problem, and run another ECG.

14. Procedural Step. Inform the patient that you are finished and he or she can now talk or move. Turn the machine off. Disconnect the lead wires. Remove and discard the electrodes.

15. Procedural Step. Assist the patient in stepping down from the table.

16. Procedural Step. Sanitize your hands. Chart the procedure. Include the date and time and the name of the procedure (12-lead ECG). Place the recording in the patient's medical record, and put the record in the appropriate place to be reviewed by the physician.

17. Procedural Step. Return all equipment to its proper storage place.

CHARTING EXAMPLE

Date	
6/12/08	10:30 a.m. Completed a 12-lead ECG.
	Recording to physician for review.
	J. Canterbury, CMA

PROCEDURE 12-1

HOLTER MONITOR ELECTROCARDIOGRAPHY

A Holter monitor is a portable ambulatory monitoring system for recording the cardiac activity of a patient for 24 hours. The system is designed so that the patient is able to maintain his or her usual daily activities with minimal inconvenience while being monitored. Holter monitor electrocardiography is an important noninvasive procedure used to diagnose cardiac rhythm and conduction abnormalities. Specifically, it is most frequently used to evaluate patients with unexplained syncope, to discover intermittent cardiac dysrhythmias not picked up on a routine 12-lead ECG, to assess the effectiveness of antidysrhythmic medications (e.g., digitalis and antianginal medications), and to assess the effectiveness of an artificial pacemaker.

The Holter monitor consists of electrodes placed on the patient's chest and a special portable recorder that continually monitors the heart's activity. The portable recording device is available in two formats: a magnetic tape recorder that uses a cassette tape to record the heart's activity (Figure 12-13), and a newer computerized digital recorder that uses a compact flash memory card to document the heart's activity.

The lightweight, battery-powered recorder is held in a protective case, which is worn on a belt around the patient's waist or hung over the patient's shoulder by a strap. Throughout the 24-hour period, the system continuously records the patient's heartbeat on a magnetic cassette tape or the compact flash memory card.

Some physicians have Holter monitors in their medical offices. The medical assistant is responsible for preparing the patient, applying and removing the monitor, and instructing the patient for the procedure (see the box *Holter Monitor Patient Guidelines*).

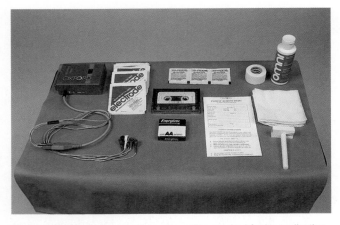

Figure 12-13. Holter monitor and supplies required for its application.

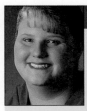

Memories *from* Externship

Janet Canterbury: During my externship, I was at an office where electrocardiograms were one of the many procedures that were performed. For my first electrocardiogram, the patient was a man who had a lot of hair on his chest, and I would need to shave the electrode placement sites on his chest. I was very nervous, but the procedure went well. When the electrocardiogram was run, he told me that I did a wonderful job and that it did not hurt at all to have his chest shaved. I realized then that it was not so bad after all. That patient made me feel so good about what I do and helped me feel confident in the procedures I had ahead of me. ■

Holter Monitor Patient Guidelines

The following guidelines must be relayed to the patient to ensure an accurate and reliable electrocardiographic recording.

1. Keep the electrodes and monitor dry to ensure an accurate recording and prevent damage to the recorder. Do not shower, bathe, or swim while wearing the monitor.
2. Do not touch or move the electrodes during the monitoring period to prevent artifacts from appearing in the recording.
3. Do not handle the monitor or take it out of its carrying case.
4. Depress the event marker only momentarily when a significant symptom or event occurs. Try not to overuse the event marker; overuse of the marker can cause masking of the ECG signals that are being relayed from the electrodes.
5. Do not use an electric blanket while wearing the monitor.
6. Record your activities in the diary. With each entry, note the time that the activity occurred. The following activities should be recorded:
   - Physical exercise
   - Walking up or down stairs
   - Smoking
   - Bowel movements
   - Meals (including alcohol and caffeinated beverages)
   - Sexual intercourse
   - Medications consumed
   - Sleep periods
7. Record emotional states (e.g., relaxed, anger, excitement) and physical symptoms (e.g., chest pain, nausea, dizziness) experienced during each activity. ■

Electrode Placement

A special type of electrode is used with the Holter monitor. It consists of a plastic disposable electrode plate with an adhesive backing and a central sponge pad that contains an electrolyte gel (Figure 12-14). This type of electrode is disposable and must be discarded after use.

Holter monitors used in the medical office are typically dual-channel systems, which means that two leads are recorded at one time. A dual-channel monitor requires five electrodes, one of which is the ground electrode. Some dual-channel monitors have the ground built into the monitor, in which case only four electrodes are required. The electrodes must be properly placed to ensure an accurate recording. Figure 12-15 shows the electrode positions

for the dual-channel Holter monitor. When one is learning to place these leads, it may help to mark their location on the patient's chest with a felt-tipped pen.

The monitor's effectiveness should be checked after hooking up the patient to ensure that a clear signal is being relayed from the electrodes to the recorder. This check is performed by attaching one end of an accessory device known as a *test cable* to the recorder and the other end to an electrocardiograph machine. A short baseline strip is recorded and observed for correct waveforms and the absence of artifacts. If the waveforms are incorrect or if artifacts are present, the patient may not be hooked up properly, or a cable or lead malfunction may exist. The medical assistant should reconnect the leads and reposition the electrodes. If a problem still exists, the monitor may be malfunctioning and need repair.

Activity Diary

An important aspect of the Holter monitor procedure is the completion of an *activity diary* by the patient (Figure 12-16). All activities (e.g., physical exercise, meals, sleep periods) and emotional states (e.g., stress, anger, excitement) must be recorded during the monitoring period, along with the time of their occurrence. In addition, any physical symptoms experienced by the patient, such as dizziness, fainting, palpitations, chest pain, dyspnea, and nausea, must be recorded, along with the time of their occurrence. As a result, any dysrhythmia recorded on the magnetic tape or flash memory card can

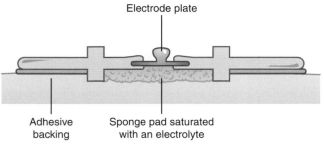

Electrode plate

Adhesive backing   Sponge pad saturated with an electrolyte

Figure 12-14. Electrode used with a Holter monitor.

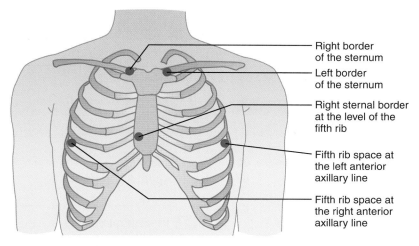

Figure 12-15. Holter monitor electrode positions.

PATIENT ACTIVITY DIARY		
TIME	**ACTIVITY**	**SYMPTOM**
AM PM	*Start recording*	
8:30 AM	Ate breakfast Smoked cigarette	Relaxed
9:15 AM	Driving freeway	Chest pounding
10:35 AM	Argued with boss	Chest pounding
10:45 AM	Took medication	Relaxed
12:30 PM	Ate lunch	Relaxed
1:15 PM	Walked up two flights of stairs	Stomach burning Pain in left arm

Page 1

PATIENT ACTIVITY DIARY		
TIME	**ACTIVITY**	**SYMPTOM**

Page 2

Figure 12-16. Patient's activity diary while wearing a Holter monitor.

be compared with reports in the patient's diary to correlate patient symptoms with cardiac activity.

Event Marker

Most monitors have an *event marker* mounted on one end of the recorder; the event marker is used along with the patient diary for patient evaluation. The patient should be told to depress the event marker momentarily when experiencing a symptom. Depressing the marker places an electronic signal on the recording. This signal later alerts the technician to a significant event on the recording.

Evaluating Results

At the end of the 24-hour period, the Holter monitor system is removed from the patient, and the recording is evaluated by displaying and analyzing it on a special Holter scanning screen or by computer analysis. Printouts of any portion of the electrocardiographic recording can be obtained for further study. The recording must be analyzed where a trained technician and Holter scanner or computer are available. This may involve transferring the recording and patient diary to the cardiac department of a hospital for evaluation. The physician is provided with a written data report of the 24-hour period along with selected printouts of the patient's cardiac activity, including samples of any abnormal cardiac activity exhibited by the patient, such as dysrhythmias. Procedure 12-2 describes how to apply a Holter monitor.

Text continued on p. 512

MEDICAL PRACTICE *and the* LAW

Cardiopulmonary procedures are frightening for many patients because of the potential for unfavorable results. These results must never be given to the patient by the medical assistant. Only a physician can interpret results of electrocardiographic and pulmonary function tests. If results indicate a life-threatening condition, your duty is to calmly to notify the physician at once, without alarming the patient. All offices have emergency supplies; be sure you know where they are and how to use them. While you are attending to the machinery and technology, remember the human dignity of the patient, and attend to all of his or her needs for privacy, comfort, respect, and caring. ∎

What Would You Do? What Would You *Not* Do? RESPONSES

Case Study 1
Page 499
What Did Janet Do?
- ❏ Tried to reduce Camilla's fears by talking with her calmly and quietly.
- ❏ Explained to Camilla that an ECG is the best screening test available to check for heart problems.
- ❏ Reassured Camilla that she would be draped during the procedure and that she would be exposed as little as possible.
- ❏ Told Camilla that the wires may look a little scary, but there is no chance of being shocked by it. Explained that she won't feel anything when the test is being run.
- ❏ Told Camilla that she could talk with the billing clerk about setting up a payment plan for the test. Provided her with information about community resources that might help her pay for the test.

What Did Janet Not *Do?*
- ❏ Did not tell Camilla that she was too young to have heart problems.
- ❏ Did not tell Camilla that she needed to act more mature about being tested.

What Would You Do?/What Would You *Not* Do? Review Janet's response and place a checkmark next to the information you included in your response. List additional information you included in your response.

_____

_____

_____

_____

Case Study 2
Page 516
What Did Janet Do?
- ❏ Commended Joel on his weight loss and positive lifestyle changes.
- ❏ Shared a positive story with Joel about a patient who stopped smoking and did not gain weight.
- ❏ Asked Joel whether he would like any of the latest information on smoking cessation.

What Did Janet Not *Do?*
- ❏ Did not agree that Joel's positive lifestyle changes would counteract the bad effects of smoking.

- ❏ Did not lecture Joel on the dangers of smoking because if he has been smoking since age 17 and has been trying to quit, he already knows what they are.

What Would You Do?/What Would You *Not* Do? Review Janet's response and place a checkmark next to the information you included in your response. List additional information you included in your response.

_____

_____

_____

_____

Case Study 3
Page 518
What Did Janet Do?
- ❏ Removed the nose clips and empathized with Mr. Conrad that the test is hard to do and that the nose clips do fit very snugly.
- ❏ Explained to Mr. Conrad that it is normal to feel dizzy and that it is only temporary.
- ❏ Allowed Mr. Conrad to rest for awhile. Tried to relax and calm him by talking with him about his family and interests.
- ❏ Talked to Mr. Conrad about the importance of performing the test. Told him that detecting a problem early would help him get the treatment he needs as soon as possible so that his condition will not get worse.
- ❏ Asked Mr. Conrad whether he would try the test one more time.

What Did Janet Not *Do?*
- ❏ Did not criticize Mr. Conrad for not being able to perform the test.
- ❏ Did not force Mr. Conrad to stay if he did not want to, but scheduled another pulmonary function test for him before he left the office.

What Would You Do?/What Would You *Not* Do? Review Janet's response and place a checkmark next to the information you included in your response. List additional information you included in your response.

_____

_____

_____

_____

APPLY YOUR KNOWLEDGE

Choose the best answer to each of the following questions.

1. McCabe Waller, 45 years old, has come to the office for a physical examination. Dr. Cardiac has ordered an ECG. Mr. Waller has never had an ECG and asks Janet Canterbury, CMA, what it is. An appropriate response to Mr. Waller would be:
   A. It is a tracing of the muscular activity of the heart.
   B. It is a tracing of the electrical activity of the brain.
   C. It is an imaging test used to visualize the chambers of the heart.
   D. It is a tracing of the electrical activity of the heart.

2. Janet uses proper technique while preparing to run the ECG. Janet does all of the following *except:*
   A. Positions the electrocardiograph on Mr. Waller's left side.
   B. Tells Mr. Waller there will be some slight discomfort during the recording.
   C. Asks Mr. Waller to lie still and not to talk during the recording.
   D. Makes sure the lead wires follow his body contour and do not dangle.

3. Janet applies the 10 disposable adhesive electrodes to Mr. Waller. Just before running the ECG, she rechecks the electrodes and finds that two of the chest electrodes have come loose. What is the best step for Janet to take to correct this situation?
   A. Remove all of the electrodes, and reapply a new set of electrodes.
   B. Use nonallergenic tape to secure the loose electrodes.
   C. Replace the disposable electrodes with reusable metal electrodes.
   D. Ask Mr. Waller to hold the loose electrodes in place while she runs the ECG.

4. Janet realizes that it is important for the electrodes to be firmly attached to prevent:
   A. Muscle artifacts.
   B. Mr. Waller from escaping.
   C. A wandering baseline.
   D. Atrial fibrillation.

5. After running the ECG, Janet reviews the recording and notices that it contains three premature ventricular contractions. Janet should:
   A. Shout for help and immediately start CPR on Mr. Waller.
   B. Check that all the leads are hooked up correctly.
   C. Ask Mr. Waller whether he has a living will.
   D. Inform Dr. Cardiac that the recording shows a dysrhythmia.

6. Mariana Bertilla has come to the office with complaints of an irregular heartbeat, dizziness, and shortness of breath. Dr. Cardiac asks Janet Canterbury, CMA, to run an ECG on Mrs. Bertilla. While recording the ECG, Janet notices that Mrs. Bertilla is shivering, and the recording has a fuzzy, irregular baseline. An appropriate action to eliminate this problem would be to:
   A. Cover Mrs. Bertilla with a blanket and rerun the ECG.
   B. Unplug all electrical equipment in the room and rerun the ECG.
   C. Check that the patient cable is not twisted or dangling.
   D. Give Mrs. Bertilla a swig of whiskey to calm her down.

7. After running the recording on Mrs. Bertilla, Janet checks to make sure the electrocardiograph machine is properly standardized. This is accomplished by:
   A. Checking the recording to ensure there are no artifacts.
   B. Checking the recording to make sure the standardization mark is 10 mm high.
   C. Checking the machine to make sure no warning lights are flashing.
   D. Checking the recording to ensure it shows a normal sinus rhythm.

8. Clement Cooper, 64 years old, has been having some fainting spells lately. His ECG showed a normal sinus rhythm. Dr. Cardiac decides to order a Holter monitor test. To prepare Mr. Cooper for the procedure, Janet Canterbury, CMA, would:
   A. Determine which medications Mr. Cooper should not take during the testing period.
   B. Instruct Mr. Cooper to depress the event marker when a significant symptom occurs.
   C. Tell Mr. Cooper to take a shower instead of a bath during the testing period.
   D. Interpret the recording after the test is completed.

9. Mr. Cooper's Holter monitor report indicates that he had intervals of paroxysmal atrial tachycardia (PAT) during the testing period. The Holter monitor recorded four episodes in 24 hours. Dr. Cardiac checks Mr. Cooper's activity diary to see whether he had symptoms at the time of the PAT episodes. Of the following, what symptom would be associated with PAT?
   A. Chest pain.
   B. Hiccups.
   C. Weakness and breathlessness.
   D. Severe headache.

APPLY YOUR KNOWLEDGE—cont'd

10. Albert Newsome, 58 years old, has come to the office. He has a 40-year history of smoking and has mild COPD. Dr. Cardiac wants to assess his lung functioning and asks Janet Canterbury, CMA, to perform spirometry on Mr. Newsome. Which of the following should Janet do during the test?
    A. Ask Mr. Newsome when he last ate.
    B. Instruct Mr. Newsome to loosen his necktie.
    C. Apply a nose clip to Mr. Newsome's nose.
    D. Instruct Mr. Newsome to seal his lips tightly around the mouthpiece.
    E. All of the above.

11. Janet instructs Mr. Newsome in the spirometry breathing maneuver. All of the following would be included in her explanation *except:*
    A. Relax and take in the deepest breath possible.
    B. Seal your lips tightly around the mouthpiece.
    C. Blow out as hard as you can into the mouthpiece.
    D. Blow out all of your air for no more than 3 seconds.

12. Mr. Newsome performs the first breathing maneuver, but does not perform it correctly. Janet should:
    A. Explain to Mr. Newsome what he did wrong and have him perform the test again.
    B. Remove the nose clips and have Mr. Newsome try again.
    C. Tell Mr. Newsome that if he doesn't do better, he won't get a sticker.
    D. Reschedule Mr. Newsome for another appointment.

CERTIFICATION REVIEW

❏ **The electrocardiograph** records the heart's electrical activity. An electrocardiogram (ECG) is the graphic representation of this activity.

❏ **The heart consists of four chambers:** the right and left atria and the right and left ventricles. The SA node consists of a knot of modified myocardial cells that have the ability to send out an electrical impulse, which initiates and regulates the heartbeat. The AV node delays the impulse momentarily to give the ventricles a chance to fill with blood. The impulse is transmitted to the bundle of His, and the Purkinje fibers distribute the impulse evenly to the right and left ventricles, causing them to contract.

❏ **The cardiac cycle** represents one complete heartbeat. It consists of the contraction of the atria, the contraction of the ventricles, and the relaxation of the entire heart. The electrocardiograph records the electrical activity that causes these events in the cardiac cycle.

❏ **The ECG cycle** consists of a P wave, a QRS complex, and a T wave. The P wave represents the contraction of the atria, the QRS complex represents the contraction of the ventricles, and the T wave represents the electrical recovery of the ventricles.

❏ **The electrocardiograph must be standardized** when recording an ECG. This ensures an accurate and reliable recording. A normal standardization mark should be 10 mm high. If it is more or less than this, the electrocardiograph machine must be adjusted.

❏ **The standard ECG consists of 12 leads.** Each lead records the heart's activity from a different angle. The 12 leads are I, II, III, aVR, aVL, aVF, V_1, V_2, V_3, V_4, V_5, and V_6.

❏ **The electrical impulses** given off by the heart are picked up by electrodes and conducted into the machine through lead wires. An electrolyte assists in transmission of the heart's electrical impulses. An electrolyte consists of a chemical substance that promotes conduction of an electrical current.

❏ **An electrocardiograph** with a three-channel recording capability can record three leads simultaneously. An electrocardiograph with telephone transmission capabilities can transmit a recording over a telephone line to an ECG data interpretation site. An electrocardiograph with interpretive capabilities has a built-in computer program that analyzes the recording as it is being run.

❏ **Artifacts** represent additional electrical activity that is picked up by the electrocardiograph. A muscle artifact has a fuzzy, irregular baseline and is caused by voluntary and involuntary muscle movement. A wandering

Continued

CERTIFICATION REVIEW—cont'd

baseline artifact can be caused by electrodes that are too loose and by body creams, oils, or lotions on the skin. An alternating current artifact is caused by electrical interference and is characterized by small, straight spiked lines on the ECG. An interrupted baseline is caused by the metal tip of a lead wire becoming detached or by a broken patient cable.

❑ **Holter monitor electrocardiography** monitors and records the cardiac activity of a patient for 24 hours. It is used to evaluate patients with unexplained syncope, to discover intermittent cardiac dysrhythmias, and to assess the effectiveness of antiarrhythmic medications.

❑ **Normal sinus rhythm** refers to an ECG that is within normal limits. Cardiac abnormalities known as *dysrhythmias* include extra beats, an abnormal rhythm, and an abnormal heart rate. Cardiac dysrhythmias include atrial premature contraction, paroxysmal atrial tachycardia, atrial flutter, atrial fibrillation, premature ventricular contraction, ventricular tachycardia, and ventricular fibrillation.

❑ **The purpose of a pulmonary function test** is to assess lung functioning, assisting in the detection and evaluation of pulmonary disease. The most frequently performed pulmonary function test is spirometry; an instrument known as a *spirometer* is used to conduct the test. A spirometer measures how much air is pushed out of the lungs and how fast that occurs.

❑ **The most important parameters obtained from spirometry testing** are FVC, FEV_1, and the FEV_1/FVC ratio. The measured values are compared with the predicted values to detect the presence of pulmonary disease. To obtain accurate spirometry test results, it is essential that the following be performed: proper patient preparation, proper calibration of the spirometry machine, and correct performance of the breathing maneuver. Post-bronchodilator spirometry assists the physician in determining how treatment would work for patients with obstructive lung disease.

TERMINOLOGY REVIEW

Amplitude Refers to amount, extent, size, abundance, or fullness.

Artifact Additional electrical activity picked up by the electrocardiograph that interferes with the normal appearance of the ECG cycles.

Atherosclerosis Buildup of fibrous plaques of fatty deposits and cholesterol on the inner walls of the coronary arteries.

Baseline The flat horizontal line that separates the various waves of the ECG cycle.

Cardiac cycle One complete heartbeat.

Dysrhythmia An irregular heart rhythm; also termed *arrhythmia*.

ECG cycle The graphic representation of a heartbeat.

Electrocardiogram (ECG) The graphic representation of the electrical activity of the heart.

Electrocardiograph The instrument used to record the electrical activity of the heart.

Electrode A conductor of electricity, which is used to promote contact between the body and the electrocardiograph.

Electrolyte A chemical substance that promotes conduction of an electrical current.

Interval The length of a wave or the length of a wave with a segment.

Ischemia Deficiency of blood in a body part.

Normal sinus rhythm Refers to an ECG that is within normal limits.

Segment The portion of the ECG between two waves.

Spirometer An instrument for measuring air taken into and expelled from the lungs.

Spirometry Measurement of an individual's breathing capacity by means of a spirometer.

ON THE WEB

For Information on Heart Disease:

American Heart Association: www.americanheart.org

National Heart, Lung, and Blood Institute: www.nhlbi.nih.gov

American Association of Cardiovascular and Pulmonary Rehabilitation: www.aacvpr.org

Health Centers Online: www.healthcentersonline.com

Heart Information Network: www.heartinfo.org

Cardiology Channel: www.cardiologychannel.com

American College of Cardiology: www.acc.org

The National Coalition for Women with Heart Disease: www.womenheart.org

For Information on Lung Disease:

American Lung Association: www.lungusa.org

Pulmonary Channel: www.pulmonarychannel.com

Lung Cancer Online: www.lungcanceronline.org

American Association for Respiratory Care: www.aarc.org

For Information on Smoking Cessation:

The Foundation for a Smokefree America: www.anti-smoking.org

Quit Net: www.quitnet.com

Habitrol Support Program: www.habitrol.com

National Center for Tobacco-free Kids: www.tobaccofreekids.org

Why Quit.com: www.whyquit.com

Quit Smoking Now: www.smokefree.gov

The Quit Smoking Company: www.quitsmoking.com

The prostate gland surrounds the urethra and is located just below the bladder and in front of the rectum (Figure 13-3). It is approximately the size and shape of a walnut, and its function is to secrete fluid that transports sperm.

In the early stages, prostate cancer often causes no symptoms. Symptoms that occur when the cancer is more developed include the following:

• Difficulty in urinating
• Weak or interrupted urinary flow
• Pain or burning during urination
• Frequent urination, especially at night
• Blood in the urine
• Pain in the lower back, pelvis, or upper thighs

When prostate cancer is diagnosed early, the chances for a cure are very good. Because of this, the American Cancer Society recommends that men older than age 50 undergo annual prostate screening. The primary screening tests for prostate cancer are the digital rectal examination (DRE) and the prostate-specific antigen (PSA) test. The American Cancer Society recommends that both of these tests be offered annually to men older than 50 so that if cancer does develop, it is found at an early stage.

Digital Rectal Examination

The digital rectal examination (DRE) is a quick and simple procedure that causes only momentary discomfort. During the examination, the physician inserts a lubricated gloved finger into the patient's rectum. Because the prostate gland is located in front of the rectum, the physician is able to palpate the surface of the prostate gland through the rectal wall (see Figure 13-3). The physician palpates the gland to determine whether it is enlarged or has an abnormal consistency. Normally, the prostate gland should feel soft, whereas malignant tissue is firm and hard. The

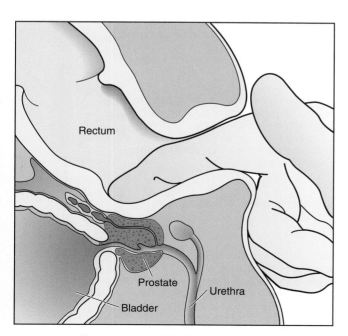

Figure 13-3. Digital rectal examination.

sensitivity of the DRE is limited, however, because the physician can palpate only the posterior and lateral aspects of the prostate gland.

Prostate-Specific Antigen Test

The PSA test is a screening test that measures the amount of PSA in the blood. PSA is a protein normally produced by the cells of the membrane that covers the prostate gland. The normal range for PSA is 0 to 4 ng/ml of blood. The PSA level becomes elevated in men who have a benign or malignant growth in the prostate. A PSA level of 4 to 10 ng/ml is considered slightly elevated; levels between 10 to 20 ng/ml are considered moderately elevated; and a value greater than 20 ng/ml is considered highly elevated. The higher the PSA level, the more likely that cancer is present.

The PSA level may normally increase after vigorous exercise, such as jogging or biking. The medical assistant should instruct the patient to engage only in normal activity for 2 days before having blood drawn for a PSA test. The patient also should be instructed not to have sexual intercourse for 2 days before the test because it can change the PSA level.

If the physician determines the likelihood of cancer through prostate screening, further testing is performed to determine whether prostate cancer is present and, if so, the type of cancer and its location and stage of development. To make this assessment, one or more of the following tests may be performed: transrectal ultrasound (TRUS), biopsy of the prostate gland, bone scan, and computed tomography (CT) scan.

TESTICULAR SELF-EXAMINATION

The purpose of testicular self-examination (TSE) is early detection of testicular cancer. In the past 40 years, testicular cancer among young Caucasian men has more than doubled. Although testicular cancer can develop at any age, it is most common in males 15 to 34 years old. If detected early, it has a very high cure rate. Most cases of testicular cancer are detected by men themselves, either by accident or when

What Would You Do? | **What Would You *Not* Do?**

Case Study 3

Peter Bota, a 62-year-old retired Caucasian male, came to the medical office 1 week ago for a physical examination. The physician performed a DRE but did not palpate anything abnormal. At that visit, Mr. Bota's blood was drawn for a PSA test, and the results came back as slightly elevated (8 ng/ml). Mr. Bota has returned to the office and is waiting to talk with the physician about his test results and possible follow-up testing. Mr. Bota is extremely worried that he has cancer and wants to know the symptoms of prostate cancer. He also wants to know whether there's anything he did to cause prostate cancer. He says he does not smoke and drinks very little and that he walks his dog twice a day for exercise. ∎

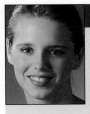

Memories *from* **Externship**

Megan Baer: While on externship in an office specializing in internal medicine, I had an experience that made me feel that all my schooling and hard work were worthwhile. A patient who had a colostomy had an embarrassing "accident." I took her into a room and cleaned her up, rinsed her colostomy bag, and helped her put it back on. She apologized profusely and asked me if I minded or felt repulsed. I replied that I was learning and getting experience in helping people. She told me that at the nursing home where she lived, she overheard some of the aides saying that it was disgusting and that it made them sick. She said she could not help it and that she felt very ashamed. I reassured her that it was nothing to be ashamed about. She then told me that she wished I could be the one to take care of her all the time. When I reached out to shake her hand and say goodbye, she pulled me down and whispered in my ear that she loved me. I was very moved and knew at that moment that I had chosen the right profession. ■

performing a TSE. Certain factors increase a man's chance of getting testicular cancer, including the following:

- A history of cryptorchidism (undescended testicles)
- Family history of testicular cancer
- Cancer of the other testicle
- Caucasian race (testicular cancer is five times more common in Caucasian men than in African-American men)

The TSE should be performed monthly starting at 15 years of age. A good idea is for the patient to choose an easy-to-remember date each month, such as the first day of the month. The best time to perform the examination is after taking a warm bath or shower. Heat allows the scrotal skin to relax and become soft, making it easier to palpate the underlying testicular tissues.

The most common sign of testicular cancer is a small, hard, painless lump (about the size of a pea) located on the front or side of the testicle. Any abnormalities should be reported to the physician immediately. It does not mean that the patient has cancer, however; the physician must make that determination. Figure 13-4 outlines the procedure for a TSE.

TESTICULAR SELF-EXAMINATION

1
Take a warm bath or shower.

2
Stand in front of a mirror. Look for any swelling of the skin of the scrotum.

3
Place the index and middle fingers of both hands on the underside of one testicle and the thumbs on top of the testicle.

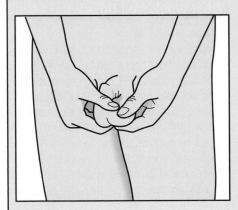

4
Apply a small amount of pressure and gently roll the testicle between the thumb and fingers of both hands, feeling for lumps, swelling, or any change in the size, shape, or consistency of the testicle. A normal testicle should feel smooth, egg-shaped and rather firm. It is also normal for one testicle to be larger or hang lower than the other testicle.

5
Find the epididymis so that you do not confuse it with a lump. The epididymis is a soft tubular cord, located behind the testicle, that functions in storing and carrying sperm.
(Note: Tenderness in the area of the epididymis is considered normal.)

6
Repeat the examination outlined above on the other testicle.

7
Report any of the following abnormalities to the physician: any unusual lump, a feeling of heaviness in the scrotum, a dull ache in the lower abdomen or groin, enlargement of one of the testicles, tenderness or pain in a testicle, or any change in the way the testicle feels.

Figure 13-4. Testicular self-examination.

MEDICAL PRACTICE and the LAW

Colon procedures can be embarrassing for the patient. Most colon procedures can be diagnostic for cancer. This combination makes these procedures very stressful for the patient. Professionalism, compassion, and a caring attitude can alleviate many fears. Many invasive procedures require a written informed consent.

While assisting with a flexible sigmoidoscopy, assist the patient and maintain proper positioning as comfortably as possible. Be aware of the patient's condition, and inform the physician if the patient is not tolerating the procedure well.

Malpractice

Malpractice laws require a minimal level of care and of doing good, or beneficence. Malpractice is a type of negligence, which is a tort, or wrong. Torts can be done intentional or accidental (negligently) and can be caused by something that was done or by something that was omitted. ■

What Would You Do? What Would You *Not* Do? RESPONSES

Case Study 1
Page 529
What Did Megan Do?

❑ Relayed to Mrs. Bernard that this is not the most fun test to perform, but that if colon cancer is detected early, the cure rate is very high.

❑ Explained to Mrs. Bernard that colon cancer increases after age 40, and that an individual can develop colon cancer without a family history of it.

❑ Told Mrs. Bernard that during the early stages of colon cancer, there are no symptoms, so it is possible to feel fine but still have a problem.

❑ Explained to Mrs. Bernard in more detail the reason for not eating red meat or taking aspirin during the testing period.

❑ Told Mrs. Bernard that disposable gloves could be given to her to take home to wear when she collected the specimens.

❑ Explained to Mrs. Bernard that the physician talks with patients every day about these types of things, and it is important to talk with him about all aspects of her health so that she receives the best care possible.

❑ Told Mrs. Bernard that the office would call her in 3 days to see whether she has any questions or is having any problems with the test.

What Did Megan Not *Do?*

❑ Did not tell Mrs. Bernard that she is getting older and needs to be more concerned about performing health screening tests.

What Would You Do?/What Would You *Not* Do? Review Megan's response and place a checkmark next to the information you included in your response. List additional information you included in your response.

_____

_____

_____

_____

Case Study 2
Page 536
What Did Megan Do?

❑ Told Dr. Mitchell that the physician cannot perform a sigmoidoscopy unless the colon has been properly prepared.

❑ Explained that the colon needs to be cleaned out so that the physician can see the wall of the colon to check for abnormalities.

❑ Went over the preparation instructions with Dr. Mitchell again and gave him another instruction sheet to take home.

❑ Rescheduled his appointment and told him that he would be called the day before the examination to be reminded of his appointment and to see whether he has any questions regarding the preparation.

What Did Megan Not *Do?*

❑ Told Dr. Mitchell that an entire office hour had been scheduled for his examination and that other patients could have been seen during this time.

What Would You Do?/What Would You *Not* Do? Review Megan's response and place a checkmark next to the information you included in your response. List additional information you included in your response.

_____

_____

_____

_____

Case Study 3
Page 537
What Did Megan Do?

❑ Listened patiently and tried to reassure and calm Mr. Bota. Told him that physicians do not yet know what causes prostate cancer.

Continued

What Would You Do? What Would You *Not* Do? RESPONSES—cont'd

- ❑ Explained that the PSA test is a screening test and that he should not jump to conclusions about the results.
- ❑ Told Mr. Bota that the physician would talk with him about his test results in a short while.
- ❑ Commended Mr. Bota on his healthy lifestyle habits and encouraged him to continue with them.
- ❑ Gave Mr. Bota some brochures on male reproductive health to read while he waited to be seen by the physician.

What Did Megan Not Do?

- ❑ Did not tell Mr. Bota that there was nothing to worry about.

What Would You Do?/What Would You *Not* Do? Review Megan's response and place a checkmark next to the information you included in your response. List additional information you included in your response.

_____

_____

_____

_____

APPLY YOUR KNOWLEDGE

Choose the best answer to each of the following questions.

1. Tess Terrell, a 52-year-old woman, comes to the medical office for a complete physical examination. As part of the examination, she is given a Hemoccult test to perform at home. Tess asks Megan Baer, CMA, why she has to do this test. Megan explains to her that the purpose of a Hemoccult test is to:
   A. Screen for the presence of blood in the stool.
   B. Detect the presence of parasites in the stool.
   C. Detect the presence of polyps in the large intestine.
   D. Diagnose colorectal cancer.

2. Megan instructs Tess in how to prepare for the Hemoccult test. Megan relays all of the following information to her *except:*
   A. Discontinue taking vitamin supplements that contain iron.
   B. Eat moderate amounts of broccoli and melon.
   C. Start the diet modifications 2 days before collecting the first stool specimen.
   D. Do not eat any red meat.

3. Tess asks Megan why she must consume a high-fiber diet during the testing period. Megan explains that a high-fiber diet:
   A. Prevents the occurrence of a false-negative test result.
   B. Prevents gastrointestinal irritation during the test.
   C. Encourages bleeding from intestinal lesions.
   D. Prevents constipation during the testing period.
   E. All of the above.

4. Tess completes the Hemoccult test and returns it to the medical office. Megan develops the slides. After applying the developing solution to the first slide, Megan observes a trace of blue at the edge of the slide. Megan records this as:
   A. Slide 1: Positive.
   B. Slide 1: Negative.
   C. Slide 1: No reaction.
   D. Slide 1: Invalid.

5. Dr. Polyp instructs Megan to schedule Tess for a flexible sigmoidoscopy and to instruct Tess in proper bowel preparation. Megan instructs Tess to perform all of the following *except:*
   A. Take a laxative the evening before the examination.
   B. Eat a light, low-residue meal the evening before the examination
   C. Fast for 12 hours before the examination.
   D. Perform a Fleet's enema the evening before the examination.

6. Tess arrives at the medical office for the flexible sigmoidoscopy. Megan prepares Tess for the procedure by positioning her in:
   A. Fowler's position.
   B. Sims position.
   C. Knee-chest position.
   D. Prone position.

APPLY YOUR KNOWLEDGE—cont'd

7. During the flexible sigmoidoscopy procedure, Megan assists Dr. Polyp by:
   A. Lubricating Dr. Polyp's gloved finger for the digital rectal examination.
   B. Lubricating the distal end of the sigmoidoscope.
   C. Assisting with suction equipment.
   D. Holding a specimen container to accept a biopsy specimen.
   E. All of the above.

8. After the sigmoidoscopy, Megan cleans up the examining room. She removes the flexible sigmoidoscope to the back work area and cleans it by:
   A. Rinsing it with hot water.
   B. Sanitizing and disinfecting it.
   C. Sterilizing it in the autoclave.
   D. Soaking it in gasoline.

9. Ted Wright, 50 years old, comes to the medical office for a physical examination. Dr. Polyp recommends that he have a DRE and a PSA test. Ted asks Megan Baer, CMA, the purpose of this type of screening. Megan responds by telling Ted that it is:
   A. For the early detection of colorectal cancer.
   B. To determine the cause of infertility.
   C. To assist in the diagnosis of colitis.
   D. For the early detection of prostate cancer.

10. Megan draws a blood specimen from Ted for a PSA test. Ted asks Megan what the normal range is for this test. Megan tells him:
    A. 0 to 4 ng/ml.
    B. 0 to 10 ng/ml.
    C. 5 to 10 ng/ml.
    D. 10 to 20 ng/ml.

11. Matt Coleman, 22 years old, comes to the medical office for an employment physical. Dr. Polyp asks Megan Baer, CMA, to instruct Matt in the procedure for a testicular self-examination. All of the following are included in Megan's discussion *except:*
    A. Perform the examination once each month.
    B. Refrain from sexual intercourse for 2 days before performing the examination.
    C. Take a warm shower before performing the examination.
    D. Palpate each testicle for lumps using both hands.

12. While taking Matt's medical history, Megan obtains the following information. Which of the following puts Matt at higher risk for testicular cancer?
    A. Matt was born with undescended testicles.
    B. Matt collects old coins.
    C. Matt is a vegetarian.
    D. Matt is of African-American heritage.

CERTIFICATION REVIEW

❑ **Blood in the stool** may indicate many conditions, including hemorrhoids, diverticulosis, polyps, upper gastrointestinal ulcers, and colorectal cancer. Hidden, or nonvisible, blood in the stool is termed *occult blood,* and its presence can be determined through fecal occult blood testing.

❑ **Fecal occult blood testing** is routinely performed in the medical office using the guaiac slide test (e.g., Hemoccult and ColoScreen). Patient preparation for the test is important to ensure accurate test results. A positive test result warrants further diagnostic procedures, such as flexible sigmoidoscopy, colonoscopy, and a double-contrast barium enema radiographic study.

❑ **Flexible sigmoidoscopy** is the visual examination of the mucosa of the rectum and sigmoid colon via a flexible fiberoptic sigmoidoscope. Sigmoidoscopy may be performed to detect the presence of lesions, polyps, hemorrhoids, fissures, infection, and inflammation or to determine the cause of rectal bleeding. It is especially valuable in the early detection of colorectal cancer.

❑ **A digital rectal examination** is performed by the physician before the sigmoidoscopy to palpate the rectum for tenderness, hemorrhoids, polyps, or tumors. The digital examination also helps relax the sphincter muscles of the anus for the insertion of the sigmoidoscope.

❑ **The prostate gland** surrounds the urethra and secretes fluid that transports sperm. Beginning at age 50, men should undergo annual prostate screening for the early detection of prostate cancer. The primary screening tests for prostate cancer are the digital rectal examination (DRE) and the PSA test. If the test results indicate the possibility of cancer, further testing is done, which may include one or more of the following: transrectal ultrasound (TRUS), biopsy of the prostate gland, bone scan, and CT scan.

❑ **The purpose of the testicular self-examination (TSE)** is to detect testicular cancer early. Testicular cancer is most common between 15 and 34 years of age. The TSE should be performed monthly beginning at age 15. Any abnormality should be reported to the physician immediately.

TERMINOLOGY REVIEW

Biopsy The surgical removal and examination of tissue from the living body. Biopsies generally are performed to determine whether a tumor is benign or malignant.

Colonoscopy The visualization of the entire colon using a colonoscope.

Endoscope An instrument that consists of a tube and an optical system that is used for direct visual inspection of organs or cavities.

Insufflate To blow a powder, vapor, or gas (e.g., air) into a body cavity.

Melena The darkening of the stool caused by the presence of blood in an amount of 50 ml or greater.

Occult blood Blood in such a small amount that it is not detectable by the unaided eye.

Peroxidase (as it pertains to the guaiac slide test) A substance that is able to transfer oxygen from hydrogen peroxide to oxidize guaiac, causing the guaiac to turn blue.

Sigmoidoscope An endoscope that is specially designed for passage through the anus to permit visualization of the rectum and sigmoid colon.

Sigmoidoscopy The visual examination of the rectum and sigmoid colon using a sigmoidoscope.

ON THE WEB

For Information on Colorectal Cancer:

American Cancer Society: www.cancer.org

National Cancer Institute: www.cancer.gov

Colorectal Cancer Network: www.colorectalcancer.net

Colon Cancer Alliance: www.ccalliance.org

Oncology Channel: www.oncologychannel.com

For Information on Prostate Cancer:

Prostate Health: www.prostatehealth.com

Prostate Information: www.prostateinfo.com

Prostate.com: www.prostate.com

Prostate.org: www.prostatitis.org

Male Health: www.malehealthcenter.com

14

Radiology and Diagnostic Imaging

LEARNING OBJECTIVES

Radiology

1. State the function of radiographs in medicine.
2. Explain the importance of proper patient preparation for a radiographic examination.
3. Describe each of the following positions used for radiographic examinations:
   - Anteroposterior
   - Posteroanterior
   - Right and left lateral
   - Supine
   - Prone
4. Explain the function of a contrast medium.
5. Describe the purpose of a fluoroscope.
6. Explain the purpose of each of the following types of radiographic examinations:
   - Mammography
   - Upper gastrointestinal
   - Lower gastrointestinal
   - Intravenous pyelography

Diagnostic Imaging

1. Explain the purpose of each of the following diagnostic imaging procedures:
   - Ultrasonography
   - Computed tomography
   - Magnetic resonance imaging
   - Nuclear medicine

2. Explain how nuclear medicine is used to produce an image of a body part or organ.
3. State the guidelines that may be required for nuclear medicine.

Digital Radiology

1. Explain the advantages of digital radiology.

PROCEDURES

Instruct a patient in the proper preparation necessary for each of the following types of radiographic examinations:
- Mammography
- Upper gastrointestinal
- Lower gastrointestinal
- Intravenous pyelography

Instruct a patient in the purpose and advance preparation for each of the following diagnostic imaging procedures:
- Ultrasonography
- Computed tomography
- Magnetic resonance imaging
- Nuclear medicine

NATIONAL COMPETENCIES

General Competencies
Patient Instruction
Instruct individual patients according to their needs.
Provide instruction for health maintenance and disease prevention.

KEY TERMS

contrast medium
echocardiogram (EK-oh-KAR-dee-oh-gram)
enema (EN-em-ah)
fluoroscope (FLOOR-oh-skope)
fluoroscopy (floor-OS-koe-pee)
radiograph (RAY-dee-oh-graf)
radiography (ray-dee-OG-rah-fee)

radiologist (ray-dee-AH-lah-jist)
radiology (ray-dee-AH-lah-jee)
radiolucent (ray-dee-oh-LOO-sent)
radiopaque (ray-dee-oh-PAYK)
sonogram (SON-oh-gram)
ultrasonography (ul-trah-son-AH-grah-fee)

Introduction to Radiology

Wilhelm Konrad Roentgen, a German physicist, discovered x-rays on November 8, 1895, while working with a cathode ray tube. He noticed that these rays could pass through solid materials, such as paper, wood, and human skin. Because he did not know what they were, he named them *x-rays*. The rays have since been renamed *roentgen rays* after their discoverer; however, they are better known as "x-rays."

X-rays are high-energy electromagnetic waves that are invisible and have a short wavelength that enables them to penetrate solid materials. A special radiographic film is placed behind the part being examined, and a shadow or image of the internal body structure photographed is produced on the film. **Radiograph** is the term for the permanent record of the picture produced on the radiographic film.

X-rays are used to visualize internal organs and structures and serve as a diagnostic aid in determining the presence of disease. They also are used therapeutically in the treatment of disease conditions, such as malignant neoplasms.

Radiology is the branch of medicine that deals with the use of radiant energy in the diagnosis and treatment of disease. A **radiologist** is a physician who specializes in the di-

agnosis and treatment of disease with any of various forms of radiant energy, such as x-rays, radium, and radioactive material.

A medical office may have its own radiograph machine, but more often radiographs are taken in a hospital by radiology personnel. Some radiographs, such as a chest x-ray, require no advance preparation, whereas others, such as a lower gastrointestinal (GI) study, require a great deal of special preparation. Medical assistants are usually responsible for patient instruction in the type of preparation necessary for a particular radiographic examination and for ensuring that the patient understands the importance of the preparation. If the patient does not prepare properly, the radiograph may be of poor quality, and the procedure may need to be rescheduled. This section provides an introduction to the study of radiographs, with a focus on the patient preparation necessary for common radiographs.

CONTRAST MEDIA

Radiography relies on differences in density between various body structures to produce shadows of varying intensities on the radiographic film. There is a difference in density between bone and flesh (bone is denser than flesh). The bone absorbs more x-rays and does not allow them to reach the radiographic film. This leaves that part of the film unexposed and causes white areas to appear on the processed film. If the x-rays penetrate an organ or structure, a black area appears on the film. Because the lungs contain air, x-rays are able to penetrate them easily. As a result, the lungs appear black on the processed film. The ribs absorb the x-rays and appear as white shadows on the film (Figure 14-1). A structure, such as lung tissue, that permits the passage of x-rays is **radiolucent.** A structure, such as bone, that obstructs the passage of x-rays and causes an image to be cast on the film is **radiopaque.**

In many cases, the natural densities of two adjacent organs or structures are similar. In this instance, a **contrast medium** must be used to make a particular structure visible on the radiograph. Contrast media are usually radiopaque chemical compounds that cause the body tissue or organ to absorb more radiation. This absorption provides a contrast in density between the tissue or organ and the surrounding area. The tissue or organ becomes visible and appears white on the processed radiograph. Substances used as contrast media must be able to be ingested or injected into the body tissues or organs without causing harm to the patient.

Barium sulfate and inorganic iodine compounds are commonly used radiopaque contrast media. Barium sulfate is a chalky compound that is water-insoluble and does not allow penetration by x-rays. It is frequently used for examination of the GI tract because barium is not absorbed into the body through the GI tract and does not alter its normal function. Iodine salts are radiopaque and are combined with other compounds for radiographic examination of structures such as the gallbladder and kidneys. Iodine sometimes may produce an allergic reaction, and before administration, patients should be asked whether they have an allergy to iodine or foods containing iodine. Patients with known allergies may be given an iodine-sensitivity test as a precautionary measure.

Another type of contrast medium causes the structure to become less dense than the surrounding area. The x-rays can easily penetrate the structure, which appears as a darker area on the radiograph. This type of contrast medium includes substances such as air and carbon dioxide.

What Would You Do? What Would You *Not* Do?

Case Study 1

Jose Ramirez is a 7-year-old boy with episodes of unexplained abdominal pain and vomiting during the past 6 months. The physician has scheduled an upper GI at the local hospital. Mrs. Ramirez wants to know how best to prepare Jose for the procedure so that he will not be so afraid of the radiograph room and equipment. She asks what she can do so that he will drink the barium solution. She says he will not drink milk, and if the barium tastes anything like milk, it will be hard to get him to drink the barium. Mrs. Ramirez wants to know whether Jose can hold his favorite toy (a Tonka truck) during the procedure to help comfort him. She also wants to know whether the barium solution will make him feel sick afterward. ∎

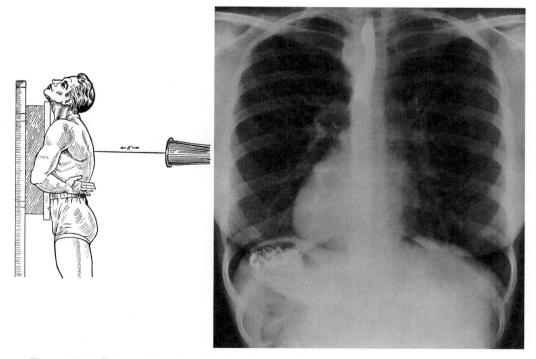

Figure 14-1. Posteroanterior view of the chest. Position of patient and radiograph. (From Meschan I: *Synopsis of radiologic anatomy with computed tomography,* Philadelphia, 1980, Saunders.)

MEDICAL PRACTICE and the LAW

Radiology and diagnostic imaging involve high-technology equipment and procedures that can be frightening and uncomfortable to the patient. Be aware of the patient's reactions, and provide assistance and comfort whenever possible. Be specific in providing the patient with instructions to ensure the best imaging results.

Procedures that involve injectable contrast media or that are invasive usually require written informed consent. Check office policy for procedures that require signed consent forms.

With procedures that use radiation, federal laws regulate usage and exposure testing and record keeping. The acronym ALARA (As Low As Reasonably Able) reminds workers to minimize exposure to themselves and patients. Ask female patients whether they may be pregnant before starting any radiologic procedure. ■

What Would You Do? What Would You *Not* Do? RESPONSES

Case Study 1
Page 545

What Did Michelle Do?

❑ Told Mrs. Ramirez that a role-playing game with Jose might help. Suggested that she play the "doctor" and pretend she is taking a radiograph of Jose.

❑ Told Mrs. Ramirez that the barium will have a flavoring in it but that it does taste chalky. Suggested that she explain to Jose why he needs to drink the barium—to help the doctor find what is wrong with him so that he will not get sick anymore.

❑ Told Mrs. Ramirez that Jose's truck is made of metal and would interfere with a good radiograph. Suggested that she bring the truck and tell Jose he could have it after the procedure.

❑ Told Mrs. Ramirez that the barium solution should not make Jose sick, but if it does, she should call the office. Explained that the barium might cause constipation and would cause Jose's next bowel movement to be lighter in color. Told her that she should encourage Jose to drink water after the procedure to help prevent constipation.

What Did Michelle Not *Do?*

❑ Did not tell Mrs. Ramirez that the barium solution would taste good and that she should not have any trouble getting Jose to drink it.

What Would You Do?/What Would You *Not* Do? Review Michelle's response and place a checkmark next to the information you included in your response. List additional information you included in your response.

_____

_____

_____

_____

Case Study 2
Page 550

What Did Michelle Do?

❑ Told Sara-Jayne that the procedure uses sound waves to visualize the heart. Explained that the procedure does not use a dye injected into the veins. Gave her an educational brochure on ultrasound imaging.

❑ Reassured Sara-Jayne that no pain is involved with an echocardiogram.

❑ Told Sara-Jayne that an ultrasound is normally safe during pregnancy because radiation is not used. The physician would be informed that she is pregnant, however, and if there is a change in his order, Sara-Jayne would be notified.

What Did Michelle Not *Do?*

❑ Did not allow Sara-Jayne to go ahead with the procedure without checking with the physician.

What Would You Do?/What Would You *Not* Do? Review Michelle's response and place a checkmark next to the information you included in your response. List additional information you included in your response.

_____

_____

_____

_____

Case Study 3
Page 553

What Did Michelle Do?

❑ Explained to Michael that an MRI does not use radiation, so he would not be exposed to any radiation during the procedure.

Continued

What Would You Do? What Would You *Not* Do? RESPONSES—cont'd

❑ Told Michael that he would not be able to play his Game Boy during the procedure. Explained that the MRI works with a strong magnet that might damage the Game Boy and also interfere with a good image of the shoulder. Told Michael that he also would need to lie still during the procedure.

❑ Told Michael the physician would be informed of his problem with claustrophobia. Explained that the physician may want to give him something to help him relax during the procedure.

❑ Told Michael that it was fine to eat before the procedure.

What Did Michelle Not *Do*?

❑ Did not overlook or minimize Michael's concern about claustrophobia.

What Would You Do?/What Would You *Not* Do? Review Michelle's response and place a checkmark next to the information you included in your response. List additional information you included in your response.

_____

_____

_____

_____

APPLY YOUR KNOWLEDGE

Choose the best answer to each of the following questions.

1. Joyce Langley, a 45-year-old woman, comes to the office for her gynecologic examination. Dr. Radiolucent asks Michelle Shockey, CMA, to schedule Mrs. Langley for a mammogram at Grant Hospital's radiology department. Michelle provides Mrs. Langley with the following instructions on how to prepare for the examination by telling her to:
   A. Not wear any lotions, powders, or deodorants to the examination.
   B. Fast for 12 hours before the examination.
   C. Take a mild sedative before the examination.
   D. Cleanse her breasts with isopropyl alcohol the morning of the examination.

2. Mrs. Langley returns to the office. Dr. Radiolucent has determined from the results of Mrs. Langley's mammogram that she has fibrocystic breast disease and wants to discuss this condition with her. Mrs. Langley asks Michelle why her breasts were compressed during the mammography procedure. Michelle responds by telling her it was to:
   A. Prevent her from moving during the procedure.
   B. Protect her from a radiation burn.
   C. Obtain a clear radiograph of her breasts.
   D. Make the procedure more comfortable for her.

3. James Whitmore, a 62-year-old man, comes to the office with a burning pain that occurs right before he eats. Dr. Radiolucent suspects that James may have a peptic ulcer. He asks Michelle Shockey, CMA, to schedule James for an upper GI radiographic examination at Grant Hospital. Michelle in-

structs James in the preparation necessary for the radiograph by telling him to:
   A. Perform a cleansing enema on the morning of the examination.
   B. Take a laxative the evening before the examination.
   C. Not eat or drink anything after midnight on the day before the examination.
   D. Take special dye tablets with his evening meal.

4. Michelle explains to James that he will be asked to drink a mixture of barium and water before the upper GI examination. Michelle tells James that the barium mixture will be in his stool the next day and will cause his stool to be:
   A. Dark and tarlike.
   B. Streaked with mucus.
   C. Radioactive.
   D. Lighter in color.

5. Susan March comes to the office with cramping pain in her lower left side. Dr. Radiolucent suspects that Mrs. March may have diverticulitis. He asks Michelle Shockey, CMA, to schedule a lower GI radiographic examination at Grant Hospital. Michelle relays the patient preparation for this examination to Mrs. March. She tells her to do all of the following *except*:
   A. Consume only clear liquids the day before the examination.
   B. Eat a breakfast high in fat on the morning of the examination.
   C. Take a laxative on the day before the examination.
   D. Perform a cleansing enema on the morning of the examination.

APPLY YOUR KNOWLEDGE—cont'd

6. Beth Carroll, a 35-year-old woman, comes to the office with severe pain in her left side, nausea and vomiting, and blood in her urine. Dr. Radiolucent suspects that Beth may have a kidney stone. He asks Michelle Shockey, CMA, to schedule an IVP at Grant Hospital. An important question for Michelle to ask Beth would be:
   A. Are you allergic to shellfish or iodine?
   B. What is the date of your last menstrual period?
   C. Is there a history of kidney stones in your family?
   D. How much water do you drink every day?

7. Michelle instructs Beth in how to prepare for the IVP. Michelle tells her to:
   A. Take a laxative the day before the examination.
   B. Perform a cleansing enema the morning of the examination.
   C. Not eat or drink anything after 9:00 PM the day before the examination.
   D. All of the above.

8. Megan McCoy, a 35-year-old pregnant woman, comes to the office for an obstetric ultrasound. She is in her fourth month of pregnancy. Megan asks Michelle Shockey, CMA, what kinds of things can be determined from the ultrasound. Michelle responds by saying that it can be used to:
   A. Determine the gestational age of her baby and confirm the due date.
   B. Detect certain birth defects.
   C. Detect whether or not there is more than one fetus.
   D. Determine the position of the fetus in the uterus.
   E. All of the above.

9. Charles Morrison comes to the office with indigestion and nausea after eating fried foods. Dr. Radiolucent suspects that Charles may be having a problem with his gallbladder. He asks Michelle Shockey, CMA, to schedule an ultrasound of the gallbladder at Grant Hospital's diagnostic imaging department. Michelle relays information to Charles regarding this procedure. She includes all of the following *except:*
   A. Charles must fast for 12 hours before the examination.
   B. Charles will be required to lie still during the procedure.
   C. Charles will hear a metallic clacking sound during the procedure.
   D. It is a safe and painless procedure.

10. Sarah Strong has been diagnosed with colorectal cancer. Dr. Radiolucent asks Michelle Shockey, CMA, to schedule a CT scan at Grant Hospital to determine the extent of the cancer. Michelle explains the preparation required for the examination by telling Sarah to:
   A. Discontinue all medications 2 days before the scan.
   B. Not wear any jewelry.
   C. Consume four glasses of water an hour before the scan.
   D. Perform a cleansing enema on the morning of the scan.
   E. All of the above.

CERTIFICATION REVIEW

❑ **X-rays are used to visualize internal organs and structures** and serve as a diagnostic aid in determining of the presence of disease. They also are used therapeutically in the treatment of malignant neoplasms. *Radiograph* is the term for the permanent record of the picture produced on the radiographic film. Radiology is the branch of medicine that deals with the use of radiant energy in the diagnosis and treatment of disease.

❑ **A structure that permits the passage of x-rays is radiolucent.** A structure that obstructs the passage of x-rays is radiopaque. A contrast medium is used to make a particular structure visible on the radiograph. A fluoroscope is an instrument used to view internal organs and structures of the body directly on a display screen.

❑ **The position of the patient** is determined by the purpose of the examination and the area examined. Different types of radiographic views include anteroposterior (AP), posteroanterior (PA), lateral, oblique, supine, and prone.

❑ **Mammography** is a radiographic examination of the breasts used to detect breast disease. Mammography can be used to detect a breast tumor when the growth is less than 1 cm in diameter.

Continued

CERTIFICATION REVIEW—cont'd

❑ **An upper GI** is an examination of the upper digestive tract with fluoroscopy and radiography. It is used in the diagnosis of disorders of the esophagus, stomach, duodenum, and small intestine.

❑ **A lower GI** involves filling the colon with a barium sulfate mixture with a tube inserted into the colon. The examination is used in the diagnosis of disorders of the lower intestine, such as polyps, tumors, lesions, and diverticulosis.

❑ **An intravenous pyelogram (IVP)** is a radiograph of the kidneys and urinary tract. It is used to assist in the diagnosis of kidney stones, blockage or narrowing of the urinary tract, and growths within or near the urinary system.

❑ **Ultrasonography** uses high-frequency sound waves to study soft tissue structures. It is frequently used in the

diagnosis of conditions of the abdominal and pelvic organs, particularly the liver, gallbladder, spleen, pancreas, kidneys, uterus, and ovaries. An ultrasound examination of the heart is called an *echocardiogram*. Ultrasound shows movement and allows for continuous viewing of a structure. Obstetric ultrasound is used to determine gestational age of a fetus and to confirm date of delivery.

❑ **CT** is used to view the bones and organs of the head and body in fine detail. CT scans are used in the detection and evaluation of tumors and other abnormalities and in the monitoring of the effects of surgery, radiation therapy, or chemotherapy on tumors.

❑ **MRI** is used to assist in the diagnosis of intracranial and spinal lesions and of cardiovascular and soft tissue abnormalities.

TERMINOLOGY REVIEW

Contrast medium A substance used to make a particular structure visible on a radiograph.

Echocardiogram An ultrasound examination of the heart.

Enema An injection of fluid into the rectum to aid in the elimination of feces from the colon.

Fluoroscope An instrument used to view internal organs and structures directly.

Fluoroscopy Examination of a patient with a fluoroscope.

Radiograph A permanent record of a picture of an internal body organ or structure produced on radiographic film.

Radiography The taking of permanent records (radiographs) of internal body organs and structures by passing x-rays through the body to act on a specially sensitized film.

Radiologist A physician who specializes in the diagnosis and treatment of disease using radiant energy, such as x-rays, radium, and radioactive material.

Radiology The branch of medicine that deals with the use of radiant energy in the diagnosis and treatment of disease.

Radiolucent Describing a structure that permits the passage of x-rays.

Radiopaque Describing a structure that obstructs the passage of x-rays.

Sonogram The record obtained with ultrasonography.

Ultrasonography The use of high-frequency sound waves to produce an image of an organ or tissue.

ON THE WEB

For Information on Radiography and Diagnostic Imaging:

BrighamRAD: www.brighamrad.harvard.edu

Society for Computer Applications in Radiology: www.scarnet.org

Whole Brain Atlas: www.med.harvard.edu/AANLIB/home.html

Radiology Information: www.radiologyinfo.org

For Information on Breast Cancer:

American Cancer Society: www.cancer.org

15

Introduction to the Clinical Laboratory

Clinical Laboratory

1. Explain the general purpose of a laboratory test.
2. List and explain specific uses of laboratory test results.
3. Describe the relationship between the medical office and an outside laboratory.
4. List the information included in a laboratory directory.

5. Identify the purpose of a laboratory request form. List and explain the function of each type of information included on the form.
6. Identify the use of each of the following profiles, and list the tests included in each:
    Comprehensive metabolic profile
    Electrolyte profile
    Hepatic profile
    Renal profile
    Lipid profile
    Thyroid profile
    Rheumatoid profile
    Prenatal profile
    Hepatitis profile
7. Identify the purpose of the laboratory report form, and list the information included on it.

Collecting, Transporting, and Handling Specimens

1. Explain the purpose of advance patient preparation for the collection of a laboratory specimen.
2. List examples of specimens.
3. Identify and explain the guidelines that should be followed during specimen collection.
4. Explain why specimens must be handled and stored properly.
5. Identify the proper handling and storage techniques for each of the following specimens: blood, urine, microbiologic specimen, and stool specimen.

Physician's Office Laboratory

1. Identify and define the eight categories of a laboratory test on the basis of function. List examples of tests included under each category.
2. List the six basic steps involved in testing a specimen.
3. Describe the methods that are used to test a specimen.
4. Explain the purpose of quality control in the laboratory, and list quality control methods that should be used for each of the following: advance patient preparation; specimen collection, handling, and transportation; and laboratory testing.
5. List the laboratory safety guidelines that should be followed in the medical office to prevent accidents.

Use a laboratory directory.
Complete a laboratory request form.
Read a laboratory report.
Instruct a patient in the preparation necessary for a laboratory test that requires fasting.

Collect a specimen.

Handle and store a specimen.

Use quality control methods.

Practice laboratory safety.

NATIONAL COMPETENCIES

Clinical Competencies
Diagnostic Testing
Screen and follow-up test results.
Use methods of quality control.

General Competencies
Patient Instruction
Instruct individual patients according to their needs.
Instruct and demonstrate the use and care of patient equipment.
Provide instruction for health care maintenance and disease prevention.
Identify community resources.

KEY TERMS

automated method
fasting
homeostasis (hoe-mee-oh-STAY-sis)
in vivo (in-VEE-voe)
laboratory test
manual method
normal range

plasma (PLAZ-ma)
profile
quality control
routine test
serum (SERE-um)
specimen (SPES-i-men)

Introduction to the Clinical Laboratory

Clinical laboratory test results are often used along with a thorough health history and physical examination to provide essential data needed by the physician for accurate diagnosis and management of a patient's condition. Clinical **laboratory tests** provide objective and quantitative information regarding the status of body conditions and functions. When the body is healthy, its systems function normally, and a state of equilibrium of the internal environment is said to exist; this is termed **homeostasis.** When the body is in a state of homeostasis, the physical and chemical characteristics of the body substances (e.g., fluids, secretions, excretions) are within an acceptable range known as the **normal range** or reference range.

When a pathologic condition exists, biologic changes occur within the body, altering the normal physiology or functioning of the body and resulting in an imbalance. These changes cause the patient to experience the symptoms of that particular pathologic condition. Iron deficiency anemia usually causes the patient to experience weakness, fatigue, pallor, irritability, and, in some cases, shortness of breath on exertion. In addition, these changes in the body's biologic processes may cause an alteration in the characteristics of body substances, such as an alteration of the chemical content of the blood or urine, an alteration in the antibody level, or an alteration in cell counts or cellular morphology.

The physical and chemical alterations of body substances become evident through abnormal values or results in laboratory tests—in other words, values outside the accepted normal range or limit for that particular test. Just as certain pathologic conditions cause specific symptoms to occur, certain pathologic conditions cause abnormal values to occur for specific laboratory tests. Iron deficiency anemia causes an alteration in normal red blood cell morphology and a decreased hemoglobin level.

An important realization is that an abnormal value for a particular test may be seen with more than one pathologic condition. A decrease in the hemoglobin level is found with hyperthyroidism and cirrhosis of the liver. In this regard, the physician cannot rely solely on laboratory test results to make a final diagnosis, but rather must rely also on the combination of the data obtained from the health history, the physical examination, and diagnostic and laboratory test results.

LABORATORY TESTS

The number of laboratory tests ordered for a patient varies depending on the physician's clinical findings. A clinical diagnosis of a urinary tract infection usually necessitates only a urine culture for confirmation. Many diseases cause more than one alteration in the physical and chemical characteristics of body substances, however, and a series of laboratory tests is often necessary to establish the pattern of abnormalities characteristic of a particular disease.

The medical assistant should realize that not all pathologic conditions necessitate the use of laboratory test results for arrival at a final diagnosis; the information obtained from the patient's clinical signs and symptoms can be sufficient for a final diagnosis of some conditions. In these instances, the physician is so certain of the clinical diagnosis that therapy can be instituted without laboratory confirmation. Most physicians diagnose acute purulent otitis media with the information obtained from patient symptoms (earache, fever, feeling of fullness in the ear) and from an otoscopic examination of the tympanic membrane (the tympanic membrane is red and bulging). The information obtained through the clinical signs and symptoms is sufficiently specific to otitis media to allow the physician to make a final diagnosis and to prescribe treatment.

The medical assistant must acquire knowledge and skill in basic clinical laboratory methods and techniques. It is important that the medical assistant have knowledge of the laboratory tests that are performed most often, including the purpose of these tests; the normal value or range for each test; any advance patient preparation or special instructions; and any substances that might interfere with accurate test results, such as food or medication.

The medical assistant frequently works with this information when collecting, handling, and storing specimens; performing laboratory tests; typing health histories; and receiving and filing laboratory reports. It is essential that the medical assistant understand the value of laboratory tests and alert the physician to any abnormal results as soon as the test is performed or the laboratory report is received.

This chapter serves as an introduction to the clinical laboratory by providing an overview of methods and general guidelines to follow and by focusing on the relationship between the medical office and an outside laboratory. Specific information for collection, handling, storing, and testing of biologic specimens is presented in subsequent chapters.

PURPOSE OF LABORATORY TESTING

The most frequent use of laboratory test results is to assist in the diagnosis of a patient's condition. Laboratory test results also have many other significant medical uses. A summary of the purpose and function of laboratory testing follows:

1. Laboratory tests are most frequently ordered by the physician *to assist in the diagnosis of pathologic conditions.* Along with the health history and the physical examination, laboratory test results provide the physician with essential data needed to arrive at the final diagnosis and prescribe treatment. After obtaining the health history and performing the physical examination, the physician may order laboratory tests for these reasons:

   - *To confirm a clinical diagnosis.* The patient's signs and symptoms may provide a strong clinical diagnosis of a particular condition, and the physician may order laboratory tests simply to confirm that diagnosis. For example, the patient may have the typical signs and symptoms of diabetes mellitus, which would provide the physician with a fairly certain clinical diagnosis. In this instance, a glucose tolerance test (GTT) would be ordered to confirm the diagnosis and to institute therapy.

   - *To assist in the differential diagnosis of a patient's condition.* Two or more diseases may have similar signs and symptoms; the physician orders laboratory tests to assist in the differential diagnosis of the patient's condition. A final diagnosis of streptococcal sore throat must be made with a laboratory test to differentiate it from other pathologic conditions with similar signs and symptoms, such as pharyngitis.

   - *To obtain information regarding a patient's condition* when not enough concrete evidence exists to support a clinical diagnosis. The patient sometimes may have vague signs and symptoms, and laboratory tests are ordered to provide information on what may be causing the patient's problem. For example, the patient may have nonspecific abdominal pain, and the physical examination may not yield enough information to support a clinical diagnosis. In this case, the physician may order a series of laboratory and diagnostic tests to assist in pinpointing the cause of the patient's problems.

2. When the final diagnosis has been made, laboratory testing may be performed *to evaluate the patient's progress and to regulate treatment.* On the basis of the laboratory results, the therapy may need to be adjusted or further treatment prescribed. A patient undergoing iron therapy for iron deficiency anemia should have a complete blood count (CBC) performed every month to assess response to the treatment and to ensure the condition is improv-

ing. Another example is a patient with thrombophlebitis who is taking warfarin (Coumadin), an anticoagulant used to inhibit blood clotting. The patient must have a prothrombin time test at regular intervals to assess the clotting ability of the blood. On the basis of the test results, the medication may need to be adjusted to ensure the dosage is at a safe level. A patient with diabetes who measures the blood glucose level each day to regulate insulin dosage provides another example of laboratory tests used to regulate treatment.

3. On the basis of such factors as age, gender, race, and geographic location, individuals have different normal levels within the established normal range for a particular test. In this respect, laboratory tests also can serve *to establish each patient's baseline or normal level* with which future results can be compared. A patient who is going to receive warfarin (Coumadin) therapy should have a blood specimen drawn for a prothrombin time test before administration of this anticoagulant. The results serve as a baseline recording for that particular patient with which future prothrombin time test results can be compared.

4. Laboratory tests also can help *to prevent or reduce the severity of disease* by early detection of abnormal findings. Certain conditions, such as high cholesterol, anemia, and diabetes, are relatively common disorders and sometimes may exist undetected in a patient, especially early in the development of the disease. Laboratory tests known as **routine tests** are performed on a routine basis on apparently healthy patients (usually as part of a general physical examination) to assist in the early detection of disease. These tests are relatively easy to perform and present a minimal hazard to the patient. The most commonly used routine tests are urinalysis, CBC, and routine blood chemistries.

5. Another reason for a laboratory test is its *requirement by state law.* The statutes of most states require a gonorrhea and syphilis test to be performed on pregnant women. The purpose of these tests is to protect the mother and fetus from harm by screening for the presence of these venereal diseases.

TYPES OF CLINICAL LABORATORIES

The medical office may use an outside laboratory for testing, or the office may contain its own laboratory, known as a *physician's office laboratory* (POL), in which the medical assistant performs various tests. Most medical offices use a combination of the two to fulfill the physician's needs for test results.

Physician's Office Laboratory

Generally, laboratory tests that are convenient to perform and commonly required, such as a glucose determination and urinalysis, are performed in the POL. Most physicians consider it too time-consuming and expensive in terms of equipment, supplies, medical laboratory personnel, and

quality control to perform highly sophisticated and complex tests, such as serologic studies and microbiologic studies, in the medical office. These tests are usually performed at an outside laboratory. These laboratories use automated equipment to perform the tests, providing the medical offices with fast and reliable test results.

Outside Laboratories

Because the medical assistant usually works closely with an outside laboratory, a basic knowledge of the relationship between the medical office and the laboratory, as described in the following paragraphs, is important. Outside laboratories include hospital and privately owned commercial laboratories, which employ individuals specifically trained in clinical laboratory techniques and methods. If the specimen is collected at the medical office, the laboratory provides the medical office with the supplies and forms necessary to collect the specimen and prepare it for transport to the laboratory. The medical assistant is responsible for checking these supplies periodically and for reordering them from the laboratory as needed.

Laboratory Directory

The outside laboratory provides the medical office with a laboratory directory that serves as a valuable reference source for the proper collection and handling of specimens in the medical office for transport to the outside laboratory. Directories vary in organization, depending on the laboratory. The following information is generally included, however: names of the tests performed by the laboratory, the normal range for each test, instructions on completion of forms, patient preparation necessary for each test, supplies necessary for the collection of each specimen, amount and type of specimen required for each test, techniques to use for the collection of the specimen, proper handling and storage of the specimen, and instructions for transporting specimens.

Table 15-1 is a sample of representative tests taken from a laboratory directory. If the medical assistant has a question regarding any aspect of the collection and handling of the specimen, the laboratory should be called before proceeding.

Collection and Testing Categories

Collection and testing of a specimen can be categorized as follows: (1) the specimen is collected and tested at the medical office, (2) the specimen is collected at the medical office and transferred to an outside medical laboratory for testing, or (3) the patient is given a laboratory request to have the specimen collected and tested at an outside laboratory. The medical assistant's responsibilities depend on which of these methods is used in the medical office. For example, a specimen collected at the medical office and transferred to an outside laboratory for testing involves a series of individual steps different from the steps followed when it is collected and tested at the medical office. The following clinical laboratory methods are presented in the

kit. To assist individuals in keeping up with new waived test additions and new methodologies for waived tests, the Centers for Disease Control and Prevention (CDC) maintains the following website: www.cms.hhs.gov/clia. The following tests are examples of waived tests:

- Dipstick or tablet reagent urinalysis
- Fecal occult blood testing
- Ovulation testing with visual color comparisons
- Urine pregnancy tests with visual color comparisons
- Erythrocyte sedimentation rate, nonautomated
- Hemoglobin using a CLIA-waived analyzer
- Spun microhematocrit
- Blood glucose determination using a Food and Drug Administration–approved blood glucose
- Rapid streptococcus testing

2. *Moderate-complexity tests.* Moderate-complexity tests account for 75% of the estimated 10,000 laboratory tests performed in the United States every day. Examples of moderate-complexity tests performed in the medical office include hematology and blood chemistry tests performed on automated blood analyzers that are not CLIA-waived and microscopic analysis of urine sediment.

3. *High-complexity tests.* High-complexity tests include all procedures related to cytogenetics, histopathology, histocompatibility, and cytology (includes Pap testing). These tests are not usually performed in medical offices; most of these tests are done in laboratories already subject to federal regulation.

Requirements for Moderate-Complexity and High-Complexity Testing

Laboratories that perform moderate-complexity or high-complexity tests or both must meet the CLIA regulations and are subject to unannounced inspections every 2 years by CMS. The major components of the CLIA 1988 regulations relating to laboratory standards are as follows:

1. *Patient test management.* A system must be established to maintain the optimal integrity and identification of patient specimens throughout the testing process. This system must also ensure accurate reporting of results.

2. *Quality control.* To ensure accurate and reliable test results, each laboratory must establish and follow written quality control procedures that monitor and evaluate the quality of each testing process. These include:
   - Developing a laboratory procedures manual, following the manufacturer's instructions for each product
   - Performing calibration procedures at least every 6 months and documenting results
   - Performing two levels of controls daily and documenting results
   - Performing and documenting actions taken when problems or errors are identified
   - Documenting all quality control activities.

3. *Quality assurance.* Each laboratory must establish and follow written policies and procedures to monitor and evaluate the overall quality of the total testing process to

ensure the accuracy and reliability of patient test results.

4. *Proficiency testing.* Proficiency testing (PT) is a form of external quality control in which laboratory specimens are prepared by an approved proficiency testing agency. Three times a year, the POL must test a shipment of these unknown specimens with the same procedure as for testing a patient's specimen. The results are forwarded to the PT agency for evaluation.

5. *Personnel requirements.* The CLIA regulations specify qualifications and responsibilities for personnel for laboratory directors, technical consultants, clinical consultants, and testing personnel. The regulations list specific education and training qualifications for the various positions and define the responsibilities for the persons who fill these positions. Personnel requirements are most stringent for high-complexity testing.

PHYSICIAN'S OFFICE LABORATORY

As previously discussed, a POL consists of an in-house medical office laboratory. The testing of a specimen in a POL involves following a series of steps to measure or identify the presence of a specific substance in the specimen, such as the measurement of a chemical or the identification of a microorganism. The medical assistant may be responsible for performing the laboratory tests and recording the results, or the physician may employ a medical laboratory technologist or a medical technician to perform the tests. The decision is based on the number of tests performed in the medical office, the complexity of these tests, and the CLIA regulations. The medical assistant is qualified to perform waived laboratory tests; more sophisticated tests require the knowledge and skill of the medical laboratory technologist or technician.

Laboratory tests can be classified by function into one of the following categories: hematology, clinical chemistry, serology and blood banking, urinalysis, microbiology, parasitology, cytology, and histology. Table 15-4 lists the

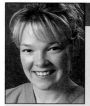

Memories *from* Externship

Korey McGrew: One of my most difficult situations as a medical assisting student was taking the temperature of a patient who went into seizures. I was scared because I was only a student, and I had never been in a situation like that before. I knew I had to act immediately, and luckily one of the Certified Medical Assistants (CMAs) was nearby. We immediately put the patient on the floor and moved things away from him to prevent him from hurting himself. We then notified the physician, who was with a patient in another examining room. The seizures lasted only about 4 minutes, and the patient was fine. The CMA told me that the patient had a history of seizures and that I was not to be alarmed. That surely was a difficult but valuable learning experience for me. ■

Table 15-4 Categories of Laboratory Tests*

Category	Definition and Commonly Performed Tests	Category	Definition and Commonly Performed Tests
Hematology	Hematology is science dealing with study of blood and blood-forming tissues. Laboratory analysis in hematology deals with examination of blood for detection of abnormalities and includes areas such as blood cell counts, cellular morphology, clotting ability of blood, and identification of cell types White Blood Cell Count (WBC) Red Blood Cell Count (RBC) Differential White Blood Cell Count (Diff) Hemoglobin (Hgb) Hematocrit (Hct) Platelet Count Reticulocyte Count Prothrombin Time (PT) Erythrocyte Sedimentation Rate (ESR) Platelet Count	Serology and blood banking	Laboratory analysis in serology and blood banking deals with studying antigen-antibody reactions to assess presence of substance or to determine presence of disease Syphilis Tests (VDRL, RPR) C-Reactive Protein (CRP) ABO Blood Typing Rh Typing Rh Antibody Test Antinuclear Antibody (ANA) Rheumatoid Factor (RF) Latex Mononucleosis Test Hepatitis Tests HIV Tests Antistreptolysin O (ASO) Pregnancy Test
Clinical chemistry	Laboratory analysis in clinical chemistry determines the amount of chemical substances present in body fluids, excreta, and tissues (e.g., blood, urine, cerebrospinal fluid). The largest area in clinical chemistry is blood chemistry Glucose Blood Urea Nitrogen (BUN) Creatinine Total Protein Albumin Globulin Calcium Inorganic Phosphorus Chloride Sodium Potassium Bilirubin Cholesterol Triglycerides Uric Acid Lactate Dehydrogenase (LDH) Aspartate Aminotransferase (AST) Alanine Aminotransferase (ALT) Alkaline Phosphatase (ALP) Amylase Carbon Dioxide Gamma-Glutamyltranspeptidase Thyroxine (T_4) Triiodothyronine (T_3) Uptake Creatine Phosphokinase (CPK)	Urinalysis	Urinalysis involves physical, chemical, and microscopic analysis of urine A. Tests included in physical analysis of urine: Color Appearance Specific Gravity B. Tests included in chemical analysis of urine: pH Specific Gravity Glucose Protein Ketones Blood Bilirubin Urobilinogen Nitrite Leukocytes C. Tests included in microscopic analysis of urine: Red Blood Cells White Blood Cells Epithelial Cells Casts Crystals

definitions of each of these categories and provides examples of commonly performed tests in each. Use of these classifications makes it easier to refer to laboratory tests.

Specimens can be analyzed with the **manual method** or the **automated method.** The method the physician uses to test biologic specimens in the medical office is based on the number and type of laboratory tests performed in the office. Regardless of the method used, a series of basic steps must be followed in testing each specimen, as follows:

1. The specific amount of the specimen necessary for the test method is measured from the specimen sample.
2. The necessary chemical reagents necessary for the test are combined with the specimen.

Table 15-4 Categories of Laboratory Tests*—cont'd

Category	Definition and Commonly Performed Tests	Category	Definition and Commonly Performed Tests

Microbiology	Microbiology is scientific study of microorganisms and their activities. Laboratory analysis in microbiology deals with identification of pathogens present in specimens taken from body (e.g., urine, blood, throat, sputum, wound, urethra, vagina, cerebrospinal fluid). Examples of infectious diseases diagnosed through identification of pathogen present in specimen include:
	   Candidiasis
	   Chlamydia
	   Diphtheria
	   Gonorrhea
	   Meningitis
	   Pertussis
	   Pharyngitis
	   Pneumonia
	   Streptococcal Sore Throat
	   Tetanus
	   Tonsillitis
	   Tuberculosis
	   Urinary Tract Infection
		Cytology	Laboratory analysis in cytology deals with detection of presence of abnormal cells
			   Chromosome Studies
			   Pap Test

Parasitology	Laboratory analysis in parasitology deals with detection of presence of disease-producing human parasites or eggs present in specimens taken from body (e.g., stool, vagina, blood). Examples of human diseases caused by parasites include:
	   Amebiasis
	   Ascariasis
	   Hookworms
	   Malaria
	   Pinworms
	   Scabies
	   Tapeworms
	   Toxoplasmosis
	   Trichinosis
	   Trichomoniasis
		Histology	Histology is microscopic study of form and structure of various tissues that comprise living organisms. Laboratory analysis in histology deals with detection of diseased tissues
			   Tissue Analysis
			   Biopsy Studie

*Categories of laboratory tests are listed, including definitions of each and commonly performed tests or pathologic condition in each category. Tests that are commonly known by their abbreviations are listed that way.

3. The specimen/reagents may require further processing, such as centrifugation, incubation, air drying, or heat fixing.
4. The substance undergoing assessment is manually or automatically measured or identified.
5. The results of the laboratory testing are obtained from a direct readout or with a mathematic calculation.
6. The results are recorded on a laboratory report form or in the patient's chart. The entry includes the patient's name, the date, the time, the name of each laboratory test, the results of the tests, and the name of the individual performing the tests.

These steps are stated in general terms, but a basis is provided for understanding the process of laboratory testing. Textbooks such as this one and the manufacturer's instructions included with testing equipment should be consulted as reference sources to obtain the procedure for performing specific tests. The medical assistant must follow the procedure exactly to ensure accurate and reliable test results.

Manual Method

The manual method of laboratory testing involves performing the series of steps included in the test method by hand, rather than using a self-operating system that performs them automatically. Testing kits are available to speed up the process, making it more convenient to perform the procedure with the manual method. Testing kits are available to perform urinalysis, strep-testing, mononucleosis testing, and urine pregnancy testing. Because each step in the procedure necessitates a physical manipulation and the application of clinical laboratory theory, the manual method requires a more thorough knowledge and skill in testing procedures than does the automated method. The medical assistant must be especially careful to avoid errors in technique that may lead to inaccurate test results.

Automated Analyzers

Tremendous growth has been seen in the development of automated analyzer systems for performing laboratory tests, especially in the area of blood chemistry. Automated systems also are available for certain tests in the areas of hematology, blood banking, serology, urinalysis, and microbiology. Highly sophisticated automated analyzers are almost always confined to an outside laboratory setting because the smaller laboratory workload of the medical office does not justify the expense of such systems. Automated systems have been developed, however, that are more practical and economical for the medical office.

Automated systems designed for use in the medical office permit the processing of a specimen in a short time with accurate test results. Automated instruments take less time and provide greater precision than the manual method because the steps in the testing procedure are automated. Such procedures include the measurement of the amount of the specimen necessary, the use of premeasured chemical reagents, measurement of the reaction, and calculation of results. The test results are obtained with a direct (digital display or printed) readout.

The ease in operating automated systems should not lead to a false sense of security because these systems have limitations that must be recognized—the most critical one being the mechanical failure of the equipment. One of the most important aspects of use of an automated system is the ability to recognize signs that indicate the system is malfunctioning because the malfunctioning may lead to inaccurate test results.

Numerous automated systems are available for the medical office; they are continually growing in number and are being modified as new technology becomes available. The manufacturer of each automated system provides a detailed operating manual with the instrument that includes the information needed to collect, handle, perform quality control procedures on, and test the specimen. In addition, the manufacturer has personnel available for on-site training and service. It is important that the medical assistant become completely familiar with all aspects of any automated system used to perform laboratory tests in the medical office. Some examples of automated analyzer systems include the QBC hematology analyzer (Becton-Dickinson), the Reflotron blood chemistry analyzer (Roche Diagnostics), and the Clinitek urine analyzer (Bayer Corporation).

QUALITY CONTROL

The ultimate goal in the clinical laboratory is to ensure the laboratory test accurately measures what it is supposed to measure; this involves practicing and maintaining a quality control program. **Quality control** may be defined as the application of methods and means to ensure that test results are reliable and valid and errors that may interfere with obtaining accurate test results are detected and eliminated. Quality control is an ongoing process that encompasses every aspect of patient preparation and specimen collection, handling, transport, and testing. The quality control methods that should be used to obtain precision and accuracy in these areas have already been presented in this chapter under their respective headings, with the exception of testing, which is discussed here.

Quality control methods used in testing the specimen include the following:
1. Using standards to check the precision and accuracy of laboratory equipment
2. Using controls to identify reagents that are outdated or have been improperly stored or to detect any errors in technique of the individual performing the test
3. Discarding outdated reagents
4. Following the procedure exactly to test the specimen
5. Performing tests in duplicate
6. Periodically checking the accuracy of the test results with a reference laboratory (PT)
7. Maintaining equipment by having it checked periodically for proper working order

Practicing quality control methods ensures that the test results represent the true status of the patient's condition and body functions and provides the physician with reliable information with which to make a diagnosis and prescribe treatment.

LABORATORY SAFETY

Laboratory safety is an important aspect of clinical laboratory testing in the medical office. Many of the laboratory tests performed in the medical office involve the use of strong chemical reagents, the handling of specimens that may contain pathogens, and the use of laboratory equipment. Practicing good techniques in testing laboratory specimens and recognizing potential hazards help reduce accidents in the laboratory. Some areas specifically related to laboratory safety in the medical office are described here.

The careful handling and storing of glassware to prevent breakage should be performed as follows:
1. Carefully arrange glassware in storage cabinets to prevent breakage.
2. Carefully remove glassware from storage cabinets.
3. If glassware does break, dispose of it in a puncture-resistant container to protect trash handlers from the shards.

The medical assistant should handle all chemical reagents carefully by adhering to the following instructions:
1. Ensure that all reagent containers are clearly and properly labeled.
2. If a label is loose, reattach it immediately.
3. Recap reagent containers immediately after use to prevent spills.

Laboratory specimens should be handled carefully as follows:
1. Follow the OSHA Bloodborne Pathogens Standard in collecting and handling of laboratory specimens.

2. Wash hands immediately if some of the material contained in the specimen is accidentally touched.
3. Avoid hand-to-mouth contact while working with specimens.
4. Immediately clean up any specimen spilled on the worktable, and cleanse the table with a disinfectant.
5. Properly dispose of all contaminated needles, syringes, specimen containers, and infectious waste.
6. Cover any break in the skin, such as a cut or scratch, with a bandage.

7. Ensure that all specimen containers are tightly capped to prevent leakage.
8. Handle all laboratory equipment and supplies properly and with care as indicated by the manufacturer. For example, wait until the centrifuge comes to a complete stop before opening it.

 *Check out the **Companion CD** bound with the book to access additional interactive activities.*

MEDICAL PRACTICE and the LAW

Laboratory procedures must be performed with precision to obtain accurate test results. Pay particular attention to each step in the procedure. Inaccurate laboratory results may cause the physician to incorrectly diagnose a patient's condition, which could lead to the wrong treatment. This situation could lead to a lawsuit.

Certain federal regulations govern laboratory testing, including those from CLIA and OSHA. These regulations help ensure standardization of laboratory tests and safe handling of reagents, blood, and body fluids to prevent contamination of specimens and infection of health care workers. Know and follow all regulations. Failure to do so could result in a legal liability. ∎

What Would You Do? What Would You *Not* Do? RESPONSES

Case Study 1
Page 565
What Did Korey Do?
❑ Told Hildy that the laboratory cannot release test results. Explained that they are experts in performing tests but do not have the medical knowledge to know their meanings.
❑ Told Hildy that the physician needed to give her the test results. Explained that the physician was out of town today but that an appointment could be made for her for tomorrow with the physician to discuss the results.

What Did Korey Not Do?
❑ Did not give Hildy the test results.
❑ Did not alarm Hildy that something might be wrong.

What Would You Do?/What Would You *Not* Do? Review Korey's response and place a checkmark next to the information you included in your response. List additional information you included in your response.

_____
_____
_____
_____

Case Study 2
Page 569
What Did Korey Do?
❑ Told Hans that the term "clinical diagnosis" means what the physician "thinks" is wrong before the laboratory tests are performed. Explained that when the test results are returned, the physician would be able to make a final diagnosis and then he would determine what treatment is needed.
❑ Told Hans that a lipid profile includes several tests, and one of those tests is a cholesterol test. Explained that the tests in a lipid profile all help to determine whether someone is at risk for heart disease.
❑ Told Hans that he could not have any coffee until after his blood was drawn because it would affect the test results. Told him that his test could be scheduled first thing in the morning if that would help.

What Did Korey Not Do?
❑ Did not tell Hans he could have a cup of coffee before the laboratory tests.
❑ Did not tell Hans that he should not be eating doughnuts if he was concerned about his heart.

Continued

What Would You Do? What Would You *Not* Do? RESPONSES—cont'd

What Would You Do?/What Would You *Not* Do? Review Korey's response and place a checkmark next to the information you included in your response. List additional information you included in your response.

_____
_____
_____
_____

Case Study 3
Page 570
What Did Korey Do?
❑ Stressed to Kathleen that if the laboratory test results are abnormal, it is better to know so that the physician can help make her better.
❑ Told Kathleen that many patients feel the same way about having blood drawn, so she is not alone. Relayed to her that her fear is normal, and she has no reason to be embarrassed.
❑ Told Kathleen that she should tell the laboratory about her last experience so that they could make it easier for her. Explained that they would probably put her in a reclining position to draw her blood so that she would not get light-headed.

❑ Gave Kathleen some suggestions on how to relax during the venipuncture. Told her to turn her head when the blood was drawn.
❑ Asked Kathleen whether she had any additional symptoms.
❑ Checked with the physician to see whether he wanted to keep her appointment for today or have her appointment rescheduled after the laboratory work is completed.

What Did Korey Not *Do?*
❑ Did not ignore or minimize Kathleen's concerns and fears.
❑ Did not tell Kathleen that her test results would probably be fine.

What Would You Do?/What Would You *Not* Do? Review Korey's response and place a checkmark next to the information you included in your response. List additional information you included in your response.

_____
_____
_____
_____

APPLY YOUR KNOWLEDGE

Choose the best answer to each of the following questions.

1. Jennifer Keyes, an 18-year-old woman, comes to the office with a painful sore throat, extreme fatigue, fever, and swollen glands. After taking a health history and performing an examination, Dr. Invivo suspects that Jennifer may have infectious mononucleosis. He asks Korey McGrew, CMA, to run a Monospot test. The purpose of Dr. Invivo ordering this test is to:
   A. Confirm his clinical diagnosis.
   B. Ensure Jennifer is not allergic to antibiotics.
   C. Regulate Jennifer's treatment.
   D. Comply with state regulations.

2. Korey performs the Monospot test in the office laboratory. The name given to this type of laboratory is:
   A. CLIA
   B. Reference laboratory
   C. POL
   D. HIPAA

3. Because Jennifer also has paleness and shortness of breath, Dr. Invivo decides to order a CBC to rule out iron deficiency anemia. Korey is getting ready to draw the blood specimen to send to Outside Laboratory for testing. Korey wants to be sure that she uses the correct color stopper blood tube. The best way to obtain this information is to:
   A. Send an email to Outside Laboratory requesting this information.
   B. Look at a laboratory report from Outside Laboratory.
   C. Look in the *Farmer's Almanac*.
   D. Refer to Outside Laboratory's laboratory directory.

4. Korey completes the laboratory request form to accompany the blood specimen to Outside Laboratory. Korey is careful to ensure she includes Jennifer's age on the request form because Korey realizes:
   A. The laboratory needs this information for third-party billing.
   B. The normal range for some tests varies based on the age of the patient.
   C. The type of test procedure the laboratory uses to analyze the specimen depends on the age of the patient.
   D. Outside Laboratory will want to send Jennifer balloons on her next birthday.

APPLY YOUR KNOWLEDGE—cont'd

5. Jennifer's test results are returned by Outside Laboratory's courier service the next day. The hemoglobin value on the report is 10 g/dL. To determine whether this value is normal, Korey should compare this value with:
    A. Jennifer's social security number.
    B. The normal range published in a laboratory reference text.
    C. The normal range for hemoglobin on the laboratory report from Outside Laboratory.
    D. Jennifer's last hemoglobin test result listed in her medical record.

6. After receiving Jennifer's laboratory report and highlighting values outside the normal range, Korey takes the following action:
    A. Files the laboratory report in Jennifer's medical record.
    B. Calls Jennifer to inform her of the abnormal test results.
    C. Makes a tentative diagnosis of Jennifer's condition.
    D. Places the report on Dr. Invivo's desk for his review.

7. Keith Thompson comes to the medical office for a complete physical examination. Keith has a history of heart disease in his family. Dr. Invivo wants to have a lipid profile performed. Korey McGrew, CMA, explains to Keith the patient preparation necessary for this test. Keith returns to the office the next morning to have blood drawn. Which of the following statements would indicate that Keith did not prepare properly for this test?
    A. My last meal was at 6 PM last night, but I had a glass of water when I got up this morning.
    B. I had a cup of black coffee this morning with low-fat milk.
    C. I ran 5 miles this morning before coming to the office.
    D. I rinsed out my mouth with mouthwash this morning.

8. Dr. Invivo tells Korey to review the patient preparation instructions again with Keith and have him return the next day. Keith tells Korey that he does not understand why his blood cannot be drawn now. The most appropriate response for Korey to make would be:
    A. If you would have listened the first time, you would not have to come back.
    B. The laboratory will refuse to test your blood specimen if you have not prepared properly.
    C. It is beyond me; Dr. Invivo has a habit of making strange requests.
    D. If your blood is drawn now, the test results may be inaccurate, and you will not receive proper care.

9. Dr. Invivo purchases a blood chemistry analyzer for the office. Korey McGrew, CMA, realizes that the tests run on this analyzer are considered moderate-complexity tests; the following will need to be performed to comply with CLIA requirements:
    A. Calibration of the analyzer every 6 months.
    B. Two levels of controls run each day.
    C. Documentation of when errors occur and what actions are taken to correct them.
    D. All of the above.

10. Korey is spinning a blood tube in the centrifuge so that she can obtain serum for laboratory tests. What is an important safety practice to follow with a centrifuge?
    A. Waiting until the centrifuge comes to a complete stop before removing the blood tube.
    B. Opening the centrifuge while it is spinning to see whether the blood is separating properly.
    C. Using her hand to help the centrifuge come to a complete stop after the timer goes off.
    D. Placing the centrifuge on a Mayo stand so that it is easily accessible.

CERTIFICATION REVIEW

❑ **The purpose of laboratory testing** is to assist in the diagnosis of pathologic conditions, to evaluate a patient's progress, to regulate treatment, to establish a patient's baseline, to prevent or reduce the severity of disease, and to comply with state law if necessary. A routine test is a laboratory test performed on a routine basis on an apparently healthy patient to assist in the early detection of disease.

❑ **POL** consists of an in-house medical office laboratory. Laboratory tests that are convenient to execute and commonly required are often performed in the POL. Outside laboratories include hospital and privately owned commercial laboratories.

❑ **A laboratory request** is a printed form that contains a list of the most frequently ordered laboratory tests. The laboratory request includes the physician's name and address; the patient's name, age, and gender; the date and time of collection of the specimen; the laboratory tests desired; the source of the specimen; the clinical diagnosis; and medications taken by the patient. A profile consists of numerous laboratory tests that provide related information used to determine the health status of a patient.

❑ **The purpose of the laboratory report** is to relay the results of the laboratory tests to the physician. Information included on a laboratory report is as follows: the name, address, and telephone number of the laboratory; the physician's name and address; the patient's name, age, and gender; the patient accession number; the date the specimen was received by the laboratory; the date the results were reported by the laboratory; the names of the tests performed; the results of the tests; and the normal range for each test performed. The normal range is a certain established and acceptable parameter or reference range within which the laboratory test results of a healthy individual are expected to fall.

❑ **Laboratory safety** is an important aspect of clinical laboratory testing in the medical office. Practicing good techniques in testing laboratory specimens and recognizing potential hazards helps reduce accidents in the laboratory.

❑ **Some laboratory tests** require advance patient preparation to obtain a quality specimen suitable for testing. A specimen obtained from a patient who has not prepared properly may invalidate the test results and necessitate calling the patient back to collect a specimen again. The specific type of preparation necessary for a particular test depends on the test ordered and the method used to perform it. A common patient preparation requirement for laboratory testing is fasting. Fasting means that the patient must abstain from food or fluids (except water) for a specified amount of time (usually 12 to 14 hours) before the collection of a specimen.

❑ **A specimen** is a small sample taken from the body to represent the nature of the whole. Examples of specimens include blood, urine, feces, sputum, a cervical and vaginal scraping of cells, and a sample of a secretion or discharge taken from various parts of the body such as the nose, throat, wound, ear, eye, vagina, or urethra.

❑ **The purpose of CLIA** is to improve the quality of laboratory testing in the United States. CLIA consists of federal regulations governing all facilities that perform laboratory tests for health assessment or for the diagnosis, prevention, or treatment of disease.

❑ **CLIA regulations** establish three categories of laboratory testing—waived tests, moderate-complexity tests, and high-complexity tests. Laboratories that perform moderate-complexity or high-complexity tests must meet the CLIA regulations. Laboratories that perform only waived tests must apply for a certificate of waiver from HCFA, which exempts them from many of the CLIA requirements.

❑ **Quality control** is the application of methods to ensure that test results are reliable and valid and that errors are detected and eliminated. Quality control is an ongoing process that encompasses every aspect of patient preparation and specimen collection, handling, transport, and testing.

TERMINOLOGY REVIEW

Automated method *(for testing laboratory specimens)* A method of laboratory testing in which the series of steps in the test method is performed with an automated analyzer.

Fasting Abstaining from food or fluids (except water) for a specified amount of time before the collection of a specimen.

Homeostasis The state in which body systems are functioning normally, and the internal environment of the body is in equilibrium; the body is in a healthy state.

In vivo Occurring in the living body or organism.

Laboratory test The clinical analysis and study of materials, fluids, or tissues obtained from patients to assist in diagnosis and treatment of disease.

Manual method A method of laboratory testing in which the series of steps in the test method is performed by hand.

Normal range *(for laboratory tests)* A certain established and acceptable parameter or reference range within which the laboratory test results of a healthy individual are expected to fall.

Plasma The liquid part of the blood, consisting of a clear, yellowish fluid that comprises approximately 55% of the total blood volume.

Profile Numerous laboratory tests providing related or complementary information used to determine the health status of a patient.

Quality control The application of methods to ensure that test results are reliable and valid and that errors are detected and eliminated.

Routine test A laboratory test performed routinely on apparently healthy patients to assist in the early detection of disease.

Serum The clear, straw-colored part of the blood (plasma) that remains after the solid elements and the clotting factor fibrinogen have been separated out of it.

Specimen A small sample of something taken to show the nature of the whole.

ON THE WEB

For Information on Aging:

National Institute on Aging: www.nia.nih.gov

Administration on Aging: www.aoa.dhhs.gov

American Association of Retired Persons: www.aarp.org

Social Security Administration: www.ssa.gov

Centers for Medicare and Medicaid Services: www.cms.hhs.gov

Growth House: www.growthhouse.org

The AGS Foundation for Health in Aging: www.healthinaging.org

The Institute for Geriatric Social Work: www.bu.edu/igsw

Geriatrics at Your Fingertips: www.geriatricsatyourfingertips.org

Family Caregiver Alliance: www.caregiver.org

Maturity Health Matters: www.fda.gov/cdrh/healthmatters

Senior Citizens Resources: www.firstgov.gov

Medicare: www.medicare.gov

Aging Statistics: www.agingstats.gov

Alzheimer's Foundation of America: www.alzfdn.org

Urinalysis

Clinical Competencies

Specimen Collection
Instruct patients in the collection of a clean-catch midstream
    urine specimen.

Diagnostic Testing
Use methods of quality control.
Perform urinalysis.
Screen and follow-up test results.

General Competencies

Patient Instruction
Instruct individual patients according to their needs.
Instruct and demonstrate the use and care of patient equipment.
Provide instruction for health care maintenance and disease pre-
    vention.

KEY TERMS

agglutination (ah-gloo-tih-NAY-shun)
bilirubinuria (bill-ih-roo-bin-YUR-ee-ah)
bladder catheterization
glycosuria (glie-koe-SOO-ree-ah)
ketonuria (kee-toe-NOO-ree-ah)
ketosis (kee-TOE-sis)
micturition (mik-tur-ISH-un)
nephrons (NEF-ron)
oliguria (oh-lig-YUR-ee-ah)
pH (PEE-AYCH)

polyuria (pol-ee-YUR-ee-ah)
proteinuria (proe-ten-YUR-ee-ah)
refractive index
refractometer (reh-frak-TOM-ih-tur)
renal threshold (REE-nul-THRESH-hold)
specific gravity
supernatant (soo-per-NAY-tent)
suprapubic aspiration
urinalysis (yur-in-AL-ih-sis)
void (VOYD)

Structure and Function of the Urinary System

The function of the urinary system is to regulate the fluid and electrolyte balance of the body and to remove waste products. The urinary system consists of the kidneys, the ureters, the urinary bladder, and the urethra (Figure 16-1). The *kidneys* are bean-shaped organs approximately 4.5 inches (11.5 cm) long and 2 to 3 inches (5 to 8 cm) wide; they are located in the lumbar region of the body. Urine drains from the kidneys into the urinary bladder through two tubes known as *ureters*. Each ureter is approximately 10 to 12 inches long and ½ inch in diameter. The urine produced by the kidneys is propelled into the urinary bladder by the force of gravity and the peristaltic waves of the ureters. The *urinary bladder* is a hollow, muscular sac that can hold approximately 500 ml of urine. Its function is to store and expel urine. The *urethra* is a tube that extends from the urinary bladder to the outside of the body. The *urinary meatus* is the external opening of the urethra. In males, the urethra functions in transporting urine and reproductive secretions. In females, the urethra functions in urination only.

Each kidney contains approximately 1 million smaller units known as **nephrons** (Figure 16-2). The nephron is the functional unit of the kidney. It filters waste substances from the blood and dilutes them with water to produce urine. Another function of the nephron is reabsorption. Some substances filtered by the nephron, such as water,

glucose, and electrolytes, are needed by the body and are reabsorbed or returned to the body for future use.

COMPOSITION OF URINE

A physiologic change in the body caused by disease can create a disturbance in one or more of the functions of the kidney. Detection of such a disturbance can be made with the examination of urine and other body fluids such as blood.

Urine is composed of 95% water and 5% organic and inorganic waste products. Organic waste products consist of urea, uric acid, ammonia, and creatinine. Urea is present in the greatest amounts and is derived from the breakdown of proteins. Inorganic waste products include chloride, sodium, potassium, calcium, magnesium, phosphate, and sulfate.

A normal adult excretes approximately 750 to 2000 ml of urine per day. This amount varies according to the amount of fluid consumed and the amount of fluid lost through other means, such as perspiration, feces, and water vapor from the lungs. An excessive increase in urine output is known as **polyuria,** with the urine volume exceeding 2000 ml in 24 hours. Polyuria may be caused by the excessive intake of fluids or the intake of fluids that contain caffeine (e.g., coffee, tea, cola), which is a mild diuretic. Certain drugs, such as diuretics, and the pathologic conditions of diabetes mellitus, diabetes insipidus, and renal disease also may result in polyuria. A decreased or scanty urine output is known as **oliguria.** In the case of oliguria, the urine volume is less than 400 ml in 24 hours. Oliguria may

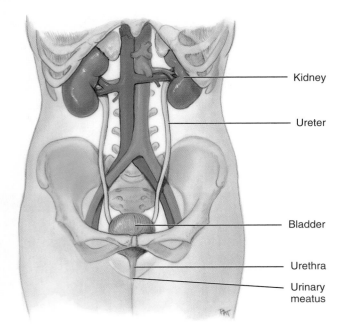

Figure 16-1. Structures that make up the urinary system. (Modified from Applegate EJ: *The anatomy and physiology learning system,* ed 2, Philadelphia, 2000, Saunders.)

occur with decreased fluid intake, dehydration, profuse perspiration, vomiting, diarrhea, or kidney disease. The normal act of voiding urine is known as **micturition.**

Terms Relating to the Urinary System

The medical assistant should have a thorough knowledge of the following terms used to describe symptoms associated with the urinary system:

Anuria   Failure of the kidneys to produce urine.

Diuresis   Secretion and passage of large amounts of urine.

Dysuria   Difficult or painful urination.

Frequency   The condition of having to urinate often.

Hematuria   Blood present in the urine.

Nocturia   Excessive (voluntary) urination during the night.

Nocturnal enuresis   Inability of an individual to control urination at night during sleep (bedwetting).

Oliguria   Decreased output of urine.

Polyuria   Increased output of urine.

Pyuria   Pus present in the urine.

Retention   The inability to empty the bladder. The urine is being produced normally but is not being voided.

Urgency   The immediate need to urinate.

Urinary incontinence   The inability to retain urine.

COLLECTION OF URINE

The advantage of urine testing is that urine is readily available and does not require an invasive procedure or the use of special equipment to obtain. For accurate test results,

however, the medical assistant must adhere to proper urine collection procedures to obtain the proper specimen as ordered by the physician.

Guidelines for Urine Collection

The guidelines listed should be followed in collection of a urine specimen:

1. The medical assistant must obtain an adequate volume of urine as necessary for the type of test (usually 30 to 50 ml of urine).
2. Each specimen must be labeled properly with the patient's name, the date and time of collection, and the type of specimen (i.e., urine) to avoid any mix-ups in specimens.
3. Any medication the patient is taking should be recorded on the laboratory requisition and in the patient's chart because some medications may interfere with the accuracy of the test results.
4. If possible, the collection of a urine specimen should be avoided in women during menstruation and for several days thereafter because the specimen may become contaminated with blood. This results in a false-positive test result for blood in the urine.
5. The medical assistant should take into consideration that voiding may be difficult for patients under stress and anxiety. In these instances, understanding and patience should be conveyed to the patient.
6. A urine specimen may be difficult to obtain from a child, even with the assistance of a parent. In this case, the physician should be informed because another collection method may be used, such as a urine collection bag, suprapubic aspiration, or catheterization of the patient.

Urine Specimen Collection Methods

The type of test to be performed often dictates the method used to collect the urine specimen. A first-voided morning specimen is recommended for pregnancy testing, and a clean-catch midstream specimen is necessary for identification of the presence of a urinary tract infection (UTI).

Most offices use disposable plastic urine specimen containers. These containers are available in different sizes and

What Would You Do? What Would You *Not* Do?

Case Study 1

Yusuke Urameshi is at the office with fever and chills, dysuria, frequency, and difficulty urinating. The physician suspects that Mr. Urameshi has prostatitis and orders a clean-catch urine specimen for a complete urinalysis, including a microscopic examination of the sediment. Mr. Urameshi tries to collect the specimen but is able to collect only 5 ml of urine. He says that he is worried about what is wrong with him and that he thinks his nervousness is making it hard to get a specimen. Mr. Urameshi says that it is probably just as well because he did not understand how to cleanse himself, and he is not sure that he did it right. ■

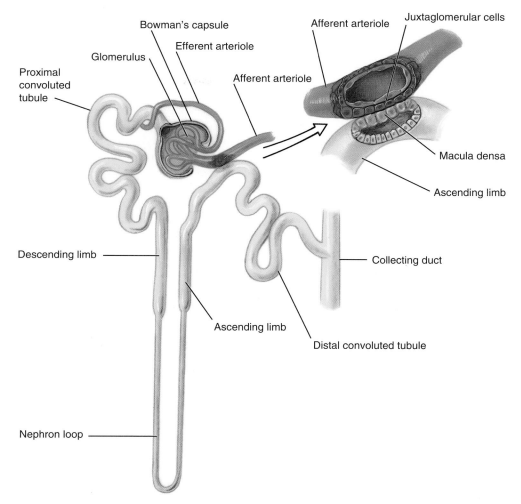

Figure 16-2. Nephron. (From Applegate EJ: *The anatomy and physiology learning system,* ed 2, Philadelphia, 2000, Saunders.)

come with lids to prevent spillage and to reduce bacterial and other types of contamination.

Random Specimen

Urine testing in the medical office is often performed on freshly voided, random specimens. The medical assistant instructs the patient to **void** into a clean, dry, wide-mouthed container, and the urine is tested immediately at the medical office.

First-Voided Morning Specimen

In many cases, a first-voided morning specimen may be desired for testing because it contains the greatest concentration of dissolved substances, and a small amount of an abnormal substance that is present would be more easily detected. The patient should be instructed to collect the first specimen of the morning after rising and to preserve the specimen by refrigerating it until it is brought to the medical office. It is important to provide the patient with a specimen container to prevent the patient's use of a container from home that might harbor contaminants and affect the test results.

Clean-Catch Midstream Specimen

The urinary bladder and most of the urethra are normally free of microorganisms, whereas the distal urethra and urinary meatus normally harbor microorganisms. If the urine is being cultured and examined for bacteria, a clean-catch midstream specimen is necessary to prevent contamination of the specimen with these normally present microorganisms. Only microorganisms that may be causing the patient's condition are desired in the urine specimen. A clean-catch midstream collection may be ordered for the detection of a UTI and the evaluation of the effectiveness of drug therapy in a patient undergoing treatment for such an infection.

The purpose of the clean-catch midstream collection is the removal of microorganisms from the urinary meatus and the distal urethra. This is accomplished by instructing the patient to thoroughly cleanse the area surrounding the meatus and to void a small amount of urine into the toilet,

The urine becomes yellow-brown or greenish, and a yellow foam appears when the urine is shaken.

Urobilinogen

Normally, bilirubin is excreted by the liver into the intestinal tract. Bacteria present in the intestines convert it to urobilinogen. Approximately 50% of the urobilinogen is reabsorbed into the body for reexcretion by the liver. Small amounts may appear in the urine, but most of the urobilinogen is excreted in the feces. An increase in the production of bilirubin increases the amount of urobilinogen excreted in the urine. Conditions such as excessive hemolysis of red blood cells, infectious hepatitis, cirrhosis, congestive heart failure, and infectious mononucleosis may increase the level of urobilinogen in the urine.

Blood

Blood is considered an abnormal constituent of urine, unless it is present as a contaminant during menstruation. The condition in which blood is found in the urine is termed *hematuria.* Hematuria may be the result of injury or disorders such as cystitis, tumors of the bladder, urethritis, kidney stones, and certain kidney disorders.

Nitrite

Nitrite in the urine indicates the presence of a pathogen in the (normally sterile) urinary tract, which results in a UTI. The pathogen possesses the ability to convert nitrate, which normally occurs in the urine, to nitrite, which is normally absent. The nitrite test must be performed with urine that has been in the bladder for at least 4 to 6 hours to ensure that bacteria have converted nitrate to nitrite. Therefore, use of a first-voided morning specimen is recommended. The test should *not* be performed on specimens that have been left standing out because a false-positive result may occur from bacterial contamination from the environment. The nitrite test is a screening test and is usually followed by a quantitative culture and identification of the invading pathogen.

Leukocytes

The presence of leukocytes in the urine is known as *leukocyturia* and accompanies inflammation of the kidneys and the lower urinary tract. Examples of specific conditions include acute and chronic pyelonephritis, cystitis, and urethritis. Reagent strips are available that contain a reagent area that permits the chemical detection of intact and lysed leukocytes in the urine. The advantage of detecting lysed leukocytes is that these cells cannot be observed during a microscopic examination of urine sediment and would otherwise remain undetected. The recommended urine specimen, particularly for women, is a clean-catch midstream collection to prevent contamination of the specimen with leukocytes from vaginal secretions leading to false-positive test results.

Reagent Strips

In the medical office, reagent strips are the most commonly used diagnostic urine testing kit. Reagent strips consist of disposable plastic strips on which separate reagent areas are affixed for testing specific chemical constituents that may be present in the urine during pathologic conditions. The results provide the physician with information to assist in the diagnosis of the following:
- Conditions affecting kidney function (e.g., kidney stones)
- Urinary tract infections
- Conditions affecting carbohydrate metabolism (e.g., diabetes mellitus)
- Conditions affecting liver function (e.g., hepatitis)

The test results also provide the physician with information related to the status of the patient's acid-base balance and urine concentration. Reagent strips are considered qualitative tests, and a positive result necessitates further testing. Table 16-2 presents an outline of reagent strip parameters and the diagnoses in which they assist.

The number and type of reagent areas included on the reagent strip depend on the particular brand of reagent strips. Multistix 10 SG (Bayer Corporation, Tarrytown, NY) contains 10 reagent areas for testing pH, protein, glucose, ketones, bilirubin, blood, urobilinogen, nitrite, specific gravity, and leukocytes. Other brands and the tests included for each are listed in Table 16-1.

The reagent strip procedure in this chapter (Procedure 16-5) is specifically for Multistix 10 SG; however, the procedure can be followed for the chemical testing of urine with most reagent strips. In all instances, the medical assistant should read the manufacturer's instructions before performing the test.

Guidelines for Reagent Strip Urine Testing

Testing urine with reagent strips is a relatively easy procedure to perform. Specific guidelines must be used, however, to obtain accurate test results.
1. *Type of specimen.* The best results are obtained with a freshly voided and thoroughly mixed urine specimen. If the medical assistant is unable to test the specimen within 1 hour of voiding, the specimen should be refrigerated immediately and then allowed to return to room temperature before testing.
2. *Type of collection.* Most reagent strips are designed to be used with a random specimen collection; however, clean-catch midstream and first-voided morning specimens are suggested for specific tests. The nitrite test results are optimized with a first-voided morning specimen, whereas a clean-catch midstream collection is recommended for the leukocyte test.
3. *Specimen container.* The specimen container used must be thoroughly clean and free from any detergent or disinfectant residue because cleansing agents contain oxidants that react with the chemicals on the reagent strip, leading to inaccurate test results. The container should be large enough to allow for complete immersion of all reagent strip areas.
4. *Interpretation of results.* Of particular importance is the comparison of the reagent strip with the color chart. The reagent strip must be compared with the color chart in

Text continued on p. 602

Table 16-2 Urine Test Strip Parameters and the Diagnoses They Assist*

System/Source	Leukocytes	Nitrite	Urine pH		Protein
Genitourinary	Renal infection or inflammation • Acute/chronic pyelonephritis • Glomerulonephritis • Urolithiasis • Tumors • Lower urinary tract infection (cystitis, urethritis, prostatitis)	Bacteriuria • Urinary tract infection (cystitis, urethritis, prostatitis, pyelonephritis)	Up (greater than 6) in: • Renal failure • Bacterial infection (e.g., *Proteus* bacteriuria) • Renal tubular acidosis		Renal, glomerular, or tubular disease • Glomerulonephritis • Glomerulosclerosis (e.g., in diabetes) • Nephrotic syndrome • Pyelonephritis • Renal tuberculosis
Hepatobiliary					
Gastrointestinal			Up in: • Pyloric obstruction	Down in: • Diarrhea • Malabsorption	
Cardiovascular					Congestive heart failure
Hormonal, metabolic, and other systems			Up in: • Alkalosis (metabolic, respiratory)	Down in: • Acidosis (metabolic, respiratory, diabetic) • Pulmonary emphysema • Dehydration	Gout Hypokalemia Preeclampsia Severe febrile infection
Environmental (diet, drugs, stress)	Phenacetin-induced nephritis		Up in: • Diet high in vegetables, citrus fruits • Alkalizing drug use (sodium bicarbonate, acetazolamide)	Down in: • Diet high in meats or other protein, cranberries • Acidifying drug use (e.g., ammonium chloride, methenamine mandelate therapy)	Nephrotoxic drugs

*Reagent strip detection of abnormal urine constituent or concentration characteristic of disease (e.g., glycosuria in diabetes mellitus) may provide useful screen or monitor, but requires confirmation with other laboratory and clinical evidence.

Courtesy Boehringer-Mannheim Diagnostics, Indianapolis, Ind.

Modified from Conn HF, Conn RB (eds): *Current diagnosis 5,* Philadelphia, 1977, Saunders; Davidson I, Henry JB (eds): *Todd-Stanford clinical diagnosis by laboratory methods,* ed 15, Philadelphia, 1974, Saunders; Raphael SS, et al: *Lynch's medical laboratory technology,* ed 3, Philadelphia, 1976, Saunders; Wallach J: *Interpretation of diagnostic tests,* ed 2, Boston, 1974, Little, Brown; Widmann FK: *Goodale's clinical interpretation of laboratory tests,* ed 7, Philadelphia, 1973, Davis.

Table 16-2 Urine Test Strip Parameters and the Diagnoses They Assist*—cont'd

Glucose	Ketones	Urobilinogen	Bilirubin	Blood, Erythrocytes (Hematuria)	Hemoglobin
Renal glycosuria (e.g., during pregnancy Renal tubular disease (e.g., in Fanconi's syndrome) Decreased renal glucose threshold (e.g., in old age)				Renal infection, inflammation, or injury • Renal tuberculosis • Renal infarction • Calculi (urethral, renal) • Polycystic kidneys • Tumors (bladder, renal pelvis, prostate) • Salpingitis • Cystitis	Renal intravascular Hemolysis Acute glomerulonephritis
		Liver cell damage Chronic liver stasis Cirrhosis Dubin-Johnson syndrome Note: May be 0 or down in biliary obstruction	Biliary dysfunction • Gallstones Obstructive jaundice Hepatitis (viral toxic) Dubin-Johnson syndrome	Cirrhosis	
	Vomiting Diarrhea	Note: May be negative with inhibition of intestinal flora by antimicrobial agents		Colon tumor Diverticulitis	
Myocardial infarction				Bacterial endocarditis	
Diabetes mellitus Hemochromatosis Hyperthyroidism Cushing's syndrome Pheochromocytomas	Diabetic ketosis Glycogen storage disease Preeclampsia Acute fever	Sickle cell anemia Hemolytic disease • Pernicious anemia Leptospirosis	Hemolytic disease Leptospirosis	Blood dyscrasias • Hemophilia • Thrombocytopenia • Sickle cell anemia Disseminated lupus erythematosus Malignant hypertension	Hemolytic disease Plasmodium (malaria) Clostridium (tetanus)
Sudden shock or pain Steroid therapy	Weight-reducing diet Ketogenic diet (e.g., in anticonvulsant therapy) Starvation			Hemorrhagenic drugs (e.g., anticoagulant, salicylate) Nephrotoxic agents Internal injury or foreign body Vitamin C or K deficiency	Overexertion Exposure to cold Incompatible blood transfusion Drug-induced hemolysis

good lighting to obtain a good visual match of the color reactions with the color chart provided with the test kit.

5. *Storage of reagent strips.* The reagents on the strips are sensitive to light, heat, and moisture, and the bottle containing the strips must be stored in a cool, dry area with the cap tightly closed to maintain reactivity of the reagent. The bottle may contain a desiccant that should not be removed because its purpose is to promote dryness by absorbing moisture. The bottle of reagent strips must be stored at a temperature less than 86°F (less than 30°C) but should not be stored in the refrigerator or freezer. A tan-to-brown discoloration or darkening on the reagent areas indicates deterioration of the chemical reagent strips, in which case the strips should not be used because the test results would be inaccurate.

Quality Control

Quality control should be used in a chemical examination of urine with a reagent strip. Quality control ensures the reliability of test results by (1) determining whether the reagent strips are reacting properly and (2) confirming that the test is being properly performed and accurately interpreted.

To check the reliability of Multistix reagent strips, the Chek-Stix control (Bayer Corporation) should be used. Each Chek-Stix control consists of a firm plastic strip to which are affixed seven synthetic ingredients (Figure 16-6). The control strip is reconstituted by immersing it in distilled water for 30 minutes, which allows the ingredients on the strip to dissolve in the water. After reconstitution, the resulting solution is tested in the same manner as a urine specimen. The values to be expected are outlined on a reference sheet that accompanies the control strips. If the expected values are not obtained, the cause of the problem must be determined and corrected. Factors that can cause a problem include outdated reagent strips, improper storage of the strips, or an error in testing technique. The quality control test should be performed when each bottle of strips is opened for the first time or when there is a question of reliability regarding the testing strips.

Urine Analyzer

Urine analyzers are used to perform an automatic chemical examination of urine with reagent strips. They offer the advantage of the ability to perform the chemical analysis quickly and to interpret results automatically. These analyzers are used most often in medical offices that perform moderate-volume to large-volume urine testing.

The Clinitek Analyzer (Bayer Corporation) is an example of a urine analyzer that automatically reads Multistix SG and other (Bayer) urinalysis reagent strips (Figure 16-7A). The results are printed out, and abnormal results are flagged to call attention to them (Figure 16-7B). Different models are available; some can be used to perform a color and appearance analysis and a microscopic examination of the urine.

Text continued on p. 605

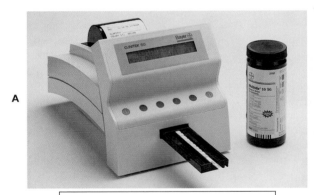

A

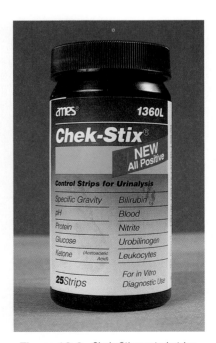

Figure 16-6. Chek-Stix control strips.

B

```
ID: ____Erika Seager____
        11-16-06    5:37 PM
CLARITY: ____Clear_____
COLOR: YELLOW

MULTISTIX 10 SG

GLU     NEGATIVE
BIL     NEGATIVE
KET     NEGATIVE
SG      1.025
BLO*    TRACE-LYSED
pH      5.5
PRO     NEGATIVE
URO     0.2 E.U./dl
NIT     NEGATIVE
LEU     NEGATIVE
```

Figure 16-7. **A,** Clinitek Urine Analyzer. **B,** Clinitek printout.

PROCEDURE 16-5   Chemical Testing of Urine with the Multistix 10 SG Reagent Strip

Outcome Perform a chemical assessment of a urine specimen.

Equipment/Supplies

- Disposable gloves
- Multistix 10 SG reagent strips
- Urine container
- Timer
- Laboratory report form

---

1. **Procedural Step.** Obtain a freshly voided urine specimen from the patient with a clean container. The specimen should be uncentrifuged and at room temperature.
   Principle. The best results are obtained with a freshly voided specimen. The container should be clean because contaminants could affect the results. Uncentrifuged specimens ensure a homogeneous sample.

2. **Procedural Step.** Sanitize your hands.

3. **Procedural Step.** Assemble the equipment. Check the expiration date of the reagent strips.
   Principle. Outdated reagent strips may lead to inaccurate test results.

4. **Procedural Step.** Apply gloves. Remove a reagent strip from its plastic container, and recap the container immediately. Do not touch the test areas with your fingers or lay the strip on the table. It is permissible, however, to lay the reagent strip on a clean, dry paper towel.
   Principle. Recapping the container is necessary to prevent exposing the strips to environmental moisture, light, and heat, which cause altered reagent reactivity. Contamination of the test areas by the hands or table surface may affect the accuracy of the test results.

5. **Procedural Step.** Thoroughly mix the urine specimen and remove the lid from the container. Using the dominant hand, completely immerse the reagent strip in the urine specimen, and remove it immediately.

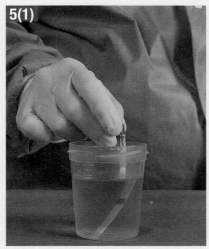
Completely immerse the reagent strip in the urine.

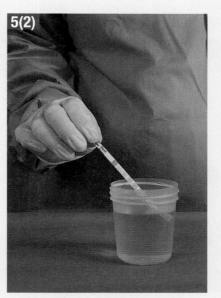
Run the edge of the strip against the urine container.

While removing, run the edge of the strip against the rim of the urine container to remove excess urine.
Principle. The strip should be completely immersed to ensure that all test areas are moistened for accurate test results. Prolonged immersion of the reagent strip and failure to remove excess urine may cause the reagents to dissolve and leach onto adjacent test areas, affecting the accuracy of the test results.

6. **Procedural Step.** With the nondominant hand, start the timer, pick up the reagent strip container and rotate it to the color chart. Hold the reagent strip in a horizontal position and place it as close as possible to the corresponding color blocks on the color chart. Do not lay the strip directly on the color chart because this would result in the urine soiling the chart. Read the results carefully and at the exact reading times specified on the color chart and as indicated here:

Glucose, 30 seconds	Bilirubin, 30 seconds
Ketones, 40 seconds	Specific gravity, 45 seconds
Blood, 60 seconds	pH, 60 seconds
Protein, 60 seconds	Urobilinogen, 60 seconds
Nitrite, 60 seconds	Leukocytes, 2 minutes

Principle. Holding the strip in a horizontal position avoids soiling your gloves with urine and prevents

Continued

PROCEDURE 16-5

PROCEDURE 16-5 **Chemical Testing of Urine with the Multistix 10 SG Reagent Strip—cont'd**

reagents from running over into the adjacent testing areas, causing inaccurate test results. The strip must be read at the proper time to avoid dissolving out reagents, leading to inaccurate test results.

7. **Procedural Step.** Dispose of the strip in a regular waste container.

8. **Procedural Step.** Remove gloves, and sanitize your hands.

9. **Procedural Step.** Chart the results. The results should be charted following the interpretation guide provided above each color block on the color chart. Most offices use a preprinted reporting form to make it easier to record results. The recording should include the date and time, the brand name of the test used (Multistix 10 SG), and the results.

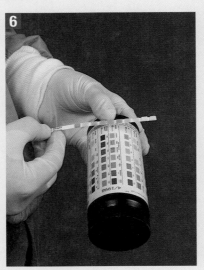

Hold the strip horizontally and read the results.

CHARTING EXAMPLE

Multistix® 10 SG *Reageant Strips for Urinalysis*

PATIENT   Annette Ross

DATE   3/22/08   TIME   9:45 a.m.

TEST							
LEUKOCYTES	NEGATIVE ☑		TRACE ☐	SMALL ☐ +	MODERATE ☐ ++	LARGE ☐ +++	
NITRITE	NEGATIVE ☑		POSITIVE ☐	POSITIVE ☐	(Any degree of uniform pink color is found)		
UROBILINOGEN	NORMAL ☑ 0.2	NORMAL ☐ 1	mg/dL ☐ 2	4 ☐	8 ☐ (1mg = approx. 1 BU)		
PROTEIN	NEGATIVE ☐	TRACE ☑	mg/dL ☐ 30 *	100 ☐ ++	300 ☐ +++	2000 OR MORE ☐	
pH	5.0 ☑	6.0 ☐	6.5 ☐	7.0 ☐	7.5 ☐	8.0 ☐	8.5 ☐
BLOOD	NEGATIVE ☑	NON-HEMOLYZED TRACE ☐	NON-HEMOLYZED MODERATE ☐	HEMOLYZED TRACE ☐	SMALL ☐ +	MODERATE ☐ ++	LARGE ☐ +++
SPECIFIC GRAVITY	1.000 ☐	1.006 ☐	1.010 ☐	1.015 ☑	1.020 ☐	1.025 ☐	1.030 ☐
KETONE	NEGATIVE ☑	mg/dL	TRACE ☐ 5	SMALL ☐ 15	MODERATE ☐ 40	LARGE ☐ 80	LARGE ☐ 160
BILIRUBIN	NEGATIVE ☑		SMALL ☐ +	MODERATE ☐ ++	LARGE ☐ +++		
GLUCOSE	NEGATIVE ☑	g/L (%) mg/dL	1/10 tr.) ☐ 100	1/6 ☐ 250	1/2 ☐ 500	1 ☐ 1000	2 or more ☐ 2000 or more

(Modified and printed by permission of Siemens Medical Solutions Diagnostics, Tarrytown, NY, 10591.)

BAYER   **2161**

Multistix® 10 SG

Reagent Strips for Urinalysis
For In Vitro Diagnostic Use

COLOR CHART

Bayer BAYER

READ PRODUCT INSERT BEFORE USE.
IMPORTANT: Do not expose to direct sunlight.
Do not use after 4/01.

TESTS AND READING TIME

TEST							
LEUKOCYTES 2 minutes	NEGATIVE		TRACE	SMALL +	MODERATE ++	LARGE +++	
NITRITE 60 seconds	NEGATIVE		POSITIVE	POSITIVE	(Any degree of uniform pink color is positive)		
UROBILINOGEN 60 seconds	NORMAL 0.2	NORMAL 1	mg/dL 2	4	8 (1 mg = approx. 1EU)		
PROTEIN 60 seconds	NEGATIVE	TRACE	mg/dL 30 +	100 ++	300 +++	2000 or more ++++	
pH 60 seconds	5.0	6.0	6.5	7.0	7.5	8.0	8.5
BLOOD 60 seconds	NEGATIVE	NON-HEMOLYZED TRACE	NON-HEMOLYZED MODERATE	HEMOLYZED TRACE	SMALL +	MODERATE ++	LARGE +++
SPECIFIC GRAVITY 45 seconds	1.000	1.005	1.010	1.015	1.020	1.025	1.030
KETONE 40 seconds	NEGATIVE	mg/dL	TRACE 5	SMALL 15	MODERATE 40	LARGE 80	LARGE 160
BILIRUBIN 30 seconds	NEGATIVE		SMALL +	MODERATE ++	LARGE +++		
GLUCOSE 30 seconds	NEGATIVE	g/dL (%) mg/dL	1/10 (tr.) 100	1/4 250	1/2 500	1 1000	2 or more 2000 or more

Do not use this chart for interpreting test results.

Microscopic Examination of Urine

Urine sediment is the solid material contained in the urine. A microscopic examination of the urine sediment helps clarify results of the physical and chemical examinations. A first-voided morning specimen is generally preferred because it is more concentrated and contains more dissolved substances; small amounts of abnormal substances are more likely to be detected. Use of a fresh specimen is important because changes occur in a specimen left standing out, as previously discussed. These changes affect the reliability of the test results. Procedure 16-6 presents the procedures for preparation of a urine specimen for microscopic examination and examination of the sediment under a microscope. Structures that may be found in a microscopic examination of urine are described next. Tables 16-3 to 16-6 provide an outline of these structures and of the possible causes of their presence.

Red Blood Cells

Red blood cells appear as round, colorless, biconcave discs that are highly refractile. The presence of 0 to 5 per high-power field (HPF) is considered normal. More than this amount may indicate bleeding somewhere along the urinary tract. Table 16-3 lists the possible causes of an abnormal number of red blood cells in the urine. Concentrated urine causes the red blood cells to become shrunken or *crenated,* whereas dilute urine causes them to swell and become rounded, which may cause them to hemolyze. If the red blood cells have hemolyzed, they cannot be seen under the microscope. The presence of blood in the urine still can be identified, however, with a reagent strip, such as Multistix, designed to detect free hemoglobin.

White Blood Cells

White blood cells are round and granular and have a nucleus. They are approximately 1.5 times as large as a red blood cell. The presence of 0 to 8 per HPF is considered normal. More than this amount may indicate inflammation of the genitourinary tract. Table 16-3 lists the possible causes of an abnormal number of white blood cells in the urine.

Epithelial Cells

Most structures that make up the urinary system are composed of several layers of epithelial cells. The outer layer is constantly sloughed off and replaced by the cells underneath it. *Squamous epithelial cells* are large, clear, flat cells with an irregular shape. They contain a small nucleus and come from the urethra, bladder, and vagina. Squamous epithelial cells are normally present in small amounts in the urine. *Renal epithelial cells* are round and contain a large nucleus. They come from the deeper layers of the urinary tract, and their presence in the urine is considered abnormal. Table 16-3 lists the types of epithelial cells and possible causes of the presence of abnormal amounts in the urine.

Casts

Casts are cylindric structures formed in the lumen of the tubules that make up the nephron. Materials in the tubules harden, are flushed out, and appear in the urine in the form of casts. Various types of casts may be present in the urine. Their presence generally indicates a diseased condition.

Casts are named according to what they contain. *Hyaline casts* are pale, colorless cylinders with rounded edges that vary in size. *Granular casts* are hyaline casts that contain granules and are described as "coarsely granular" or "finely granular," depending on the size of the granules. *Fatty casts* are hyaline casts that contain fat droplets. *Waxy casts* are light yellow and have serrated edges; their name is derived from the fact that they appear to be made of wax. *Cellular casts* contain organized structures and are named according to what they contain. Examples include red blood cell casts, which are hyaline casts containing red blood cells; white blood cell casts, which are hyaline casts containing white blood cells; epithelial casts, which are hyaline casts containing epithelial cells; and bacterial casts, which are hyaline casts containing bacteria. Table 16-4 lists the types of casts and possible causes of their presence in urine.

Crystals

A variety of crystals may be found in the urine. The type and number vary with the pH of the urine. Abnormal crystals include leucine, tyrosine, cystine, and cholesterol. Crystals that commonly appear in acid urine include amorphous urates, uric acid, and calcium oxalate. Crystals that commonly appear in alkaline urine include amorphous phosphate, triple phosphate, calcium phosphate, and ammonium urate crystals. Table 16-5 lists the types of urine crystals and their significance when found in urine.

Miscellaneous Structures

Mucous threads are normally present in small amounts in the urine. They appear as long, wavy, threadlike structures with pointed ends.

Bacteria should not normally exist in the urinary tract. The presence of more than a few bacteria may indicate either contamination of the specimen during collection or a

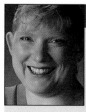

Memories *from* Externship

Linda Proffitt: My main problem as a student on externship was that I was a little shy. I learned that when your patient is relaxed, he or she is more likely to give you additional and important information about what is wrong. If your patient tenses up during a procedure, it can cause pain for the patient and make the procedure more difficult. When I started to make myself talk more to the patients and staff, things went more smoothly. ■

UTI. Bacteria are small structures and may be rod-shaped or round.

Yeast cells are smooth, refractile bodies with an oval shape. A distinguishing feature of yeast cells is small buds that project from the cells involved with reproduction. Yeast cells in the urine of female patients are usually a vaginal contaminant caused by the yeast *Candida albicans* and produce the vaginal infection known as *candidiasis*. They also may be present in the urine of patients with diabetes mellitus.

Parasites may be present in the urine sediment as a contaminant from fecal or vaginal material. *Trichomonas vaginalis* is a parasite that causes trichomoniasis vaginitis.

Spermatozoa may be present in the urine of a man or woman after intercourse. The spermatozoa have round heads and long, slender, hairlike tails.

Table 16-6 lists the miscellaneous structures that may be present in the urine and the significance when found.

Text continued on p. 618

PATIENT TEACHING   Urinary Tract Infections

Answer questions patients may have about UTIs.

What is a UTI?
UTI is a general term for the presence of bacteria in any portion of the urinary tract. UTIs, particularly those involving the bladder (cystitis) and urethra (urethritis), are common and treatable. A UTI is usually treated with an antibiotic. Use of all of the antibiotic for the full number of days prescribed by the physician is important, even if the symptoms disappear. If the medication is stopped too soon, the infection may recur and be more difficult to treat than the original infection.

What are the symptoms of a UTI?
The symptoms of a simple UTI (cystitis) commonly include the frequent need to urinate, urgency (meaning the immediate need to urinate), a burning sensation during urination, and sometimes blood in the urine. The symptoms of a more complicated UTI involving the kidneys (pyelonephritis) include the above symptoms as well as lower abdominal discomfort, low back pain, fever, cloudy or foul-smelling urine, and blood in the urine.

Why do women have UTIs more frequently than do men?
Women are more prone to the type of UTI called *cystitis* than are men because the urethra of a woman is much shorter than that of a man, which makes travel up the urethra and into the bladder easier for bacteria. The most common source of infection is bacteria *(Escherichia coli)*. This organism is normally found in the large intestine but can travel from the anal area to the urinary bladder, often as the result of poor hygienic practices. Cystitis occurs if *E. coli* organisms are able to overcome the body's natural defenses when the bacteria reach the urinary bladder and set up an infection.

What can women do to prevent a UTI?
Women prone to development of UTIs should practice include the following prevention measures:

Practice good hygienic measures by always cleaning the genital area from front to back after a bowel movement.

Avoid possible irritants, such as bubble baths, perfumed soaps, feminine hygiene sprays, or the use of strong powders and bleaches for washing underclothes.

Avoid clothing that traps moisture and encourages the growth of microorganisms, such as tight, constricting clothing; nylon panties; and panty hose.

Avoid activities that can contribute to irritation of the urinary meatus, such as prolonged bicycling, motorcycling, horseback riding, and traveling that involves prolonged sitting.

Urinate as soon as possible when you feel the urge. Holding urine in the bladder gives the bacteria more time to grow, which can cause more infection. The more often you urinate, the quicker the bacteria are removed from the bladder.

Seek prompt treatment if you experience any of the symptoms of a UTI.

- Encourage the patient with a UTI to drink plenty of water to help flush the bacteria out of the urinary tract.
- Emphasize to the patient the importance of taking all of the antibiotic for the duration of time prescribed by the physician.
- Emphasize the importance of practicing preventive measures to prevent the occurrence of UTIs.
- Provide the patient with educational materials on UTIs. ∎

Table 16-3 Cells in Urine Sediment

Type	Presence in Normal Urine	Possible Causes of Abnormal Amounts of Cells in Urine	Microscopic Appearance
Red blood cells	0-5 cells per high-power field (depending on preparation of urine sediment)	Inflammatory diseases Acute glomerulonephritis Pyelonephritis Hypertension Renal infarction Trauma Stones Tumor Bleeding diseases Use of anticoagulants	 Red blood cells
White blood cells	0-8 cells per high-power field (depending on preparation of urine sediment)	Pyelonephritis Cystitis Urethritis Prostatitis Transplant rejection (manifested by lymphocytes in urine) Tissue injury accompanied by severe inflammation (manifested by monocytes in urine) Inflammation, immune mechanisms, and other host defense mechanisms (manifested by histiocytes in urine)	 White blood cells
Squamous epithelial cells	Often present, depending on collection technique	Vaginal contamination	 Squamous epithelial cells
Transitional epithelial cells	Moderate number of cells present	Disease of the bladder or renal pelvis Catheterization	 Transitional epithelial cells
Renal tubular epithelial cells	Present in small numbers, higher numbers in infants	Acute tubular necrosis Glomerulonephritis Acute infection Renal toxicity Viral infection	 Renal tubular epithelial cells

Text courtesy Boehringer Mannheim Diagnostics, Indianapolis, Ind.
Photomicrographs courtesy Bayer Corporation, Elkhart, Ind.

Continued

PROCEDURE 16-7   Performing a Rapid Urine Culture Test

Outcome   Perform a rapid urine culture test.

Equipment/Supplies

- Disposable gloves
- Rapid urine culture kit
- Urine specimen (clean-catch midstream specimen)
- Incubator
- Biohazard waste container

Preparing the Specimen

1. Procedural Step. Sanitize your hands, and assemble the equipment. Check the expiration date on the rapid culture test. It should not be used if the expiration date has passed. Label the vial with the patient's name and the date and time of inoculation.
Principle. An expired urine culture test may produce inaccurate test results.

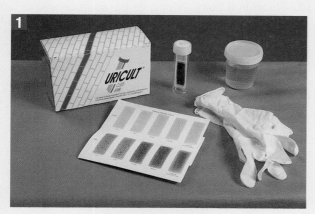

Assemble the equipment.

2. Procedural Step. Apply gloves. Remove the slide from its protective vial by unscrewing the cap of the vial; do not touch the culture media.

3. Procedural Step. Dip the agar-coated slide into the urine specimen; it must be completely immersed. If the urine volume is not sufficient to immerse the agar slide fully, the urine may be poured over the agar surfaces.

4. Procedural Step. Allow excess urine to drain from the slide.

5. Procedural Step. Immediately replace the inoculated slide in its protective vial. Screw the cap on loosely.

6. Procedural Step. Place the vial upright in an incubator for 18 to 24 hours at 93°F to 100°F (35°C to 38°C).
Principle. Incubation for more than 24 hours may cause erroneous test results.

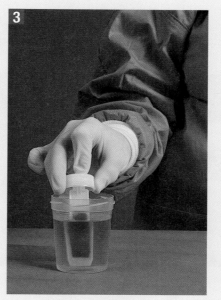

Dip the slide into the urine specimen.

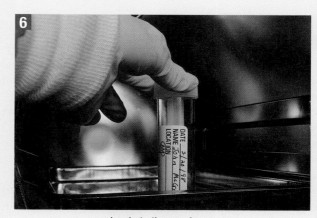

Incubate the specimen.

Continued

PROCEDURE 16-7   *Performing a Rapid Urine Culture Test—cont'd*

Reading Test Results

7. Procedural Step. Apply gloves. Remove the vial from the incubator after the incubation period. Remove the slide from its protective vial, and compare the bacterial colony count density on the agar surface with the colony density reference chart provided by the manufacturer. The bacterial colony density on the agar surface should be matched with the printed example it most closely resembles on the colony density chart. (No actual bacterial colony counting is necessary.)

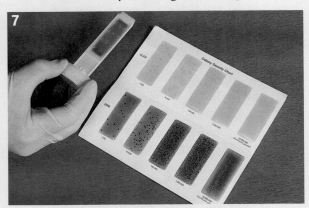

Compare the slide with the reference chart.

8. Procedural Step. Interpret results. The results of rapid urine tests are interpreted as follows:
Normal: Less than 10,000 bacteria/ml of urine.
Significance: A normal result indicates the absence of infection.

Borderline: 10,000 to 100,000 bacteria/ml of urine.
Significance: A borderline result may be caused by chronic and relapsing infections, and it is recommended that the test be repeated.
Positive:
a. More than 100,000 bacteria/ml of urine.
b. Confluent growth, or complete coverage of the agar surface with bacterial colonies, which may occur occasionally when a colony count is more than 100,000 bacteria/ml.
Significance: A positive result indicates that a bacterial infection is present.

9. Procedural Step. Return the slide to the vial, and screw on the cap. (*Note:* To aid in the safe disposal of inoculated slides, it is recommended that the slide be immersed in a disinfectant solution, such as 3% phenol solution or Cidex, before placing the slide in the vial.)

10. Procedural Step. Dispose of the rapid culture test in a biohazard waste container. Remove the gloves, and sanitize the hands.

11. Procedural Step. Chart the results. Include the date and time, the name of the test (e.g., Uricult), and the results.

CHARTING EXAMPLE	
Date	
3/21/08	10:00 a.m. Uricult: Normal. —— L. Proffitt, CMA

URINE PREGNANCY TESTING

The diagnosis of pregnancy can be accomplished several ways. By the eighth week after fertilization, pregnancy can be confirmed with the medical history and physical examination. The physician may desire an earlier diagnosis, however, with a pregnancy test to initiate early prenatal care. A pregnancy test also may be necessary before certain medications are ordered or procedures are performed that may cause injury to a fetus.

In the medical office, immunologic tests are often used for pregnancy testing. These tests are performed on a concentrated urine specimen and rely on the presence of a hormone known as *human chorionic gonadotropin* (HCG) for a positive reaction.

Human Chorionic Gonadotropin

HCG is produced by the developing fertilized egg, and small amounts of it are secreted into the urine and blood. Immediately after conception and implantation of the fertilized egg, the plasma level of HCG increases rapidly and can be used to detect pregnancy with a serum pregnancy test as early as 6 days before the first missed menstrual period . The highest plasma levels of HCG occur at about 8 weeks after conception. After this time, the production of HCG declines and remains at a lower level for the duration of the pregnancy. Within 72 hours of delivery, HCG disappears entirely from the plasma. As a result, pregnancy tests are more sensitive during the first trimester and may show a negative reaction when the level of HCG begins to decline during the second and third trimesters.

Testing Methods

The two main types of urine pregnancy tests are immunoassay enzyme tests and agglutination tests. These tests are used in the medical office because they are convenient to perform and provide immediate test results. Positive and negative reactions are evidenced by a specific visible reaction that is observed and interpreted by the individual performing the test.

Urine pregnancy tests are commercially available in kits that contain all the required reagents and supplies to perform the test. Each kit can be used to perform a specific number of tests, ranging from 10 to 50. The manufacturer's instructions should be followed carefully to prevent inaccurate test results. When performed correctly, urine pregnancy tests are 97% accurate with low occurrences of false-positive test results.

Agglutination Tests

The slide **agglutination** test is sometimes used to perform pregnancy testing in the medical office. Positive test results are based on the inhibition of latex particle agglutination. The test takes place in two steps and can be performed in only 2 minutes. In the first step, a drop of the urine specimen is placed on a specially provided glass slide that comes with the kit. An HCG antiserum reagent (antibody) is added to the urine specimen. If the patient's urine contains HCG, the antiserum combines with the HCG (antigen) in the urine specimen, resulting in an antigen-antibody reaction.

The next step involves the addition of an antigen reagent containing latex particles coated with HCG. If the antigen-antibody reaction has previously occurred in the first step of the procedure, no available HCG antiserum is left in the specimen to react with the latex particles. The absence of agglutination on the slide test, known as *agglutination inhibition*, indicates a positive reaction for pregnancy. If agglutination occurs on the slide, the results are interpreted as negative (Figure 16-8). Coating the HCG with latex permits visible agglutination that can be observed and interpreted as a negative reaction by the individual performing the test. Without the latex, agglutination would be invisible when the HCG antigen and antibody combine.

Immunoassay Tests

Immunoassay tests provide for the rapid, qualitative detection of HCG in a urine specimen; brand names include QuickVue, Clearview, OSOM, and ICON. Early prediction pregnancy tests tests may be able to detect pregnancy 1 week after implantation, or 4 to 5 days before a first missed menstrual period. Urine pregnancy tests performed this early, however may show a false-negative result and should be repeated later to confirm the results. Accurate results are much more probable if the urine is tested 1 week after a missed period.

Immunoassay tests take approximately 5 minutes to perform and are easier to read than agglutination tests because the results are easily observed as a color change. Specific instructions for the test are included with each commercially available testing kit. The procedure for performing an immunoassay test with QuickVue (Quidel) is outlined in Procedure 16-8.

Guidelines for Urine Pregnancy Testing

Specific guidelines must be followed in a urine pregnancy test to ensure accurate test results:

1. Use clean, preferably disposable, urine containers to collect the specimen. Traces of detergent in the specimen container may cause inaccurate test results.
2. The preferred specimen for a urine pregnancy test is a first-voided morning specimen because it contains the highest concentration of HCG. If the urine specimen cannot be tested immediately after voiding, it should be preserved in the refrigerator. A patient who collects the specimen at home should be given instructions on preserving the specimen.
3. The specific gravity of the urine specimen should be determined before the test is performed. A specific gravity of less than 1.010 is considered too dilute for pregnancy testing because it may lead to a false-negative test result.
4. The urine specimen should be at room temperature before the procedure is performed.

Slide agglutination method

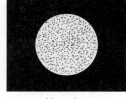
Negative

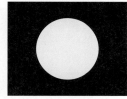
Positive

Figure 16-8. Urine pregnancy test results: slide agglutination method.

What Would You Do? What Would You *Not* Do?

Case Study 3

Rita Lavelle is 8½ months pregnant and is at the clinic for a prenatal appointment. Lately, she has been having difficulty obtaining a urine specimen at the medical office because of her enlarged abdomen. At her last appointment, the office provided her with a urine specimen container so that she could obtain her specimen more easily at home. Rita brings in a first-voided urine specimen in a glass jar. She says her dog chewed up the specimen container from the office, so she used an empty peanut butter jar. The urine testing results from her specimen show that her glucose level is normal, but her protein level is +4. Until this time, her urine test results all have been normal. Rita is concerned about her baby. She says that she was cleaning her bathroom cabinet yesterday and came across a pregnancy test; just for the fun of it, she decided to run the test. The results were negative, and now she is worried that something is wrong. Rita says that she has not been sleeping as well at night, and that she has noticed more Braxton Hicks contractions, but that the baby has been kicking and moving as usual. ■

5. The urine pregnancy testing kit should be stored according to the manufacturer's instructions. Most testing kits are stored at room temperature.
6. Testing kits past their expiration dates should not be used.

SERUM PREGNANCY TEST

The radioimmunoassay (RIA) for HCG is used to detect HCG in the serum of the blood. This test can detect pregnancy earlier and with more accuracy than a urine pregnancy test. A serum pregnancy test and can usually detect pregnancy at approximately the eighth day after fertilization, which is 6 days before the first missed menstrual period. This test uses a radioisotope technique and is capable of detecting minute amounts of HCG in the blood. This test is generally used to diagnose abnormalities, such as ectopic pregnancy; to follow the course of early pregnancy when abnormalities of embryonic development are suspected; and to provide an early diagnosis of pregnancy in individuals at high risk, such as patients with diabetes.

PROCEDURE 16-8   Performing a Urine Pregnancy Test

Outcome Perform a urine pregnancy test.

Equipment/Supplies

- Disposable gloves
- Urine pregnancy testing kit (QuickVue by Quidel)
- Urine specimen (first-voided morning specimen)

1. Procedural Step. Sanitize the hands, and assemble the equipment. Check the expiration date on the urine pregnancy test. It should not be used if the expiration date has passed. When a new testing kit is opened, an external positive and negative control should be performed according to the manufacturer's instructions. If the control does not produce the expected results, the testing kit should not be used.

Principle. An expired pregnancy test may produce inaccurate test results. Running positive and negative test results ensures that the test results are valid and reliable.

2. Procedural Step. Apply gloves. Rotate the urine specimen cup to mix the urine. Remove the test cassette from its foil pouch, and place it on a clean, dry, level surface.

3. Procedural Step. Add 3 drops of urine to the round sample well on the test cassette with a disposable pipet

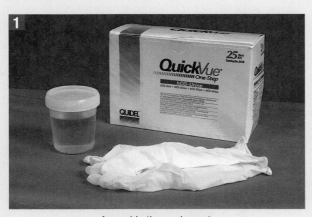

Assemble the equipment.

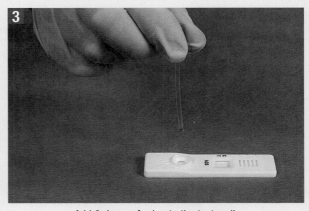

Add 3 drops of urine to the test well.

supplied with the kit. The test cassette should not be handled again until the test is ready for interpretation. Dispose of the pipet in a regular waste container.

4. Procedural Step. Wait 3 minutes, and read the results by observing the result window.

5. Procedural Step. Interpret the test results as follows:

Negative: The appearance of the blue procedural control line next to the letter "C" only and no pink-to-purple test line next the letter "T."

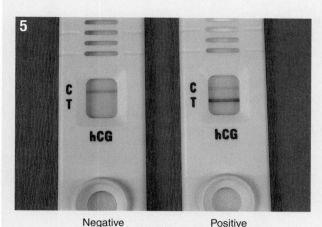

5

C
T

hCG

Negative

C
T

hCG

Positive

Interpret the results.

Positive: The appearance of any pink-to-purple line next to the letter "T" along with a blue procedural control line next to the letter "C."

No result: If no blue procedural control line appears, the test result is invalid, and the specimen must be re-tested. The blue procedural control line is an internal quality-control indicator designating that the test is working properly and the result is valid and reliable.

6. Procedural Step. Dispose of the test cassette in a regular waste container. Remove gloves, and sanitize your hands.

7. Procedural Step. Chart the results. Include the date and time of the patient's last menstrual period (LMP), the name of the test, and the results recorded as either positive or negative.

CHARTING EXAMPLE

Date	
3/25/08	10:30 a.m. LMP: 2/20/08.
	QuickVue preg test: Positive. _____
	_____ L. Proffitt, CMA

 Check out the **Companion CD** bound with the book to access additional interactive activities.

MEDICAL PRACTICE *and the* LAW

In collection and analysis of patient urine, meticulous attention should be paid to patient instructions, such as cleansing and collecting first morning, midstream, or 24-hour specimens. Patients are often embarrassed to have someone else see their urine, so handle urine specimens in a professional, matter-of-fact manner, with universal precautions to protect yourself. As with all diagnostic procedures, care must be taken to perform the test correctly and treat results confidentially.

Civil versus Criminal Law

Civil law involves a conflict with another person, and if found guilty by a preponderance of evidence (greater than 50%), the loser may lose money or property. Malpractice is a type of civil law. Civil law is divided into *torts,* or wrongs, and *contracts,* or promises. Malpractice is a tort, and nonpayment for services is a contract.

Criminal law involves a conflict with society as a whole (local, state, or federal law). If found guilty beyond a reasonable doubt, the loser may lose money, property, freedom (jail), or life (execution). Violation by the physician of licensure laws and failure to report child abuse are criminal suits. ■

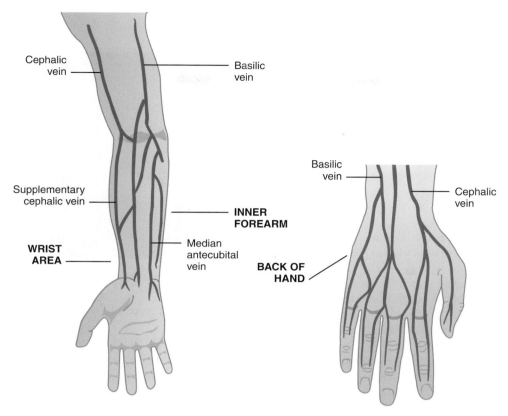

Figure 17-5. Alternative venipuncture sites: the inner forearm, the wrist area above the thumb, and the back of the hand.

2. **Serum.** Serum is obtained from clotted blood by allowing the specimen to stand and then centrifuging it. Centrifuging a blood specimen that does not contain an anticoagulant causes the blood to separate into the following layers (Figure 17-6A):
   - Top layer—serum
   - Bottom layer—clotted blood cells
3. **Whole blood.** Whole blood is obtained by using a tube that contains an anticoagulant. The anticoagulant prevents clotting of the blood cells. It is important to mix the anticoagulant with the blood by gently inverting the tube back and forth 8 to 10 times after collection.
4. **Plasma.** Plasma is obtained from whole blood that has been centrifuged. Centrifuging a blood specimen that contains an anticoagulant causes the blood to separate into the following layers (Figure 17-6B):
   - Top layer—plasma
   - Middle layer—**buffy coat** (contains white blood cells and platelets)
   - Bottom layer—red blood cells

OSHA Safety Precautions

The OSHA Bloodborne Pathogens Standard presented in Chapter 2 must be carefully followed during the venipuncture procedure to avoid exposure to bloodborne pathogens. The following OSHA requirements apply specifically to the

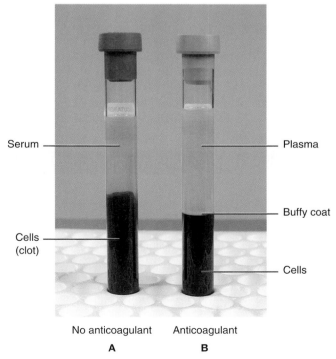

Figure 17-6. Layers into which the blood separates when there is no anticoagulant **(A)** and when an anticoagulant is present **(B)**.

venipuncture procedure and to separation of serum or plasma from whole blood (see later):

1. Wear gloves when it is reasonably anticipated that you will have hand contact with blood.
2. Wear a face shield or mask in combination with an eye protection device whenever splashes, spray, splatter, or droplets of blood may be generated.
3. Perform all procedures involving blood in a manner so as to minimize splashing, spraying, splattering, and generating droplets of blood.
4. Bandage cuts and other lesions on the hands before gloving.
5. Sanitize hands as soon as possible after removing gloves.
6. If your hands or other skin surfaces come in contact with blood, wash the area as soon as possible with soap and water.
7. If your mucous membranes (e.g., eyes, nose, mouth) come in contact with blood, flush them with water as soon as possible.
8. Do not bend, break, or shear contaminated venipuncture needles.
9. Do not recap a contaminated venipuncture needle.
10. Locate the sharps container as close as possible to the area of use. Immediately after use, place the contaminated venipuncture needle (and plastic holder) in the biohazard sharps container.
11. Place blood specimens in containers that prevent leakage during collection, handling, processing, storage, transport, and shipping.
12. If you are exposed to blood, report the incident immediately to your physician-employer.

VACUUM TUBE METHOD OF VENIPUNCTURE

The vacuum tube method is frequently used to collect venous blood specimens. This method is considered ideal for collecting blood from normal healthy antecubital veins that are adequate in size to withstand the pressure of the vacuum in the evacuated tube. Procedure 17-1 outlines the veni-

What Would You Do? What Would You *Not* Do?

Case Study 1
Angela Castillo is 21 years old and comes to the office at 9:00 AM to have her blood drawn for a CBC and a thyroid profile. She has brought a friend along with her. Angela seems nervous, and her voice is shaking. She says this is the first venipuncture she has ever had. Angela asks whether her friend could stay with her to give her moral support while her blood is being drawn. Angela says that the blood has to be taken out of her left arm. She says she is right-handed and has a softball game this evening. When the veins of Angela's left arm are examined, a suitable vein cannot be located; however, she has a good median cubital vein in her right arm. Angela then wants to know whether the blood could be drawn from her left hand like they do on hospital television shows. ■

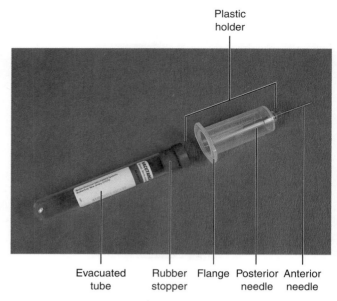

Figure 17-7. Vacuum tube system.

puncture vacuum tube method. The vacuum tube system consists of a collection needle, a plastic holder, and an evacuated tube (Figure 17-7). One commercially available vacuum tube system is the Vacutainer (Becton Dickinson, Tarrytown, NY).

Needle

The needle used with the vacuum tube method consists of a double-pointed stainless steel needle with a threaded hub near its center (Figure 17-8). The needle is coated with silicon, enabling it to penetrate the skin smoothly. The threaded hub of the needle screws into the plastic holder.

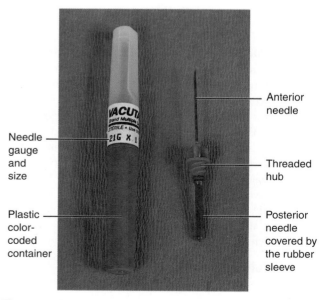

Figure 17-8. Vacuum tube needle in its container showing the gauge and size of the needle. The gauge of this needle is 21 G, and the size is 1 inch.

Vacuum tube needles are packaged in sealed twist-apart plastic containers. The needle gauge and length are printed on the paper seal on the container (see Figure 17-8). A needle should not be used if the seal has been broken.

The double-pointed needle consists of an anterior needle and a posterior needle. The *anterior needle* is longer and has a beveled point designed to facilitate entry into the skin and the vein. The *posterior needle* is shorter, and its purpose is to pierce the rubber stopper of the evacuated tube. The posterior needle has a rubber sleeve that functions as a valve. Pushing the tube stopper of an evacuated tube onto the posterior needle compresses this rubber sleeve and exposes the opening of the needle, allowing blood to enter the tube. When a tube is removed, the sleeve slides back over the needle opening and stops the flow of blood.

Vacuum tube needles are available in sizes 20 G to 22 G, with 21 G needles used most often for a routine venipuncture. Vacuum tube needles come in two lengths, 1 inch and 1½ inch. The length used is based on individual preference; most medical assistants prefer the 1-inch needle for routine venipunctures. A 1-inch needle is less intimidating to the patient and tends to offer more control because it allows the medical assistant to rest the fourth and fifth fingers on the patient's arm for stability. A 1½-inch needle allows more room for stabilizing the vein.

Safety Engineered Venipuncture Devices

OSHA stipulates requirements to reduce needlestick and other sharps injuries among health care workers. As discussed in Chapter 2, employers are required to evaluate and implement commercially available safer medical devices that reduce occupational exposure to the lowest extent feasible.

Safer medical devices include safety engineered venipuncture devices. These devices incorporate a built-in safety feature to reduce risk of a needlestick injury. Figure 17-9

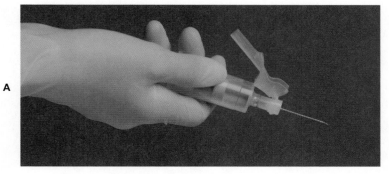

A, Perform the venipuncture with the shield in a downward position.

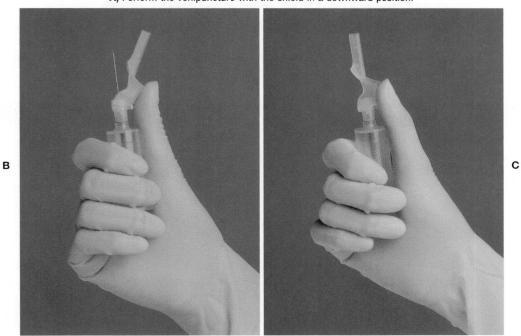

B, After performing the venipuncture, push the shield forward.

C, Continue pushing until the needle tip is fully covered by the shield. Discard the needle and holder in a biohazard sharps container.

Figure 17-9. Safety engineered venipuncture device.

illustrates a safety engineered venipuncture device and method for using it.

Plastic Holder

The plastic holder consists of a plastic cylinder with two openings. The small opening is used to secure the double-pointed needle, and the large opening is used to hold the evacuated tube. The large opening has a plastic extension known as the *flange*. The flange assists in the insertion and removal of evacuated tubes and prevents the plastic holder from rolling when it is placed on a flat surface.

The plastic holder has an indentation about ½ inch from the hub of the needle. This marks the point at which the posterior needle starts to enter the rubber stopper of the tube. If a tube stopper is inserted past this point before the vein is entered, the tube fills with air, which prevents blood from entering the tube.

Evacuated Tubes

Evacuated tubes consist of a glass tube with a rubber stopper. The tube contains a premeasured vacuum that creates suction to pull the blood specimen into the tube. Evacuated tubes use a color-coded stopper system for ease in identifying the additive (or no additive) content of the tube. The additive content of evacuated tubes is described in the box *Additive Content of Evacuated Tubes* and illustrated in Figure 17-10. A tube additive must not alter the blood components or affect the laboratory test to be performed.

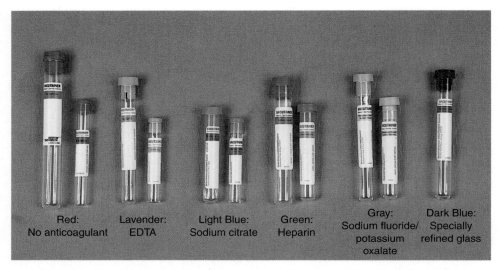

| Red: No anticoagulant | Lavender: EDTA | Light Blue: Sodium citrate | Green: Heparin | Gray: Sodium fluoride/ potassium oxalate | Dark Blue: Specially refined glass |

Figure 17-10. Vacutainer evacuated tubes. The stoppers of the evacuated tubes are color-coded for ease in identifying the additive content. The lavender, light-blue, green, gray, and dark-blue stoppered tubes contain an anticoagulant and are used to obtain whole blood or plasma. The red stoppered tube contains no additive and is used to obtain clotted blood or serum.

Additive Content of Evacuated Tubes

The vacuum tube method uses a color-coded system for ease in identifying the additive content of each type of tube. The most frequently used vacuum tubes are classified here according to the color of the stopper and additive content.

1. **Red.** Red stoppered tubes do not contain an anticoagulant and are used to obtain clotted blood or serum. Serum is required for serologic tests and most blood chemistries.
2. **Red/gray** (gold if using Hemoguard tubes). These tubes do not contain an anticoagulant and are used to obtain serum. Red/gray and gold stoppered tubes contain a gel that separates the cells from the serum when the tube is centrifuged.
3. **Lavender.** Lavender stoppered tubes contain the anticoagulant ethylenediaminetetraacetic acid (EDTA) and are used to obtain whole blood or plasma. The most common use is to collect a blood specimen for a complete blood count (CBC).
4. **Light blue.** Light blue stoppered tubes contain the anticoagulant sodium citrate and are used to obtain whole blood or plasma; the most common use is for coagulation tests, such as the prothrombin time.
5. **Green.** Green stoppered tubes contain the anticoagulant heparin and are commonly used to collect blood specimens to perform blood gas determinations and pH assays.
6. **Gray.** Gray stoppered tubes contain the anticoagulant sodium fluoride/potassium oxalate and are used to obtain whole blood or plasma; the most common use is to collect blood specimens to perform a glucose tolerance test (GTT).
7. **Dark blue.** Dark blue stoppered tubes contain either heparin or no additive at all. These tubes are made of a specially refined glass and rubber stopper and are used for the detection of trace elements, such as lead, zinc, arsenic, and copper, which are contracted through occupational or environmental exposure.

The color of the tube stopper used depends on the type of test to be performed. The medical assistant must determine the correct stopper color to use for each collection. The color-coded stoppered tubes must not be substituted for one another because inaccurate test results could occur. If a CBC has been ordered by the physician, a lavender stoppered tube must be used and a different color stoppered tube cannot be substituted for it.

Evacuated tubes are available in varying capacities, the most common being the 2-, 3-, 5-, 7-, 10-, and 15-ml sizes (Figure 17-11). The capacity of the tube used depends on the amount of the specimen required for the test. If the medical assistant is working with an outside laboratory, information on the amount of specimen required for a laboratory test and the stopper color of the tube required is indicated in the laboratory directory. If the test is being performed in the medical office, this information is indicated in the instructions accompanying the blood analyzer or testing kit.

Information regarding additive content, expiration date, and tube capacity is on the label of each box of evacuated tubes. In addition, evacuated tubes have a label affixed to them indicating the additive content, expiration date, tube capacity, and a fill indicator to indicate when the vacuum has been exhausted and the tube is full.

Hemogard closure tubes, manufactured by Becton Dickinson, are a newer type of evacuated tube (see Figure 17-10). A Hemogard tube consists of a special rubber stopper and a plastic closure that overhangs the outside of the tube. Together, these components act as a single unit to reduce the likelihood of coming in contact with the contents of the tube. After collecting a blood specimen, the medical assistant may need to gain access to the blood in the tube for

testing it or for further processing, such as in separating serum from whole blood. A regular evacuated tube "pops" as the top is removed, which may result in splattering of blood. The design of the Hemogard tube works to prevent splattering of blood when the top is removed. In addition, closure tubes are made of plastic, which reduces the possibility of tube breakage under normal conditions. The color coding of Hemogard stoppers is similar to that of rubber stoppered tubes (refer to Figure 17-10).

Order of Draw for Multiple Tubes

When using the vacuum tube system, and when multiple tubes of blood are to be drawn, the following order of draw is recommended by the Clinical Laboratory Standards Institute:

1. **Blood culture tube** (and other tests that require sterile specimens)
   * *Rationale:* To prevent contamination of the specimen by other tubes, which may lead to inaccurate test results.
2. **Coagulation tube:** Light blue stoppered tube for coagulation tests.
   * *Rationale:* To prevent additives from other tubes from getting into the tube.
   * *Note:* When the needle penetrates the patient's skin, thromboplastin, a clotting factor, is released because of tissue trauma. It was previously thought that thromboplastin entering the blood specimen could alter coagulation test results. To avoid this problem, it was recommended that a red stoppered tube be drawn first to collect the thromboplastin, followed by the collection of the blue stoppered tube. Current studies show that tissue thromboplastin entering the blood specimen does not affect coagulation test results. Further studies show, however, that a modification in technique is required when a butterfly setup is used to obtain the specimen for a coagulation test. The tubing

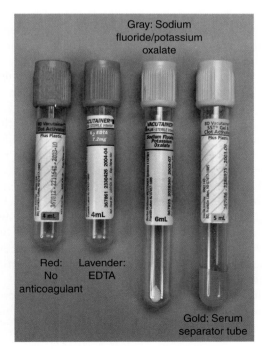

Figure 17-11. Hemogard tubes.

What Would You Do? What Would You *Not* Do?

Case Study 2

Buzz Braydon had a heart attack 4 weeks ago and is taking the anticoagulant warfarin (Coumadin). He is at the office for a checkup and to have his prothrombin time tested. Blood is collected from a small vein in Buzz's left arm using the butterfly method. After the specimen is collected, Buzz wants to know why a red stoppered tube was used to draw blood from him and then thrown away. Buzz says that they used something called a Vacutainer to draw his blood in the hospital and wants to know if a Vacutainer is ever used in the medical office. Buzz says that he is going on vacation in North Carolina for 2 weeks. He says that they explained to him at the hospital why he should have his blood tested every week, but he's not sure where to go to get his blood tested while he's on vacation. Buzz wants to know if as long as he takes his medication exactly as he should, it would be all right to skip his weekly prothrombin test during that time. ■

of the butterfly setup contains 0.3 to 1 cc of air. If a blue stoppered tube is the first or only tube to be drawn, a 5-ml red stoppered tube must be drawn first and discarded. This is because some of the tube's vacuum is exhausted by the air in the tubing (rather than blood), resulting in underfilling of the tube. If the blue stoppered tube is filled first, the underfilled tube results in an incorrect anticoagulant-to-blood ratio. An incorrect ratio when performing a coagulation test leads to inaccurate coagulation test results.

3. **Serum tubes:** Tubes with or without a clot activator and serum separator tubes (e.g., red stoppered tube and red/slate-gray stoppered tube)
   - *Rationale:* To prevent contamination of nonadditive tubes by tubes with an anticoagulant.

4. **Anticoagulant tubes** in this order of stopper color: green, lavender, gray
   - *Rationale:* To prevent cross-contamination between different types of anticoagulants, which may lead to inaccurate test results.

Evacuated Tube Guidelines

Certain guidelines should be followed when using evacuated tubes, as follows:

1. Select the proper evacuated tubes according to the tests to be performed and amount of specimen required.
2. Check to ensure the tube is not cracked. A cracked tube no longer has a vacuum.
3. Check the expiration date of each tube. Outdated tubes may no longer contain a vacuum, and, as a result, they would not be able to draw blood into the tube.
4. Label each tube with the patient's name, the date, and your initials. Proper labeling avoids mixing up specimens. Advances in specimen identification include the use of computer bar codes to identify specimens (Figure 17-12). The laboratory instruments that do the testing are able to read the bar codes and automatically record results onto the laboratory report form.
5. Before using tubes that contain powdered additives (e.g., gray stoppered tube), gently tap the tube just below the stopper so that all of the additive is dislodged from the stopper. If an additive remains trapped in the stopper, erroneous test results may occur.
6. Take precautions to avoid premature loss of the tube's vacuum. Premature loss of vacuum can occur from the following:
   - Dropping the tube
   - Pushing the posterior needle through the tube stopper before puncturing the vein
   - Partially pulling the needle out of the vein after penetrating the patient's vein
7. Use a continuous, steady motion to make the puncture. Performing the puncture with a slow, timid motion or a rapid, jabbing motion is painful for the pa-

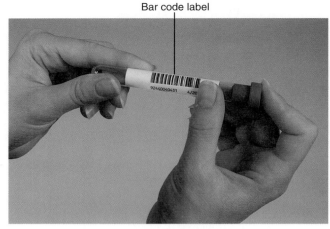

Bar code label

Figure 17-12. Identifying a blood specimen using a computer bar code.

tient. In addition, a rapid motion could cause the needle to go completely through the vein, resulting in a failure to obtain blood and possibly a hematoma.

8. When multiple tubes are to be drawn, follow the proper *order of draw.* This prevents contamination of nonadditive tubes by additive tubes and cross-contamination between different types of additive tubes, which could lead to inaccurate test results.
9. Fill evacuated tubes until the vacuum is exhausted, as evidenced by the cessation of the blood flow into the tube. The tube is almost, but not quite, full when the vacuum is exhausted. If the evacuated tube is removed before the vacuum is exhausted, a rush of air enters the tube, damaging the red blood cells. A tube that contains an anticoagulant must be filled completely to ensure the proper ratio of anticoagulant to the blood specimen.
10. Remove the last tube from the plastic holder before removing the needle from the patient's vein. This prevents blood from dripping out of the tip of the needle after it is withdrawn from the patient's skin.
11. Mix tubes that contain an anticoagulant immediately after drawing by gently inverting the tube back and forth 8 to 10 times. This provides adequate mixing without causing **hemolysis,** or breakdown of blood cells. Inadequate mixing or not mixing the tubes immediately after drawing them may result in clotting of the blood, leading to inaccurate test results.
12. After the venipuncture, the top of the stopper may contain residual blood. Take precautions following the OSHA standard when handling these tubes.

Text continued on p. 645

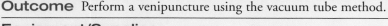

PROCEDURE 17-1   Venipuncture—Vacuum Tube Method

Outcome Perform a venipuncture using the vacuum tube method.

Equipment/Supplies

- Disposable gloves
- Tourniquet
- Antiseptic wipe
- Double-pointed needle
- Plastic holder
- Evacuated tubes with labels
- Sterile 2 × 2 gauze pad
- Adhesive bandage
- Biohazard sharps container
- Biohazard specimen bag
- Laboratory request form

1. **Procedural Step.** Sanitize your hands.
2. **Procedural Step.** Greet the patient and introduce yourself. Identify the patient by asking the patient to state his or her full name and date of birth. Compare this information with the demographic data in the patient's chart. If the patient was required to prepare for the test (e.g., fasting, medication restriction), determine whether he or she has prepared properly. If the patient has not followed the patient preparation requirements, notify the physician for instructions on handling this situation.

   Principle. It is important to confirm that you have the correct patient to avoid collecting a specimen on the wrong patient. The patient must prepare properly to obtain a quality specimen that would lead to accurate test results.

3. **Procedural Step.** Assemble the equipment. Select the proper evacuated tubes for the tests to be performed. Check the expiration date of the tubes. Label each tube using one of the following methods: (a) attaching a computer bar code label to each tube to be drawn and labeling it with your initials, or (b) manually labeling each tube with the patient's name, the date, and your initials. If the specimen is to be tested at an outside laboratory, complete a laboratory request form.

   Principle. Outdated tubes may no longer contain a vacuum, and, as a result, they may not be able to draw blood into the tube. Proper labeling of blood specimens avoids a mixup of specimens.

4. **Procedural Step.** Prepare the vacuum tube system. Remove the cap from the posterior needle using a twisting and pulling motion. Insert the posterior needle into the small opening on the plastic holder. Screw the plastic holder onto the Luer adapter, and tighten it securely.

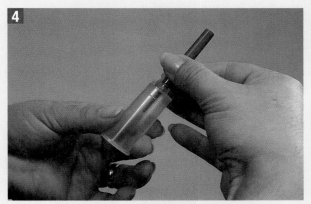

Insert the posterior needle into the plastic holder.

   Principle. An unsecured needle can fall out of its plastic holder.

5. **Procedural Step.** Open the sterile gauze packet, and lay it flat to allow the gauze pad to rest on the inside

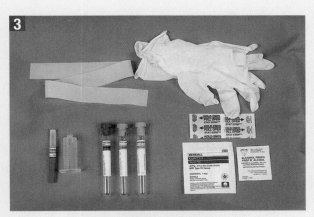

Assemble the equipment.

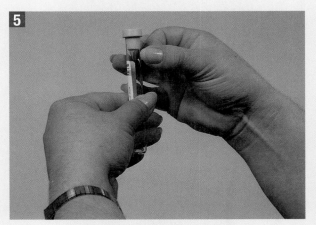

Tap tubes with powdered additives.

Continued

of its wrapper. Position the evacuated tubes in the correct order of draw. If the evacuated tube contains a powdered additive, tap the tube just below the stopper to release any additive adhering to the stopper.

Principle. If an additive remains trapped in the stopper, erroneous test results may occur.

6. **Procedural Step.** Place the first tube loosely in the plastic holder.

7. **Procedural Step.** Explain the procedure to the patient, and reassure the patient. Perform a preliminary assessment of both arms to determine the best vein to use. It also is helpful to ask the patient which arm has been used in the past to obtain blood.

Principle. Venipuncture is often a frightening experience for the patient, and reassurance should be offered to reduce apprehension.

8. **Procedural Step.** Apply the tourniquet. Position the tourniquet 3 to 4 inches above the bend in the elbow. The tourniquet should be snug but not tight. Ask the patient to clench the fist of the arm to which the tourniquet has been applied.

Principle. The combined effect of the pressure of the tourniquet and the clenched fist should cause the antecubital veins to stand out so that accurate selection of a puncture site can be made.

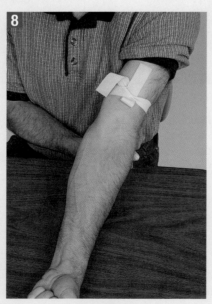

Apply the tourniquet.

9. **Procedural Step.** With a tourniquet in place, thoroughly assess the veins of first one arm and then the other to determine the best vein to use.

10. **Procedural Step.** Position the patient's arm. The arm with the vein selected for the venipuncture should be extended and placed in a straight line from the shoulder to the wrist with the antecubital veins facing anteriorly. The arm should be supported on the armrest by a rolled towel or by having the patient place the fist of the other hand under the elbow.

Principle. This position allows easy access to the antecubital veins.

11. **Procedural Step.** Thoroughly palpate the selected vein. Gently palpate the vein with the fingertips to determine the direction of the vein and to estimate its size and depth. Never leave the tourniquet on an arm for more than 1 minute at a time. (*Note:* If you need to perform several assessments to locate the best vein, the tourniquet must be removed and reapplied after a 2-minute waiting period.)

Principle. Leaving the tourniquet on for more than 1 minute is uncomfortable for the patient and may alter the test results.

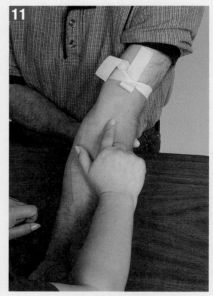

Palpate the vein.

12. **Procedural Step.** Remove the tourniquet and cleanse the site with an antiseptic wipe. Cleansing should be done in a circular motion, starting from the inside and moving away from the puncture site. Allow the site to air dry; after cleansing, do not touch the area, wipe the area with gauze, or fan the area with your hand. Place the remaining supplies within comfortable reach of your nondominant hand.

Principle. Using a circular motion helps carry foreign particles away from the puncture site. The site must be allowed to air dry to allow the alcohol enough time to destroy microorganisms on the patient's skin. Residual alcohol entering the blood specimen can cause hemolysis, leading to inaccurate test results. In addition, residual alcohol causes the patient to experience a stinging sensation when the puncture is made. Touching or fanning the area causes contamination of the puncture site, and the cleansing process must be repeated. Items used during the procedure should be positioned so that you do not have to reach over the patient and possibly move the needle, resulting in pain, injury, or both.

13. **Procedural Step.** Reapply the tourniquet. Apply gloves. If you are using a needle with a safety shield, rotate the shield backwards toward the holder (refer to Figure 17-9A). Remove the cap from the needle using a twisting and pulling motion. Hold the vacuum tube system by placing the thumb of the dominant hand on top of the plastic holder and the pads of the first three fingers underneath the holder and evacuated tube. The needle should be positioned with the bevel facing up. Position the evacuated tube so that the label is facing down.

    Principle. Gloves provide a barrier against blood-borne pathogens. Positioning the needle with the bevel up allows easier entry into the skin and the vein, resulting in less pain for the patient. With the label facing down, you would be able to observe the blood as it fills the tube, which allows you to know when the tube is full.

14. **Procedural Step.** Anchor the vein. Grasp the patient's arm with the nondominant hand. Your thumb should be placed 1 to 2 inches below and to the side of the puncture site. Using your thumb, draw the skin taut over the vein in the direction of the patient's hand.

    Principle. The thumb helps hold the skin taut for easier entry and helps stabilize the vein to be punctured. Placing the thumb to the side keeps it out of the way of the vacuum tube setup so that you can maintain a 15-degree angle when entering the vein.

15. **Procedural Step.** Position the needle at a 15-degree angle to the arm. Rest the backs of the fingers on the patient's forearm. Ensure that the needle points in the same direction as the vein to be entered. The needle should be positioned so that it enters the vein approximately ⅛ inch below the place where the vein is to be entered.

    Principle. An angle of less than 15 degrees may cause the needle to enter above the vein, preventing puncture. An angle of more than 15 degrees may cause the needle to go through the vein by puncturing the posterior wall. This could result in a hematoma.

16. **Procedural Step.** Tell the patient that he or she will "feel a small stick," and with one continuous steady motion, enter the skin and then the vein. You will feel a sensation of resistance followed by a "release" as the vein is entered. When the "release" is felt, you have entered the vein and should not advance the needle any further.

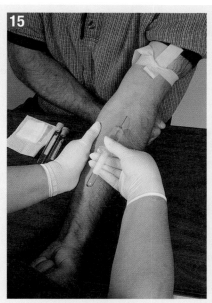

Position the needle.

Principle. Using one continuous steady motion helps to prevent tissue damage.

17. **Procedural Step.** Stabilize the vacuum tube setup by firmly grasping the holder between the thumb and the underlying fingers to prevent the needle from moving. Do *not* change hands during the procedure.

    Principle. Stabilizing the holder helps prevent the needle from moving when a tube is inserted or removed. Changing hands may cause the needle to move, which is painful for the patient.

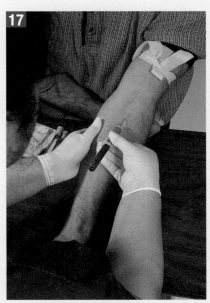

Make the puncture.

Continued

PROCEDURE 17-1

18. **Procedural Step.** With the nondominant hand, place the first two fingers on the underside of the flange on the plastic holder, and with the thumb, slowly push the tube forward to the end of the holder. This allows the posterior needle to puncture the rubber stopper. Blood begins flowing into the tube if the (anterior) needle is in a vein.

    Principle. Not using the flange may cause the needle to advance forward and go completely through the vein, resulting in failure to obtain blood; internal bleeding also may occur, resulting in a hematoma.

19. **Procedural Step.** Allow the evacuated tube to fill to the exhaustion of the vacuum, as indicated by the cessation of the blood flow into the tube. The suction of the evacuated tube automatically draws the blood into the tube.

    Principle. If the evacuated tube is removed before the vacuum is exhausted, a rush of air enters the tube, damaging the red blood cells. Also, a tube containing an additive, such as an anticoagulant, must be filled completely to ensure accurate test results.

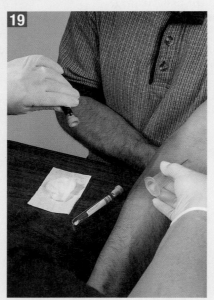
Invert tubes with additives back and forth 8 to 10 times.

20. **Procedural Step.** Remove the tube from the holder by grasping the tube with the fingers, placing the thumb or index finger against the flange, and pulling the tube off the posterior needle. Do not change the position of the needle in the vein. If the tube contains an anticoagulant, gently invert the tube back and forth 8 to 10 times before laying it down.

    Principle. The rubber sheath covers the point of the needle, stopping the flow of blood until the next tube is inserted. Not using the flange to remove the tube can

cause the needle to come out of the vein prematurely, resulting in blood being forced out of the puncture site. A tube containing an anticoagulant must be inverted immediately to prevent the blood from clotting. Careful mixing of the blood with the anticoagulant prevents hemolysis.

21. **Procedural Step.** Using the flange, carefully insert the next tube into the holder. Continue in this manner until the last tube has been filled.

22. **Procedural Step.** Remove the tension from the tourniquet by pulling upward on one of the flaps of the tourniquet. Ask the patient to unclench the fist.

    Principle. The tourniquet tension must be removed before the needle. Otherwise, the pressure on the vein from the tourniquet could cause internal and external bleeding around the puncture site.

23. **Procedural Step.** Remove the last tube from the holder. Immediately invert the tube back and forth 8 to 10 times if it contains an anticoagulant.

    Principle. Removing the last tube prevents blood from dripping out of the tip of the needle after it is removed from the patient's arm.

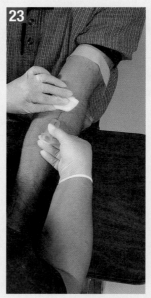
Remove the tourniquet, and withdraw the needle.

24. **Procedural Step.** Place a sterile gauze pad slightly above the puncture site, and carefully withdraw the needle at the same angle as that for penetration. Immediately move the gauze over the puncture site, and apply firm pressure. (Do not apply any pressure to the puncture site until the needle is completely removed.) If you are using a needle with a safety shield, push the shield forward with your thumb until you hear an audible click, which indicates the shield has locked into

place. Do not push the shield forward by pressing it against a hard surface. (Refer to Figure 17-9B,C.)

Principle. Placing the gauze pad above the puncture helps prevent tissue movement as the needle is withdrawn and reduces patient discomfort. Careful withdrawal prevents further tissue damage.

25. **Procedural Step.** Immediately discard the plastic holder and attached needle in a biohazard sharps container. Do not remove the needle from the holder; the holder must be discarded and not reused.

    Principle. Immediate disposal of the needle and holder unit is required by the OSHA standard to prevent a needlestick injury; even if a safey shield has been activated to encase the anterior needle, a needlestick injury can still occur from the posterior needle, which is only covered with a rubber sleeve. Plastic holders are often contaminated with blood and must not be reused.

26. **Procedural Step.** Continue to apply pressure with the gauze pad. Cooperative patients can be asked to assist by applying pressure with the gauze pad for 1 to 2 minutes. The arm can be elevated to facilitate clot formation. Do not allow the patient to bend the arm at the elbow because this increases blood loss from the puncture site.

    Principle. Applying pressure reduces the leakage of blood from the puncture site externally or internally. Internal leakage of blood into the tissues could result in a hematoma.

27. **Procedural Step.** Stay with the patient until the bleeding has stopped. Remove the gauze, and inspect the puncture site to ensure that the opening is sealed with a clot. Apply an adhesive bandage to the puncture site. As an alternative, the gauze pad can be folded into quarters and taped on the puncture site to be used as a pressure bandage. Instruct the patient not to pick up anything heavy for about an hour. (*Note:*

If swelling or discoloration occurs, apply an ice pack to the site after bandaging it.)

Principle. Lifting a heavy object causes pressure on the puncture site, which could result in bleeding.

28. **Procedural Step.** Remove the gloves, and sanitize your hands.

29. **Procedural Step.** Chart the procedure. Include the date and time, which arm and vein were used, unusual patient reaction, and your initials.

30. **Procedural Step.** Test the specimen or prepare the specimen for transport to an outside laboratory for testing according to the medical office policy. If the specimen is to be transported to an outside laboratory, perform the following:

    a. Place the specimen tube in a biohazard specimen bag.

    b. Place the laboratory request in the outside pocket of the specimen bag.

    c. Properly handle and store the specimen while awaiting pick-up by a laboratory courier.

    d. Chart the date the specimen was transported to the laboratory in the patient's record.

    Principle. The biohazard bag protects the laboratory courier from the possibility of an exposure incident. The outside laboratory must have the completed request form to know which laboratory tests have been ordered by the physician. The specimen must be handled and stored properly to maintain the in vivo characteristics of the specimen.

CHARTING EXAMPLE	
Date	
4/5/08	9:00 a.m. Venous blood specimen collected from Ⓛ arm. Picked up by Medical Center Laboratory on 4/5/08.——— D. Glover, CMA

BUTTERFLY METHOD OF VENIPUNCTURE

The butterfly method of venipuncture also is called the *winged infusion method.* This is because a winged infusion set is used to perform the procedure. The term *butterfly* is derived from the plastic "wings" located between the needle and the tubing of the winged infusion set (Figure 17-13).

The butterfly method is used to collect blood from patients who are difficult to stick by conventional methods because it provides better control when making the puncture and also less pressure is exerted on the vein wall from the evacuated tube. The butterfly method is recommended for adults with small antecubital veins and children, who typically have small antecubital veins. The butterfly method also is used when the antecubital veins are unavailable, and the veins in the forearm, wrist area, or back of the hand are used, as may occur with elderly and obese patients. These alternative veins are usually smaller

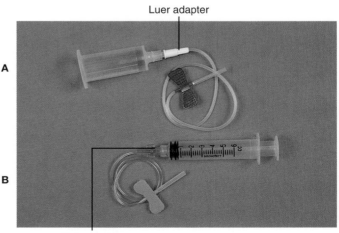

Figure 17-13. Winged infusion set. **A,** Luer adapter with evacuated tube. **B,** Hub adapter with syringe.

pressure should be applied to the puncture site until the bleeding stops.

Hemolysis

The blood specimen should be handled carefully at all times. Blood cells are fragile, and rough handling may cause hemolysis, or breakdown of the blood cells. Hemolyzed blood specimens produce inaccurate test results. To prevent hemolysis, these guidelines should be followed:

1. Store the vacuum tubes at room temperature because chilled tubes can result in hemolysis.
2. Allow the alcohol to air dry completely before performing the venipuncture. Alcohol entering a blood specimen can cause hemolysis.
3. Use an appropriate-gauge needle to collect the specimen; a needle with a gauge between 20 G and 22 G should be used. Using a small-gauge needle (e.g., 25 G) can cause the blood cells to rupture as they pass through the lumen of the needle.
4. Practice good technique in collecting the specimen; excessive trauma to the blood vessel can result in hemolysis.
5. Always handle the blood tube carefully; do not shake it or handle it roughly.

Fainting

Occasionally, a patient experiences dizziness or fainting during or after a venipuncture. Should this occur, the most immediate concern is to protect the patient from injury; for example, by preventing the patient from falling. The pa-tient should be placed in a position that promotes blood flow to the brain, and the physician should be notified for further treatment; see the box *Highlight on Vasovagal Syncope (Fainting)*.

OBTAINING A SERUM SPECIMEN

Serum

Serum is plasma from which the clotting factor fibrinogen has been removed. A brief discussion of serum is presented here, and a thorough discussion of plasma is presented later in this chapter.

Serum contains many dissolved substances, such as glucose, cholesterol, sodium, potassium, chloride, antibodies, hormones, and enzymes. As a result, many laboratory tests require a serum specimen to determine whether these substances are within normal limits and to detect substances that should not normally be in the serum, and that, if present, indicate a pathologic condition. To perform laboratory tests on serum, it must be separated from the blood specimen, which is usually the responsibility of the medical assistant.

Tube Selection

A tube without an anticoagulants (red stoppered) must be used to collect the blood specimen, to allow the specimen to separate into serum and clotted blood cells. Because the amount of serum recovered is only a portion of the specimen, a blood specimen must be drawn that is 2.5 times the amount required for the test. If 2 ml of serum is required, a

Highlight on Vasovagal Syncope (Fainting)

Most people experience no change in their sense of well-being when they have blood taken. A very small percentage of individuals experience a type of fainting, however, known as *vasovagal syncope.*

Cause and Symptoms

Vasovagal syncope is caused by unpleasant physical or emotional stimuli, such as pain, fright, and the sight of blood. A sudden pooling of blood occurs, which results in a sudden decrease in the blood pressure. This momentarily deprives the brain of blood, causing a temporary loss of consciousness, usually lasting only 1 to 2 minutes. Vasovagal syncope usually occurs when an individual is in an upright position, as in standing or sitting. Before fainting, the patient usually experiences some warning signals, such as sudden lightheadedness, nausea, weakness, yawning, paleness, blurred vision, a feeling of warmth, and sweating followed by drooping eyelids, weak, rapid pulse, and finally unconsciousness.

Treatment

A person who is about to faint should be placed in a position that facilitates blood flow to the brain and told to breathe deeply. The preferred position is lying down (supine) with the legs elevated and the collar and clothing loosened. This position may not al-ways be possible, such as when a patient is seated and the venipuncture needle has already been inserted. In this case, the tourniquet and then the needle should be removed, and the patient's head should be lowered between the legs. An individual who has fainted should be protected from injury by falling and be placed in a position that facilitates blood flow to the brain, as just described.

Prevention

Fainting during or after venipuncture is more likely in the following individuals: patients having a venipuncture for the first time, young patients, thin patients, patients with a low diastolic or high systolic blood pressure, patients with a history of fainting, nervous and apprehensive patients, and patients who are very quiet or very talkative. Fainting often can be prevented by identifying and closely observing individuals who are more likely to faint (as described). Talking to the patient often helps relax the patient and divert attention from the venipuncture procedure. If a patient has a history of fainting, he or she should be in a semi-Fowler's position for the venipuncture procedure because people rarely faint in this position. Other factors that contribute to fainting and that should be avoided include fatigue, lack of sleep, hunger, and environmental factors, such as a noisy, crowded, or overheated room. ■

5-ml red stoppered tube of blood must be collected; if 4 ml of serum is required, a 10-ml red stoppered tube is collected, and if 6 ml of serum is required, a 15-ml red stoppered tube is needed.

Preparation of the Specimen

After the blood specimen has been collected, the tube must be allowed to stand upright at room temperature for 30 to 45 minutes before being centrifuged. This allows clot formation, which yields more serum from the specimen. If the specimen is centrifuged immediately after collection, the clotting factors do not have an opportunity to settle down into the cell layer to form a whole blood clot. The result of this is the formation of a *fibrin clot* in the serum layer. A fibrin clot is a spongy substance that occupies space, interfering with adequate serum collection. The blood specimen should not be allowed to stand for longer than 1 hour, however, because leaching of substances from the cell layer into the serum may occur. This leaching of substances changes the integrity of the serum, leading to inaccurate test results.

Removal of Serum

After the blood cells have clotted by allowing the specimen to stand, the specimen is centrifuged. The serum is removed from the clot using a pipet and placed in a separate transfer tube. It is important that proper technique be employed in removing the serum, to avoid disturbing the cell layer of the clot and drawing red blood cells into the serum layer. If cells do enter the serum, the entire specimen must be recentrifuged.

When the serum has been removed from the blood specimen, the medical assistant should hold the specimen in the transfer tube up to good light. The serum specimen should be inspected for the presence of intact red blood cells or hemolyzed blood; in both cases, the specimen has a reddish appearance. A specimen having a reddish appearance must be recentrifuged. If the specimen contains intact red blood cells, they settle to the bottom of the tube, and the serum can be removed. If the blood is hemolyzed, recentrifugation would not make the red color disappear because the red blood cells have ruptured and released hemoglobin into the serum. Hemolyzed serum is unsuitable for laboratory tests because the results would be inaccurate; another blood specimen must be collected. Procedure 17-4 presents the method for separating serum from whole blood using a conventional evacuated tube.

Serum Separator Tubes

A serum separator tube (SST) is an evacuated tube specially designed to facilitate the collection of a serum specimen.

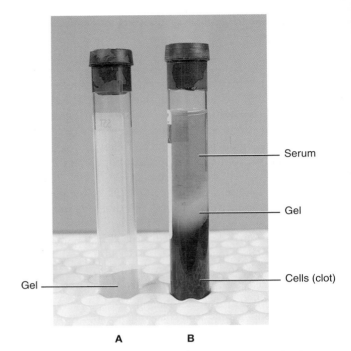

Gel

Serum

Gel

Cells (clot)

A   B

Figure 17-17. Serum separator tubes. **A,** An unused tube that contains the thixotropic gel in the bottom of the tube. **B,** A tube that has been used to collect a blood specimen. During centrifugation, the gel temporarily becomes fluid and moves to the dividing point between the serum and blood cells in a fibrin clot.

The SST glass tube is identified by a red/gray stopper (or gold stopper if using Hemoguard tubes) and is used for collection and separation of blood. The serum separator tube contains a thixotropic gel, which is in a solid state in the bottom of the unused tube (Figure 17-17A).

The blood specimen is collected and processed following the appropriate venipuncture method. The specimen must be allowed to stand in an upright position for 30 to 45 minutes for proper clot formation and centrifuged as previously described. During centrifugation, the gel temporarily becomes fluid and moves to the dividing point between the serum and clotted cells, where it reforms into a solid gel, serving as a physical and chemical barrier between the serum and clot (Figure 17-17B).

The serum can be transported or stored in the separator tube; the medical assistant must inspect the tube carefully to ensure that the gel barrier is firmly attached to the glass wall. If a complete barrier has not formed, the serum specimen must be removed and placed in a transfer tube to prevent leaching of substances from the cell layer into the serum, affecting the accuracy of the test results.

Text continued on p. 661

PROCEDURE 17-4   Separating Serum from Whole Blood

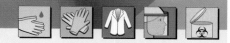

Outcome Separate serum from whole blood.

Equipment/Supplies

- Red stoppered evacuated tube venipuncture setup
- Test tube rack
- Disposable pipet
- Transfer tube and label

- Disposable gloves
- Face shield or mask and an eye protection device
- Centrifuge
- Biohazard sharps container

1. Procedural Step. Collect the blood specimen following the venipuncture procedure. Use a tube containing no additives (red stoppered) to collect the specimen. The tube selected should have a capacity of 2½ times the amount of serum required. Label the red stoppered tube and the transfer tube with the patient's name, the date, and your initials. In addition, the transfer tube should bear the word "serum." Allow the tube to fill until the vacuum is exhausted.

Principle. To obtain serum, a tube containing no additives must be used. The tube must be allowed to fill completely to obtain the proper amount of serum. Several types of specimen, such as serum, plasma, and urine, are straw-colored; the transfer tube containing serum must be labeled as such to avoid confusion and mixup among these specimens.

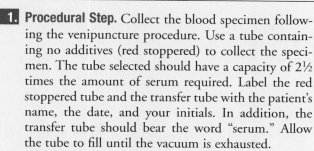

Label the tubes.

2. Procedural Step. Place the blood specimen tube in an upright position for 30 to 45 minutes at room temperature. To prevent evaporation of the serum sample, do not remove the tube's stopper.

Principle. Specimens must be placed in an upright position and allowed to stand to permit clot formation, which yields more serum from the specimen. Evaporation of the sample leads to falsely elevated test results.

3. Procedural Step. Place the specimen in the centrifuge, stopper end up. Balance the specimen with the same type and weight of tube or another specimen tube. Make sure the tube is stoppered to prevent

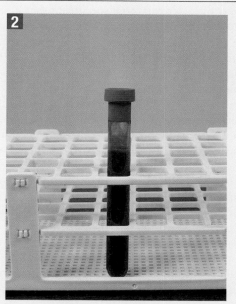

Allow the specimen to stand for 30 to 45 minutes.

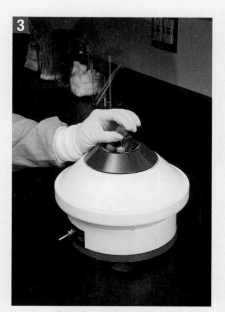

Centrifuge the specimen.

Continued

PROCEDURE 17-4   Separating Serum from Whole Blood—cont'd

evaporation of the sample during centrifugation. Centrifuge the specimen for 10 to 15 minutes.

Principle. Centrifuging packs the cells and causes them to settle at the bottom of the tube, yielding more serum. If the centrifuge is not balanced, it may vibrate and move across the table top. An unbalanced centrifuge also can cause specimen tubes to break.

4. **Procedural Step.** Put on a face shield or a mask and an eye protection device such as goggles or glasses with solid side-shields. Apply gloves. Carefully remove the tube from the centrifuge without disturbing the contents.

Principle. The OSHA standard requires the use of personal protective equipment whenever spraying or splashing of blood might be generated. Disturbing the contents may cause the cells to enter the serum, and the specimen will need to be recentrifuged.

5. **Procedural Step.** Using a twisting and pulling motion, carefully remove the stopper from the tube, pointing the stopper away from you. Squeeze the bulb of the pipet to push the air out, then insert it into the serum. Place the tip of the pipet against the side of the tube approximately ¼ inch above the cell layer. Release the bulb to suction serum into the pipet. Do not allow the tip of the pipet to touch the cell layer.

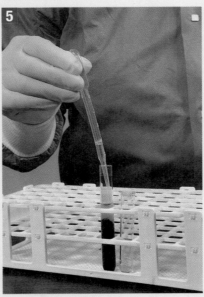

Pipet the serum.

Principle. Pointing the stopper away prevents accidental spraying or splashing of the specimen onto the medical assistant. The air should be removed from the bulb before inserting the pipet into the serum to pre-

vent disturbance of the cell layer. If the cell layer is disturbed, red blood cells would enter the serum, and the specimen would need to be recentrifuged.

6. **Procedural Step.** Transfer the serum in the pipet to the transfer tube. Continue pipetting until as much serum as possible is removed without disturbing the cell layer. Tightly cap the transfer tube to prevent sample evaporation.

7. **Procedural Step.** Hold the serum specimen up to the light, and examine it for the presence of hemolysis. Ensure that the proper amount of serum has been obtained.

Principle. Hemolyzed serum is unsuitable for laboratory testing.

8. **Procedural Step.** Properly dispose of equipment. Fol-

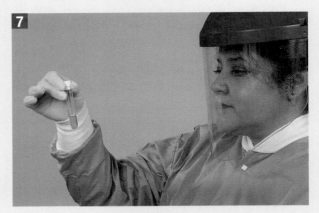

Examine the serum.

lowing the OSHA standard, the evacuated tube (containing the blood specimen) and the disposable pipet must be discarded in a biohazard sharps container.

9. **Procedural Step.** Remove the gloves, and sanitize your hands.

10. **Procedural Step.** Test the specimen, or prepare the specimen for transport to an outside laboratory for testing according to the medical office policy. If the specimen is to be transported to an outside laboratory, perform the following:

  a. Place the specimen tube in a biohazard specimen bag.

  b. Place the laboratory request in the outside pocket of the biohazard bag.

  c. Properly store the specimen while awaiting pickup by a laboratory courier.

  d. Chart the date the specimen was transported to the laboratory in the patient's record.

OBTAINING A PLASMA SPECIMEN

Plasma

Plasma is the straw-colored liquid portion of the blood. It serves as a transportation medium in which various substances are dissolved and blood cells are suspended for circulation through the body. Approximately 92% of plasma consists of water; the remaining 8% is dissolved solid substances (solutes) that are carried by the blood to and from the tissues.

The solutes present in greatest amounts are the *plasma proteins,* which include serum albumin, globulins, fibrinogen, and prothrombin. Serum albumin is synthesized in the liver and regulates the volume of plasma in the blood vessels. Globulins play an important role in the immunity mechanism of the body, and fibrinogen and prothrombin are essential for proper blood clotting.

Various *electrolytes* are carried by the plasma and are needed for normal cell functioning and the maintenance of the normal fluid and acid-base balance of the body. Some of these electrolytes are sodium, chloride, potassium, calcium, phosphate, bicarbonate, and magnesium. *Nutrients* derived from the breakdown of food substances are carried by the plasma to nourish the tissues of the body and include glucose, amino acids, and lipids. *Waste products* formed as the by-products of metabolism are carried by the plasma to be excreted and include urea, uric acid, lactic acid, and creatinine. *Respiratory gases* are dissolved in and carried by the plasma and include carbon dioxide and a small amount of oxygen. Substances in the plasma that help regulate and control body functions include hormones, antibodies, enzymes, and vitamins.

Tube Selection

Sometimes a plasma specimen is required for a laboratory test. The procedure for separating plasma from whole blood is essentially the same as that for separating serum from whole blood with minor variances, which are described here.

A tube containing an anticoagulant must be used to obtain plasma. The medical assistant should check the laboratory directory or the medical office laboratory procedures manual to determine the type of anticoagulant to be used, which is specified by the color of the tube stopper. The tube used to collect the specimen *and* the transfer tube should be properly labeled with the patient's name, the date, and the medical assistant's initials. In addition, the transfer tube should bear the word "plasma."

Preparation and Removal of the Specimen

As with serum, a blood specimen must be collected that is 2.5 times the amount required for the test. Before collecting the specimen, evacuated tubes containing a powdered additive (e.g., gray-stoppered tube) should be tapped just below the stopper to release any of the anticoagulant that may have adhered to the stopper. It is important to allow the specimen to fill to the exhaustion of the vacuum to ensure the proper ratio of anticoagulant to blood, which ensures accurate test results.

Immediately after the specimen is drawn, the tube should be gently inverted back and forth 8 to 10 times to mix the anticoagulant with the blood specimen. The specimen is placed in a centrifuge with the stopper on for 10 to 15 minutes. (The specimen does not need to stand before it is centrifuged.) Centrifuging the specimen packs the blood cells and causes the blood to separate into three layers: a top layer of plasma, a middle layer (the buffy coat), and a bottom layer of red blood cells. The plasma is separated from the blood specimen using the same procedure as that outlined for the separation of serum from whole blood.

SKIN PUNCTURE

A skin puncture is used to obtain a capillary blood specimen and is also called a *capillary puncture.* Laboratory testing of a capillary blood specimen is usually performed at the medical office. Examples of such tests are hemoglobin, hematocrit, blood glucose, mononucleosis, and prothrombin time.

A skin puncture is performed when a test requires only a small blood specimen. Skin puncture is the method preferred for obtaining blood from infants and young children. Collecting blood in this age group by venipuncture is often difficult and may damage veins and surrounding tissues. In addition, infants and young children have such a small blood volume that removing large quantities of blood may cause anemia. A skin puncture also might be performed as a last resort on an adult when a blood specimen is needed and there are no acceptable veins. Before collecting a capillary blood specimen, the medical assistant must (1) select a puncture site, (2) select the skin puncture device, and (3) obtain the proper microcollection device to collect the specimen.

PUNCTURE SITES

The puncture site varies depending on the age of the patient. The fingertip of the third or fourth finger is the preferred site for a skin puncture on an adult. In the past, the earlobe also was recommended as a skin puncture site for an adult. This is no longer true. Blood obtained by puncturing the earlobe has been found to contain a higher concentration of hemoglobin than fingertip blood. In addition, the earlobe produces a slower flow of blood, making it more difficult to obtain a blood specimen.

In an infant (birth to 1 year old), the skin puncture should be performed on the plantar surface of the heel. A finger puncture should *never* be performed on infants. The amount of tissue between skin surface and bone is so small that an injury to the bone is likely. After a child is walking, the skin puncture can be performed on the fingertip.

SKIN PUNCTURE DEVICES

According to OSHA, a skin puncture should be performed in the medical office using either a disposable or reusable semiautomatic retractable lancet device. The device used to perform the skin puncture is a matter of personal preference, and the technique for performing the puncture depends on the device that is used. A description of skin puncture devices is presented next, and the procedures for using them are presented at the end of this section.

Regardless of the skin puncture device, the puncture must not penetrate deeper than 3.1 mm on adults and 2.4 mm on infants and children. If the puncture is deeper than this, the bone may be penetrated, which could result in the painful and serious conditions of osteochondritis or osteomyelitis. **Osteochondritis** is inflammation of bone and cartilage, and **osteomyelitis** is an inflammation of the bone caused by bacterial infection. To avoid these complications, skin puncture devices are used with a spring-loaded blade available in different lengths to control the depth of puncture. The blade length used to perform a skin puncture is based on the size of the patient's fingers and the amount of blood specimen required. Adults with thin fingers and children require a shorter blade to avoid penetrating the bone. A longer blade must be used to obtain enough blood to fill a microcollection device, whereas a shorter blade can be used if only a drop of blood is needed.

OSHA does not recommend the use of lancets that are not retractable. A lancet that is not retractable increases the possibility that the medical assistant will stick himself or herself accidentally, resulting in an exposure incident. A disadvantage of a lancet that is spring loaded and does not retract automatically is that some patients may become apprehensive and flinch when they see the point of the lancet coming. Children might pull their hands out of the medical assistant's grasp.

Disposable Semiautomatic Lancet

A disposable semiautomatic retractable lancet consists of a spring-loaded plastic holder with a metal blade inside the holder. Disposable lancets are available in different lengths of blades to control the depth of the puncture. The plastic holder is color coded by the manufacturer for ease in identifying the blade length of the lancet device. The plastic holder conceals the blade so that the patient cannot see it during the puncture. One such lancet device is the Microtainer Brand Safety Flow Lancet (Becton Dickinson) (Figure 17-18A). Another example is the Tenderlette (International Technidyne Corporation, Edison, NJ), which is used for heel punctures on infants.

To perform the skin puncture, the lancet device is placed on the patient's skin, and the device is activated. Depending on the brand, this is accomplished by one of the following methods:

- Depressing an activation button located on the top or side of the lancet until an audible click is heard (Microtainer BD Genie Lancet)
- Pushing the lancet firmly onto the puncture site until an audible click is heard (e.g., Surgilance Safety Lancet)

When the device is activated, the spring forces the blade into the skin and retracts the blade into the holder. The concealed blade and automatic puncture tend to result in less patient apprehension. After the puncture, the entire lancet device is discarded in a biohazard sharps container. Procedure 17-5 describes the skin puncture procedure using a disposable semiautomatic lancet.

Reusable Semiautomatic Lancet

A wide variety of reusable semiautomatic lancets are commercially available; however, not all are appropriate for use in the medical office. Some of these devices are suitable for use only by an individual patient to perform home blood glucose

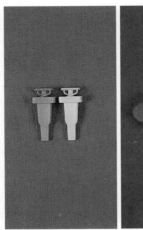

A. Microtainer Brand
Safety Flow Lancet

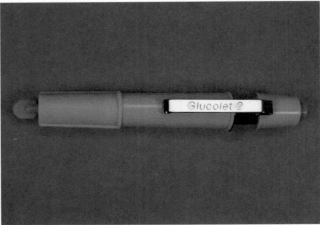

B. Glucolet II

Figure 17-18. Lancet devices. **A,** Microtainer Brand Safety Flow Lancet. **B,** Glucolet II.

monitoring. When used by more than one patient in the medical office, they have been associated with the transmission of hepatitis B. The safest reusable device is one in which the part that becomes contaminated is retractable and can be disposed of easily. This type of device reduces the risk of a sharps injury and infection from a contaminated sharp. An example of a reusable lancet that is safe to use in the medical office is the Glucolet II (Bayer Corporation).

The Glucolet II consists of a plastic spring-loaded lancet holder and a retractable lancet/endcap (Figure 17-18B). The lancet holder is reusable, whereas the lancet/endcap is retractable and disposable and meant for only one use. To perform the puncture, the lancet/endcap is placed on the patient's skin, and a release button is depressed. The spring forces the blade into the skin and retracts the blade into the endcap. After the procedure, the lancet/endcap is discarded in a biohazard sharps container (Procedure 17-6).

MICROCOLLECTION DEVICES

After the skin has been punctured, a capillary blood specimen must be collected. The blood specimen can be collected directly onto a reagent strip, such as occurs with blood glucose monitors. It also can be collected in a small container known as a *microcollection device*. The device depends on the laboratory equipment running the test. Common microcollection devices are capillary tubes and microcollection tubes.

Capillary Tubes

A capillary tube consists of a disposable glass or plastic tube (see Figure 17-19). Depending on the size of the tube, it can hold 5 to 75 μl of blood. In the medical office, a capillary tube is used to collect a blood specimen for a hematocrit determination. This procedure is presented in Chapter 18.

Microcollection Tubes

A microcollection tube consists of a small plastic tube with a removable blood collector tip. The tip is designed to collect capillary blood from a skin puncture and results in a relatively large blood specimen. After the specimen has been collected, the collector tip is removed, discarded, and replaced by a plastic plug. Microcollection tubes are available with or without additives. The plugs are color-coded and correspond to the color-coded evacuated tube system used in venipuncture. One such device is the Microtainer (Becton-Dickinson) (Figure 17-19).

GUIDELINES FOR PERFORMING A FINGER PUNCTURE

1. If a laboratory test requires advance preparation, before you perform the finger puncture, verify that the patient has prepared properly. If not, do not collect the specimen unless directed otherwise by the physician. If the finger puncture is to be rescheduled, carefully review the preparation requirements with the patient.

2. The patient should be seated comfortably in a chair. The arm should be firmly supported and extended with the palmar surface of the hand facing up. Never perform a skin puncture with the patient sitting on a stool or standing. The patient may faint and injure himself or herself.

3. Instruct the patient to remain still during the procedure. Explain to the patient that the procedure should be relatively quick and only slightly uncomfortable. Just before making the puncture, tell the patient that he or she will "feel a small stick." This prevents startling the patient, which could cause the patient to move.

4. Use the lateral part of the tip of the third or fourth finger (middle or ring finger) of the nondominant hand for the puncture site. The capillary bed in these fingers is large, and the skin is easy to penetrate. The puncture site should be free of lesions, scars, bruises, and edema. The index finger is not recommended as puncture site. The index finger is more calloused, which makes it harder to penetrate than the other fingers. Also, the patient uses that finger more and would notice the pain longer. The little finger should also not be used as a puncture site. The amount of tissue between the skin surface and the bone is so small that using this finger as a puncture site could result in an injury to the bone.

5. After selecting the puncture site, warm the site to increase the blood flow to the capillary bed. Warming the site can be accomplished by gently massaging the finger five or six times from base to tip or by placing the hand in warm water for a few minutes (105°F [40°C]). Warming the site promotes bleeding after an effective puncture.

6. Cleanse the site with an antiseptic wipe, and allow it to dry thoroughly. The site must be dry to allow a round drop of blood to form on the finger. Otherwise, the drop would leach out onto the skin of the patient's finger and be difficult to collect. In addition, alcohol entering the capillary specimen contaminates it, leading to

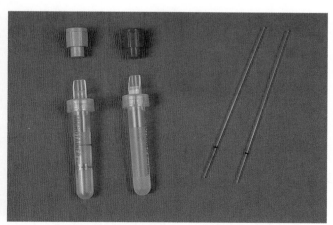

A. Microcollection tubes   B. Capillary tubes

Figure 17-19. Microcollection devices.

TERMINOLOGY REVIEW

Antecubital space The surface of the arm in front of the elbow.

Anticoagulant A substance that inhibits blood clotting.

Buffy coat A thin, light-colored layer of white blood cells and platelets that lies between a top layer of plasma and a bottom layer of red blood cells when an anticoagulant has been added to a blood specimen.

Evacuated tube A closed glass or plastic tube that contains a premeasured vacuum.

Hematoma A swelling or mass of coagulated blood caused by a break in a blood vessel.

Hemoconcentration An increase in the concentration of the nonfilterable blood components in the blood vessels, such as red blood cells, enzymes, iron, and calcium, as a result of a decrease in the fluid content of the blood.

Hemolysis The breakdown of blood cells.

Osteochondritis Inflammation of bone and cartilage.

Osteomyelitis Inflammation of the bone as a result of bacterial infection.

Phlebotomist A health care professional trained in the collection of blood specimens.

Phlebotomy Incision of a vein for the removal of blood; the collection of blood.

Plasma The liquid part of the blood consisting of a clear, straw-colored fluid that comprises approximately 55% of the blood volume.

Serum Plasma from which the clotting factor fibrinogen has been removed.

Venipuncture Puncturing of a vein.

Venous reflux The backflow of blood (from an evacuated tube) into the patient's vein.

Venous stasis The temporary cessation or slowing of the venous blood flow.

ON THE WEB

For Information on Phlebotomy:

Clinical Laboratory Standards Institute: www.clsi.org

National Accrediting Agency for Clinical Laboratory Sciences: www.naacls.org

Lab Explorer: www.labexplorer.com

American Society for Clinical Laboratory Science (ASCLS): www.ascls.org

American Society for Clinical Pathology (ASCP): www.ascp.org

American Society of Phlebotomy Technicians (ASPT): www.aspt.org

Becton Dickinson: www.bd.com

National Phlebotomy Association (NPA): www.nationalphlebotomy.org

The Safety Lady: www.safetylady.com

My Blood Draw: www.myblooddraw.com

Phlebotomy Pages: www.phlebotomypages.com

18

Hematology

LEARNING OBJECTIVES

Hematology Tests
1. List the tests included in a complete blood count.
2. Describe the shape of an erythrocyte, and explain how it acquires this shape.
3. Describe the composition of hemoglobin, and explain its function.
4. Describe the normal appearance of leukocytes, and explain how they fight infection in the body.
5. State the normal value or range for each of the following hematologic tests:
   Hemoglobin
   Hematocrit
   Red and white blood cell counts
   Differential cell count
   Platelet count
6. State the purpose of the hematocrit, and list the layers into which the blood separates after it has been centrifuged.
7. Explain the purpose of the differential cell count.
8. Describe the appearance of the five types of white blood cells.

PROCEDURES

Perform a hemoglobin determination using an automated analyzer and the manufacturer's operating manual.
Perform a hematocrit determination.
Prepare a blood smear.

CHAPTER OUTLINE

Introduction to Hematology
Components and Function of Blood
   Erythrocytes
   Leukocytes
   Thrombocytes
Hemoglobin Determination
Hematocrit

White Blood Cell Count
Red Blood Cell Count
White Blood Cell Differential Count
   Automated Method
   Manual Method
   Types of White Blood Cells

NATIONAL COMPETENCIES

Clinical Competencies
Diagnostic Testing
Perform hematology testing.

Patient Care
Screen and follow-up test results.

General Competencies
Patient Instruction
Provide instruction for health maintenance and disease prevention.

Operational Functions
Use methods of quality control.

ameboid movement (ah-MEE-boid-MOVE-ment)
anemia (ah-NEE-mee-ah)
bilirubin (bill-ih-ROO-bin)
diapedesis (die-ah-pah-DEE-sis)
hematology (hee-mah-TOL-oe-jee)
hemoglobin (HEE-moe-gloe-bin)

hemolysis (hee-MOL-oe-sis)
leukocytosis (loo-koe-sie-TOE-sis)
leukopenia (loo-koe-PEE-nee-ah)
oxyhemoglobin (ok-see-HEE-moe-gloe-bin)
phagocytosis (fay-goe-sie-TOE-sis)
polycythemia (pol-ee-sie-THEE-mee-ah)

Introduction to Hematology

Hematology is the study of blood, including the morphologic appearance and function of blood cells and diseases of the blood and blood-forming tissues. Laboratory analysis in hematology is concerned with the examination of blood for the purpose of detecting pathologic conditions. It includes performing blood cell counts, evaluating the clotting ability of the blood, and identifying cell types. These tests are valuable tools that allow the physician to determine whether each blood component falls within its normal value or range.

Examples of hematologic tests include the hemoglobin, hematocrit, white blood cell count, red blood cell count, differential white blood cell count, prothrombin time, erythrocyte sedimentation rate, and platelet count. Table 18-1 summarizes common hematologic tests, including specimen requirements, normal values, and conditions that cause abnormal test results.

Hematologic laboratory tests may be performed in the medical office. Advances in automated blood analyzers designed for use in the medical office have made this possible. Automated blood analyzers perform laboratory tests with accurate test results in a short time. Each automated analyzer is accompanied by a detailed operating manual that explains its operation, test parameters, care, and maintenance.

The most frequently performed hematologic laboratory test is the *complete blood count* (CBC). A CBC is routinely performed on new patients and on patients with a pathologic condition. The test results provide valuable information to assist the physician in making a diagnosis, evaluating the patient's progress, and regulating treatment. The tests included in a CBC are as follows:

- White blood cell (WBC) count
- Red blood cell (RBC) count
- Platelet count
- Hemoglobin (Hgb)
- Hematocrit (Hct)
- Differential white blood cell count (diff)
- Red blood cell indices

COMPONENTS AND FUNCTION OF BLOOD

Blood consists of two parts—liquid and solid. Plasma, the liquid portion of the blood, consists of a clear yellowish fluid that makes up approximately 55% of the blood volume. The plasma transports nutrients to the tissues of the body to nourish and sustain them, and it picks up wastes from the tissues. These wastes are eliminated through the kidneys. The plasma also transports antibodies, enzymes, and hormones to help regulate normal body functioning.

The solid portion of the blood consists of three types of cells: erythrocytes, leukocytes, and thrombocytes. The solid portion of the blood accounts for 45% of the total blood volume. The average adult body contains 10 to 12 pints (5 to 6 L) of blood.

Erythrocytes

In an adult, erythrocytes, or red blood cells, are formed in the red bone marrow of the ribs, sternum, skull, and pelvic bone and in the ends of the long bones of the limbs. The immature form of an erythrocyte contains a nucleus. As the cell develops and matures, however, it loses its nucleus and acquires the shape of a biconcave disc, thicker at the rim than at the center. This shape provides the erythrocyte with a greater surface area for the exchange of substances. An erythrocyte is approximately 7 to 8 μm in diameter. The average number of erythrocytes ranges from 4 to 5.5 million per cubic millimeter of blood in a woman and from 4.5 to 6.2 million per cubic millimeter of blood in a man.

A major portion of the erythrocyte consists of **hemoglobin,** a complex compound that transports oxygen and is responsible for the red color of the erythrocyte. The amount of hemoglobin in the blood averages 12 to 16 g/dL for a woman and 14 to 18 g/dL for a man. A hemoglobin molecule consists of a globin, or protein, and an iron-containing pigment called *heme.* One hemoglobin molecule loosely combines with four oxygen molecules in the lungs to form a substance called **oxyhemoglobin.** Oxyhemoglobin is transported and distributed to the tissues, where the oxygen is easily released from the hemoglobin. The blood picks up carbon dioxide, a waste product, and transports it back to the lungs to be expelled. When oxygen combines with hemoglobin, a bright

Table 18-1 Common Hematologic Tests

Name of Test (Abbreviation)	Purpose	Normal Range	Increased with	Decreased with
White blood cell count (WBC)	Assist in diagnosis and prognosis of disease	4,500-11,000/mm^3 (or 10^9 cells/L)	**Leukocytosis** Acute infections (appendicitis, chickenpox, diphtheria, infectious mononucleosis, meningitis, pneumonia, rheumatic fever, smallpox, tonsillitis) Hemorrhaging Trauma Malignant disease Leukemia Polycythemia vera	**Leukopenia** Viral infections Hypersplenism Bone marrow depression Infectious hepatitis Cirrhosis Chemotherapy Radiation therapy
Red blood cell count (RBC)	Assist in diagnosis of anemia and polycythemia	*Male:* 4.5-6.2 million/mm^3 (or 10^{12} cells/L) *Female:* 4-5.5 million/mm^3 (10^{12} cells/L) MCV 80-100 fL MCH 27-34 pg MCHC 1-36% RDW 11.5-14.5%	Polycythemia vera Secondary polycythemia Severe diarrhea Dehydration Acute poisoning Pulmonary fibrosis Severe burns	Iron deficiency anemia Hodgkin's disease Multiple myeloma Leukemia Hemolytic anemia Pernicious anemia Lupus erythematosus Addison's disease
Hemoglobin (Hgb or Hb)	To screen for anemia, determine its severity, monitor response to treatment	*Male:* 14-18 g/dL (SI units: 2.17-2.79 mmol/L) *Female:* 12-16 g/dL (SI units: 1.86-2.48 mmol/L)	Severe burns Chronic obstructive pulmonary disease Congestive heart failure	Anemia Hyperthyroidism Cirrhosis Severe hemorrhage Hemolytic reactions Hodgkin's disease Leukemia
Hematocrit (Hct)	Assist in diagnosis and evaluation of anemia	*Male:* 40-54% *Female:* 37-47%	Polycythemia vera Severe dehydration Shock Severe burns	Anemia Leukemia Hyperthyroidism Cirrhosis Acute blood loss Hemolytic reactions
Differential white blood cell count (diff)	Assist in diagnosis and prognosis of disease	Neutrophils 50-70% Eosinophils 1-4% Basophils 0-1% Lymphocytes 20-35% Monocytes 3-8%	**Neutrophilia** Acute bacterial infections Parasitic infections Liver disease **Eosinophilia** Allergic conditions Parasitic infections Addison's disease Lung and bone cancer **Basophilia** Leukemia Chronic inflammation Polycythemia vera Hemolytic anemia Hodgkin's disease	**Neutropenia** Acute viral infections Blood diseases Hormone diseases Chemotherapy **Eosinopenia** Infectious mononucleosis Hypersplenism Congestive heart failure Aplastic and pernicious anemia **Basopenia** Acute allergic reactions Hyperthyroidism Steroid therapy

Table 18-1 Common Hematologic Tests—cont'd

Name of Test (Abbreviation)	Purpose	Normal Range	Increased with	Decreased with
			Lymphocytosis Acute and chronic infections Hematopoietic disorders Addison's disease Carcinoma Hyperthyroidism	**Lymphopenia** HIV infection Cardiac failure Cushing's disease Hodgkin's disease Leukemia
			Monocytosis Viral infections Bacterial and parasitic infections Collagen diseases Cirrhosis Polycythemia vera Polycythemia	**Monocytopenia** Prednisone treatment Hairy cell leukemia
Prothrombin time (PT)	Screen for coagulation disorders and regulate treatment of patients taking oral anticoagulant therapy with warfarin sodium (Coumadin)	11-16 sec	**Thrombocytosis** Prothrombin deficiency Vitamin K deficiency Hemorrhagic disease of the newborn Liver disease Anticoagulant therapy Biliary obstruction Acute leukemia Polycythemia vera	**Thrombocytopenia** Acute thrombophlebitis Diuretics Multiple myeloma Pulmonary embolism Vitamin K therapy
Erythrocyte sedimentation rate (ESR)	Nonspecific test for connective tissue diseases, malignancy, and infectious diseases; also used to evaluate progress of inflammatory diseases (elevated test results warrant further testing)	Westergren's method *Male:* younger than age 50, 0-20 mm/hr; age 50 or older, 0-20 mm/hr *Female:* younger than age 50, 0-20 mm/hr; age 50 or older, 0-30 mm/hr	Collagen diseases Infections Inflammatory diseases Carcinoma Cell or tissue destruction Rheumatoid arthritis	Polycythemia vera Sickle cell anemia Congestive heart failure
Platelet count (Plt)	Assist in evaluation of bleeding disorders that occur with liver disease, thrombocytopenia, uremia, and anticoagulant therapy	150,000-400,000/mm³ (SI units: 150-400 × 10⁹/L)	**Thrombocytosis** Cancer Leukemia Polycythemia vera Splenectomy Acute blood loss Rheumatoid arthritis Trauma (fractures)	**Thrombocytopenia** Pernicious anemia Aplastic anemia Hemolytic anemia Pneumonia Allergic conditions Infection Bone marrow–depressant drugs

red color results that is characteristic of arterial blood. Venous blood is darker red, owing to its lower oxygen content.

The average life span of a red blood cell is 120 days. Toward the end of this time, it becomes more and more fragile and eventually ruptures and breaks down; this process is known as **hemolysis.** Hemoglobin, liberated from the red blood cell, also breaks down. The iron is stored and later reused to form new hemoglobin, and the protein is metabolized by the body. **Bilirubin** is formed by metabo-

lism of the heme units and transported to the liver, where it is eventually excreted as a waste product in the bile.

Leukocytes

Leukocytes, or white blood cells, are clear, colorless cells that contain a nucleus. The number of leukocytes in the healthy adult ranges from 4500 to 11,000 per cubic millimeter of blood. **Leukocytosis** is the condition of having an abnormal increase in the number of leukocytes (greater

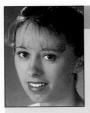

than 11,000 per cubic millimeter), and **leukopenia** is the condition of having an abnormal decrease in the number of leukocytes (less than 4500 per cubic millimeter).

The function of leukocytes is to defend the body against infection. Pathogens can gain entrance to the body in a variety of ways (review the infection process cycle in Chapter 2). Leukocytes attempt to destroy the invading pathogens and remove them from the body. In contrast to erythrocytes, leukocytes do their work in the tissues; they are transported to the site of infection by the circulatory system. During inflammation, the blood vessels in the infected area dilate, resulting in an increased blood supply. More oxygen, nutrients, and white blood cells can be delivered to the infected area to aid in the healing process. The cells in the capillary walls spread apart, enlarging the pores between the cells. White blood cells squeeze through the pores by **ameboid movement** and move out into the tissues to fight the infection. This movement of the leukocytes through the pores of the capillaries and out into the tissues is known as **diapedesis.**

Leukocytes (especially the granular forms) are phagocytic, and when they arrive at the site of infection they begin the process of **phagocytosis,** the engulfing and destruction of pathogens and damaged cells. In some conditions, pus forms in the infected area (suppuration); pus contains dead leukocytes, dead bacteria, and dead tissue cells.

Thrombocytes

Platelets, also known as *thrombocytes,* are small, clear, and disc-shaped. They lack a nucleus and are formed in the red bone marrow from giant cells known as *megakaryocytes.* Platelets function by participating in the blood-clotting mechanism. The number of platelets in a healthy adult ranges from 150,000 to 400,000 per cubic millimeter of blood.

HEMOGLOBIN DETERMINATION

Hemoglobin (Hgb) is a major component of red blood cells. Hemoglobin transports oxygen to the tissue cells of the body and is responsible for the color of the red blood cell.

The hemoglobin determination is used to measure indirectly the oxygen-carrying capacity of the blood. The normal range for a woman is 12 to 16 g/dL, and the normal range for a man is 14 to 18 g/dL. A hemoglobin determination is performed as an individual test or as part of the CBC. A hemoglobin determination is often performed as a routine test on individuals, such as children younger than 2 years of age and pregnant women, who are at risk for developing anemia.

A decreased hemoglobin level occurs with **anemia** (especially iron deficiency anemia), hyperthyroidism, cirrhosis of the liver, severe hemorrhaging, hemolytic reactions, and certain systemic diseases such as leukemia and Hodgkin's disease. Increased levels of hemoglobin are present with **polycythemia,** chronic obstructive pulmonary disease, and congestive heart failure.

The hemoglobin determination can be performed on capillary or venous blood. The most accurate and reliable method for measuring hemoglobin concentration involves the use of a blood analyzer. An office blood analyzer permits the processing of the specimen in a short time, allowing the physician to evaluate the condition while the patient is still at the medical office.

HEMATOCRIT

The hematocrit (Hct) is a simple, reliable, and informative test that is frequently performed in the medical office. The word *hematocrit* means "to separate blood." The solid or cellular elements are separated from the plasma by centrifuging an anticoagulated blood specimen. The heavier red blood cells become packed and settle to the bottom of a tube. The top layer contains the clear, straw-colored plasma. Between the plasma and the packed red blood cells is a small, thin,

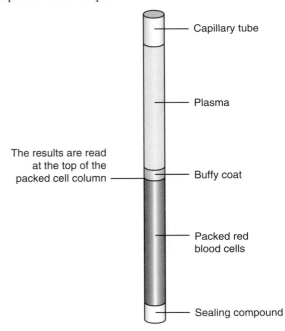

Figure 18-1. Hematocrit test results. The blood cells are separated from the plasma by centrifuging an anticoagulated blood specimen, and the results are read at the top of the packed cell column.

- **Blood consists of plasma and cells.** The function of plasma is to transport nutrients to the tissues of the body and to pick up wastes from the tissues.
- **The three types of cell in the blood** are erythrocytes, leukocytes, and thrombocytes. Erythrocytes are formed in the red bone marrow. The average number of erythrocytes in a woman is 4 to 5.5 million per cubic millimeter of blood; in a man, 4.5 to 6.2 million per cubic millimeter of blood.
- **Hemoglobin transports oxygen** and is responsible for the red color of the erythrocyte. The amount of hemoglobin in the blood averages 12 to 16 g/dL for a woman and 14 to 18 g/dL for a man. The average life span of a red blood cell is 120 days.
- **Leukocytes are clear, colorless cells** that contain a nucleus. The number of leukocytes in a healthy adult ranges from 4500 to 11,000 per cubic millimeter of blood. Leukocytosis is an abnormal increase in the number of leukocytes, and leukopenia is an abnormal decrease in the number of leukocytes. The function of leukocytes is to defend the body against infection.
- **Thrombocytes, or platelets,** participate in the blood-clotting mechanism. The normal number of platelets in an adult is 150,000 to 400,000 per cubic millimeter.
- **The hemoglobin determination** measures indirectly the blood's oxygen-carrying capacity. A hemoglobin determination is often performed as a routine test on individuals at risk for developing anemia, such as children younger than 2 years old and pregnant women.
- **The purpose of the hematocrit** is to measure the percentage volume of packed red blood cells in whole blood. The normal hematocrit range for a woman is 37% to 47%; for a man, 40% to 54%. A low hematocrit reading may indicate anemia, whereas a high reading may indicate polycythemia.
- **The white blood cell count** assists in the diagnosis and prognosis of disease. Leukocytosis is most commonly seen in acute infection. Conditions that result in leukopenia include viral infections, chemotherapy, and radiation therapy.
- **The red blood cell count** is a measurement of the number of red blood cells in whole blood. Conditions that cause a decrease in red blood cells include anemia, Hodgkin's disease, and leukemia. Conditions that cause an increase include polycythemia, dehydration, and pulmonary fibrosis.
- **The purpose of the differential cell count** is to identify and count the five types of white blood cell in a representative blood sample, which assists the physician in making a diagnosis. An increase or decrease in one or more types can occur in pathologic conditions.
- **The five types of white blood cell** are neutrophils, eosinophils, basophils, lymphocytes, and monocytes. Neutrophils are the most numerous of the white blood cells. An increase in the number of neutrophils is generally seen during an acute infection. Basophils are the least numerous of the white blood cells. Lymphocytes are the smallest white blood cells and are involved with the immune system and the production of antibodies. An increase in lymphocytes generally occurs with certain viral diseases. Monocytes are the largest white blood cells.

TERMINOLOGY REVIEW

Ameboid movement Movement used by leukocytes that permits them to propel themselves from the capillaries into the tissues.

Anemia A condition in which there is a decrease in the erythrocytes or amount of hemoglobin in the blood.

Bilirubin An orange-colored bile pigment produced by the breakdown of heme from the hemoglobin molecule.

Diapedesis The ameboid movement of blood cells (especially leukocytes) through the wall of a capillary and out into the tissues.

Hematology The study of blood and blood-forming tissues.

Hemoglobin The iron-containing pigment of erythrocytes that transports oxygen in the body.

Hemolysis The breakdown of erythrocytes with the release of hemoglobin into the plasma.

Leukocytosis An abnormal increase in the number of white blood cells (greater than 11,000 per cubic millimeter of blood).

Leukopenia An abnormal decrease in the number of white blood cells (less than 4500 per cubic millimeter of blood).

Oxyhemoglobin Hemoglobin that has combined with oxygen.

Phagocytosis The engulfing and destruction of foreign particles, such as bacteria, by special cells called *phagocytes.*

Polycythemia A disorder in which there is an increase in the red blood cell mass.

ON THE WEB

For Information on Stress and Stress Management:

American Institute of Stress: www.stress.org

The Medical Basis of Stress, Depression, Anxiety, Sleep Problems, and Drug Use: www.teachhealth.com

The Anxiety Panic Internet Resource: www.algy.com/anxiety

Stress Tips: www.stresstips.com

19

Blood Chemistry and Serology

LEARNING OBJECTIVES

Blood Chemistry

1. Explain the purpose of a blood chemistry test.
2. Describe the function of LDL cholesterol and HDL cholesterol in the body.
3. State the desirable ranges for each of the following tests: total cholesterol, LDL cholesterol, and HDL cholesterol.
4. State the patient preparation for a triglyceride test.
5. Explain the functions of glucose and insulin in the body.
6. State the patient preparation for a fasting blood sugar.
7. Identify the normal range for a fasting blood sugar.
8. State the purpose of each of the following tests: fasting blood sugar, 2-hour postprandial glucose test, and glucose tolerance test.
9. Describe the procedure for a 2-hour postprandial blood sugar test.
10. Identify the patient preparation required for a glucose tolerance test.
11. State the restrictions that must be followed by the patient during a glucose tolerance test.
12. List three advantages of self-monitoring of blood glucose by diabetic patients.
13. Explain the purpose of the hemoglobin A_{1c} test.
14. State the A_{1C} level for an individual without diabetes.
15. State the recommended blood glucose level and hemoglobin A_{1c} percentage for an individual with diabetes.
16. Explain the storage requirements for blood glucose reagent strips.

Serology

1. Explain the purpose of each of the following serologic tests: hepatitis tests, syphilis tests, mononucleosis test, rheumatoid factor, antistreptolysin test, C-reactive protein, cold agglutinins, ABO and Rh blood typing, and Rh antibody titer.
2. List the symptoms of infectious mononucleosis.
3. Identify the location of the blood antigens and antibodies.
4. Explain how the blood antigen-antibody reaction is used for blood typing in vitro.
5. List the antigens and antibodies in the following blood types: A, B, AB, and O.
6. Explain the difference between Rh-positive and Rh-negative blood.

PROCEDURES

Perform blood chemistry testing, using an automated blood chemistry analyzer and operating manual.

Perform a fasting blood sugar using a glucose monitor.

Instruct a patient in how to measure blood glucose using a glucose monitor.

Demonstrate the proper care and maintenance of a glucose monitor.

Perform a rapid mononucleosis test.

NATIONAL COMPETENCIES

Clinical Competencies

Diagnostic Testing
Use methods of quality control.
Perform chemistry testing.
Perform immunology testing.
Screen and follow-up test results.

General Competencies

Patient Instruction
Instruct individuals according to their needs.
Provide instruction for health maintenance and disease prevention.

KEY TERMS

agglutination (ah-gloo-ti-NAY-shun)
antibody (AN-ti-bod-ee)
antigen (AN-ti-jen)
antiserum (AN-ti-sere-um)
blood antibody
blood antigen
donor
gene (jeen)
glycogen (GLIE-koe-jen))
glycosylation

HDL cholesterol
hemoglobin A_{1c}
hyperglycemia (hie-per-glie-SEE-me-ah)
hypoglycemia (hie-poe-glie-SEE-me-ah)
in vitro (in-VEE-troe)
in vivo (in-VEE-voe)
LDL cholesterol
lipoprotein (lie-poe-PROE-teen)
recipient (ree-SIP-ee-ent)

Introduction to Blood Chemistry and Serology

Blood chemistry and serologic laboratory tests are often performed in the medical office. Advances in automated blood analyzers designed for use in the medical office have made this possible. Automated blood analyzers perform laboratory tests in a short time with accurate test results. Each automated analyzer is accompanied by a detailed operating manual explaining its operation, test parameters, care, and maintenance.

This chapter is divided into two units. The first presents blood chemistry laboratory tests, and the second presents serologic tests. The material in this chapter about blood testing is intended to serve only as a basic guide for the medical assistant and should be supplemented by much well-supervised practice in a classroom laboratory, the medical office, or both.

BLOOD CHEMISTRY

Blood chemistry testing involves the quantitative measurement of chemical substances in the blood. These chemicals are dissolved in the liquid portion of the blood; most blood chemistry tests require a serum specimen for analysis. There are numerous types of blood chemistry tests; the type of test (or tests) the physician orders depends on the clinical diagnosis. Table 19-1 lists common blood chemistry tests with specimen requirements, normal values, and conditions that cause abnormal test results. The blood chemistry tests that are most frequently performed are described in more detail in this chapter.

AUTOMATED BLOOD CHEMISTRY ANALYZERS

In the medical office, automated blood chemistry analyzers may be used to perform blood chemistry testing. A blood chemistry analyzer consists of a reflectance photometer that

Text continued on p. 697

Table 19-1 Common Blood Chemistry Tests

Name of Test (Abbreviation)	Purpose	Normal Range	Increased with	Decreased with
Alanine amino-transferase (ALT)	To detect liver disease	45 U/L or less	Hepatocellular disease Active cirrhosis Metastatic liver tumor Obstructive jaundice Pancreatitis	
Alkaline phos-phatase (ALP)	Assists in diagnosis of liver and bone diseases	25-140 U/L	Liver disease Bone disease Hyperparathyroidism Infectious mononucleosis	Hypophosphatasia Malnutrition Hypothyroidism Chronic nephritis
Aspartate amino-transferase (AST)	To detect tissue damage	40 U/L or less	Myocardial infarction Liver disease Acute pancreatitis Acute hemolytic anemia	Beriberi Uncontrolled diabetes mellitus with acidosis
Blood urea nitro-gen (BUN)	Screens for renal disease, especially glomerular functioning	7-25 mg/dl (SI units: 2.5-6.4 mmol/L)	Kidney disease Urinary obstruction Dehydration Gastrointestinal bleeding	Liver failure Malnutrition Impaired absorption
Calcium (Ca)	To assess parathyroid functioning and calcium metabolism and evaluate malignancies	8.5-10.8 mg/dl (SI units: 2.13-2.76 mmol/L)	**Hypercalcemia** Hyperparathyroidism Bone metastases Multiple myeloma Hodgkin's disease Addison's disease Hyperthyroidism	**Hypocalcemia** Hypoparathyroidism Acute pancreatitis Renal failure
Chloride (Cl)	Assists in diagnosing disorders of acid-base and water balance	96-109 mmol/L	Dehydration Cushing's syndrome Hyperventilation Preeclampsia Anemia	Severe vomiting Severe diarrhea Ulcerative colitis Pyloric obstruction Severe burns Heat exhaustion

Continued

Table 19-1 Common Blood Chemistry Tests—cont'd

Name of Test (Abbreviation)	Purpose	Normal Range	Increased with	Decreased with
Cholesterol (Chol)	To screen for atherosclerosis related to coronary heart disease; secondary aid in study of thyroid and liver functioning	**Total Cholesterol** Less than 200 mg/dl (SI units: less than 5.18 mmol/L)—*desirable* 200-239 mg/dl (SI units: 5.18-6.19 mmol/L)—*borderline high* 240 mg/dl or greater (≥6.22 mmol/L or greater)—*high* **LDL Cholesterol** Less than 100 mg/dl (SI units: less than 2.6 mmol/L)—*optimal* 100-129 mg/dl (SI units: 2.6-3.34 mmol/L)—*near optimal* 130-159 mg/dl (SI units: 3.4-4.14 mmol/L)—*borderline high* 160-189 mg/dl (SI units: 4.14-4.9 mmol/L)—*high* 190 mg/dl or greater (SI units: 4.92 mmol/L or greater)—*very high* **HDL Cholesterol** 60 mg/dl or greater (SI units: 1.55 mmol/L or greater)—*optimal* 45-59 mg/dl (SI units: 1.16-1.53 mmol/L)—*desirable* 40-45 mg/dl (SI units: 1.04-1.17 mmol/L)—*borderline low* Less than 40 mg/dl (SI units: less than 1.04 mmol/L)—*increased risk for coronary heart disease*	Atherosclerosis Cardiovascular disease Obstructive jaundice Hypothyroidism Nephrosis	Malabsorption Liver disease Hyperthyroidism Anemia
Creatinine (Creat)	Screening test of renal functioning	0.6-1.5 mg/dl (SI units: 46-115 μmol/L)	Impaired renal function Chronic nephritis Obstruction of urinary tract Muscle disease	Muscular dystrophy
Globulin (Glob)	To identify abnormalities in rate of protein synthesis and removal	2-3.5 g/dl (SI units: 20-35 g/L)	Brucellosis Chronic infections Rheumatoid arthritis Dehydration Hepatic carcinoma Hodgkin's disease	Agammaglobulinemia Severe burns

Table 19-1 Common Blood Chemistry Tests—cont'd

Name of Test (Abbreviation)	Purpose	Normal Range	Increased with	Decreased with
Glucose	To detect disorders of glucose metabolism		**Hyperglycemia**	**Hypoglycemia**
Fasting blood sugar (FBS)		**FBS:** 70-110 mg/dl (SI units: 3.9-6.1 mmol/L)	Diabetes mellitus	Excess insulin
2-hour post-prandial blood sugar (2-hr PPBS)		**2-hr PPBS:** less than 140 mg/dl (SI units: less than 7.8 mmol/L)	Hepatic disease	Addison's disease
Glucose tolerance test (GTT)		**GTT** **FBS:** 70-110 mg/dl (SI units: 3.9-6.1 mmol/L)—*normal* **FBS:** greater than 120 mg/dl (SI units: greater than 6.7 mmol/L)—*diabetic* **30 min:** 150-160 mg/dl (SI units: 8.4-8.9 mmol/L)—*normal* **30 min:** greater than 200 mg/dl (SI units: greater than 11.1 mmol/L)—*diabetic* **1 hr:** 160-170 mg/dl (SI units: 8.9-9.5 mmol/L)—*normal* **1 hr:** greater than 200 mg/dl (SI units: greater than 11.1 mmol/L)—*diabetic* **2 hr:** 120 mg/dl (SI units: 6.7 mmol/L)—*normal* **2 hr:** greater than 140 mg/dl (SI units: greater than 7.8 mmol/L)—*diabetic* **3 hr:** 70-110 mg/dl (SI units: 3.9-6.1 mmol/L)—*normal* **3 hr:** greater than 140 mg/dl (SI units: greater than 7.8 mmol/L)—*diabetic*	Brain damage Cushing's syndrome	Bacterial sepsis Pancreatic carcinoma Hepatic necrosis Hypothyroidism
Lactate dehydrogenase, 30°C (LD)	Assists in confirming myocardial or pulmonary infarction; also used in differential diagnosis of muscular dystrophy and pernicious anemia	240 U/L or less	Acute myocardial infarction Acute leukemia Muscular dystrophy Pernicious anemia Hemolytic anemia Hepatic disease Extensive cancer	

Continued

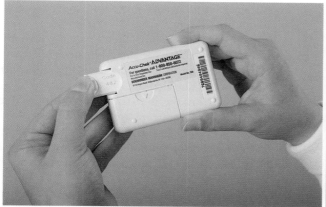

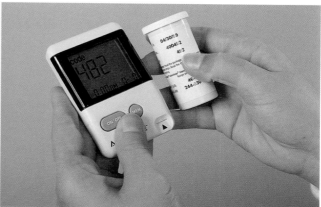

A, The code key is inserted into the monitor.

B, The code number must match the code number of the vial of reagent strips.

Figure 19-3. Accu-Chek Advantage code key calibration procedure.

PATIENT TEACHING   Obtaining a Capillary Blood Specimen

The medical assistant may need to instruct the patient in the procedure for obtaining and testing a capillary blood specimen for blood glucose measurement. Properly educating the patient to perform the procedure is the most important factor in obtaining accurate test results.

1. **Obtaining the capillary blood specimen.** Inform the patient of the sites available for obtaining the blood specimen, including the fingers and the side of the hand where there are no calluses. Most patients prefer to use an automatic lancet to perform the skin puncture. Using such a device makes the puncture less painful, and the preset puncture depth generally ensures a successful stick. For a finger puncture, instruct the patient to obtain the blood specimen from the lateral side of the fingertip because this area contains fewer nerve endings, and less pain results. If the patient's hands are cold, tell him or her to rub them together or place them in warm water, which improves the blood flow to the area. Instruct the patient in the proper procedure for obtaining enough blood to ensure accurate test results.

2. **Performing the blood glucose test.** The patient performs the test with a reagent strip using a glucose meter. Instruct the patient in the proper procedure for performing the test, making sure he or she understands that accurate test results assist in greater glucose control. Patients also should be given detailed instructions on the proper care and maintenance of the glucose meter.

3. **Recording results.** Instruct the patient to record each test result in a log book to provide a permanent record between office visits. In addition, most glucose meters are equipped with a memory system that stores test results for later retrieval. Keeping track of these factors helps explain a shift in the blood glucose level and provides the basis for sound self-management decisions. The following information should be included with each recording:
   - Date and time
   - Number of hours since the patient last ate
   - Time of the last insulin injection or oral hypoglycemic medication
   - Any feeling of physical or emotional stress
   - Amount of exercise the patient has had

The control solution can then be used for 3 months from that date or until the manufacturer's expiration date (stamped on the container) is reached, whichever comes first. The control solution is sensitive to heat, light, and moisture and must be stored in a cool, dry area at room temperature (less than 90°F [32°C]) with the cap tightly closed.

A control check should be performed under the following circumstances:
1. When the meter is new
2. Daily, before using the meter for the first time
3. When a new container of reagent strips is opened
4. If the cap is left off the vial of reagent strips for any length of time

5. If the meter is dropped
6. If a test has been repeated, and the blood glucose result is still lower or higher than expected

The control procedure outlined next should be followed to run a control check:
1. Turn the meter on. Check that the code number displayed matches the code number on the container of test strips.
2. Gently insert the end of the test strip with the silver-colored bars into the test strip guide with the yellow target area facing up.
3. Roll the Level 1 (low) control solution between your hands to mix it.

4. Wait until the flashing drop appears on the display. Remove the cap of the control solution, and squeeze one drop of the solution onto a paper towel.
5. Apply the control solution to the strip as follows:
   a. Accu-Chek Advantage Test Strip: Invert the container, and hold it over the yellow target area of the test strip. Squeeze the container, and touch and hold the drop of control solution to the center of the yellow target area.
   b. Accu-Chek Comfort Curve Test Strips. Hold the container at an angle to the edge of the yellow target area of the test strip. Squeeze the container, and touch and hold a drop of control solution to the edge (not the top) of the yellow target area.
6. Promptly replace the lid on the control solution.
7. After a short time, the control value is displayed on the screen of the glucose meter.
8. If the control value is within acceptable range, it will fall within the acceptable control ranges listed on the label of the test strip container.

9. Repeat the control check procedure using a Level 2 (high) control solution.
   If the Level 1 or Level 2 control results are not within the acceptable range, the following should be performed:
1. Check the expiration dates of the test strips and control solution to make sure they are not outdated.
2. Determine whether the test strips and control solution were stored at room temperature.
3. Make sure the container lids were tight on the test strip container and control solution container.
4. Check to make sure the code on the meter matches the code on the test strip vial.
5. Review the technique used to run the control to make sure it was followed correctly.
   Any errors should be corrected and the control should be run again. If the results are still not within acceptable range, the manufacturer of the glucose meter should be contacted.

Text continued on p. 710

PROCEDURE 19-1 Blood Glucose Measurement Using the Accu-Chek Advantage Glucose Meter

Outcome Perform a fasting blood sugar.

Equipment/Supplies

- Disposable gloves
- Accu-Chek Advantage glucose meter
- Accu-Chek Advantage reagent strips
- Check strip
- Code key
- Control solution
- Lancet
- Antiseptic wipe
- Gauze pad
- Biohazard sharps container

1. Procedural Step. Sanitize your hands. Assemble the equipment. Check the expiration date on the container of reagent strips.
Principle. Outdated reagent strips can cause inaccurate test results.

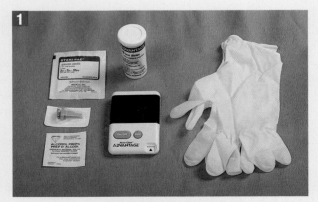

Assemble the equipment.

2. Procedural Step. If the meter requires calibration with a check strip, calibrate the glucose meter using the check strip (refer to page 706).
Principle. Calibrating with the Check Strip ensures that the glucose meter is functioning properly.
3. Procedural Step. If necessary, calibrate the glucose meter using the code key that accompanies the container of reagent strips (refer to page 706).
Principle. Calibrating with the Code Key compensates for variables that occur in the manufacturing process of the reagent strips and must be performed before using strips from a new container.
4. Procedural Step. Run a Level 1 (low) and Level 2 (high) control check on the glucose meter using Accu-Chek Advantage control solutions (refer to page 707).
Principle. Running a low and high control check ensures that the test results are reliable and valid.
5. Procedural Step. Greet and identify the patient. Introduce yourself, and explain the procedure.

6. **Procedural Step.** If a fasting specimen is required, ask the patient whether he or she has had anything to eat or drink (besides water) for the past 12 hours.
Principle. Consumption of food or fluid increases the blood glucose level, leading to inaccurate interpretation of FBS test results.

7. **Procedural Step.** Turn the meter on. Check that the code number displayed matches the code number on the vial of test strips that you are using. When the test strip symbol flashes on the display, the meter is ready to accept a test strip.

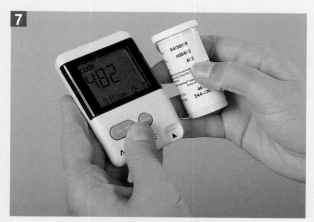

Check the code number.

8. **Procedural Step.** Remove a test strip from the container. Promptly replace the lid of the container to prevent the strips from being exposed to moisture.
Principle. The reagent pads are moisture sensitive and could be affected by environmental moisture, leading to inaccurate test results.

9. **Procedural Step.** Within 30 seconds, gently insert the end of the test strip with the silver-colored bars into the test strip guide with the yellow target area facing up. When the strip is correctly inserted, a blood drop symbol flashes on the display.

10. **Procedural Step.** Cleanse the puncture site with an antiseptic wipe, and allow it to dry. Apply gloves, and perform a finger puncture. Dispose of the lancet in a biohazard sharps container.
Principle. The antiseptic must be allowed to dry to prevent it from reacting with the chemicals on the reagent pad, which would lead to inaccurate test results. Gloves provide a barrier against bloodborne pathogens.

11. **Procedural Step.** After the puncture has been made, wipe away the first drop of blood with a gauze pad. Place the hand in a dependent position (palm facing down), and gently squeeze the finger around the puncture site until a large drop of blood forms.

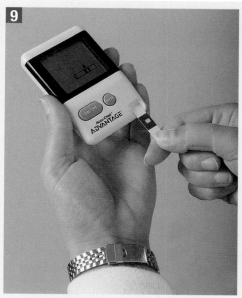

Insert the test strip into the meter.

Principle. The first drop of blood contains a large amount of serum, which dilutes the specimen and leads to inaccurate test results. A large drop of blood is needed to cover the target area of the reagent strip completely.

12. **Procedural Step.** Apply the drop of blood to the test strip as follows:
a. Accu-Chek Advantage Test Strip: Touch and hold the drop of blood to the center of the yellow target area.
b. Accu-Chek Comfort Curve Test Strips. Touch and hold a drop of blood to the edge (not the top) of the yellow target area.
Completely fill the yellow target area. If any yellow mesh is visible after you have applied the initial drop of blood, a second drop of blood may be applied to the target area within 15 seconds of the first drop. If more than 15 seconds has passed, the test result may

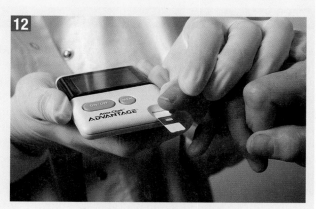

Touch the blood to the target area.

Continued

PROCEDURE 19-1   Blood Glucose Measurement Using the Accu-Chek Advantage Glucose Meter—cont'd

be erroneous, and you should discard the test strip and repeat the test.

When the blood is correctly applied to the strip, a box rotates on the display until the measurement is completed.

Principle. The entire yellow target area must be completely covered with blood to ensure accurate and reliable test results.

13. **Procedural Step.** Have the patient hold a gauze pad over the puncture site and apply pressure until the bleeding stops.

14. **Procedural Step.** After a short time, the glucose value is displayed in milligrams per deciliter (mg/dL). If the

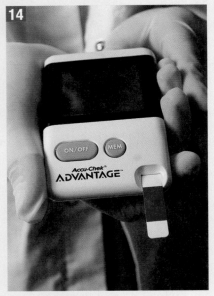

Read the glucose value on the display screen.

glucose value is higher or lower than expected, or if the screen displays something other than the glucose value, see the Troubleshooting Guide section of the operator's manual to obtain instructions for correcting the problem. (The glucose result indicated on this glucose meter is 89 mg/dL.)

15. **Procedural Step.** Remove the reagent strip from the meter, and discard it in a biohazard waste container. Turn the meter off.

16. **Procedural Step.** Remove the gloves, and sanitize your hands. Chart the results. Include the date and time, when the patient last ate, the type of test (e.g., FBS, random), the glucose test result, and your initials. If the patient has diabetes mellitus, also record the time of his or her last insulin injection or last consumption of oral hypoglycemic medication.

17. **Procedural Step.** Properly store the glucose meter according to the manufacturer's instructions.

CHARTING EXAMPLE

Date	
5/18/08	8:30 a.m. FBS: 89 mg/dL. Pt last ate on
	5/17 @ 7:00 p.m. ——— M. Villers, CMA

SEROLOGY

Serology is the scientific study of the serum of the blood. More specifically, serology deals with the study of antigen and antibody reactions. An **antigen** is a substance that is capable of stimulating the formation of antibodies in an individual. Antigens may consist of protein, glycoprotein, complex polysaccharides, or nucleic acid. Specific examples of antigens include bacteria and viruses, bacterial toxins, allergens, and blood antigens. An **antibody** is a substance that is capable of combining with an antigen, resulting in an antigen-antibody reaction.

Laboratory testing in serology deals with studying antigen-antibody reactions to assess the presence of a substance (e.g., ABO blood typing) or to assist in the diagnosis of disease (e.g., mononucleosis testing). Serologic tests are often used for the early diagnosis of disease and are used to follow the course of the disease.

SEROLOGIC TESTS

Specific examples of serologic tests are described next.

Hepatitis Tests

Hepatitis testing is performed to detect viral hepatitis. There are five types of viral hepatitis—A, B, C, D, and E—which are described in detail in Chapter 2. Hepatitis testing not only detects the presence of viral hepatitis, but it also determines the type of hepatitis present.

Syphilis Test

Syphilis is a sexually transmitted disease (STD) caused by the microorganism *Treponema pallidum*. The most common tests to detect the presence of syphilis are the Venereal Disease Research Laboratories (VDRL) test and the rapid plasma reagin (RPR) test. The test results are reported as nonreactive, weakly reactive, or reactive. Weakly reactive and reactive results are considered positive for the presence of syphilis antibodies. These tests are screening tests, and a positive result warrants more specific testing to arrive at a diagnosis of syphilis.

Mononucleosis Test

The mononucleosis test ("mono test") is used to detect the presence of infectious mononucleosis. The theory and procedure for this test are discussed in detail in this chapter.

Rheumatoid Factor

Rheumatoid arthritis is a chronic inflammatory disease that affects the joints of the body. The blood of patients with rheumatoid arthritis contains a type of antibody called *rheumatoid factor* (RF). This test detects the presence of rheumatoid factor antibodies and assists in the diagnosis of rheumatoid arthritis.

Antistreptolysin O Test

The antistreptolysin O (ASO) test is used to detect ASO antibodies in the serum. It is the most widely used serologic test for the detection of conditions resulting from streptococcal infections and diseases that occur secondary to a streptococcal infection. This test is useful in assisting in the diagnosis of rheumatic fever, glomerulonephritis, bacterial endocarditis, and scarlet fever.

C-Reactive Protein

During inflammation and tissue destruction, an abnormal protein called *C-reactive protein* (CRP) appears in the blood. Patients with inflammatory conditions or disorders accompanied by tissue destruction have positive results to this test. Because of this, the CRP test is used to assist in diagnosing or charting the progress of rheumatoid arthritis, acute rheumatic fever, widespread malignancy, and bacterial infections.

Cold Agglutinins

The cold agglutinins test is used to detect the presence of antibodies called *cold agglutinins.* This test is performed by incubating the patient's serum with erythrocytes at cold temperatures. If cold agglutinins are present, this causes **agglutination** of the erythrocytes. Cold agglutinins are found in patients with infectious mononucleosis, mycoplasmal pneumonia, chronic parasitic infections, and lymphoma.

ABO and Rh Blood Typing

Blood typing is performed to determine an individual's ABO and Rh blood type. Knowledge of blood type helps to prevent transfusion and transplant reactions and to identify problems such as hemolytic disease of the newborn. The theory and procedure for ABO and Rh blood typing are presented in this chapter.

Rh Antibody Titer

The Rh antibody titer test detects the amount of circulating Rh antibodies in the blood. These antibodies can occur in a pregnant woman who is Rh-negative and is carrying an Rh-positive fetus. This test is most frequently used to detect the presence of an Rh incompatibility problem with a mother and her unborn child.

RAPID MONONUCLEOSIS TESTING

Infectious mononucleosis is an acute infectious disease caused by the Epstein-Barr virus (EBV). Infectious mononucleosis most frequently affects children and young adults. It is transmitted through saliva by direct oral contact, and because of this, it is often called the "kissing disease." Symptoms of infectious mononucleosis include mental and physical fatigue, fever, sore throat, severe weakness, headache, and swollen lymph nodes.

The rapid mono test is often performed in the medical office and is used to assist in the diagnosis of infectious mononucleosis. Rapid mono tests are easy to perform and provide reliable results in a short time. Patients with infectious mononucleosis produce an antibody called *heterophile antibody,* usually by 6 to 10 days into the illness. Rapid mono tests detect this antibody. The presence of the heterophile antibody along with patient symptoms can provide the basis for the diagnosis of infectious mononucleosis. Figure 19-4 outlines the procedure for performing a rapid mono test using the QuickVue+ Mononucleosis Test (Quidel Corporation, San Diego, CA).

BLOOD TYPING

Blood Antigens

Each individual has a blood type. Blood type depends on the presence of certain factors, or antigens, on the surface of the red blood cells. **Blood antigens** consist of protein and are inherited through **genes,** which program the body to produce a particular antigen. If a blood antigen is present, it appears on the surface of all the red blood cells in the body.

Many types of antigen can appear in the blood. These antigens can be grouped into categories known as *blood group systems.* The blood group systems that are most likely to cause problems in blood transfusions and in Rh disease of the newborn are the ABO and Rh blood group systems. These are the blood group systems most commonly tested for in the medical laboratory.

Within the ABO blood group system, there are four main blood types—A, B, AB, and O. The blood type depends on which antigens are present on the surface of the red blood cells.

- If the A antigen is present, the blood type is A.
- If the B antigen is present, the blood type is B.
- If A and B antigens are present, the blood type is AB.
- If neither the A nor the B antigen is present, the blood type is O.

Figure 19-5 illustrates this principle.

Blood Antibodies

Blood antibodies are proteins that are naturally present in the plasma of the blood. An antibody is a substance that is

Text continued on p. 714

QuickVue + Mononucleosis Test

FOR INFORMATIONAL USE ONLY ■ FOR INFORMATIONAL USE ONLY ■ FOR INFORMATIONAL USE ONLY

Not to be used for performing assay. Refer to most current package insert accompanying your test kit.

TEST PROCEDURE – WHOLE BLOOD

Read all of the procedural instructions before running patient samples.

Remove the Reaction Unit from the pouch and place it on a well lit and level surface.

The "Read Result" window contains a horizontal blue line pre-printed on the membrane.

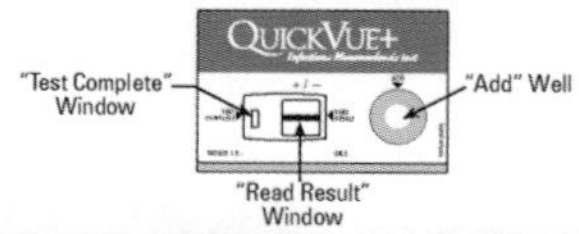

"Test Complete" Window — "Add" Well — "Read Result" Window

Capillary Tube Procedure

For fingertip blood, fill the capillary tube (50 μL) to line.

Dispense all blood into the "Add" well.

FILL TO LINE

(50μL)

OR

Venipuncture Procedure

For whole blood samples in tubes, use the sample pipette provided.

Place one drop of sample in the "Add" well.

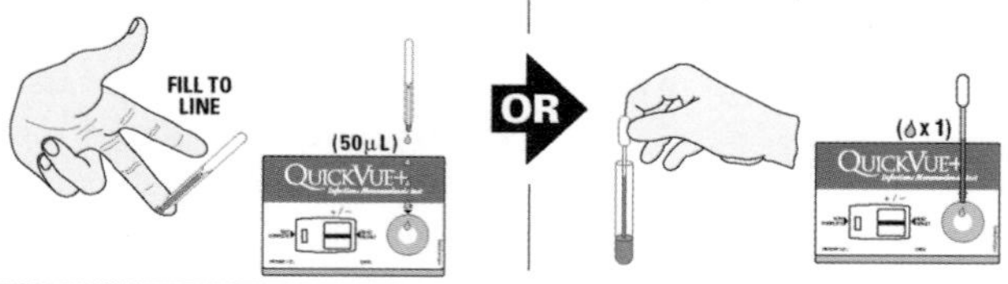

(◊ x 1)

Hold the Developer bottle vertically.

Add 5 drops of Developer to the "Add" well.

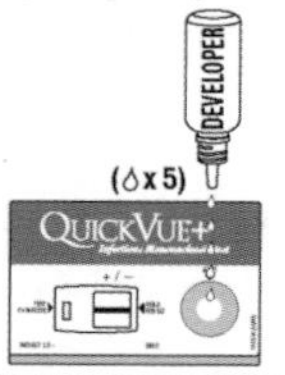

(◊ x 5)

Read results at 5 minutes.

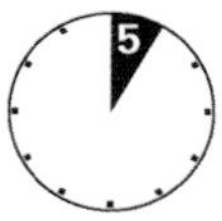

5

"Test Complete" line must be visible by 10 minutes.

INTERPRETATION OF RESULTS
FOR PATIENT SAMPLES, POSITIVE AND NEGATIVE CONTROLS

Positive Result

Any shade of a blue vertical line forming a (+) sign in the "Read Result" window along with the blue "Test Complete" line, is a positive result. **Even a faint blue vertical line should be reported as a positive.**

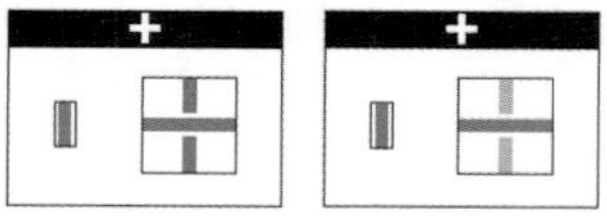

+   **+**

Negative Result

No blue vertical line in the "Read Result" window along with the blue "Test Complete" line, is a negative result.

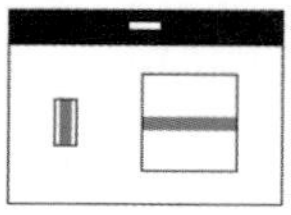

−

Invalid Result

Test results are invalid:
■ If after 10 minutes no signal is observed in the "Test Complete" window. (View #1.)
■ If after 10 minutes a blue color fills the "Read Result" window. (View #2.)

An invalid result indicates either the test was not performed correctly or the reagents are not working properly.

Should an invalid result occur, re-test the sample using a new Reaction Unit.

If the problem continues, contact Technical Support toll-free in the U.S. at (800) 874-1517. Outside the USA, contact your local representative.

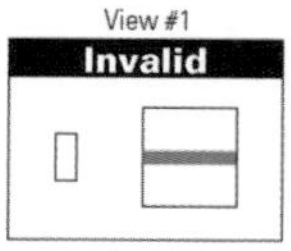

View #1
Invalid

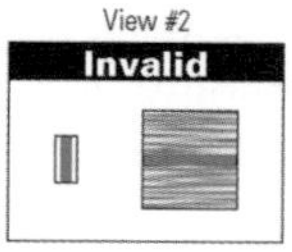

View #2
Invalid

LIMITATIONS

1. As is the case of any other diagnostic procedure, the results obtained by this kit yield data that must be used in addition to other information available to the physician.
2. QuickVue+ Infectious Mononucleosis test is a qualitative test for the detection of IM heterophile antibodies.
3. A negative result may be obtained from patients at the onset of the disease due to antibody concentration below the sensitivity of this test kit. If symptoms persist or increase in intensity, the test should be repeated.
4. Some segments of the population who contract Infectious Mononucleosis do not produce measurable levels of heterophile antibodies. Approximately 50% of children under 4 years of age who have IM may test as IM heterophile antibody negative.[4]

Figure 19-4. Procedure for performing the QuickVue+ Mononucleosis Test. (Courtesy of and modified from Quidel Corporation, San Diego, Calif.)

Highlight on Blood Donor Criteria

Every year, approximately 5 million Americans require blood transfusions, resulting in 13.5 million units of blood being transfused. A safe, readily available blood supply is essential for lifesaving medical procedures, such as replacing blood loss from hemorrhages or surgical procedures, replacing plasma in burn and shock victims, and providing platelets to control bleeding. In an average population, 75% of the people are physically and medically eligible to donate blood; only 5% of those eligible donate.

Basic blood donor criteria have been established on a national basis to ensure donor safety and a quality blood donation. All blood collection facilities, such as the American Red Cross, must follow these regulations. In general, blood donors must be in good health and be of a certain age and weight.

Health History

To protect the donor and the recipient, each donor is asked to give a brief health history. The prospective donor is asked to provide information related to diseases that may be transmitted through the blood (e.g., hepatitis and AIDS) and medications being taken that could affect the quality of the blood donation. Information also is obtained related to medical conditions that might jeopardize the health of the donor if he or she were to donate.

Based on this information, a prospective donor could be *temporarily deferred* from donating blood because of the following: recent immunizations, pregnancy, a human bite, a skin infection, certain medical conditions such as a recent heart attack or tuberculosis, certain prescription medications being taken, recent tattooing, and travel to a malaria-prone area. Temporarily deferred donors are told how long they must wait and are encouraged to donate blood when the waiting period is over. The waiting period varies based on the condition or situation; there is a 1-year waiting period after a heart attack, whereas there is only a 2-day wait after the last dose of an antibiotic medication.

A prospective donor is *permanently deferred* from giving blood because of any of the following reasons: a clotting disorder, cancer that was treated with chemotherapy, certain autoimmune disease (e.g., lupus, multiple sclerosis), a history of hepatitis, infection with the AIDS virus (HIV infection), and behavior that is associated with the spread of the AIDS virus. An individual also is permanently deferred if he or she has spent 3 months or more in the United Kingdom between 1980 and 1996 (a country where "mad cow disease" is found).

Age

An individual must be at least 17 years old to donate blood. With written parental consent, however, some states permit 16-year-olds to donate blood. There is no upper age limit for blood donation as long as the individual feels well and has no restrictions or limitations on his or her activities.

Date of Last Donation

At least 56 days (8 weeks) must elapse between donations.

Weight

The donor must weigh at least 110 lb. (In some states, the minimum weight is 105 lb.) For the average individual, the total volume of blood is approximately 8% of the body weight. Underweight donors are not accepted because a full donation would result in a proportionately greater reduction in blood volume and might precipitate a reaction. There is no upper weight limit as long as the individual's weight is not higher than the weight limit of the blood donor bed being used.

Temperature

Body temperature of donors may not exceed 99.5°F (37.5°C). The primary purpose of temperature measurement is to eliminate donors who are ill.

Pulse

The acceptable range for the pulse rate is 50 to 110 beats per minute. If the pulse rate seems to be elevated because of physical exertion, the donor may be asked to remain seated for 5 to 10 minutes, with a recheck taken after the rest period.

Blood Pressure

The acceptable limit for blood pressure is a reading no higher than 180 mm Hg for the systolic pressure and a reading no higher than 100 mm Hg for the diastolic pressure.

Hemoglobin

The hemoglobin must be 12.5 g/dL or greater for men and women.

Blood-Donating Process

It takes approximately 1 hour to donate blood. The process begins with the health history, followed by a mini-physical check of temperature, pulse, blood pressure, and hemoglobin level. Next, 1 unit (1 pint) of blood is collected using a sterile needle and a sterile plastic bag that contains an additive. A donor should feel no pain during the blood collection procedure, which takes approximately 8 to 10 minutes. It is not possible to contract AIDS or any other infectious disease by donating blood. After the collection of the unit of blood, the donor is encouraged to have refreshments to begin replenishing the fluids and nutrients temporarily lost during the donation.

Processing the Blood

Each blood donation is tested for AIDS, hepatitis, and syphilis. Any unit of blood that tests positive is rejected for transfusion. The unit of blood is typed and labeled with its ABO and Rh blood type. It is then available for distribution to hospitals for transfusing. ■

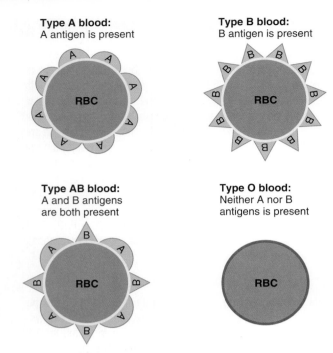

Type A blood:
A antigen is present

Type B blood:
B antigen is present

Type AB blood:
A and B antigens
are both present

Type O blood:
Neither A nor B
antigens is present

Figure 19-5. Blood type depends on which antigens are present on the surface of the red blood cells (RBCs).

Table 19-4 ABO Blood Group System		
Blood Type	Antigen Present on Red Blood Cell	Antibody Present in Plasma
A	A	B
B	B	A
AB	A, B	Neither A nor B
O	Neither A nor B	A, B

capable of combining with an antigen. The body never produces an antibody to combine with its own blood antigen. If the blood type is A, the plasma does not contain the A antibody. The B antibody naturally occurs in that plasma, however. The B antibody cannot combine with the A antigen. If a blood antigen and its corresponding antibody combine (in this case, the A antigen combining with the A antibody), a serious antigen-antibody reaction occurs that could be life-threatening.

- If the blood type is A, the plasma contains the B antibody.
- If the blood type is B, the plasma contains the A antibody.
- If the blood type is AB, neither the A nor the B antibody appears in the plasma.
- If the blood type is O, the A and B antibodies appear in the plasma. Type O blood has neither the A nor the B antigen on the surface of its red blood cells. The A and B antibodies in the plasma would not have an A or B antigen to combine with them (Table 19-4).

Rh Blood Group System

In 1940, Landsteiner and Wiener discovered the Rh blood group system while working with rhesus monkeys. Most people in the United States have the Rh antigen present on the red blood cells and have type Rh-positive blood. The remaining 15% of the Caucasian population and 7% of the African-American population do not have the Rh antigen

present on the red blood cells and have type Rh-negative blood. In contrast to the A and B antibodies, the Rh antibodies do not normally occur in the plasma.

BLOOD ANTIGEN AND ANTIBODY REACTIONS

When a blood antigen and its corresponding antibody unite, the result is the clumping, or agglutination, of red blood cells. Agglutination of red blood cells can be serious and fatal if it occurs **in vivo** (in the living body). The clumped red blood cells cannot pass through the small tubules of the kidneys, and this may lead to kidney failure. Also, the clumping of the red blood cells eventually leads to hemolysis, or breakdown of the red blood cells.

Blood antigen-antibody reactions can occur if the wrong blood type is administered to a patient during a blood transfusion. If an individual with type A blood is given a transfusion of type B blood, the B antibody of the **recipient** (person receiving the blood) would combine with the B antigen of the **donor** (person donating the blood), and an

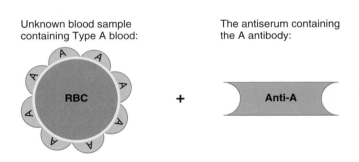

Unknown blood sample containing Type A blood:

The antiserum containing the A antibody:

+   **Anti-A**

The bridge forming between the antigen and antibody represents the antigen-antibody reaction. This reaction leads to agglutination of red blood cells, which is visible to the naked eye.

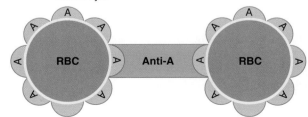

Figure 19-6. The antigen-antibody reaction that occurs in vitro when the unknown blood sample is type A.

antigen-antibody reaction would occur, resulting in agglutination of red blood cells. We say that type A blood is incompatible with type B blood.

AGGLUTINATION AND BLOOD TYPING

Agglutination of red blood cells is the basis for the ABO and Rh blood typing procedure. The antigen-antibody reaction occurs **in vitro,** or "in glass" in the laboratory, so there is no threat to life.

To test for the ABO blood group system, a commercially prepared antiserum is used. An antiserum is a serum that contains antibodies. An **antiserum** containing the A antibody is added to an unknown blood specimen. If the A antigen is present, it combines with the A antibody, result-

ing in agglutination. An antiserum containing the B antibody is added to another sample of the unknown blood. If the B antigen is present, it combines with the B antibody, resulting in agglutination. If agglutination occurs in both instances, the sample is type AB. If no agglutination occurs, this indicates the absence of blood antigens, or type O blood. Agglutination that occurs in vitro is visible to the naked eye. The antigen-antibody reaction that occurs when the unknown blood sample is type A is diagrammed in Figure 19-6.

 *Check out the **Companion CD** bound with the book to access additional interactive activities.*

MEDICAL PRACTICE and the LAW

When running laboratory tests, you must ensure that all equipment is functioning properly. This is done by the periodic calibration or running of controls on each piece of equipment. Know how and how often to calibrate or run controls, and document appropriately. Without these quality controls, results cannot be trusted to be accurate. Inaccurate results can lead to an inaccurate diagnosis and treatment. Use personal protective equipment appropriate to each test to avoid transmission of disease and cross-contamination of specimens.

Who Can Sue?

Anyone can sue for anything. The important thing to know is "can they win"? The person filing the lawsuit is called the *plaintiff,* and the one being sued is called the *defendant.* To win a malpractice lawsuit, four things are necessary:

1. The defendant must have had a duty to the plaintiff; that is, a physician-patient relationship must exist.

2. Care must have been provided that was not consistent with that of a "reasonably prudent" physician or medical assistant. In other words, a mistake was made, and the individual who made it should have known better. If you work in a specialty area, you are expected to know more about that specialty than if you worked in a general practice office. Be very familiar with your office's policy and procedures manual.
3. The plaintiff must prove proximate cause. This means the patient's problem is a direct cause of the physician's or medical assistant's actions.
4. The plaintiff must have been injured by the mistake. Damages may include pain and suffering, loss of income, and medical bills.

To avoid personal lawsuits, practice good care, document everything you do, and maintain good relationships with patients. Some patients who are hurt will sue, but most patients who are hurt and are angry *will* sue. ■

What Would You Do? What Would You *Not* Do? RESPONSES

Case Study 1
Page 698
What Did Michelle Do?
- ❏ Tried to calm and reassure Karen.
- ❏ Explained to Karen that the cholesterol results are not affected by food, so eating before the health fair should not have affected her results.
- ❏ Told Karen that before a cholesterol analyzer is used, it is usually checked to ensure it is working properly.
- ❏ Reassured Karen that the physician was checking her cholesterol again and running some additional tests to determine whether she is having any problems.
- ❏ Told Karen that if she must take medication, the physician will determine what drug is best for her.

What Did Michelle Not *Do?*
- ❏ Did not tell Karen that her cholesterol is extremely high.
- ❏ Did not tell Karen that she should be more careful about what she eats because she is overweight.
- ❏ Did not tell Karen that there was no way to know whether the cholesterol analyzer used at the health fair was calibrated and had controls run on it.

What Would You Do?/What Would You *Not* Do? Review Michelle's response and place a checkmark next to the information you included in your response. List additional information you included in your response.

_____
_____
_____
_____

Case Study 2
Page 701
What Did Michelle Do?
- ❏ Apologized to Crystal for the inconvenience. Explained to her that it takes 3 to 4 hours to run a glucose tolerance test because several specimens must be collected over time to see how her body handles sugar.
- ❏ Explained to Crystal that eating and smoking causes the test results to be inaccurate. Told her that she could eat and smoke as soon as the test was over.
- ❏ Told Crystal that she needs to sit quietly during the test, so it would not be possible for her to bring her children.
- ❏ Informed the physician of Crystal's situation to see whether he had any suggestions.

What Did Michelle Not *Do?*
- ❏ Did not become defensive or intimidated by Crystal's behavior.
- ❏ Did not tell Crystal that the staff would watch Crystal's children during the test.
- ❏ Did not tell Crystal that it was not a good idea for her to smoke around her children.

What Would You Do?/What Would You *Not* Do? Review Michelle's response and place a checkmark next to the information you included in your response. List additional information you included in your response.

_____
_____
_____

Case Study 3
Page 704
What Did Michelle Do?
- ❏ Told Dave that it would be fine for him to perform his own finger-stick.
- ❏ Made sure that his finger was cleansed with an antiseptic wipe and that he wiped away the first drop of blood.
- ❏ Explained to Dave that the air bubbles take up space that the insulin should occupy, and that if he does not get rid of them, he will not get his full dose of insulin.
- ❏ Demonstrated how to remove air bubbles, and had Dave practice it at the office.
- ❏ Told Dave he must not reuse his needle and syringe. Explained that a used needle could cause him to get an infection. Asked Dave whether he had checked to see if his insurance would cover the cost of the needles and syringes.
- ❏ Told Dave that he should put his used needles and syringes in a thick plastic container such as an empty detergent container. After the container is full, he should close it tightly with a screw lid, and then it can be thrown out with his regular trash. Explained that this will protect his family and the trash handlers from getting stuck while disposing of the trash.

What Did Michelle Not *Do?*
- ❏ Did not tell Dave he didn't need to worry about the air bubbles in the syringe.

What Would You Do?/What Would You *Not* Do? Review Michelle's response and place a checkmark next to the information you included in your response. List additional information you included in your response.

_____
_____
_____
_____

APPLY YOUR KNOWLEDGE

Blood Chemistry: **Choose the best answer to each of the following questions.**

1. Michelle Villers, CMA, supervises the running of the office laboratory. She is getting ready to run an FBS on a blood glucose meter. Which of the following must be performed to ensure accurate and reliable test results?
   A. Clean the analyzer with a mild abrasive cleaner.
   B. Run two levels of controls on the analyzer.
   C. Eat a healthy lunch.
   D. Check the warranty on the analyzer.

2. Stanley Seaver comes to the office for a general physical examination. Because he has a family history of heart disease, Dr. Donor orders a lipid profile on him. Michelle Villers, CMA, explains the patient preparation for this profile, which includes:
   A. Do not take any medications for 48 hours before the test.
   B. Consume a breakfast high in fat.
   C. Do not eat or drink anything, except water, for 12 hours before the test.
   D. Do not consume any foods containing cholesterol for 72 hours before the test.

3. Michelle performs a lipid profile on Stanley Seaver. Which of the following test results indicates an abnormal value?
   A. Total cholesterol: 260.
   B. Triglycerides: 175.
   C. LDL cholesterol: 150.
   D. HDL cholesterol: 36.
   E. All of the above.

4. Michelle is providing patient education to Stanley regarding coronary heart disease. All of the following factors are risk factors for CHD except:
   A. Cigarette smoking.
   B. Diabetes.
   C. Obesity.
   D. An elevated HDL cholesterol level.

5. Eva Marie is a 56-year-old woman with diabetes. Dr. Donor orders a 2-hour PPBS on Eva. Michelle Villers, CMA, explains the patient preparation to Eva, which includes:
   A. Do not eat or drink beginning at midnight.
   B. Consume a breakfast of 100 g of carbohydrate.
   C. Drink as much water as you desire.
   D. All of the above.

6. David Albright has come to the office for a GTT. Michelle Villers, CMA, draws a blood specimen for an FBS and determines the value to be 98 mg/dL. At this point, Michelle should:
   A. Continue with the GTT.
   B. Run another FBS.
   C. Notify the physician.
   D. Discontinue the test.

7. Pollyanna Porter is having a GTT. Michelle Villers, CMA, explains to Pollyanna that during the testing period, she is allowed to:
   A. Eat.
   B. Smoke.
   C. Drink water.
   D. Go to her health club and work out.

8. During the GTT, Pollyanna experiences some symptoms. Which of the following symptoms should Michelle report to the physician?
   A. Dizziness.
   B. Irrational speech.
   C. Weakness.
   D. Hunger.

9. Michelle Villers, CMA, receives an order of reagent strips for the Accu-Chek glucose meter. Michelle stores the strips in the:
   A. Refrigerator.
   B. Cupboard.
   C. Freezer.
   D. Fireproof safe.

10. Michelle gets ready to run a glucose test on the Accu-Chek glucose meter. She removes a test strip from the container and notices that it is discolored. Michelle should:
    A. Go ahead and run the test.
    B. Run the test, but make a notation of the color change in the patient's chart.
    C. Obtain a new container of test strips.
    D. Ask the physician what should be done.

Serology: **Choose the best answer to each of the following questions.**

1. Stephanie Carter comes to the medical office for a prenatal examination. Dr. Donor has determined that Stephanie's blood type is O-negative and wants to a run a blood test to determine whether there is

Continued

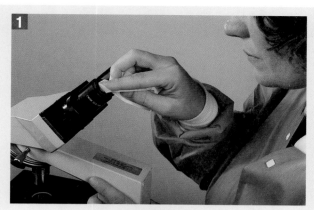

Clean the lens.

b. **Stage focus:** Lower the stage all the way down using the coarse adjustment knob.
4. **Procedural Step.** Place the slide on the stage specimen side up, and make sure it is secure.

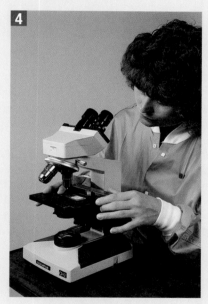

Place the slide on the stage.

5. **Procedural Step.** Position the low-power objective until it almost touches the slide using the coarse adjustment knob. Be sure to observe this step to prevent the objective from striking the slide.
6. **Procedural Step.** Look through the ocular. If a monocular microscope is being used, keep both eyes open to prevent eyestrain. With a binocular microscope, adjust the two oculars to the width between your eyes until a single circular field of vision is obtained.
7. **Procedural Step.** Bring the specimen into coarse focus as follows:
   a. **Barrel focus:** Slowly raise the objective using the coarse adjustment knob.
   b. **Stage focus:** Slowly lower the stage using the coarse adjustment knob.

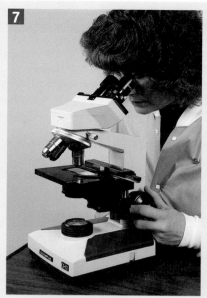

Focus the specimen.

Observe the specimen through the ocular until it comes into focus.
8. **Procedural Step.** Use the fine adjustment knob to bring the specimen into a sharp, clear focus.
9. **Procedural Step.** Adjust the light as needed, using the iris diaphragm to provide maximal focus and contrast.

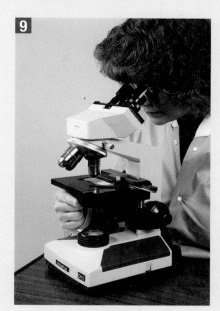

Adjust the light.

10. **Procedural Step.** Rotate the nosepiece to the high-power objective, making sure it clicks into place. Proper focusing with the low-power objective ensures that the objective does not hit the slide during this operation. Use the fine adjustment knob to bring the specimen into a precise focus. Do not use the coarse adjustment to focus the high-power objective

Continued

PROCEDURE 20-1

PROCEDURE 20-1   Using the Microscope—cont'd

to prevent the objective from moving too far and striking the slide.

11. **Procedural Step.** Examine the specimen as required by the test or procedure being performed.

12. **Procedural Step.** Turn off the light after use, and remove the slide from the stage.

13. **Procedural Step.** Clean the stage with a tissue or gauze.

14. **Procedural Step.** Properly care for and store the microscope.

Using the Oil Immersion Objective

1. **Procedural Step.** Rotate the nosepiece to the oil-immersion objective. Do not click it into place, but move it to one side.

2. **Procedural Step.** Place a drop of immersion oil on the slide directly over the center opening in the stage.

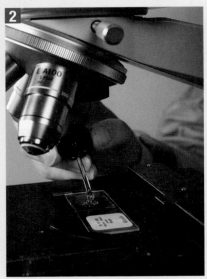

Place a drop of oil on the slide.

3. **Procedural Step.** Move the oil-immersion objective into place until a click is heard. Ensure that the objective does not touch the stage or slide.

4. **Procedural Step.** Using the coarse adjustment, slowly position the oil-immersion objective until the tip of the lens touches the oil but does not come in contact with the slide. A "pop" of light is observed. Be sure to observe carefully this step of the procedure.

5. **Procedural Step.** Look through the eyepiece, and focus slowly using the coarse adjustment until the object is visible.

6. **Procedural Step.** Use the fine adjustment to bring the object into sharp focus to view fine details.

7. **Procedural Step.** Adjust the light as needed, using the iris diaphragm to provide maximal focus and contrast. Increased light intensity is required for good visualization of the specimen with the oil-immersion objective.

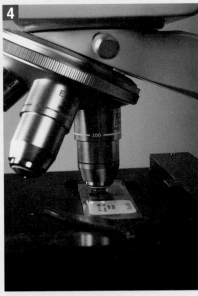

Move the lens until it just touches the oil.

8. **Procedural Step.** Examine the specimen as required by the test or procedure being performed.

9. **Procedural Step.** Turn off the light after use. Remove the slide from the stage, being careful not to get oil on the high-power objective or the stage.

10. **Procedural Step.** Using a piece of clean, dry lens paper, gently clean the oil-immersion objective. The lens must be cleaned immediately after use to prevent oil from drying on the lens surface. In addition, the oil may seep into the lens and perhaps loosen it.

11. **Procedural Step.** Clean the oil from the slide by immersing it in xylene and wiping it off with a soft cloth.

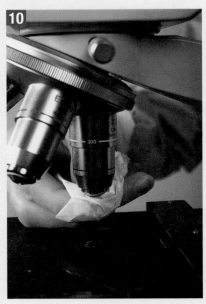

Clean the oil from the lens.

MICROBIOLOGIC SPECIMEN COLLECTION

If the physician suspects that a particular disease is caused by a pathogen, he or she may want to obtain a specimen for microbiologic examination. This examination identifies the pathogen causing the disease and aids in the diagnosis. If a urinary tract infection is suspected, a urine specimen is obtained for bacterial examination. In this instance, a clean-catch midstream collection is required to obtain a specimen that excludes the normal flora of the urethra and urinary meatus.

A **specimen** is a small sample or part taken from the body to represent the whole. The medical assistant is often responsible for collecting specimens from certain areas of the body, such as the throat, nose, and wound. The medical assistant may be responsible for assisting the physician in the collection of specimens from other areas, such as the cervix, vagina, urethra, and rectum. In most instances, a sterile swab is used to collect the specimen. A *swab* is a small piece of cotton wrapped around the end of a slender wooden or plastic stick. It is passed across a body surface or opening to obtain a specimen for microbiologic analysis.

To prevent inaccurate test results, good techniques of medical and surgical asepsis must be practiced when a specimen is obtained. The medical assistant must be careful not to contaminate the specimen with *extraneous microorganisms*. These are undesirable microorganisms that can enter the specimen in various ways; they grow and multiply and possibly obscure and prevent identification of pathogens that might be present. To prevent extraneous microorganisms (i.e., normal flora) from contaminating the specimen, all supplies used to obtain the specimen (e.g., swabs and specimen containers) must be sterile. In addition, the specimen should not contain microorganisms from areas surrounding the collection site. When obtaining a throat specimen, the swab should not be allowed to touch the inside of the mouth.

The OSHA Bloodborne Pathogens Standard presented in Chapter 2 should be carefully followed when performing microbiologic procedures. Specifically, the medical assistant must wear gloves when it is reasonably anticipated that hand contact might occur with blood or other potentially infectious materials. Eating, drinking, smoking, and applying makeup are strictly forbidden when one is working with microorganisms because pathogens can be transmitted to the medical assistant through hand-to-mouth contact. In addition, labels for specimen containers should not be licked, and any break in the skin, such as a cut or scratch, must be covered with a bandage. If the medical assistant accidentally touches some of the material in the specimen, the area of contact should be washed immediately and thoroughly with soap and water. If the specimen comes in contact with the worktable, the table should be cleaned immediately with soap and water followed by a suitable disinfectant, such as phenol. The worktable also should be cleaned with a disinfectant at the end of each day.

After collection, the specimen must be placed in its proper container with the lid securely fastened. The container must be clearly labeled with the patient's name, the date, the source of the specimen, the medical assistant's initials, and any other required information. Procedure 20-2 outlines the procedure for collecting a specimen for a throat culture.

Handling and Transporting Microbiologic Specimens

After the microbiologic specimen has been collected, care should be taken in handling and transporting it. Delay in processing the specimen may cause the death of pathogens or the overgrowth of the specimen by microorganisms that are part of the normal flora usually collected along with the pathogen from the specimen site. If the specimen is to be analyzed in the medical office, it should be examined under the microscope or cultured immediately. Otherwise, it should be preserved (if possible) with the method used by the medical office.

Specimens transported to an outside medical laboratory by a courier service are usually placed in a transport medium. The transport medium prevents drying of the specimen and preserves it in its original state until it reaches its destination. Transport media are discussed in more detail in the section on "Collection and Transport Systems."

Outside laboratories provide the medical office with specific instructions on the care and handling of specimens being transported to them. These specimens must be accompanied by a laboratory request that designates the physician's name and address; the patient's name, age, and gender; the date and time of collection; the type of microbiologic examination requested; the source of the specimen (e.g., throat, wound, urine); and the physician's clinical diagnosis. There is usually a space on the form to indicate whether the patient is receiving antibiotic therapy. Antibiotics may suppress the growth of bacteria, a factor that could produce false-negative results.

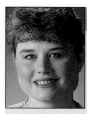

Putting It All into Practice

My Name is Natalie Moorehead, and I work for a physician who specializes in family practice. Working as a medical assistant, one can encounter many challenges. One experience that I had involved a 4-year-old boy. The patient came into the office with a very sore throat and a high fever. He did not think that his office visit had gone too badly until he found out that the physician had ordered a rapid strep test to check for strep throat. That's when he decided he did not care for me, my tongue depressor, or my swab. He decided to protest by keeping his mouth tightly shut. Rather than forcing the procedure on the child, I took my time and kept my patience. I managed to convince the child that even though the procedure was uncomfortable and tasted bad, it was the only way we would know if he was really sick or not. I also explained that the test was the only way the doctor would know what kind of medicine to prescribe so he could get well and feel like playing again. It took a while, but we got our specimen, and the patient received the right antibiotic that he needed to get better. ■

Wound Specimens

Wound specimens are collected using many of the techniques described previously. In many cases, two swabs are used to collect the specimen. The specimen is obtained by inserting the swab into the area of the wound that contains the most drainage and gently rotating the swab from side to side to allow it to absorb completely any microorganisms present. The swab is placed in the specimen container, and the process is repeated using a second swab. To obtain accurate and reliable test results, it is important to collect a specimen from within the wound, rather than from the surface.

Collection and Transport Systems

Microbiologic collection and transport systems are available to facilitate the collection of a specimen to be transported to an outside laboratory for analysis; examples include Culturette (Becton Dickinson, Franklin Lakes, NJ) and the Starswab II (Starplex Scientific, Beverly, MA) (Figure 20-5). These systems consist of a sterile swab and a plastic tube that contains a transport medium. The transport medium prevents drying of the specimen and preserves it in its original state until it reaches its destination. The collection and transport system comes packaged in a peel-apart envelope and should be stored at room temperature. The procedure for the use of a microbiologic collection and transport system is outlined next.

1. Complete a laboratory request form.
2. Sanitize your hands, and apply gloves.
3. Check the expiration date on the peel-apart envelope.

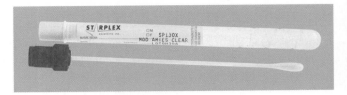

Figure 20-5. Starswab II Collection and Transport System.

4. Peel back the envelope, and remove the cap from the collection tube. Remove the cap/swab unit from the peel-apart envelope. The cap is permanently attached to the sterile swab.
5. Using aseptic technique, collect the specimen. Do not allow the swab to touch any area other than the collection site.
6. Insert the swab into the collection tube.
7. Push the cap/swab in as far as it will go to immerse the swab completely in the transport medium. Make sure the cap is tightly in place.
8. Remove gloves, and sanitize your hands.
9. Label the tube with the patient's name, the date, the source of the specimen (e.g., throat, wound), and your initials. Place the tube in a biohazard specimen transport bag. Place the laboratory request in the outside pocket of the bag.
10. Chart the procedure.
11. Transport the specimen to the laboratory within 24 hours.

Text continued on p. 734

What Would You Do? What Would You *Not* Do?

Case Study 2

Hollie Dolley, age 18, is at the medical office complaining of fatigue, fever, headache, and a terrible sore throat. She just enrolled in a medical assisting program and has been really worried about doing well in her classes. Hollie says that she stays up until midnight every night studying, and she works 30 hours at a drugstore on the weekends. The physician orders a rapid mononucleosis test on Hollie, and it is positive. Hollie says she has never felt so awful in her whole life and wants to know whether she is going to die from this. She says it hurts really bad to swallow and she cannot eat. Hollie says that she has heard one gets mono from kissing, and she does not have a boyfriend, so she does not understand how she could possibly have mono. Hollie wants to know why the physician did not prescribe an antibiotic for her so that she could get well sooner and not have to miss any of her classes. ■

PROCEDURE 20-2   Collecting a Specimen for a Throat Culture

Outcome Collect a specimen for a throat culture.

A specimen for a throat culture is obtained by using a sterile swab. It is commonly used to aid in the diagnosis of infections such as streptococcal sore throat, pharyngitis, and tonsillitis. Less frequently, it is used to diagnose whooping cough and diphtheria. These latter diseases are not prevalent today because of the availability of immunizations against them. This procedure outlines the steps necessary to obtain a throat specimen to perform a rapid streptococcus test, which is discussed later in the chapter.

Equipment/Supplies

- Disposable gloves
- Tongue depressor
- Sterile swab
- Waste container

1. **Procedural Step.** Sanitize your hands, and assemble the equipment.
2. **Procedural Step.** Greet and identify the patient. Introduce yourself, and explain the procedure.
3. **Procedural Step.** Position the patient, and adjust the light to provide clear visualization of the throat.
   Principle. The throat must be clearly visible so that the medical assistant is able to determine the proper area for obtaining the specimen.
4. **Procedural Step.** Apply gloves. Remove the sterile swab from its peel-apart package, being careful not to contaminate it.
   Principle. Contamination of the swab may lead to inaccurate test results.

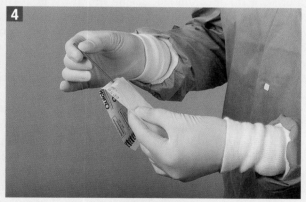

Remove the swab.

5. **Procedural Step.** Depress the tongue with the tongue depressor.
   Principle. The tongue depressor holds the tongue down and facilitates access to the throat.
6. **Procedural Step.** Place the swab at the back of the throat (posterior pharynx), and firmly rub it over any lesions or white or inflamed areas of the mucous membrane of the tonsillar area and posterior pharyngeal wall. Rotate the swab constantly as you collect the specimen, making sure there is good contact with the tonsillar area. Do not allow the swab to touch any areas other than the throat, such as the inside of the mouth.

Principle. The swab should be rubbed over suspicious-looking areas where pathogens are likely to be found. A rotating motion is used to deposit the maximal amount of material possible on the swab. Touching it to any areas other than the throat contaminates the specimen with extraneous microorganisms.

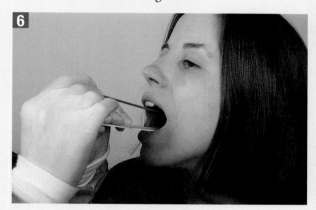

Collect the specimen.

7. **Procedural Step.** Keeping the patient's tongue depressed, withdraw the swab, and remove the tongue depressor from the patient's mouth.
8. **Procedural Step.** Properly dispose of the tongue depressor in a regular waste container to prevent transmission of microorganisms.
9. **Procedural Step.** Process the swab according to the directions accompanying the rapid strep test.
10. **Procedural Step.** Remove gloves, and sanitize your hands. Chart the test results.

CHARTING EXAMPLE

Date	
7/12/08	10:30 a.m. Throat specimen collected.
	QuickVue Strep Test: Positive. ———————
	————————————— N. Moorehead, CMA

21

Emergency Medical Procedures

LEARNING OBJECTIVES

First Aid
1. State the purpose of first aid.
2. Explain the purpose of the emergency medical services (EMS) system.
3. List the OSHA standards for administering first aid.
4. List the guidelines that should be followed when providing emergency care.

Common Emergency Situations
1. List and describe conditions that cause respiratory distress.
2. List the symptoms of a heart attack and a stroke.
3. Explain the causes of each of the following types of shock: cardiogenic, neurogenic, anaphylactic, and psychogenic.
4. Identify and describe the three classifications of external bleeding.
5. Explain the difference between an open wound and a closed wound.
6. Describe the characteristics of each of the following fractures: impacted, greenstick, transverse, oblique, comminuted, and spiral.
7. Identify the characteristics of each of the following burns: superficial, partial thickness, and full thickness.
8. Explain the difference between a partial seizure and a generalized seizure.
9. List examples of each of the following types of poisoning: ingested, inhaled, absorbed, and injected.
10. Identify factors that place an individual at higher risk for developing heat-related and cold-related injuries.
11. Describe the difference between type 1 and type 2 diabetes mellitus.
12. Explain the causes of insulin shock and diabetic coma.
13. Identify the symptoms and describe the emergency care for each of the following conditions: respiratory distress, heart attack, stroke, shock, bleeding, wounds, musculoskeletal injuries, burns, seizures, poisoning, heat and cold exposure, and diabetic emergencies.

PROCEDURES

Respond to common emergency situations.

CHAPTER OUTLINE

NATIONAL COMPETENCIES

General Competencies
Communication
Recognize and respond to verbal communications.
Recognize and respond to nonverbal communications.

KEY TERMS

burn
crash cart
crepitus (KREP-it-us)
dislocation
emergency medical services (EMS) system
first aid
fracture (FRAK-shur)
hypothermia (hie-poe-THER-mee-ah)

poison
pressure point
seizure (SEE-zhur)
shock
splint
sprain
strain
wound

Introduction to Emergency Medical Procedures

Medical emergencies often arise inside and outside of the workplace that can result in the sudden loss of life or permanent disability. If an emergency situation occurs in the medical office, the physician provides immediate medical care for the patient. Some medical offices maintain a crash cart for this purpose. In these situations, the medical assistant may be required to assist the physician in providing the emergency medical care.

The medical assistant may need to administer first aid for medical emergencies that occur outside of the medical office environment. **First aid** is defined as the immediate care administered before complete medical care can be obtained to an individual who is injured or suddenly becomes ill. The medical assistant is most likely to administer first aid to a family member or friend. The purpose of first aid is to save a life, reduce pain and suffering, prevent further injury, reduce the incidence of permanent disability, and increase the opportunity for an early recovery.

This chapter focuses on common emergency situations that the medical assistant may encounter and the first aid required for each. It is not intended, however, as a substitute for thorough first aid instruction through the American Red Cross, National Safety Council, or American Heart Association.

OFFICE CRASH CART

A **crash cart** is a specially equipped cart for holding and transporting medications, equipment, and supplies needed to perform lifesaving procedures in an emergency. A grow-ing number of physicians are incorporating crash carts into their medical offices. Patients who are injured or suddenly become ill might be brought to the medical office for emergency medical care. In addition, a patient might develop a sudden illness at the medical office that requires emergency medical care. Examples of these situations include life-threatening cardiac dysrhythmias, shock, cardiac arrest, poisoning, and traumatic injury.

The items on an office crash cart vary widely among medical offices depending on the extent of the emergency medical care that is likely to be administered. This is directly related to the time it takes for emergency medical personnel to arrive and the location of the nearest hospital. Table 21-1 is a general list of the medications, equipment, and supplies that may be included on an office crash cart. The medical assistant may be responsible for regularly checking the crash cart to replenish supplies and to check the expiration dates on medications.

EMERGENCY MEDICAL SERVICES SYSTEM

The **emergency medical services (EMS) system** is a network of community resources, equipment, and emergency medical technicians (EMTs) that provides emergency care to victims of injury or sudden illness. An *EMT-basic* (EMT-B) is a professional provider of prehospital emergency care, which includes care at the scene and during transportation to the hospital. An EMT-B has received formal training and is certified to provide basic life support measures. An *EMT-paramedic* (EMT-P) is qualified to provide advanced life support care, including advanced airway maintenance, starting intravenous drips, administration of medication, cardiac monitoring and interpretation, and cardiac defibrillation.

Text continued on p. 748

Table 21-1 Office Crash Cart

Name	Drug Category	Emergency Use
MEDICATIONS USED IN CARDIOVASCULAR EMERGENCIES		
Epinephrine (Adrenalin)	Sympathomimetic*	Helps restore cardiac rhythm in cardiac arrest
Sodium bicarbonate	Alkalinizing agent	To correct metabolic acidosis after cardiac arrest
Lidocaine (Xylocaine)	Antiarrhythmic	For rapid control of acute ventricular arrhythmias after myocardial infarction
Bretylium tosylate	Antiarrhythmic	For treatment of ventricular fibrillation or ventricular tachycardia that fails to respond to lidocaine
Procainamide (Pronestyl)	Antiarrhythmic	Alternative drug when lidocaine fails to suppress ventricular arrhythmias
Atropine	Parasympatholytic†	For treating bradycardia associated with hypotension
Isoproterenol (Isuprel)	Sympathomimetic	To increase heart rate in bradycardia that fails to respond to atropine
Dopamine (Intropin)	Sympathomimetic	For treatment of hypotension associated with cardiogenic shock
Dobutamine (Dobutrex)	Sympathomimetic	To manage congestive heart failure when increase in heart rate is not desired
Nitroprusside (Nitropress)	Antihypertensive-vasodilator	For immediate reduction of blood pressure in hypertensive crisis and cardiogenic shock
Norepinephrine (Levophed)	Sympathomimetic	To increase blood pressure in cardiogenic shock and other hypotensive emergencies
Adenosine (Adenocard)	Antiarrhythmic	To manage complex paroxysmal supraventricular tachycardia
Verapamil (Calan, Isoptin)	Antiarrhythmic	For treatment of supraventricular tachycardia that fails to respond to adenosine
Furosemide (Lasix)	Diuretic	For treatment of congestive heart failure and acute pulmonary edema
Nitroglycerin (Nitrostat)	Coronary vasodilator	For treatment of chest pain associated with angina pectoris and acute myocardial infarction
INTRAVENOUS SOLUTIONS		
5% Dextrose (D-5-W)	Glucose	Solution of 5% glucose in water used to replace fluid and nutrients
Isotonic saline	Electrolyte	Solution of sodium chloride in purified water used to replace lost fluid, sodium, and chloride
Lactated Ringer's solution	Electrolyte	Sterile solution of sodium chloride, potassium chloride, and calcium chloride in purified waters, used to replace fluids and electrolytes
MEDICATIONS USED IN BREATHING EMERGENCIES		
Epinephrine (Adrenalin)	Sympathomimetic	For symptomatic relief in acute attacks of bronchial asthma or bronchospasm associated with chronic bronchitis and emphysema
Terbutaline (Brethine)	Sympathomimetic	For symptomatic relief of bronchial asthma and reversible bronchospasm associated with bronchitis and emphysema
Aminophylline	Bronchodilator	For symptomatic relief in acute attacks of bronchial asthma or reversible bronchospasm associated with chronic bronchitis and emphysema
Albuterol (Proventil, Ventolin)	Sympathomimetic	For symptomatic relief of bronchial asthma and reversible bronchospasm associated with chronic bronchitis and emphysema
MEDICATIONS USED IN ANAPHYLACTIC REACTIONS		
Epinephrine (Adrenalin)	Sympathomimetic	For treatment of hypersensitivity reactions caused by medications, allergens, or insect stings
Diphenhydramine (Benadryl)	Antihistamine	To counteract histamine in treatment of hypersensitivity reactions
Methylprednisolone (Solu-Medrol)	Glucocorticoid	

*A drug that stimulates the sympathetic nervous system; also called an *adrenergic*.
†A drug that inhibits the action of the parasympathetic nervous system; also called an *anticholinergic*.

Continued

Table 21-1 Office Crash Cart—cont'd

Name	Drug Category	Emergency Use
MEDICATIONS USED FOR POISONING		
Ipecac syrup	Emetic	To induce vomiting of ingested poisons
Activated charcoal	Antidote, adsorbent	Used as general purpose antidote to adsorb swallowed poisons; to decrease absorption of poison or drug by binding with any unabsorbed drug from digestive tract
Naloxone (Narcan)	Narcotic antagonist	For treatment of overdoses caused by narcotics or synthetic narcotic agents
MEDICATIONS USED IN NEUROLOGIC EMERGENCIES		
Diazepam (Valium)	Anticonvulsant, antianxiety	For treatment of convulsions in major motor seizures, status epilepticus, and acute anxiety states
Phenytoin (Dilantin)	Anticonvulsant	For controlling status epilepticus; for management of generalized tonic-clonic seizures, complex partial seizures, and critical focal seizures
Phenobarbital	Anticonvulsant, sedative-hypnotic	For management of generalized tonic-clonic seizures and partial seizures, and in the control of acute convulsive episodes (status epilepticus, febrile seizures)
MEDICATIONS USED IN METABOLIC EMERGENCIES		
Glucose (e.g., orange juice)	Glucose	To provide glucose for conscious patients with hypoglycemia
50% Dextrose	Glucose	To provide glucose for unconscious patients with hypoglycemia
EQUIPMENT AND SUPPLIES		

Cardiac Equipment
Defibrillator
Defibrillator pads

Intravenous Equipment
Tourniquet
Surgical tape
IV catheters
IV cannulas
IV tubing and needles
Armboard
IV cut-down tray

Surgical Equipment
Scalpel
Curved and straight hemostats
Needle holder
Tissue forceps
Small scissors
Local anesthetic
Gauze squares

*A drug that stimulates the sympathetic nervous system; also called an *adrenergic*.
†A drug that inhibits the action of the parasympathetic nervous system; also called an *anticholinergic*.

Activating EMS is often the most important step in an emergency. The rapid arrival of EMTs increases the patient's chances of surviving a life-threatening emergency. In most urban and in some rural areas in the United States, the medical assistant can activate the local EMS by dialing 911 on the telephone. Other areas have a local seven-digit number, in which case it is important to keep the number at hand.

When calling local EMS, the medical assistant speaks with an *emergency medical dispatcher* (EMD). An EMD has had formal training in handling emergency situations over the phone. The responsibility of the EMD is to answer the emergency call, listen to the caller, obtain critical information, determine what help is needed, and send the appropriate personnel and equipment. The EMD also is responsible

Table 21-1 Office Crash Cart—cont'd

Name	Drug Category	Emergency Use
Airway Equipment		
Suction equipment		
Suction pumps		
Suction tubing		
Suction catheters		
Oral and nasal airways		
Oxygen equipment		
Oxygen		
Oxygen facemask		
Nasal cannula		
Oxygen tubing		
Laryngoscope handle and blades		
Endotracheal tubes		
Lubricant		
Miscellaneous Supplies		
Sterile gloves		
Clean gloves		
Biohazard containers		
Syringes (assorted sizes)		
Needles (assorted sizes)		
Filter needles		
Tubex syringe		
Alcohol swabs		
Betadine (povidone-iodine) swabs		
Sterile dressings		
Roller gauze (various widths)		
Adhesive tape		
Adhesive strip bandages		
Bandage scissors		
Local anesthetic (lidocaine [Xylocaine])		
Lidocaine ointment		
Lidocaine spray		
Lubricant		
Tongue blades		
Flashlight		
Cold packs		
Sphygmomanometer		
Stethoscope		

for relaying instructions to the caller about providing emergency care until the EMTs arrive.

These guidelines should be followed when calling EMS:
• Speak clearly and calmly to the EMD. Identify the problem as accurately and concisely as possible so that proper equipment and personnel can be sent. The EMD needs to know the number of victims, the condition of the victim or victims, and the emergency care that has already been administered.
• The EMD will ask you for your phone number and address. In responding, relay the exact location of the victim to the dispatcher, including the correct street name and house number, and (if applicable) the building name, the floor, and the room number. With the 911 enhanced

Musculoskeletal Injuries

The musculoskeletal system comprises all of the bones, muscles, tendons, and ligaments of the body. Injuries that affect the musculoskeletal system include fractures, dislocations, sprains, and strains.

Fracture

A **fracture** is any break in a bone. The break may range in severity from a simple chip or a crack to a complete break or shattering of the bone. Fractures can occur anywhere on the surface of the bone, including across the surface of a joint such as the wrist or ankle. Fractures result from a direct blow, a fall, bone disease, or a twisting force as may occur in a sports injury. Although fractures often cause severe pain, they are seldom life-threatening.

The two basic types of fracture are closed fractures and open fractures (Figure 21-10). A *closed fracture* is the most common type and occurs when there is a break in a bone but no break in the skin over the fracture site. An *open fracture* involves a break in the bone along with a penetration of the overlying skin surface. Open fractures are more serious owing to the risk of blood loss and contamination leading to infection.

The signs and symptoms of a fracture include pain and tenderness, deformity, swelling and discoloration, loss of function of the body part, and numbness or tingling. The patient usually guards the injured part and may relay to you that he or she heard the bone break or snap or felt a grating

sensation. This grating sensation, known as **crepitus,** is caused by the bone fragments rubbing against each other.

Fractures also can be classified according to the nature of the break: impacted, greenstick, transverse, oblique, comminuted, and spiral. Figure 21-11 illustrates and describes these types of fracture.

Dislocation

A **dislocation** is an injury in which one end of a bone making up a joint is separated or displaced from its normal position. A dislocation is caused by a violent pulling or pushing force that tears the ligaments. Dislocations usually result from falls, sports injuries, and motor vehicle accidents. The signs and symptoms of a dislocation include significant deformity of the joint, pain and swelling, and loss of function.

Sprain

A **sprain** is a tearing of ligaments at a joint. Sprains may result from a fall, a sports injury, or a motor vehicle accident. The joints most often sprained are the ankle, knee, wrist, and fingers. The signs and symptoms of a sprain include pain, swelling, and discoloration. Sprains can vary in seriousness from mild to severe, depending on the amount of damage to the ligaments.

Strain

A **strain** is a stretching and tearing of muscles or tendons. Strains are most likely to occur when an individual lifts a heavy object or overworks a muscle, as during exercise. The muscles most commonly strained are those of the neck, back, thigh, and calf. The signs and symptoms of a strain are pain and swelling. Strains do not usually cause the intense symptoms associated with fractures, dislocations, and sprains.

Emergency Care for a Fracture

It is often difficult to determine whether a patient has a fracture, dislocation, or sprain because the symptoms of these injuries are similar. Because of this, any serious musculoskeletal injury to an extremity should be treated as though it were a fracture.

The primary goal of emergency care for a fracture is to immobilize the body part. Immobilization reduces pain and prevents further damage. A **splint** is any item that immobilizes a body part. In an emergency situation, items such as a length of wood, cardboard, or rolled newspapers or magazines can be used for splinting. The splint should be padded with a soft material such as a rolled-up towel.

The body part should be splinted in the position in which you found it. Severely angulated fractures may have to be straightened before splinting, however. If you attempt to straighten an angulated fracture, be careful not to force the affected part. A dislocated bone end can become "locked" and would have to be realigned at the hospital. If you straighten an angulated bone and encounter pain, stop and splint it in the position in which you found it. The

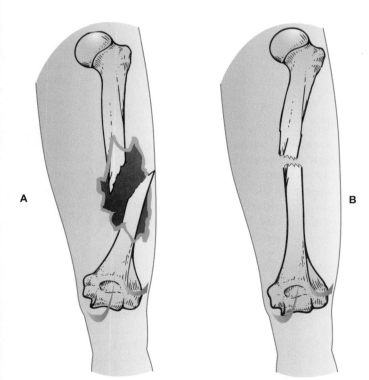

A   B

Figure 21-10. Fractures. **A,** Open fracture. **B,** Closed fracture. (From Connolly JF: *DePalma's the management of fractures and dislocations: an atlas,* Philadelphia, 1981, Saunders.)

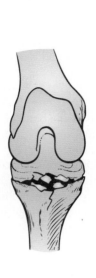 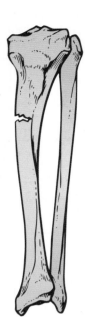 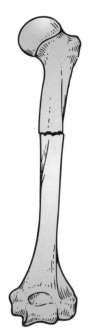 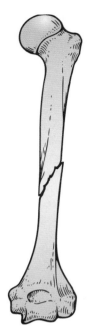 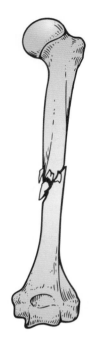 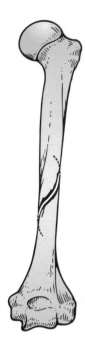

Impacted Fracture
The broken ends of the bones are forcefully jammed together.

Greenstick Fracture
The bone remains intact on one side, but broken on the other, in much the same way a that a "green stick" bends; common in children, whose bones are more flexible than those of adults.

Transverse Fracture
The break occurs perpendicular to the long axis of the bone.

Oblique Fracture
The break occurs diagonally across the bone; generally the result of a twisting force.

Comminuted Fracture
The bone is splintered or shattered into three or more fragments; usually caused by an extremely traumatic direct force.

Spiral Fracture
The bone is broken into a spiral or S-shape; caused by a twisting force.

Figure 21-11. Types of fractures.

splint also should immobilize the area above and below the injury. When splinting an injury to the wrist, the hand and forearm also should be immobilized (Figure 21-12A). When splinting an injury to the shaft of the bone, the joints above and below the injury should be immobilized. When splinting the forearm, the elbow joint and the wrist joint should be immobilized.

The splint should be held in place with a roller gauze bandage or other suitable material, such as neckties, scarves, or strips of cloth (Figure 21-12B). The splint should be applied snugly, but not so tightly that it interferes with proper circulation. After applying the splint, check the pulse below the splint to ensure the splint has not been applied too tightly. If you cannot detect a pulse, immediately loosen the splint until you can feel the pulse (Figure 21-12C).

Whenever possible, elevate an injured extremity after it has been immobilized to reduce swelling (Figure 21-12D). An ice pack also can be applied to the injured part. The cold limits the accumulation of fluid in the body tissues by constricting blood vessels and reducing leakage of fluid into the tissues. In addition, cold temporarily relieves pain because of its anesthetic or numbing effect, which reduces stimulation of nerve receptors.

After you have properly immobilized the injury, transport the patient to an emergency care facility, or if the in-

jury is serious enough, activate the local EMS. In any situation in which an injury to the spine is suspected, activate EMS.

Burns

A **burn** is an injury to the tissues caused by exposure to thermal, chemical, electrical, or radioactive agents. The severity of a burn depends on the depth of the burn, the percentage of the body involved, the type of agent causing the burn, the duration and intensity of the agent, and the part of the body. Burns are classified according to the depth of tissue injury, as illustrated in Figure 21-13.

Superficial (First-Degree) Burn

A superficial burn is the most common type of burn. It involves only the top layer of skin, the epidermis. With this type of burn, the skin appears red, is warm and dry to the touch, and is usually painful. Sunburn is a common example of a superficial burn. A superficial burn heals in 2 to 5 days of its own accord and does not cause scarring.

Partial-Thickness (Second-Degree) Burn

A partial-thickness burn involves the epidermis and extends into the dermis but does not pass through the dermis to the underlying tissues. The burned area usually appears red,

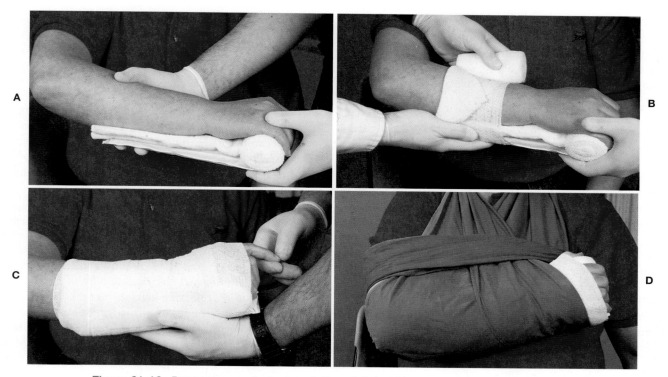

Figure 21-12. Emergency care of a fracture. **A,** The splint should immobilize the area above and below the injury. **B,** The splint is held in place with a gauze roller bandage. **C,** After the splint is applied, the pulse below the splint should be checked to ensure the splint has not been applied too tightly. **D,** A sling can be used to elevate the extremity to reduce swelling. (From Henry M, Stapleton E: *EMT prehospital care,* ed 2, Philadelphia, 1997, Saunders.)

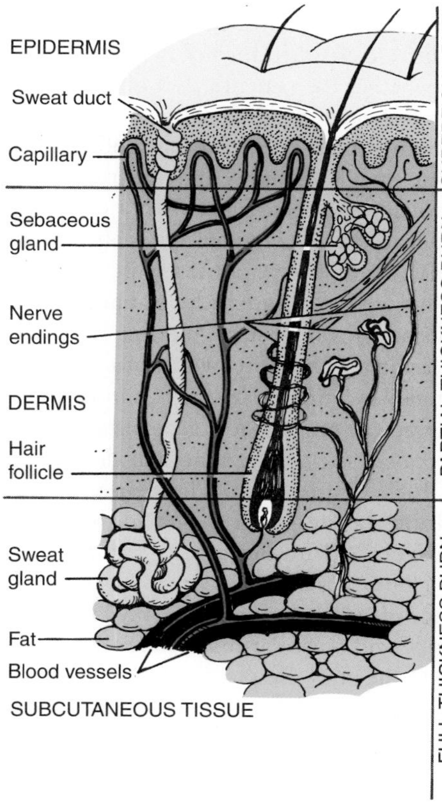

	APPEARANCE	SENSATION	COURSE
SUPERFICIAL BURN	Mild to severe erythema; skin blanches with pressure	Painful Hyperesthetic Tingling Pain eased by cooling	Discomfort lasts about 48 hours Desquamation (peeling) in 3–7 days
PARTIAL-THICKNESS BURN	Large, thick-walled blisters covering extensive area (vesiculation) Edema; mottled red base; broken epidermis; wet, shiny, weeping surface	Painful Sensitive to cold air	Superficial partial-thickness burn heals in 14–21 days Deep partial-thickness burn requires 21–28 days for healing Healing rate varies with burn depth and presence or absence of infection
FULL-THICKNESS BURN	Variable (e.g., deep red, black, white, brown) Dry surface Edema Fat exposed Tissue disrupted	Little pain Insensate	Full-thickness dead skin suppurates and liquefies after 2–3 weeks Spontaneous healing impossible Requires removal of eschar and subsequent split- or full-thickness skin grafting Hypertrophic scarring and wound contractures likely to develop without preventive measures

Labels on skin diagram:
EPIDERMIS
Sweat duct
Capillary
Sebaceous gland
Nerve endings
DERMIS
Hair follicle
Sweat gland
Fat
Blood vessels
SUBCUTANEOUS TISSUE

Figure 21-13. Types of burns. (From Polaski AL, Tatro SE: *Luckmann's core principles and practice of medical-surgical nursing,* Philadelphia, 1996, Saunders.)

mottled, and blistered. In most cases, the blisters should not be broken because they provide a protective barrier against infection. Partial-thickness burns are usually very painful, and the area often swells. This type of burn usually heals within 3 to 4 weeks and may result in some scarring.

Full-Thickness (Third-Degree) Burn

A full-thickness burn completely destroys the epidermis and the dermis and extends into the underlying tissues, such as fat, muscle, bone, and nerves. The affected area appears charred black, brown, and cherry red, with the damaged tissues underneath often pearly white. The patient may experience intense pain; however, if there has been substantial damage to the nerve endings, the patient may feel no pain at all. During the healing process, dense scars typically result. Infection is a major concern, and the patient must be carefully monitored.

Thermal Burns

Thermal burns usually occur in the home, often as a result of fire, scalding water, or coming into contact with a hot object such as a stove or curling iron.

Emergency Care for Major Thermal Burns

1. Stop the burning process to prevent further injury. If the individual is on fire, wrap him or her in a blanket, rug, or heavy coat and push him or her to the ground to help smother the flames. If a covering is unavailable, shout at the individual to drop to the ground and roll around to smother the flames.
2. Cool the burn, using large amounts of cool water from a faucet or garden hose. Do not use ice or ice water because this may result in further tissue damage; it also causes heat loss from the body. If the burn covers a large surface area (greater than 20%), do not use water. The loss of a large amount of skin surface places the patient at risk for hypothermia (generalized body cooling). With large surface area burns, you may cool the most painful areas, but not an area greater than 20% of the body (i.e., two arms, one leg).
3. Activate the local EMS.
4. Cover the patient with a clean, nonfuzzy material such as a tablecloth or sheet. The cover maintains warmth, reduces pain, and reduces the risk of contamination. Do not apply any type of ointment, antiseptic, or other substance to the burned area.

Emergency Care for Minor Thermal Burns

1. Immerse the affected area in cold water for 2 to 5 minutes. Be careful not to break any blisters because they provide a protective barrier against infection.
2. Cover the burn with a dry sterile dressing.

Chemical Burns

Chemical burns occur in the workplace and at home. The severity of the burn depends on the type and strength of the chemical and the duration of exposure to the chemi-cal. The main difference between a chemical burn and a thermal burn is that the chemical continues to burn the patient's tissues as long as it is on the skin. Because of this factor, it is important to remove the chemical from the skin as quickly as possible and then to activate the local EMS.

Liquid chemical burns should be treated by flooding the area with large amounts of cool running water until emergency personnel arrive. If a solid substance such as lime has been spilled on the patient, it should be brushed off before flooding the area with water. This is because a dry chemical may be activated by contact with water.

Seizures

A **seizure** is a sudden episode of involuntary muscular contractions and relaxation, often accompanied by a change in sensation, behavior, and level of consciousness. A seizure results when the normal electrical activity of the brain is disturbed, causing the brain cells to become irritated and overactive. Specific conditions that trigger a seizure include epilepsy, encephalitis, a recent or old head injury, high fever in infants and young children, drug and alcohol abuse or withdrawal, eclampsia associated with toxemia of pregnancy, diabetic conditions, and heatstroke.

Seizures are classified as partial or generalized according to the location of the abnormal electrical activity in the brain. *Partial seizures* are the most common type, occurring in approximately 80% of individuals who have seizures. With a partial seizure, the abnormal electrical activity is localized into specific areas of the brain; only the brain functions in those areas are affected.

Partial seizures are classified further as simple or complex, depending on whether the patient's level of consciousness is affected. The symptoms of a *simple partial seizure* include twitching or jerking in just one part of the body. This type of seizure lasts less than 1 minute, and the patient remains awake and alert during the seizure. With a *complex partial seizure,* the patient's level of consciousness is affected, and the patient has little or no memory of the seizure afterward. The symptoms of this type of seizure include abnormal behavior such as confusion, a glassy stare, aimless wandering, lip smacking or chewing, or fidgeting with clothing, which lasts from a few seconds to a minute or two. A simple and a complex partial seizure can progress to a generalized seizure.

With a *generalized seizure,* the abnormal electrical activity spreads through the entire brain. The best-known type of generalized seizure is a *tonic-clonic seizure* (formerly known as a "grand mal seizure"). With this type of seizure, the patient exhibits tonic-clonic activity followed by a postictal state. During the tonic phase, the patient suddenly loses consciousness and exhibits rigid muscular contractions, which result in odd posturing of the body. Respirations are inhibited, which may cause cyanosis around the mouth and lips. The patient may lose control of the bladder or bowels, resulting in involuntary urination and defecation. The tonic phase lasts 30 seconds, followed by the clonic phase. During the clonic phase, the patient's body jerks about violently. The patient's jaw muscles contract, which may cause the patient to bite the tongue or lips. The final phase of the seizure is the postictal state, lasting 10 to 30 minutes, in which the patient exhibits a depressed level of consciousness, is disoriented, and often has a headache. The patient generally has little or no memory of the seizure and feels confused and exhausted for several hours after the seizure.

In some instances of seizures, particularly in patients with epilepsy, an aura precedes the seizure. An *aura* is a sensation perceived by the patient that something is about to happen; examples include a strange taste, smell, or sound; a twitch; or a feeling of dizziness or anxiety. An aura provides the patient with a warning signal that a seizure is about to begin.

Although seizures are frightening to observe, they are usually not as bad as they look. Most patients fully recover within a few minutes after the seizure begins. An exception to this is *status epilepticus,* in which seizures are prolonged or come in rapid succession without full recovery of consciousness between them. Status epilepticus is a potentially life-threatening situation that requires immediate medical care.

Emergency Care for Seizures

The most important criterion in caring for a patient in a seizure is to protect the patient from harm. Remove hazards from the immediate area to prevent the patient from injury by striking a surrounding object. Do not restrain the patient. Loosen restrictive clothing that may interfere with breathing, such as collars, neckties, scarves, and jewelry. The seizure will occur no matter what you do; restraining the patient could seriously injure the patient's muscles, bones, or joints. Do not insert anything into the patient's mouth during the seizure because this could damage the teeth or mouth or interfere with breathing. In addition, it could trigger the gag reflex, causing the patient to vomit and possibly aspirate the vomitus into the lungs. If the patient vomits, roll him or her onto one side so that the vomitus can drain from the mouth.

If you are uncertain as to the cause of the seizure, or if you suspect that the patient is having status epilepticus, activate your local EMS immediately. Otherwise, transport the patient to an emergency medical care facility for further evaluation and treatment after the seizure is over.

Poisoning

A **poison** is any substance that causes illness, injury, or death if it enters the body. Most poisoning episodes occur in the home, are accidental, and occur in children younger than 5 years old. Poisoning usually involves common substances, such as cleaning agents, medications, and pesticides. For most poisonous substances, the reaction is more serious in children and the elderly than in adults. A poison can enter the body in four ways: ingestion, inhalation, absorption, or injection.

Poison control centers are valuable resources that are easily accessible to medical personnel and the community. There are more than 500 regional poison control centers across

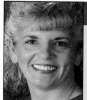

Memories *from* Externship

Judy Markins: As it turned out, one of my most terrible moments during my externship was a great learning experience. I was drawing blood (which was not my favorite procedure) and missed the vein—not once, but twice. You could see the sweat under my gloves. My stomach was in my throat, and I did not want to try again. Thank goodness my patient was understanding, and I had an excellent externship supervisor. She insisted that I try again, encouraging me that I could do it and suggesting some techniques that she had learned from her many years of experience. I got the blood specimen along with some newfound confidence.

In most situations, someone can help you if you have questions. Use your resources when you need to. Be honest, know your procedure, and have confidence in yourself. ∎

What Would You Do? What Would You *Not* Do?

Case Study 1

Beth Eaton calls the office. She says that she thinks her 3-year-old daughter, Olivia, has eaten some chewable vitamins. Beth was taking a shower and when she came out, Olivia was holding an empty vitamin bottle and saying "Good candy." Beth says she does not know how Olivia got the child-proof top off. She thinks the bottle was about a third of the way full. Beth says that Olivia is complaining that her tummy hurts. Beth says she has syrup of ipecac and wants to know whether she should give some to Olivia. ∎

the United States; most are located in the emergency departments of large hospitals. These centers are staffed by personnel who have access to information about almost all poisonous substances. Most of the centers are staffed 24 hours a day, and calls are toll-free. There also is a National Poison Control Hotline number (1-800-222-1222), which can be called 24 hours a day.

Ingested Poisons

Poisons that are ingested enter the body by being swallowed. Ingestion is the most common route of entry for poisons. Examples of poisons that are often ingested include cleaning products, pesticides, contaminated food, petroleum products (e.g., gasoline, kerosene), and poisonous plants. The abuse of drugs, alcohol, or both also can result in poisoning from an accidental or intentional overdose. The signs and symptoms of poisoning by ingestion are based on the specific substance that has been consumed but often include strange odors, burns or stains around the mouth, nausea, vomiting, abdominal pain, diarrhea, difficulty in breathing, profuse perspiration, excessive salivation, dilated or constricted pupils, unconsciousness, and convulsions.

Emergency Care for Poisoning by Ingestion

1. Acquire as much information as possible about the type of poison, the amount ingested, and when it was ingested.
2. Call your poison control center or local EMS. *Never induce vomiting unless directed to do so by a medical authority.* Vomiting is often contraindicated—when an individual is unconscious, has swallowed a petroleum product, or has swallowed a corrosive poison such as a strong acid or base. Corrosive poisons may cause more injury to the esophagus, throat, and mouth if they are vomited back up. If it is available, you may be directed by the poison control center to administer activated charcoal. Activated charcoal is used to absorb the poison that remains in the stomach and prevents absorption by the intestine.
3. If the individual vomits, collect some of the vomitus for transport with the patient to the hospital for analysis by a toxicologist, if necessary. In addition, bring along containers of any substances ingested, such as empty medication bottles and household cleaner containers, because the label of the container often lists the ingredients in the product.

Inhaled Poisons

A poison that is inhaled is breathed into the body in the form of gas, vapor, or spray. The most commonly inhaled poison is carbon monoxide, such as from car exhausts, malfunctioning furnaces, and fires. Other inhaled poisons include carbon dioxide from wells and sewers and fumes from household products such as glues, paints, insect sprays, and cleaners (e.g., ammonia, chlorine). The signs and symptoms of inhaled poisoning often include severe headache; nausea and vomiting; coughing or wheezing; shortness of breath; chest pain or tightness; facial burns; burning of the mouth, nose, eyes, throat, or chest; cyanosis; confusion; dizziness; and unconsciousness.

Emergency Care for Inhaled Poisons

1. Determine whether it is safe to approach the patient. Toxic gases and fumes also can be dangerous to individuals helping the patient.
2. Remove the individual from the source of the poison and into fresh air as quickly as possible.
3. Call your poison control center or local EMS.
4. If oxygen is available, you may be directed to administer it under the supervision of a physician. Oxygen is the primary antidote for carbon monoxide poisoning.

Absorbed Poisons

A poison that is absorbed enters the body through the skin. Examples of absorbed poisons include fertilizers and pesticides used for lawn and garden care. The signs and symptoms of absorbed poisoning are irritation, burning and itching, burning of the skin or eyes, headache, and abnormal pulse or respiration or both.

Case Study 2
Anita Alland calls the office and says that her son, Garon, was stung by a yellow jacket about an hour ago while mowing the grass. She says that his entire arm and back are red and swollen, and that he has a lot of redness and swelling around his eyes. Garon is itching all over and seems fuzzy-headed. Anita says she has never seen anyone do this after being stung. She says she had Garon take a cold shower to see if it would help. After the shower he started feeling faint and dizzy, and now he is having trouble breathing. Anita wants to know whether she can bring him to the office so that he can be seen by the physician. ■

Emergency Care for Absorbed Poisons

1. Remove the patient from the source of the poison. Avoid contact with the toxic substance.
2. Call your poison control center or local EMS. In most cases, you will be instructed to flood the area that has been exposed to the poison with water. Dry chemicals should be brushed from the skin before flooding with water.

Injected Poisons

An injected poison enters the body through bites, through stings, or by a needle. Examples of injected poisons include the venom of insects, spiders, snakes, and marine creatures such as jellyfish and the bite of rabid animals. The poison also may be a drug that is self-administered with a hypodermic needle, such as heroin. The general signs and symptoms of injected poisoning include an altered state of awareness; evidence of stings, bites, or puncture marks on the skin; mottled skin; localized pain or itching; burning, swelling, or blistering at the site; difficulty in breathing; abnormal pulse rate; nausea and vomiting; and anaphylactic shock.

Insect Stings

It is estimated that 1 of every 125 Americans is allergic to insect stings. Approximately 40 people in the United States die every year from a severe allergic reaction to insect stings. The incidence of deaths is low because most people know they need to obtain medical attention immediately if an allergic reaction begins.

Almost all of the insects whose venom can cause allergic reactions belong to a group called *Hymenoptera,* which includes honeybees and bumblebees, wasps, yellow jackets, and hornets. When a honeybee stings, its stinger remains embedded in the victim's skin, causing the bee to die as it tries to tear itself away. Wasps, yellow jackets, and hornets are more aggressive than bees and can sting repeatedly. Hornets are the most aggressive of the group and may sting even when not provoked. Yellow jackets are close behind in aggressiveness, and wasps usually sting only if someone interferes with them near their nest.

If an insect sting does not cause an allergic reaction within 30 minutes, chances are excellent that no problem will occur. A normal reaction to an insect sting includes localized pain, redness, swelling, and itching lasting 1 to 2 days. Any generalized reaction not arising directly from the area of the sting is almost certain to be an allergic reaction, which begins with symptoms such as sneezing, hives, itching, angioedema, erythema, and disorientation and progresses to difficulty in breathing, dizziness, faintness, and loss of consciousness.

Medical care should be sought immediately because these are the symptoms of an anaphylactic reaction, and most fatalities occur within 2 hours of the sting. Because time is a factor, individuals known to have a severe allergy to insect stings carry an anaphylactic emergency treatment kit containing injectable epinephrine and oral antihistamines (see Figure 21-2). With this kit, treatment for a severe allergic reaction can be started immediately.

Emergency Care for Insect Stings

1. Remove the stinger and attached venom sac. Scrape the stinger off the patient's skin with your fingernail or a plastic card such as a credit card (Figure 21-14). Do not use tweezers or forceps because squeezing the venom sac may cause more venom to be injected into the patient's tissues.
2. Wash the site with soap and water.
3. Apply a cold pack to the affected area to reduce pain and swelling.
4. Observe the patient for the signs of an anaphylactic reaction.

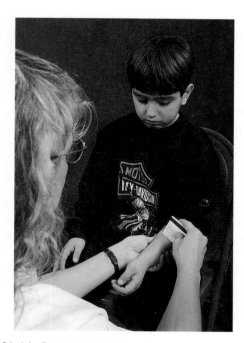

Figure 21-14. Removing a honeybee stinger and venom sac using the edge of a credit card.

Spider Bites

Although spiders are numerous throughout the United States, most do not cause injuries or serious complications. Only two spiders have bites that cause serious or life-threatening reactions: the black widow spider and the brown recluse spider. Both of these spiders prefer dark, out-of-the-way places such as in woodpiles, in brush piles, under rocks, and in dark garages and attics. Because of this, bites usually occur on the hands and arms of individuals reaching into places where the spiders are hiding. Often the individual does not know that he or she has been bitten until he or she begins to feel ill or notices swelling and a bite mark on the skin.

The black widow spider is approximately 1 inch long and is black with a distinctive bright-red hourglass shape on its abdomen. The venom injected when this spider bites an individual is toxic to the central nervous system. The signs and symptoms of a black widow bite are swelling and a dull pain at the injection site; nausea and vomiting; a rigid, boardlike abdomen; fever; rash; and difficulty in breathing or swallowing. Although the symptoms are severe, they are not usually fatal. An antivenin is available; however, because of its undesirable and frequent side effects, it is generally administered only to individuals with severe bites and to individuals who may have a heightened reaction, such as elderly individuals and children younger than 5 years old.

The brown recluse spider is light brown with a dark-brown violin-shaped mark on its back. The bite of a brown recluse causes severe local effects, including tenderness, redness, and swelling at the injection site. Systemic effects, such as difficulty in breathing or swallowing, seldom occur.

Emergency Care for Spider Bites

1. Wash the wound.
2. Apply a cold pack to the affected area to reduce pain and swelling.
3. Obtain medical help immediately if you suspect the individual has been bitten by a black widow spider or a brown recluse spider, or if a severe reaction begins to occur.

Snakebites

Snakebites kill very few people in the United States. Every year, approximately 45,000 persons are bitten by a snake; however, only 7000 of these bites involve a poisonous snake, and fewer than 15 of the individuals die. The species of snakes that are poisonous in the United States include rattlesnakes, copperheads, cottonmouths (water moccasins), and coral snakes. Individuals, zoos, or laboratories may own other poisonous species, however. Rattlesnakes account for most snakebites and nearly all fatalities from snakebites. Most snakebites occur near the home, as opposed to in the wild. Because it is often difficult to identify a snake, any unidentified snake should be considered poisonous. The general signs and symptoms of a bite from a poisonous snake include puncture marks on the skin, pain and swelling at the puncture site, rapid pulse, nausea, vomiting, unconsciousness, and convulsions.

Emergency Care for Snakebites

1. Wash the bite area gently with soap and water.
2. Immobilize the injured part, and position it below the level of the heart.
3. Call emergency personnel. Do not apply ice to a snakebite. Do not apply a tourniquet, and do not cut or suction the wound.
4. If the snake is dead, inform emergency personnel of its location so that it can be transported to the hospital for identification.

Animal Bites

Bites and other injuries from animals range in severity from minor to serious and fatal. Most people who are bitten by animals do not report the bite to a physician. Because of this factor, the incidence of animal bites in the United States each year is unknown but has been estimated at approximately 1 to 2 million for dog bites and 400,000 for cat bites.

The most serious type of bite is one from an animal with rabies. Rabies is a viral infection transmitted through the saliva of an infected animal. If the condition is not treated, rabies is generally fatal. Certain animals tend to have a higher incidence of rabies than others. These include skunks, bats, raccoons, cats, dogs, cattle, and foxes. Hamsters, gerbils, guinea pigs, chipmunks, rats, mice, gophers, and rabbits are rarely infected with the rabies virus.

An individual who has been bitten by an animal that has rabies or is suspected of having rabies must obtain medical care. To prevent rabies, a rabies vaccine, which produces antibodies to fight the rabies virus, is administered to the individual.

Emergency Care for Animal Bites

Minor Animal Bites. Wash the wound with soap and water. Apply an antibiotic ointment and a dry sterile dressing. Transport the individual to a physician so that medical care can be provided to prevent infection and to ensure that the patient's tetanus toxoid immunization is up to date.

Serious Bites. If the wound is bleeding heavily, first control the bleeding with direct pressure. Do not clean the wound because this may result in more bleeding. Transport the patient to a physician, or if the bite is serious enough, call the local EMS.

All Animal Bites. If you suspect that the animal has rabies, relay this information to the appropriate authorities, such as medical personnel, the police, or animal control personnel. If possible, try to remember what the animal looked like and the area in which you last saw it.

Heat and Cold Exposure

Exposure to excessive environmental heat or cold can result in injury to the body ranging in severity from minor to life-threatening. Heat-related injuries are most apt to occur on very hot days that are accompanied by high humidity with little or no air movement. The three conditions caused by overexposure to heat are heat cramps, heat exhaustion, and heatstroke.

The two major types of cold-related injury are frostbite and hypothermia. Although cold-related injuries are most apt to occur in the winter months, they also can occur at other times of the year, such as when an individual is exposed to cold water in a near-drowning incident.

Certain individuals are at higher risk for developing heat-related and cold-related injuries, as follows:
- Elderly individuals
- Young children, particularly infants
- Individuals who work or exercise outdoors
- Individuals with medical conditions that cause poor blood circulation, such as diabetes mellitus and cardiovascular disease
- Individuals who have had heat-related or cold-related injuries in the past
- Individuals under the influence of drugs or alcohol

Heat Cramps

Heat cramps are the least serious of the three types of heat-related injury. Heat cramps are most apt to occur when an individual is exercising or working in a hot environment and fails to replace lost fluids and electrolytes. Lost electrolytes can be replaced with a commercial sports drink (e.g., Gatorade).

The signs and symptoms of heat cramps include painful muscle spasms, particularly of the legs, calves, and abdomen; hot, sweaty skin; weakness; and a rapid pulse. These symptoms are a warning that an individual is having a problem with the heat. If the problem is ignored, heat cramps may progress to a more serious condition, such as heat exhaustion or heatstroke.

Treatment of heat cramps consists of removal of the patient to a cool environment, rest, and replacement of fluids and electrolytes. If the patient's condition does not improve, he or she should be transported to an emergency care facility for further treatment.

Heat Exhaustion

Heat exhaustion is the most common heat-related injury. It occurs most often in individuals involved in vigorous physical activity on a hot and humid day, such as athletes and construction workers. It also can occur in people who are wearing too much clothing on a hot and humid day. The signs and symptoms of heat exhaustion are similar to those of influenza: cold and clammy skin that is pale or gray, profuse sweating, headache, nausea, dizziness, weakness, and diarrhea.

Treatment of heat exhaustion consists of removal of the patient to a cool environment, replacement of fluids and electrolytes, application of a cold compress to the forehead, and rest (Figure 21-15). Tight clothing should be loosened, and excessive layers of clothing should be removed. In most cases, these measures improve the patient's condition in approximately 30 minutes. If the patient's condition does not

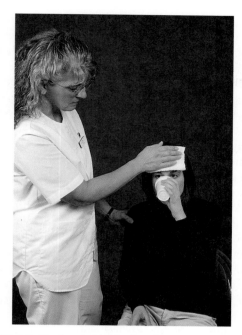

Figure 21-15. Treatment of heat exhaustion consists of removing the patient to a cool environment, replacing fluids and electrolytes, and applying a cold compress to the forehead; the patient should then rest.

improve, however, he or she should be transported to an emergency care facility.

Heatstroke

Heatstroke is the least common, but most serious, of the three heat-related injuries. Heatstroke is most apt to occur in elderly people during a heat wave and in athletes who overexert in a hot and humid environment. Heatstroke can occur in a very short time, as when a child has been left to wait in a closed car on a hot day.

During heatstroke, the body becomes so overheated that the heat-regulating mechanism breaks down and is unable to cool the body. The body temperature increases to a dangerous level, causing the destruction of tissues. The signs and symptoms of heatstroke include a body temperature of 105°F (40°C) or greater; red, hot, dry skin; a rapid, weak pulse; dizziness and weakness; rapid, shallow breathing; decreased levels of consciousness; and seizures.

Heatstroke is a life-threatening emergency and requires immediate transport of the patient to an emergency care facility by the fastest way possible. If not treated, heatstroke is always fatal. During transport, every attempt should be made to lower the body temperature, such as setting the air conditioner to its maximal capacity; covering the victim with cool, wet sheets; or fanning the victim.

Frostbite

Frostbite is the localized freezing of body tissue as a result of exposure to cold. The severity of the frostbite depends on the environmental temperature, the duration of exposure, and the wind-chill factor. Frostbite most commonly affects the hands, fingers, feet, toes, ears, nose, and cheeks. Although frostbite is not life-threatening, it can cause severe tissue damage that may require amputation of the affected body part. The signs and symptoms of frostbite include loss of feeling in the affected area; cold and waxy skin; and white, yellow, or blue discoloration of the skin.

Treatment of frostbite requires rewarming of the affected body part to prevent permanent damage. This is best accomplished in an emergency care facility because improper rewarming can result in further tissue damage. To transport the patient, loosely wrap warm clothing or blankets around the affected body part. The frozen area also can be placed in contact with another body part that is warm. It is important to handle the affected area gently. Do not rub or massage the affected area because this can damage frozen tissue further.

Hypothermia

Hypothermia is a life-threatening emergency in which the temperature of the entire body falls to a dangerously low level. Hypothermia can occur rapidly, such as when an individual falls through the ice on a frozen lake. It also can occur slowly when an individual is exposed to a cold environment for a long time, such as a hiker lost in the woods.

When the core body temperature decreases too much, the body loses its ability to regulate its temperature and to generate body heat. The signs and symptoms of hypothermia are shivering, numbness, drowsiness, apathy, a glassy stare, and decreased levels of consciousness.

Treatment of hypothermia should focus on preventing further heat loss. Remove the patient from the cold, or if this is impossible, wrap him or her in blankets. Do not attempt to rewarm the patient such as through immersion in warm water. Rapid rewarming can result in serious respiratory and cardiac problems. The patient should be transported immediately to an emergency care facility.

Diabetic Emergencies

Glucose is the end product of carbohydrate metabolism. It serves as the chief source of energy to perform normal body

---

What Would You Do? What Would You *Not* Do?

Case Study 3

David Brently has come to the medical office. He is a member of Kiwanis, and this year it was his turn to deliver Easter candy and flowers to patients at the local hospital and nursing home while wearing a bunny costume. It is a very warm day, and David says that he got really hot and sweaty in his costume and then started feeling dizzy and nauseous. He got a little worried and decided to drive himself to the medical office. David says he cannot get his costume off because the zipper is stuck. He does not want to cut it off because that would ruin it and Kiwanis would not be able to use it next year. He is hoping the physician can fix him up well enough so that he can drive home. David says he is sure his wife can get the costume off without damaging it. ∎

functions and to assist in maintaining body temperature. The body maintains a constant blood glucose level to ensure a continuous source of energy for the body. Glucose that is not needed for energy can be stored in the form of glycogen in muscle and liver tissue for later use. When no more tissue storage is possible, excess glucose is converted to fat and stored as adipose tissue.

Insulin is a hormone secreted by the beta cells of the pancreas and is required for normal use of glucose in the body. Insulin enables glucose to enter the body's cells and be converted to energy. Insulin also is needed for the proper storage of glycogen in liver and muscle cells.

Diabetes mellitus is a disease in which the body is unable to use glucose for energy because of a lack of insulin in the body. There are two types of diabetes—a severe form, usually appearing in childhood, known as *type 1 diabetes,* and a mild form, usually appearing in adulthood, known as *type 2 diabetes.* Most individuals with diabetes (90%) have type 2 diabetes. There is no cure for diabetes mellitus, but significant advances have been made in controlling the disease through a combination of drug therapy, diet therapy, and activity. The goal for the diabetic patient is to balance food intake and level of activity with the body's insulin.

A diabetic patient can experience two types of emergency: *hypoglycemia,* commonly referred to as "insulin shock", and *diabetic ketoacidosis,* commonly known as "diabetic coma." Insulin shock (hypoglycemia) occurs when there is too much insulin in the body and not enough glucose. Insulin shock can be caused by administration of too much insulin, skipping meals, and unexpected or unusual exercise. The symptoms of insulin shock are normal or rapid respirations; pale, cold, and clammy skin; sweating; dizziness and headache; full, rapid pulse; normal or high blood pressure; extreme hunger; aggressive or unusual behavior; fainting; and seizure or coma. The onset of insulin shock occurs rapidly, usually over 5 to 20 minutes, after the blood glucose level begins to decrease. Because the brain requires a constant supply of glucose for proper functioning, permanent brain damage or death can result from severe hypoglycemia.

Diabetic coma (diabetic ketoacidosis) occurs when there is not enough insulin in the body. This causes the blood glucose level to increase, resulting in hyperglycemia. When glucose cannot be used for energy, fat is broken down. This results in a buildup of acid waste products in the blood, known as *ketoacidosis.* The combined effect of the hyperglycemia and ketoacidosis causes the following symptoms: polyuria; excessive thirst and hunger; vomiting; abdominal pain; dry, warm skin; rapid, deep sighing respirations; a sweet or fruity (acetone) odor to the breath; and a rapid, weak pulse.

If the condition is not treated, diabetic coma can progress to dehydration, hypotension, coma, and death. In contrast to insulin shock, however, the onset of diabetic coma is gradual, usually developing over 12 to 48 hours. Diabetic coma can be caused by illness and infection, overeating, forgetting to administer an insulin injection, or administering an insufficient amount of insulin.

Most individuals with diabetes have a thorough knowledge of their disease and manage it effectively. Because of this, diabetic emergencies are most apt to occur when there is an unusual upset in the insulin/glucose balance in the body, such as might be caused by illness or infection. An emergency situation also may arise in an individual who has diabetes but in whom the condition has not yet been diagnosed.

It may be difficult to tell the difference between insulin shock and diabetic coma because the symptoms are similar. Often a patient with either of these conditions seems to be intoxicated. If he or she is conscious, the diabetic patient usually knows what the trouble is; you should listen carefully to the patient to determine what may have caused the problem (e.g., not eating, forgetting to administer an insulin injection). If the patient is unconscious and unable to communicate, you should observe the patient's respirations. A patient in insulin shock has normal or rapid respirations, whereas a patient in diabetic coma has deep, labored respirations. Most diabetic patients carry an emergency medical identification, such as a medical alert bracelet or necklace and a wallet card (Figure 21-16), to alert others to their condition when they cannot.

Emergency Care in Diabetes
Insulin Shock (Hypoglycemia)

A patient in insulin shock needs sugar immediately. For a conscious patient, glucose should be administered by mouth in the form of fruit juice (e.g., orange juice), non-

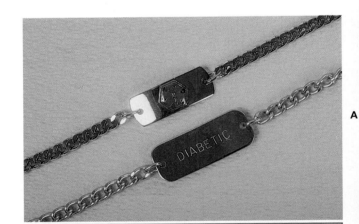

A

B

I HAVE TYPE I DIABETES
If I appear to be intoxicated or am unconscious, I may be having a reaction to diabetes or its treatment.

EMERGENCY TREATMENT
If I am able to swallow, please give me a beverage that contains sugar, such as orange juice, cola or even sugar in water. Then please send me to the nearest hospital **IMMEDIATELY.**

Figure 21-16. Diabetic medical identification. **A,** Diabetic medical alert bracelet. **B,** Diabetic wallet card.

diet soft drinks, candy, honey, or table sugar dissolved in water (Figure 21-17). Improvement is usually rapid after the glucose has been consumed. If the patient is unconscious, do not give anything by mouth because it may be aspirated into the lungs. Instead, provide the fastest possible transportation of the patient to an emergency care facility.

Diabetic Coma (Diabetic Ketoacidosis)

A patient in diabetic coma needs insulin and must be transported as soon as possible to an emergency care facility.

Doubtful Situations

If you are ever in doubt as to whether a patient is developing insulin shock or diabetic coma, give sugar, even though the final diagnosis may be diabetic coma. This is because insulin shock develops much more rapidly than diabetic coma and can quickly cause permanent brain damage or death. If you give sugar to a patient in diabetic coma, there is little risk of making the condition worse because a patient can withstand a high blood glucose level longer than he or she can tolerate a low blood glucose level.

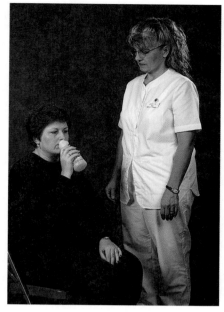

Figure 21-17. Orange juice is administered to a diabetic patient showing signs and symptoms of insulin shock.

MEDICAL PRACTICE and the LAW

Emergency medicine is one of the most litigious (lawsuit-prone) areas of health care. Owing to the nature of emergencies, there is little time to plan your actions, and one misstep could cause damage. Keep in mind that your actions would be compared in court with those of a "reasonably prudent medical assistant with similar education and experience." Do not perform procedures you are not comfortable performing.

Whenever possible, obtain written consent for all procedures. In a life-or-death situation, this is not usually possible. In this case, you are held accountable to try to save the life of the patient, even without consent.

Patients or families often become hysterical during emergencies. As a health care professional, you are expected to keep a cool head and calm the patient and family while attending to the emergency situation.

If you are out of the office and encounter an emergency situation, many states have a "Good Samaritan" law that protects you from legal action if you perform only procedures with which you are familiar, such as emergency first aid or CPR. ■

What Would You Do? What Would You *Not* Do? RESPONSES

Case Study 1
Page 763
What Did Judy Do?
❑ Gave Beth the National Poison Control hotline number (1-800-222-1222) and told her to call it immediately. Explained that was the fastest way to obtain information on what to do.
❑ Told Beth not to give the syrup of ipecac to Olivia unless she was told to do so by the poison control center.
❑ Told Beth to have the vitamin bottle in her hand when she calls. Told her that the poison control center would want to know information from the label and would especially want to know whether the vitamins contained iron.
❑ Told Beth to call the office back if she needs any more help after talking with the poison control center.

What Did Judy Not Do?
❑ Did not tell Beth she should give Olivia syrup of ipecac because some poisons can cause additional problems if they are brought back up.

What Would You Do?/What Would You *Not* Do? Review Judy's response and place a checkmark next to the information you included in your response. List additional information you included in your response.

_____

_____

_____

_____

Continued

What Would You Do? What Would You *Not* Do? RESPONSES—cont'd

Case Study 2
Page 764
What Did Judy Do?
❏ Told Anita that Garon needs to get to the hospital as soon as possible. Explained that he is having a very serious allergic reaction that could be life-threatening.
❏ Told her to stay calm and call 911 immediately.
❏ Notified the physician of the situation.

What Did Judy Not *Do?*
❏ Did not tell her to bring Garon to the office because he may need special life-support equipment available at the hospital.

What Would You Do?/What Would You *Not* **Do?** Review Judy's response and place a checkmark next to the information you included in your response. List additional information you included in your response.

_____
_____
_____
_____

Case Study 3
Page 767
What Did Judy Do?
❏ Took David to an examining room that was cool and gave him a glass of water.
❏ Told David she needed to get his costume off as soon as possible. Explained that if his condition gets worse, it could become life-threatening.
❏ Helped David out of the costume and gave him another glass of water.

What Did Judy Not *Do?*
❏ Did not let David keep the costume on.

What Would You Do?/What Would You *Not* **Do?** Review Judy's response and place a checkmark next to the information you included in your response. List additional information you included in your response.

_____
_____
_____
_____

APPLY YOUR KNOWLEDGE

Choose the best answer to each of the following questions.

1. John Adams is a 56-year-old man with a history of myocardial infarction. While at the office for a health examination, Mr. Adams starts complaining of chest pain. Dr. Cardio directs Judy Markins, CMA, to call 911 for an ambulance. Judy does all of the following when speaking to the EMS dispatcher *except:*
   A. Speaks clearly and calmly.
   B. Relays the condition of the patient.
   C. Gives the dispatcher the suite number of the office.
   D. Hangs up as soon as possible.

2. Judy Markins, CMA, is assembling a first aid kit for the medical office. Which of the following would she include in the kit?
   A. Cold packs.
   B. Pocket mask.
   C. Tourniquet.
   D. Roller gauze.
   E. All of the above.

3. Teresa Marquez is seated in the venipuncture chair. Judy Markins, CMA, is about to perform a venipuncture on Teresa. Teresa indicates that she feels warm and light-headed. Which of the following is the best step for Judy to take?
   A. Have Teresa put her head between her knees.
   B. Offer Teresa a Popsicle.
   C. Continue with the venipuncture.
   D. Have Teresa stand up and walk around slowly.

4. Timmy Tompkins is brought to the office for a recheck after recently being discharged from the hospital. He developed anaphylactic shock after being stung by a yellow jacket. Dr. Cardio explains to Timmy and his parents that any time Timmy is stung by a yellow jacket, he will develop an anaphylactic reaction. The quickest method of treating anaphylactic shock is to:
   A. Call the EMS immediately.
   B. Place a belt around the area where Timmy is stung to prevent the spread of the venom.
   C. Use an emergency treatment kit with injectable epinephrine and an oral antihistamine, and then call EMS.
   D. Timmy's parents should drive him to the emergency department after the sting because an anaphylactic reaction usually doesn't occur for several hours.

5. Sherry Walters, a 10-year-old girl, is brought to the office by her mother. Sherry fell while she was inline skating and has a deep laceration on the inner aspect of her right forearm. Sherry's mother had wrapped a clean dishtowel around the wound, but the towel was saturated with blood, and the bleeding continued. Judy Markins, CMA, should:
   A. Apply a dressing over the towel, elevate the arm, and apply direct pressure over the site.
   B. Tie a tight bandage above the site to decrease the circulation and slow the bleeding.
   C. Remove the saturated towel, and rinse the wound with warm water.
   D. Scream for help and have Sherry keep her arm below the level of her heart.

6. John Collins, 38 years old, stepped on a nail. He calls the office to ask what to do. It would be most important for Judy Markins, CMA, to ask:
   A. How Mr. Collins cleaned his wound.
   B. Whether Mr. Collins knows the signs and symptoms of infection.
   C. Whether the nail Mr. Collins stepped on was rusty.
   D. When Mr. Collins last had a tetanus toxoid immunization.

7. Beatrice Ellis is a 25-year-old woman who comes to the office because she has a sore throat and fever. She also has a history of epilepsy. While Judy Markins, CMA, is taking her chief complaint and checking vital signs, Beatrice tells Judy she is having an aura. The most appropriate response for Judy would be to:
   A. Continue taking vital signs, and reassure Beatrice that everything is okay.
   B. Have Beatrice lie down on the floor, remove all objects around her, loosen restrictive clothing, and stay with her.
   C. Run and get Dr. Cardio and make sure there is a tongue depressor in position in Beatrice's mouth.
   D. Finish taking vitals and tell Beatrice she will be back to check on her in 10 minutes.

8. Jane White calls the office and states that the 3-year-old she is babysitting has been chewing on leaves from her jade plant. She asks Judy Markins, CMA, whether jade plants are poisonous. Judy should:
   A. Recommend that Mrs. White watch the toddler closely for symptoms of poisoning.
   B. Tell Mrs. White to take the child to the local emergency department immediately.
   C. Tell Mrs. White to call the poison control center for information about the toxicity of jade plants.
   D. Call the Department of Children's Services and report Mrs. White for child endangerment.

9. Jeremy Jenkins is 6 years old and is brought to the office because he was bitten on the leg by a dog in his neighborhood. The bite is small and superficial. Appropriate actions for Judy Markins, CMA, to take would include all of the following *except:*
   A. Ask for the name and address of the owner of the dog to determine whether the animal's rabies vaccination is current.
   B. Call the local dog warden to have the animal removed and destroyed.
   C. Wash the area with soap and water, apply antibiotic ointment, and bandage.
   D. Ask Jeremy's mother whether his immunizations are up to date.

10. Judy Markins, CMA, receives a frantic phone call from her next-door neighbor's niece. She states she came to visit her aunt and found her unconscious on the floor. When Judy goes to the house, she finds Mrs. Oxford to be very warm and dry to the touch, and her pulse is rapid and weak. Her breath has a "fruity" odor, and her respirations are rapid and deep. Mrs. Oxford has been an insulin-dependent diabetic patient for many years. Judy should:
    A. Call Mrs. Oxford's physician and let him know about her condition.
    B. Give Mrs. Oxford some orange juice because she is in insulin shock.
    C. Administer 40 U of regular insulin because Mrs. Oxford is in a diabetic coma.
    D. Call the EMS to take Mrs. Oxford to the hospital because her symptoms are suggestive of ketoacidosis.

CERTIFICATION REVIEW

❑ **First aid** is the immediate care that is administered before complete medical care can be obtained to an individual who is injured or suddenly becomes ill. The emergency medical services (EMS) system is a network of community resources, equipment, and medical personnel that provides emergency care to victims of injury or sudden illness.

❑ **Respiratory distress** indicates that the patient is breathing but is having great difficulty in doing so. Asthma is a condition characterized by wheezing, coughing, and dyspnea. Emphysema is a progressive lung disorder in which the terminal bronchioles that lead into the alveoli become plugged with mucus. Hyperventilation is a manner of breathing in which the respirations become rapid and deep, causing an individual to exhale too much carbon dioxide.

❑ **A heart attack,** also known as a *myocardial infarction* (MI), is caused by partial or complete obstruction of one or both of the coronary arteries or their branches. The principal symptom of a heart attack is chest pain or discomfort. The pain is usually felt behind the sternum and may radiate to the neck, throat, jaw, both shoulders, and arms.

❑ **A stroke** results when an artery to the brain is blocked or ruptures, interrupting the blood flow to the brain. The signs and symptoms of a stroke are sudden weakness or numbness of the face, arm, or leg on one side of the body; difficulty in speaking; dimmed vision or loss of vision in one eye; double vision; dizziness; confusion; severe headache; and loss of consciousness.

❑ **Shock** is the failure of the cardiovascular system to deliver enough blood to all of the body's vital organs. Shock accompanies many types of emergency—hemorrhaging, MI, and severe allergic reaction. The five major types of shock are hypovolemic, cardiogenic, neurogenic, anaphylactic, and psychogenic. The general signs and symptoms of shock are weakness, restlessness, anxiety, disorientation, pallor, cold and clammy skin, rapid breathing, and rapid pulse.

❑ **Hypovolemic shock** is caused by a loss of blood or other body fluids. Cardiogenic shock is caused by the failure of the heart to pump blood adequately to all of the vital organs of the body. Neurogenic shock occurs when the nervous system is unable to control the diameter of the blood vessels. Anaphylactic shock is a life-threatening reaction of the body to an allergen. Psychogenic shock is caused by an unpleasant experience or emotional stimulus, such as pain, fright, or the sight of blood.

❑ **Bleeding or hemorrhaging** is the escape of blood from a severed blood vessel. External bleeding is bleeding that can be seen coming from a wound. The most effective way to control bleeding is through the application of direct pressure to the bleeding site. If bleeding cannot be controlled with direct pressure, a pressure point can be used. A pressure point is a site on the body where an artery lies close to the surface of the skin and can be compressed against an underlying bone. Internal bleeding is bleeding that flows into a body cavity, an organ, or between tissues.

❑ **A wound** is a break in the continuity of an external or internal surface caused by physical means. An open wound is a break in the skin surface or mucous membrane that exposes the underlying tissues; examples include incisions, lacerations, punctures, and abrasions.

❑ **An incision** is a clean, smooth cut caused by a sharp cutting instrument, such as a knife, a razor, or a piece of glass. A laceration is a wound in which the tissues are torn apart, rather than cut, leaving ragged and irregular edges. A puncture is a wound made by a sharp, pointed object piercing the skin layers and sometimes the underlying structures. An abrasion is a wound in which the outer layers of the skin are scraped or rubbed off.

❑ **A closed wound** involves an injury to the underlying tissues of the body without a break in the skin or mucous membrane; an example is a contusion or bruise.

❑ **A fracture** is any break of a bone. A closed fracture occurs when there is a broken bone, but no break in the skin over the fracture site. An open fracture involves a break in the bone along with a penetration of the overlying skin surface. The signs and symptoms of a fracture include pain and tenderness, deformity, swelling and discoloration, loss of function of the body part, and numbness or tingling.

❑ **A dislocation** is an injury in which one end of a bone making up a joint is separated or displaced from its normal position. A sprain is a tearing of ligaments at a joint. A strain is a stretching and tearing of muscles or tendons. A splint is any item that immobilizes a body part.

❑ **A burn** is an injury to the tissues caused by exposure to thermal, chemical, electrical, or radioactive agents. A superficial (first-degree) burn involves only the epidermis; an example is sunburn. A partial-thickness (second-degree) burn involves the epidermis and extends into the dermis. A full-thickness (third-degree) burn completely destroys the epidermis and the dermis and extends into the underlying tissues, such as fat, muscle, bone, and nerves.

❑ **A seizure** is a sudden episode of involuntary muscle contractions and relaxation often accompanied by a change in sensation, behavior, and level of consciousness. Seizures are classified as partial or generalized. In a partial seizure, the abnormal electrical activity is localized into specific areas of the brain; only the brain functions in those areas are affected. With a generalized seizure, the abnormal electrical activity spreads through the entire brain.

CERTIFICATION REVIEW—cont'd

- ❑ **A poison** is any substance that causes illness, injury, or death if it enters the body. Poisons that are ingested enter the body by being swallowed. A poison that is inhaled is breathed into the body in the form of gas, vapor, or spray. A poison that is absorbed enters the body through the skin. An injected poison enters the body through bites, through stings, or by a needle.

- ❑ **Heat cramps** are most apt to occur when an individual is exercising or working in a hot environment and fails to replace lost fluids and electrolytes. The symptoms are painful muscle spasms, particularly of the legs, calves, and abdomen; hot, sweaty skin; weakness; and a rapid pulse.

- ❑ **Heat exhaustion** occurs most often in individuals involved in vigorous physical activity on a hot and humid day. The symptoms of heat exhaustion are cold and clammy skin, profuse sweating, headache, nausea, dizziness, weakness, and diarrhea.

- ❑ **Heatstroke** is the most serious heat-related injury and is most apt to occur in elderly individuals during a heat wave and in athletes who overexert in a hot and humid environment. The symptoms of heatstroke are a body temperature of 105°F or greater; red, hot, dry skin; a rapid, weak pulse; dizziness and weakness; rapid, shallow breathing; decreased level of consciousness; and seizures.

- ❑ **Frostbite** is the localized freezing of body tissue as a result of exposure to cold. Frostbite commonly affects the hands, fingers, feet, toes, ears, nose, and cheeks. Hypothermia is a life-threatening emergency in which the temperature of the entire body falls to a dangerously low level.

- ❑ **Diabetes mellitus** is a disease in which the body is unable to use glucose for energy because the body lacks enough insulin. Insulin shock (hypoglycemia) occurs when there is too much insulin in the body and not enough glucose. Diabetic coma occurs when there is not enough insulin in the body. This causes the blood glucose level to increase in the body, resulting in hyperglycemia.

TERMINOLOGY REVIEW

Burn An injury to the tissues caused by exposure to thermal, chemical, electrical, or radioactive agents.

Crash cart A specially equipped cart for holding and transporting medications, equipment, and supplies needed for lifesaving procedures in an emergency.

Crepitus A grating sensation caused by fractured bone fragments rubbing against each other.

Dislocation An injury in which one end of a bone making up a joint is separated or displaced from its normal anatomic position.

Emergency medical services (EMS) system A network of community resources, equipment, and personnel that provides care to victims of injury or sudden illness.

First aid The immediate care administered before complete medical care can be obtained to an individual who is injured or suddenly becomes ill.

Fracture Any break in a bone.

Hypothermia A life-threatening condition in which the temperature of the entire body falls to a dangerously low level.

Poison Any substance that causes illness, injury, or death if it enters the body.

Pressure point A site on the body where an artery lies close to the surface of the skin and can be compressed against an underlying bone to control bleeding.

Seizure A sudden episode of involuntary muscular contractions and relaxation, often accompanied by a change in sensation, behavior, and level of consciousness.

Shock The failure of the cardiovascular system to deliver enough blood to all of the vital organs of the body.

Splint Any device that immobilizes a body part.

Sprain Trauma to a joint, which causes tearing of ligaments.

Strain A stretching or tearing of muscles or tendons caused by trauma.

Wound A break in the continuity of an external or internal surface, caused by physical means.

ON THE WEB

For Information on Emergency Medicine:

American Red Cross: www.redcross.org

Federal Emergency Management Agency: www.fema.gov

The Human Body—Highlights of Structure and Function

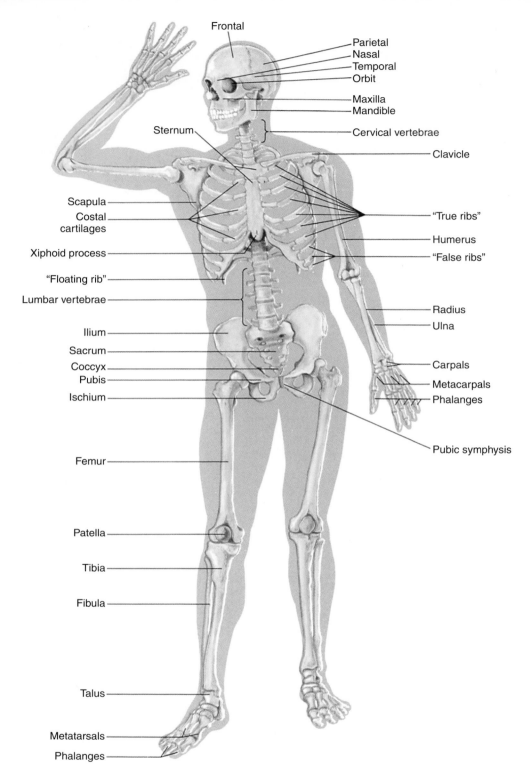

Frontal
Parietal
Nasal
Temporal
Orbit
Maxilla
Mandible
Cervical vertebrae
Clavicle
Sternum
Scapula
Costal cartilages
"True ribs"
Humerus
Xiphoid process
"False ribs"
"Floating rib"
Lumbar vertebrae
Radius
Ulna
Ilium
Sacrum
Coccyx
Carpals
Pubis
Metacarpals
Ischium
Phalanges
Pubic symphysis
Femur
Patella
Tibia
Fibula
Talus
Metatarsals
Phalanges

Plate 1. Skeletal System

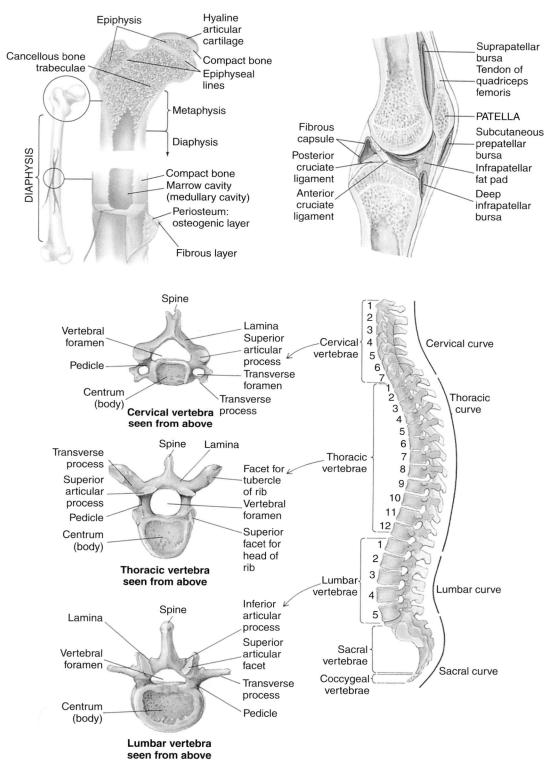

Plate 2. Skeletal System

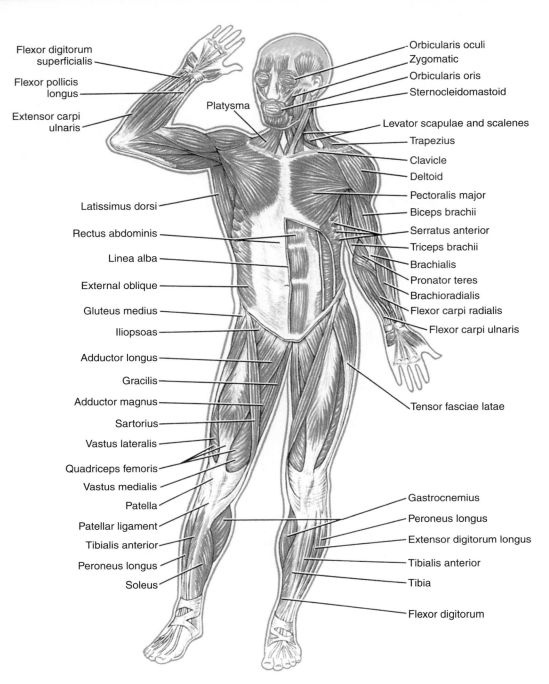

Flexor digitorum superficialis
Flexor pollicis longus
Extensor carpi ulnaris
Platysma

Orbicularis oculi
Zygomatic
Orbicularis oris
Sternocleidomastoid
Levator scapulae and scalenes
Trapezius
Clavicle
Deltoid
Pectoralis major
Biceps brachii
Serratus anterior
Triceps brachii
Brachialis
Pronator teres
Brachioradialis
Flexor carpi radialis
Flexor carpi ulnaris

Latissimus dorsi
Rectus abdominis
Linea alba
External oblique
Gluteus medius
Iliopsoas
Adductor longus
Gracilis
Adductor magnus
Sartorius
Vastus lateralis
Quadriceps femoris
Vastus medialis
Patella
Patellar ligament
Tibialis anterior
Peroneus longus
Soleus

Tensor fasciae latae

Gastrocnemius
Peroneus longus
Extensor digitorum longus
Tibialis anterior
Tibia
Flexor digitorum

Plate 3. Anterior Superficial Muscles

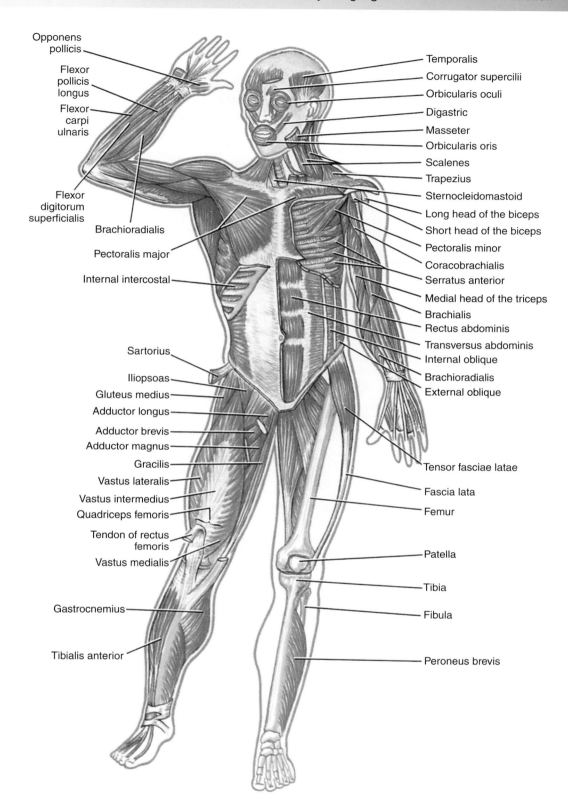

Opponens pollicis
Flexor pollicis longus
Flexor carpi ulnaris
Flexor digitorum superficialis
Brachioradialis
Pectoralis major
Internal intercostal
Sartorius
Iliopsoas
Gluteus medius
Adductor longus
Adductor brevis
Adductor magnus
Gracilis
Vastus lateralis
Vastus intermedius
Quadriceps femoris
Tendon of rectus femoris
Vastus medialis
Gastrocnemius
Tibialis anterior

Temporalis
Corrugator supercilii
Orbicularis oculi
Digastric
Masseter
Orbicularis oris
Scalenes
Trapezius
Sternocleidomastoid
Long head of the biceps
Short head of the biceps
Pectoralis minor
Coracobrachialis
Serratus anterior
Medial head of the triceps
Brachialis
Rectus abdominis
Transversus abdominis
Internal oblique
Brachioradialis
External oblique
Tensor fasciae latae
Fascia lata
Femur
Patella
Tibia
Fibula
Peroneus brevis

Plate 4. Anterior Deep Muscles

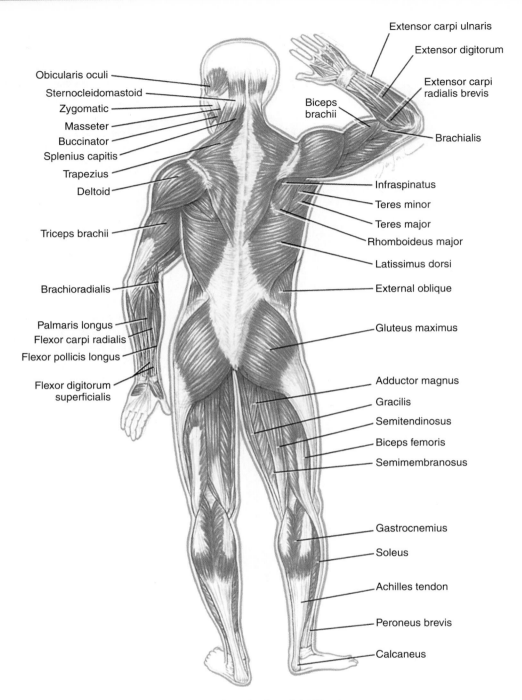

Obicularis oculi

Sternocleidomastoid

Zygomatic

Masseter

Buccinator

Splenius capitis

Trapezius

Deltoid

Triceps brachii

Brachioradialis

Palmaris longus

Flexor carpi radialis

Flexor pollicis longus

Flexor digitorum
superficialis

Extensor carpi ulnaris

Extensor digitorum

Extensor carpi
radialis brevis

Biceps
brachii

Brachialis

Infraspinatus

Teres minor

Teres major

Rhomboideus major

Latissimus dorsi

External oblique

Gluteus maximus

Adductor magnus

Gracilis

Semitendinosus

Biceps femoris

Semimembranosus

Gastrocnemius

Soleus

Achilles tendon

Peroneus brevis

Calcaneus

Plate 5. Posterior Superficial Muscles

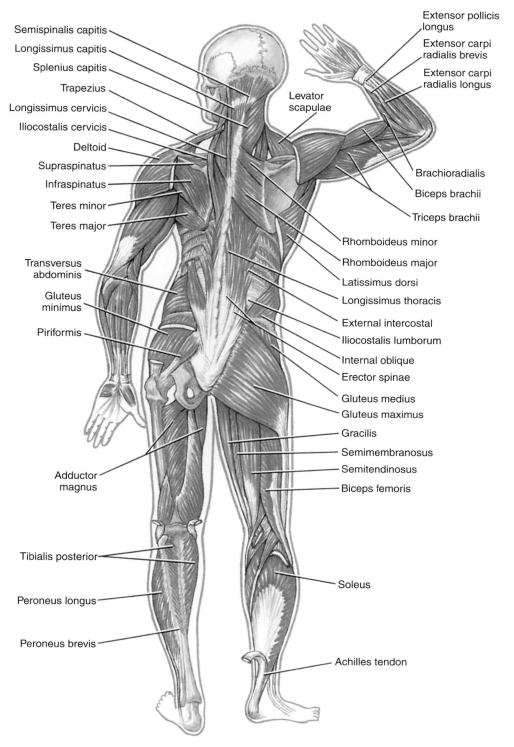

Semispinalis capitis

Longissimus capitis

Splenius capitis

Trapezius

Longissimus cervicis

Iliocostalis cervicis

Deltoid

Supraspinatus

Infraspinatus

Teres minor

Teres major

Transversus abdominis

Gluteus minimus

Piriformis

Adductor magnus

Tibialis posterior

Peroneus longus

Peroneus brevis

Levator scapulae

Extensor pollicis longus

Extensor carpi radialis brevis

Extensor carpi radialis longus

Brachioradialis

Biceps brachii

Triceps brachii

Rhomboideus minor

Rhomboideus major

Latissimus dorsi

Longissimus thoracis

External intercostal

Iliocostalis lumborum

Internal oblique

Erector spinae

Gluteus medius

Gluteus maximus

Gracilis

Semimembranosus

Semitendinosus

Biceps femoris

Soleus

Achilles tendon

Plate 6. Posterior Deep Muscles

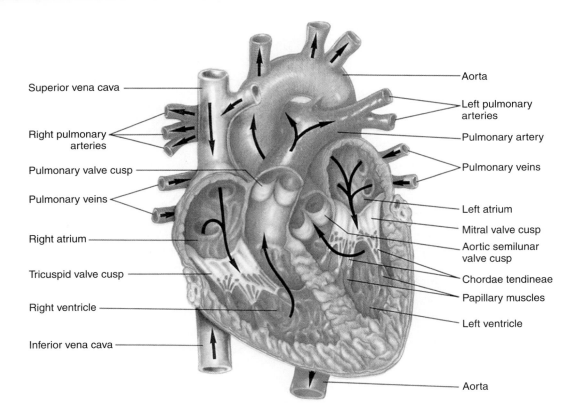

Superior vena cava

Right pulmonary arteries

Pulmonary valve cusp

Pulmonary veins

Right atrium

Tricuspid valve cusp

Right ventricle

Inferior vena cava

Aorta

Left pulmonary arteries

Pulmonary artery

Pulmonary veins

Left atrium

Mitral valve cusp

Aortic semilunar valve cusp

Chordae tendineae

Papillary muscles

Left ventricle

Aorta

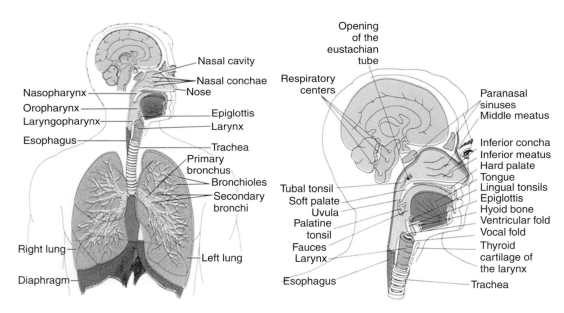

Nasal cavity

Nasal conchae

Nose

Nasopharynx

Oropharynx

Laryngopharynx

Esophagus

Epiglottis

Larynx

Trachea

Primary bronchus

Bronchioles

Secondary bronchi

Right lung

Left lung

Diaphragm

Opening of the eustachian tube

Respiratory centers

Paranasal sinuses

Middle meatus

Inferior concha

Inferior meatus

Hard palate

Tongue

Lingual tonsils

Epiglottis

Hyoid bone

Ventricular fold

Vocal fold

Thyroid cartilage of the larynx

Trachea

Tubal tonsil

Soft palate

Uvula

Palatine tonsil

Fauces

Larynx

Esophagus

Plate 7. Heart and Respiratory System

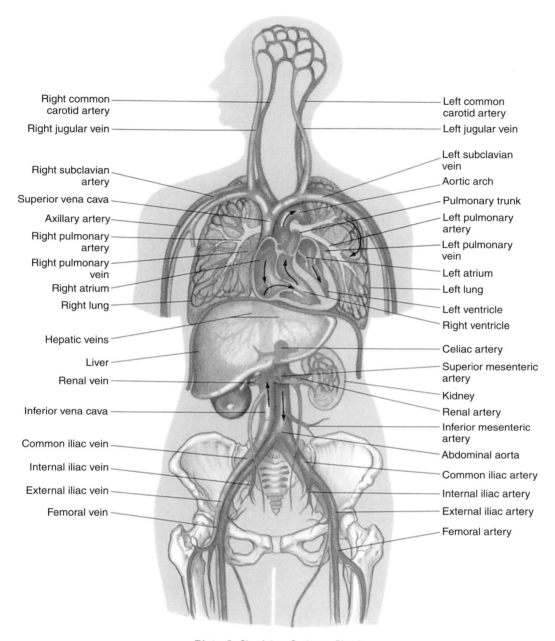

Right common carotid artery

Right jugular vein

Right subclavian artery

Superior vena cava

Axillary artery

Right pulmonary artery

Right pulmonary vein

Right atrium

Right lung

Hepatic veins

Liver

Renal vein

Inferior vena cava

Common iliac vein

Internal iliac vein

External iliac vein

Femoral vein

Left common carotid artery

Left jugular vein

Left subclavian vein

Aortic arch

Pulmonary trunk

Left pulmonary artery

Left pulmonary vein

Left atrium

Left lung

Left ventricle

Right ventricle

Celiac artery

Superior mesenteric artery

Kidney

Renal artery

Inferior mesenteric artery

Abdominal aorta

Common iliac artery

Internal iliac artery

External iliac artery

Femoral artery

Plate 8. Circulatory System—Blood

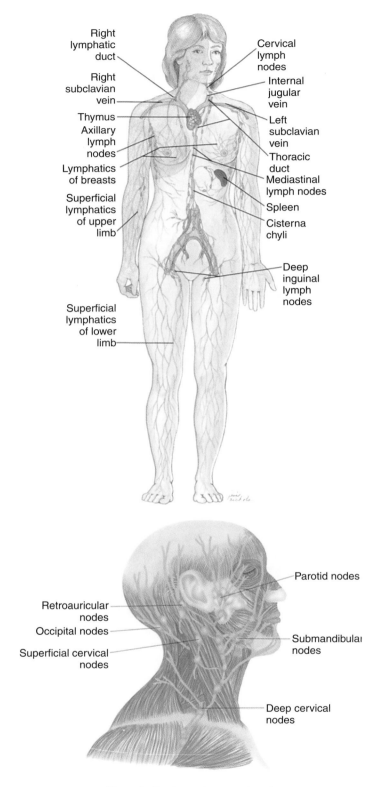

Right lymphatic duct
Right subclavian vein
Thymus
Axillary lymph nodes
Lymphatics of breasts
Superficial lymphatics of upper limb
Superficial lymphatics of lower limb

Cervical lymph nodes
Internal jugular vein
Left subclavian vein
Thoracic duct
Mediastinal lymph nodes
Spleen
Cisterna chyli
Deep inguinal lymph nodes

Retroauricular nodes
Occipital nodes
Superficial cervical nodes
Parotid nodes
Submandibular nodes
Deep cervical nodes

Plate 9. Circulatory System—Lymph

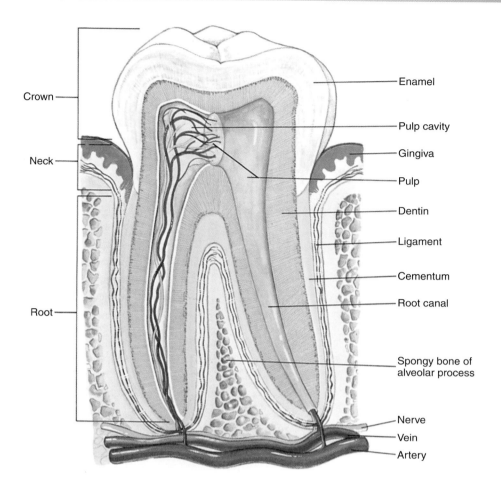

Crown

Neck

Root

Enamel

Pulp cavity

Gingiva

Pulp

Dentin

Ligament

Cementum

Root canal

Spongy bone of
alveolar process

Nerve

Vein

Artery

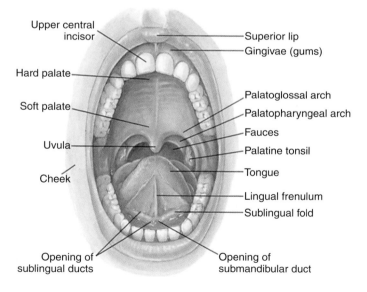

Upper central
incisor

Hard palate

Soft palate

Uvula

Cheek

Opening of
sublingual ducts

Superior lip

Gingivae (gums)

Palatoglossal arch

Palatopharyngeal arch

Fauces

Palatine tonsil

Tongue

Lingual frenulum

Sublingual fold

Opening of
submandibular duct

Plate 10. Digestive System

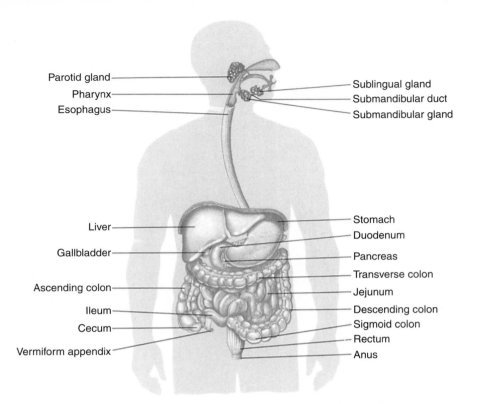

Parotid gland

Pharynx

Esophagus

Sublingual gland

Submandibular duct

Submandibular gland

Liver

Gallbladder

Ascending colon

Ileum

Cecum

Vermiform appendix

Stomach

Duodenum

Pancreas

Transverse colon

Jejunum

Descending colon

Sigmoid colon

Rectum

Anus

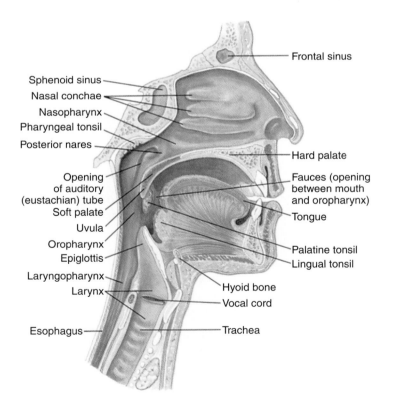

Sphenoid sinus

Nasal conchae

Nasopharynx

Pharyngeal tonsil

Posterior nares

Opening
of auditory
(eustachian) tube

Soft palate

Uvula

Oropharynx

Epiglottis

Laryngopharynx

Larynx

Esophagus

Frontal sinus

Hard palate

Fauces (opening
between mouth
and oropharynx)

Tongue

Palatine tonsil

Lingual tonsil

Hyoid bone

Vocal cord

Trachea

Plate 11. Digestive System

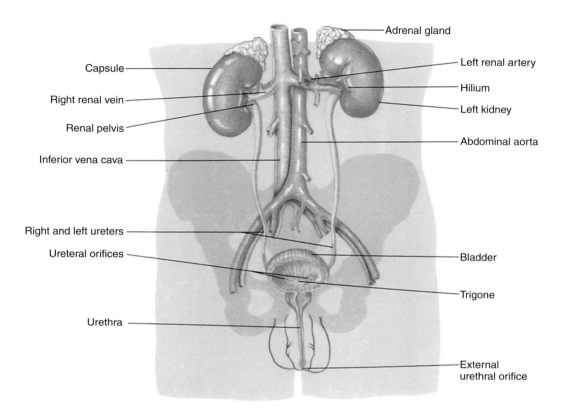

Adrenal gland

Capsule

Left renal artery

Hilium

Right renal vein

Left kidney

Renal pelvis

Abdominal aorta

Inferior vena cava

Right and left ureters

Ureteral orifices

Bladder

Trigone

Urethra

External
urethral orifice

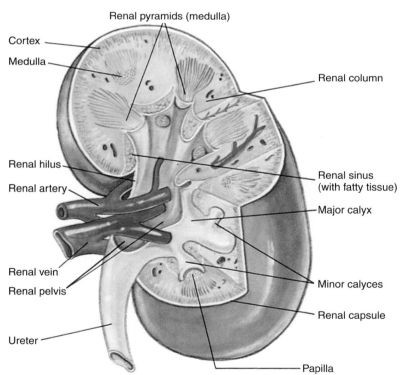

Renal pyramids (medulla)

Cortex

Medulla

Renal column

Renal hilus

Renal sinus
(with fatty tissue)

Renal artery

Major calyx

Renal vein

Renal pelvis

Minor calyces

Renal capsule

Ureter

Papilla

Plate 12. Genitourinary System

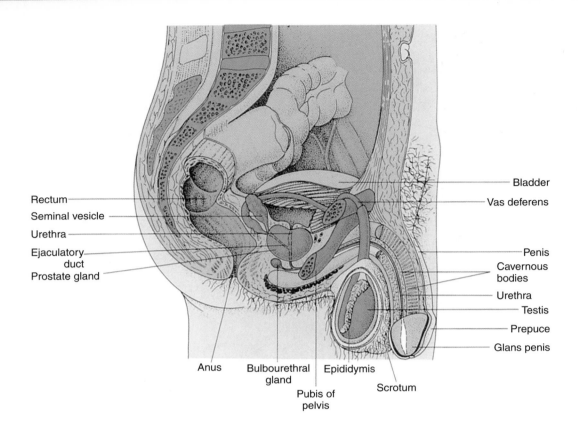

Rectum

Seminal vesicle

Urethra

Ejaculatory
duct

Prostate gland

Bladder

Vas deferens

Penis

Cavernous
bodies

Urethra

Testis

Prepuce

Glans penis

Anus   Bulbourethral   Epididymis
gland

Scrotum

Pubis of
pelvis

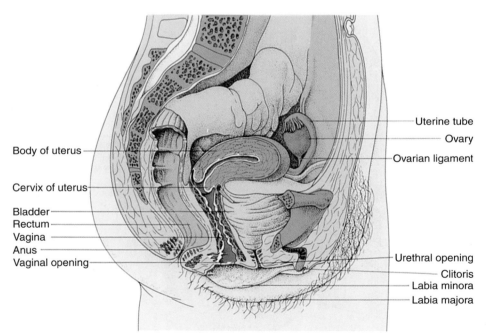

Body of uterus

Cervix of uterus

Bladder
Rectum
Vagina
Anus
Vaginal opening

Uterine tube

Ovary

Ovarian ligament

Urethral opening

Clitoris

Labia minora

Labia majora

Plate 13. Genitourinary System

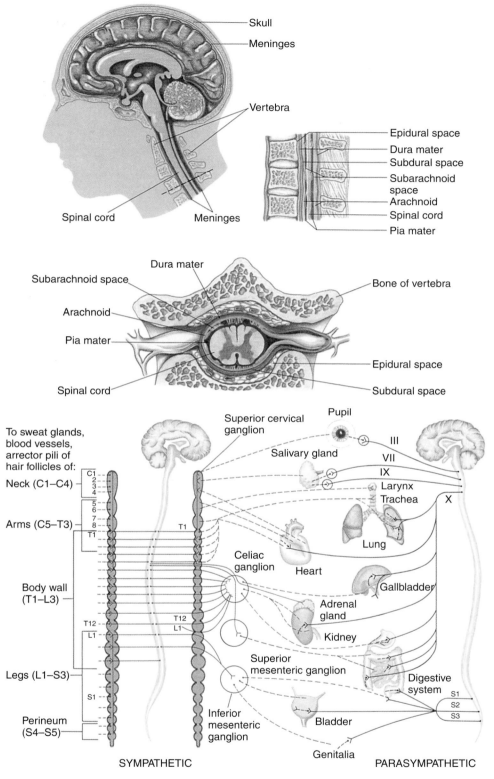

Plate 14. Nervous System

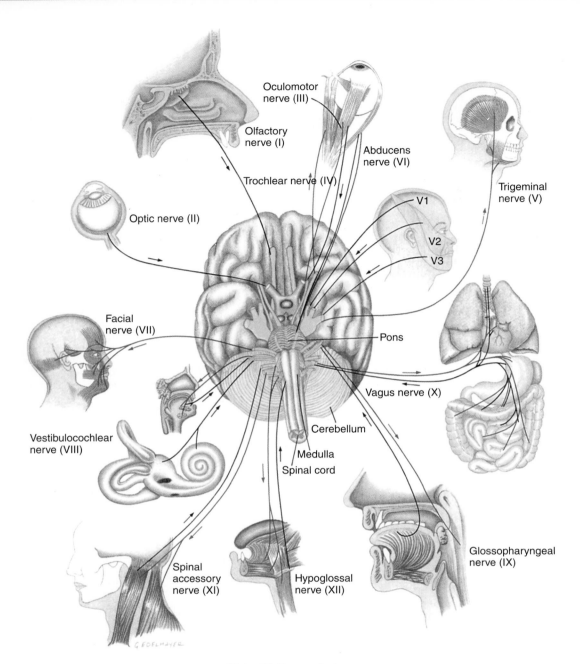

Plate 15. Nervous System

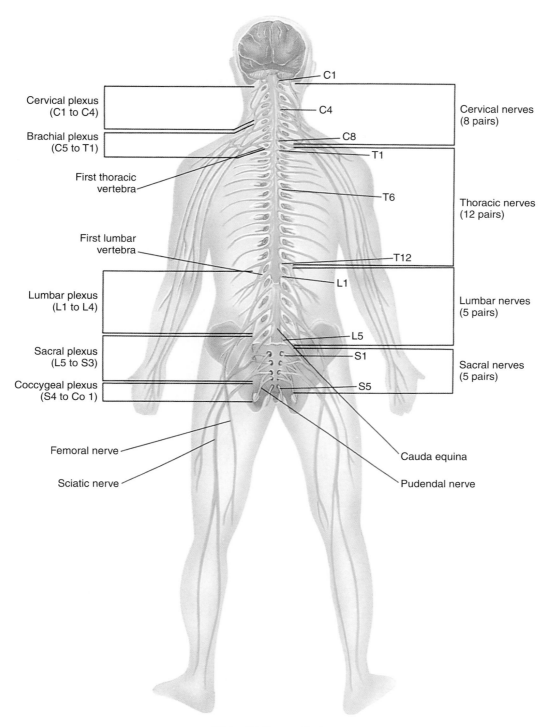

Cervical plexus (C1 to C4)

Brachial plexus (C5 to T1)

First thoracic vertebra

First lumbar vertebra

Lumbar plexus (L1 to L4)

Sacral plexus (L5 to S3)

Coccygeal plexus (S4 to Co 1)

Femoral nerve

Sciatic nerve

C1

C4

C8

T1

T6

T12

L1

L5

S1

S5

Cervical nerves (8 pairs)

Thoracic nerves (12 pairs)

Lumbar nerves (5 pairs)

Sacral nerves (5 pairs)

Cauda equina

Pudendal nerve

Plate 16. Nervous System

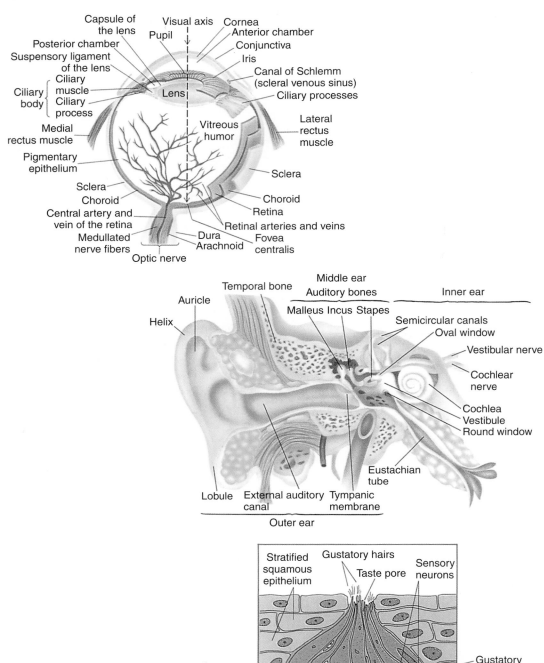

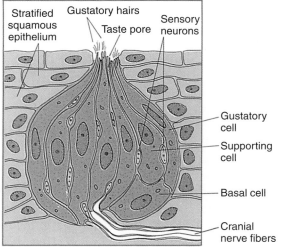

Plate 17. Organs of Special Sense

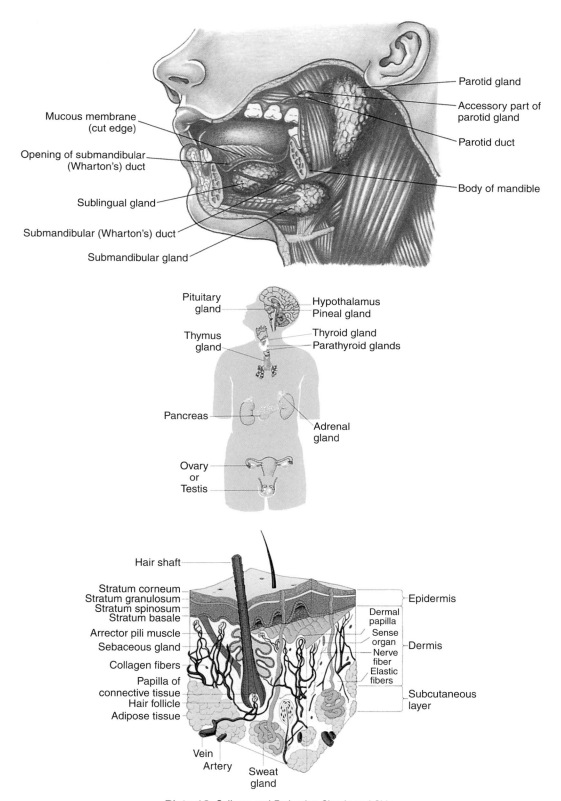

Parotid gland

Accessory part of parotid gland

Parotid duct

Body of mandible

Mucous membrane (cut edge)

Opening of submandibular (Wharton's) duct

Sublingual gland

Submandibular (Wharton's) duct

Submandibular gland

Pituitary gland

Hypothalamus
Pineal gland

Thymus gland

Thyroid gland
Parathyroid glands

Pancreas

Adrenal gland

Ovary
or
Testis

Hair shaft

Stratum corneum
Stratum granulosum
Stratum spinosum
Stratum basale

Arrector pili muscle

Sebaceous gland

Collagen fibers

Papilla of connective tissue
Hair follicle
Adipose tissue

Epidermis

Dermal papilla
Sense organ
Nerve fiber
Elastic fibers

Dermis

Subcutaneous layer

Vein
Artery
Sweat gland

Plate 18. Salivary and Endocrine Glands and Skin

Glossary

Abortion The termination of a pregnancy before the fetus reached the age of viability.

Abrasion A wound in which the outer layers of the skin are damaged; a scrape.

Abscess A collection of pus in a cavity surrounded by inflamed tissue.

Absorbable suture Suture material that is gradually digested by tissue enzymes and absorbed by the body.

Adnexal Adjacent.

Adolescent An individual 12 to 18 years old.

Adventitious sounds Abnormal breath sounds.

Adverse reaction An unintended and undesirable effect produced by a drug.

Aerobe A microorganism that needs oxygen to live and grow.

Afebrile Without fever—the body temperature is normal.

Agglutination The aggregation or uniting of separate particles into clumps or masses; the clumping of blood cells.

Allergen A substance that is capable of causing an allergic reaction.

Allergy An abnormal hypersensitivity of the body to substances that are ordinarily harmless.

Alveolus (*pl.* alveoli) A thin-walled air sac of the lungs in which the exchange of oxygen and carbon dioxide takes place.

Ambulation Walking or moving from one place to another.

Ambulatory Able to walk, as opposed to being confined to bed or a wheelchair.

Ameboid movement Movement used by leukocytes that permits them to propel themselves from the capillaries out into the tissues.

Amenorrhea The absence or cessation of the menstrual period. Amenorrhea occurs normally before puberty, during pregnancy, and after menopause.

Amplitude Refers to amount, extent, size, abundance, or fullness.

Ampule A small sealed glass container that holds a single dose of medication.

Anaerobe A microorganism that grows best in the absence of oxygen.

Anaphylactic reaction A serious allergic reaction that requires immediate treatment.

Anemia A condition in which there is a decrease in the number of erythrocytes or in the amount of hemoglobin in the blood.

Antecubital space The space located at the front of the elbow.

Antibody A substance capable of combining with an antigen, resulting in an antigen-antibody reaction.

Anticoagulant A substance that inhibits blood clotting.

Antigen A substance capable of stimulating the formation of antibodies.

Antipyretic An agent that reduces fever.

Antiseptic An agent that kills disease-producing microorganisms but not their spores. An antiseptic is usually applied to living tissue.

Antiserum (*pl.* antisera) A serum that contains antibodies.

Aorta The major trunk of the arterial system of the body. The aorta arises from the upper surface of the left ventricle.

Apnea The temporary cessation of breathing.

Approximation The process of bringing two parts, such as tissue, together through the use of sutures or other means.

Arrhythmia An irregular heart rhythm; also termed *dysrhythmia*.

Artifact Additional electrical activity picked up by the electrocardiograph that interferes with the normal appearance of the ECG cycles.

Asepsis Free from infection or pathogens; the actions practiced to make and maintain an object free from infection or pathogens.

Atherosclerosis Buildup of fibrous plaques of fatty deposits and cholesterol on the inner walls of the coronary arteries.

Attending physician The physician responsible for the care of a hospitalized patient.

Atypical Deviation from the normal.

Audiometer An instrument used to measure hearing acuity quantitatively for the various frequencies of sound waves.

Auscultation The process of listening to the sounds produced within the body to detect signs of disease.

Autoclave An apparatus for the sterilization of materials, using steam under pressure.

Autoimmune disease A condition in which the body's immune system produces antibodies that attack the body's own cells. The cause is unknown.

Automated method (for testing laboratory specimens) A method of laboratory testing in which the series of steps in the test is performed by an automated analyzer.

Axilla The armpit.

Bacilli (*sing.* bacillus) Bacteria that have a rod shape.

Bandage A strip of woven material used to wrap or cover a part of the body.

Bariatrics The branch of medicine that deals with the treatment and control of obesity including diseases associated with obesity.

Baseline The flat horizontal line that separates the various waves of the ECG cycle.

Bilirubin An orange-colored bile pigment produced by the breakdown of heme from the hemoglobin molecule.

Bilirubinuria The presence of bilirubin in the urine.

Biopsy The surgical removal and examination of tissue from the living body. Biopsies are generally performed to determine whether a tumor is benign or malignant.

Bladder catheterization The passing of a sterile catheter through the urethra and into the bladder to remove urine.

Blood antibody A protein in blood plasma that is capable of combining with its corresponding blood antigen to produce an antigen-antibody reaction.

Blood antigen A protein present on the surface of red blood cells that determines a person's blood type.

Bounding pulse A pulse with an increased volume that feels very strong and full.

Brace An orthopedic device used to support and hold a part of the body in the correct position to allow functioning and healing.

Bradycardia An abnormally slow heart rate (less than 60 beats per minute).

Bradypnea An abnormal decrease in the respiratory rate of less than 10 respirations per minute.

Braxton Hicks contractions Intermittent and irregular painless uterine contractions that occur throughout pregnancy. They occur more frequently toward the end of pregnancy and are sometimes mistaken for true labor pains.

Buffy coat A thin, light-colored layer of white blood cells and platelets that lies between a top layer of plasma and a bottom layer of red blood cells when an anticoagulant has been added to a blood specimen.

Burn An injury to the tissues caused by exposure to thermal, chemical, electrical, or radioactive agents.

Canthus The junction of the eyelids at either corner of the eye.

Capillary action The action that causes liquid to rise along a wick, a tube, or a gauze dressing.

Cardiac arrest A condition in which the heart has stopped beating or beats too irregularly to circulate blood effectively through the body.

Cardiac cycle One complete heartbeat.

Celsius scale A temperature scale on which the freezing point of water is 0° and the boiling point of water is 100°; also called the *centigrade scale*.

Cerumen Ear wax.

Cervix The lower narrow end of the uterus that opens into the vagina.

Charting The process of making written entries about a patient in the medical record.

Chemotherapy The use of chemicals to treat disease. *Chemotherapy* is most often used to refer to the treatment of cancer using antineoplastic medications.

Cilia Slender, hairlike projections that constantly beat toward the outside to remove microorganisms from the body.

Clinical diagnosis A tentative diagnosis of a patient's condition obtained through the evaluation of the health history and the physical examination, without the benefit of laboratory or diagnostic tests.

Cocci (*sing.* coccus) Bacteria that have a round shape.

Colonoscopy The visualization of the entire colon using a colonoscope.

Colony A mass of bacteria growing in a solid culture medium that have arisen from the multiplication of a single bacterium.

Colposcope A lighted instrument with a binocular magnifying lens used to examine the vagina and cervix.

Colposcopy The visual examination of the vagina and cervix using a colposcope.

Compress A soft, moist, absorbent cloth that is folded in several layers and applied to a part of the body in the local application of heat or cold.

Conduction The transfer of energy, such as heat, from one object to another by direct contact.

Consultation report A narrative report of an opinion about a patient's condition by a practitioner other than the attending physician.

Contagious Capable of being transmitted directly or indirectly from one person to another.

Contaminate To soil or to make impure.

Contrast medium A substance that is used to make a particular structure visible on a radiograph.

Controlled drug A drug that has restrictions placed on it by the federal government because of its potential for abuse.

Contusion An injury to the tissues under the skin causing blood vessels to rupture, allowing blood to seep into the tissues; a bruise.

Convection The transfer of energy, such as heat, through air currents.

Conversion Changing from one system of measurement to another.

Crash cart A specially equipped cart for holding and transporting medications, equipment, and supplies needed for performing lifesaving procedures in an emergency.

Crepitus A grating sensation caused by fractured bone fragments rubbing against each other.

Crisis (pertaining to fever) A sudden falling of an elevated body temperature to normal.

Critical item An item that comes in contact with sterile tissue or the vascular system.

Cryosurgery The therapeutic use of freezing temperatures to destroy abnormal tissue.

Cubic centimeter The amount of space occupied by 1 milliliter (1 ml = 1 cc).

Culture The propagation of a mass of microorganisms in a laboratory culture medium.

Culture medium A mixture of nutrients in which microorganisms are grown in the laboratory.

Cyanosis A bluish discoloration of the skin and mucous membranes.

Cytology The science that deals with the study of cells, including their origin, structure, function, and pathology.

DEA number A registration number assigned to physicians by the Drug Enforcement Administration for prescribing or dispensing controlled drugs.

Decontamination The use of physical or chemical means to remove, inactivate, or destroy bloodborne pathogens on a surface or item to the point where they are no longer capable of transmitting infectious particles, and the surface or item is rendered safe for handling, use, or disposal.

Detergent An agent that cleanses by emulsifying dirt and oil.

Diagnosis The scientific method of determining and identifying a patient's condition.

Diagnostic procedure A procedure performed to assist in the diagnosis, management, and treatment of a patient's condition.

Diapedesis The ameboid movement of blood cells (especially leukocytes) through the wall of a capillary and out into the tissues.

Diastole The phase in the cardiac cycle in which the heart relaxes between contractions.

Diastolic pressure The point of lesser pressure on the arterial wall, which is recorded during diastole.

Differential diagnosis A determination of which of two or more diseases with similar symptoms is producing a patient's symptoms.

Dilation (of the cervix) The stretching of the external os from an opening a few millimeters wide to an opening large enough to allow the passage of an infant (approximately 10 cm).

Discharge summary report A brief statement of the significant events of a patient's hospitalization.

Disinfectant An agent used to destroy pathogenic microorganisms but not their spores. Disinfectants are usually applied to inanimate objects.

Dislocation An injury in which one end of a bone comprising a joint is separated or displaced from its normal anatomic position.

Donor One who furnishes something such as blood, tissue, or organs to be used in another individual.

Dose The quantity of a drug to be administered at one time.

Drug A chemical used for the treatment, prevention, or diagnosis of disease.

Dysmenorrhea Pain associated with the menstrual period.

Dyspareunia Pain in the vagina or pelvis experienced by a woman during sexual intercourse.

Dysplasia The growth of abnormal cells. Dysplasia is a precancerous condition that may or may not develop into cancer.

Dyspnea Shortness of breath or difficulty in breathing.

Dysrhythmia An irregular heart rhythm; also termed *arrhythmia.*

ECG cycle The graphic representation of a heartbeat.

Echocardiogram An ultrasound examination of the heart.

Ectocervix The part of the cervix that projects into the vagina and is lined with stratified squamous epithelium.

EDD Expected date of delivery, or due date.

Edema The retention of fluid in the tissues, resulting in swelling.

Effacement The thinning and shortening of the cervical canal from its normal length of 1 to 2 cm to a structure with paper-thin edges in which there is no canal at all. Effacement occurs late in pregnancy, during labor, or both. The purpose of effacement along with dilation is to permit the passage of the infant into the birth canal.

Electrocardiogram (ECG) The graphic representation of the electrical activity of the heart.

Electrocardiograph The instrument used to record the electrical activity of the heart.

Electrode A conductor of electricity that is used to promote contact between the body and the electrocardiograph.

Electrolyte A chemical substance that promotes conduction of an electrical current.

Electronic medical record (EMR) A medical record that is stored on a computer.

Embryo The child in utero from the time of conception to the beginning of the first trimester.

Emergency medical services (EMS) system A network of community resources, equipment, and personnel that provides care to victims of injury or sudden illness.

Endocervix The mucous membrane lining the cervical canal.

Endoscope An instrument that consists of a tube and an optical system that is used for direct visual inspection of organs or cavities.

Enema An injection of fluid into the rectum to aid in the elimination of feces from the colon.

Engagement The entrance of the fetal head or the presenting part into the pelvic inlet.

Enteral nutrition The delivery of nutrients through a tube inserted into the gastrointestinal (GI) tract.

Erythema Reddening of the skin caused by dilation of superficial blood vessels in the skin.

Eupnea Normal respiration. The rate is 16 to 20 respirations per minute, the rhythm is even and regular, and the depth is normal.

Evacuated tube A closed glass or plastic tube that contains a premeasured vacuum.

Exhalation The act of breathing out.

Expected date of delivery (EDD) Projected birth date of the infant.

External os The opening of the cervical canal of the uterus into the vagina.

Exudate A discharge produced by the body's tissues.

Fahrenheit scale A temperature scale on which the freezing point of water is 32° and the boiling point of water is 212°.

False negative A test result indicating that a condition is absent when it is actually present.

False positive A test result indicating that a condition is present when it is actually absent.

Familial Occurring or affecting members of a family more frequently than would be expected by chance.

Fastidious Extremely delicate, difficult to culture, and involving specialized growth requirements.

Fasting Abstaining from food or fluids (except water) for a specified amount of time before the collection of a specimen.

Febrile Pertaining to fever.

Fetal heart rate The number of times the fetal heart beats per minute.

Fetal heart tones The sounds of the heartbeat of the fetus heard through the mother's abdominal wall.

Fetus The child in utero from the third month after conception to birth; during the first 2 months of development, it is called an *embryo*.

Fever A body temperature that is above normal. Synonym for *pyrexia*.

Fibroblast An immature cell from which connective tissue can develop.

First aid The immediate care that is administered to an individual who is injured or suddenly becomes ill before complete medical care can be obtained.

Fluoroscope An instrument used to view internal organs and structures directly.

Fluoroscopy Examination of a patient with a fluoroscope.

Forceps A two-pronged instrument for grasping and squeezing.

Fracture Any break in a bone.

Frenulum linguae The midline fold that connects the undersurface of the tongue with the floor of the mouth.

Fundus The dome-shaped upper portion of the uterus between the fallopian tubes.

Furuncle A localized staphylococcal infection that originates deep within a hair follicle; also known as a *boil*.

Gauge The diameter of the lumen of a needle used to administer medication.

Gene A unit of heredity.

Gestation The period of intrauterine development from conception to birth; the period of pregnancy. The average pregnancy lasts about 280 days, or 40 weeks, from the date of conception to childbirth.

Gestational age The age of the fetus between conception and birth.

Glycogen The form in which carbohydrate is stored in the body.

Glycosuria The presence of sugar in the urine.

Glycosylation The process of glucose attaching to hemoglobin.

Gravidity The total number of pregnancies a woman has had regardless of duration, including a current pregnancy.

Gynecology The branch of medicine that deals with diseases of the reproductive organs of women.

Hand hygiene The process of cleansing or sanitizing the hands.

HDL cholesterol A lipoprotein consisting of protein and cholesterol that removes excess cholesterol from the cells.

Health history report A collection of subjective data about a patient.

Hematology The study of blood and blood-forming tissues.

Hematoma A swelling or mass of coagulated blood caused by a break in a blood vessel.

Hemoconcentration An increase in the concentration of the nonfilterable blood components, such as red blood cells, enzymes, iron, and calcium, as a result of a decrease in the fluid content of the blood.

Hemoglobin The iron-containing pigment of erythrocytes that transports oxygen in the body.

Hemoglobin A_{1c} compound formed when glucose attaches or glycosylates to the protein in hemoglobin.

Hemolysis The breakdown of erythrocytes with the release of hemoglobin into the plasma; the breakdown of blood cells.

Hemophilia An inherited bleeding disorder caused by a deficiency of a clotting factor needed for proper coagulation of the blood.

Hemostasis The arrest of bleeding by natural or artificial means.

Home health care The provision of medical and nonmedical care in a patient's home or place of residence.

Homeostasis The state in which body systems are functioning normally and the internal environment of the body is in equilibrium; the body is in a healthy state.

Hyperglycemia An abnormally high level of glucose in the blood.

Hyperopia Farsightedness.

Hyperpnea An abnormal increase in the rate and depth of respiration.

Hyperpyrexia An extremely high fever.

Hypertension High blood pressure.

Hyperventilation An abnormally fast and deep type of breathing usually associated with acute anxiety conditions.

Hypoglycemia An abnormally low level of glucose in the blood.

Hypopnea An abnormal decrease in the rate and depth of respiration.

Hypotension Low blood pressure.

Hypothermia A body temperature that is below normal.

Hypoxemia A decrease in the oxygen saturation of the blood. Hypoxemia may lead to hypoxia.

Hypoxia A reduction in the oxygen supply to the tissues of the body.

Immune globulins A blood product that consists of pooled human plasma containing antibodies.

Immunity The resistance of the body to the effects of a harmful agent such as a pathogenic microorganism or its toxins.

Immunization (active, artificial) The process of becoming immune or of rendering an individual immune through the use of a vaccine or toxoid.

Impacted Wedged firmly together so as to be immovable.

Incision A clean cut caused by a cutting instrument.

Incubate To provide proper conditions for growth and development. In microbiology, the act of placing a culture in a chamber (incubator), which provides optimal growth requirements for the multiplication of the organisms, such as the proper temperature, humidity, and darkness.

Incubation period The interval of time between the invasion by a pathogenic microorganism and the appearance of first symptoms of the disease.

Induration An area of hardened tissue.

Infant A child from birth to 12 months of age.

Infection The condition in which the body, or part of it, is invaded by a pathogen.

Infectious disease A disease caused by a pathogen that produces harmful effects on its host.

Infiltration The process by which a substance passes into and is deposited within the substance of a cell, tissue, or organ.

Inflammation A protective response of the body in trauma and the entrance of foreign matter. The purpose of inflammation is to destroy invading microorganisms and to repair injured tissue. Symptoms at the site of the inflammation include pain, swelling, redness, and warmth.

Informed consent Consent given by a patient for a medical procedure after being informed of the nature of his or her condition, the purpose of the procedure, the risks involved with the procedure, alternative treatments or procedure available, the likely outcome of the procedure, and the risks involved with declining or delaying the procedure.

Infusion The administration of fluids, medications, or nutrients into a vein.

Inhalation The act of breathing in.

Inhalation administration The administration of medication by way of air or other vapor being drawn into the lungs.

Inoculate To introduce microorganisms into a culture medium for growth and multiplication.

Inoculum The specimen used to inoculate a medium.

Inpatient A patient who has been admitted to a hospital for at least one overnight stay.

Inscription The part of a prescription that indicates the name of the drug and the drug dosage.

Inspection The process of observing a patient to detect signs of disease.

Instillation The dropping of a liquid into a body cavity.

Insufflate To blow a powder, vapor, or gas (e.g., air) into a body cavity.

Intercostal Between the ribs.

Internal os The internal opening of the cervical canal into the uterus.

Interval The length of a wave or the length of a wave with a segment.

Intradermal injection Introduction of medication into the dermal layer of the skin.

Intramuscular injection Introduction of medication into the muscular layer of the body.

Intravenous (IV) therapy The administration of a liquid agent directly into a patient's vein, where it is distributed throughout the body by way of the circulatory system.

In vitro Occurring in glass. Refers to tests performed under artificial conditions, as in the laboratory.

In vivo Occurring in the living body or organism.

Irrigation The washing of a body canal with a flowing solution.

Ischemia Deficiency of blood in a body part.

Ketonuria The presence of ketone bodies in the urine.

Ketosis An accumulation of large amounts of ketone bodies in the tissues and body fluids.

Korotkoff sounds Sounds heard during the measurement of blood pressure that are used to determine the systolic and diastolic blood pressure readings.

Laboratory test The clinical analysis and study of materials, fluids, or tissues obtained from patients to assist in diagnosing and treating disease.

Laceration A wound in which the tissues are torn apart, leaving ragged and irregular edges.

LDL cholesterol A lipoprotein, consisting of protein and cholesterol, that picks up cholesterol and delivers it to the cells.

Length (recumbent) The measurement from the vertex of the head to the heel of the foot in a supine position.

Leukocytosis An abnormally high number of white blood cells (more than 11,000 per cubic millimeter of blood).

Leukopenia An abnormal decrease in the number of white blood cells (less than 4500 per cubic millimeter of blood).

Ligate To tie off and close a structure such as a severed blood vessel.

Lipoprotein A complex molecule consisting of protein and a lipid fraction such as cholesterol. Lipoproteins transport lipids in the blood.

Load Articles that are being sterilized.

Local anesthetic A drug that produces a loss of feeling and an inability to perceive pain in only a specific part of the body.

Lochia A discharge from the uterus after delivery, consisting of blood, tissue, white blood cells, and some bacteria.

Long arm cast A cast that extends from the axilla to the fingers, usually with a bend in the elbow.

Long leg cast A cast that extends from the midthigh to the toes.

Maceration The softening and breaking down of the skin as a result of prolonged exposure to moisture.

Malaise A vague sense of body discomfort, weakness, and fatigue that often marks the onset of a disease and continues through the course of the illness.

Manometer An instrument for measuring pressure.

Manual method A method of laboratory testing in which the series of steps in the test is performed by hand.

Material safety data sheet (MSDS) A sheet that provides information regarding a chemical, its hazards, and measures to take to prevent injury and illness when handling the chemical.

Mayo tray A broad, flat metal tray placed on a stand and used to hold sterile instruments and supplies after it has been covered with a sterile towel.

Medical asepsis Practices that are employed to reduce the number and hinder the transmission of pathogens.

Medical impressions Conclusions drawn by the physician from an interpretation of data. Other terms for impressions include *provisional diagnosis* and *tentative diagnosis.*

Medical record A written record of the important information regarding a patient, including the care of the patient and the progress of the patient's condition.

Medical record format The way a medical record is organized. The two main types of medical record format are the source-oriented record and the problem-oriented record.

Melena The darkening of the stool caused by the presence of blood in an amount of 50 ml or greater.

Meniscus The curved upper surface of liquid in a tube or container. The surface is convex if the liquid does not wet the container and concave if it does.

Menopause The permanent cessation of menstruation, which usually occurs between the ages of 35 and 58.

Menorrhagia Excessive bleeding during a menstrual period, as measured in the number of days, the amount of blood, or both; also called *dysfunctional uterine bleeding* (DUB).

Mensuration The process of measuring the patient.

Metrorrhagia Bleeding between menstrual periods.

Microbiology The scientific study of microorganisms and their activities.

Microorganism A microscopic plant or animal.

Micturition The act of voiding urine.

Mucous membrane A membrane lining body passages or cavities that open to the outside.

Multigravida A woman who has been pregnant more than once.

Multipara A woman who has completed two or more pregnancies to the age of fetal viability regardless of whether they ended in live infants or stillbirths.

Myopia Nearsightedness.

Needle biopsy A type of biopsy in which tissue from deep within the body is obtained by the insertion of a biopsy needle through the skin.

Nephron The functional unit of the kidney.

Nonabsorbable suture Suture material that is not absorbed by the body and either remains permanently in the body tissue and becomes encapsulated by fibrous tissue or is removed.

Noncritical item An item that comes into contact with intact skin but not mucous membranes.

Nonintact skin Skin that has a break in the surface. It includes, but is not limited to, abrasions, cuts, hangnails, paper cuts, and burns.

Nonpathogen A microorganism that does not normally produce disease.

Normal flora Harmless, nonpathogenic microorganisms that normally reside in many parts of the body but do not cause disease.

Normal range (for laboratory tests) A certain established and acceptable parameter or reference range within which the laboratory test results of a healthy individual are expected to fall.

Normal sinus rhythm Refers to an electrocardiogram that is within normal limits.

Nullipara A woman who has not carried a pregnancy to the point of fetal viability (20 weeks of gestation).

Objective symptom A symptom that can be observed by an examiner.

Obstetrics The branch of medicine concerned with the care of a woman during pregnancy, childbirth, and the postpartal period.

Occult blood Blood in such a small amount that it is not detectable by the unaided eye.

Oliguria Decreased or scanty output of urine.

Ophthalmoscope An instrument for examining the interior of the eye.

Opportunistic infection An infection resulting from a defective immune system that cannot defend the body from pathogens normally found in the environment.

Optimum growth temperature The temperature at which an organism grows best.

Oral administration Administration of medication by mouth.

Orthopedist A physician who specializes in the diagnosis and treatment of disorders of the musculoskeletal system, which includes the bones, joints, ligaments, tendons, muscles, and nerves.

Orthopnea The condition in which breathing is easier when an individual is sitting or standing.

Osteochondritis Inflammation of bone and cartilage.

Osteomyelitis Inflammation of the bone resulting from bacterial infection.

Otoscope An instrument for examining the external ear canal and tympanic membrane.

Oxyhemoglobin Hemoglobin that has combined with oxygen.

Palpation The process of feeling with the hands to detect signs of disease.

Paper-based patient record (PPR) A medical record in paper form.

Parenteral Taken into the body through the piercing of the skin barrier or mucous membranes, such as through needlesticks, human bites, cuts, and abrasions. Administration of medication by injection.

Parity The condition of having borne offspring regardless of the outcome.

Pathogen A disease-producing microorganism.

Patient An individual receiving medical care.

Pediatrician A physician who specializes in the care and development of children and the diagnosis and treatment of children's diseases.

Pediatrics The branch of medicine that deals with the care and development of children and the diagnosis and treatment of children's diseases.

Pelvimetry Measurement of the capacity and diameter of the maternal pelvis, which helps determine whether it would be possible to deliver the infant via the vaginal route.

Percussion The process of tapping the body to detect signs of disease.

Percussion hammer An instrument with a rubber head, used for testing reflexes.

Perimenopause Before the onset of menopause, the phase during which a woman with regular periods changes to irregular cycles and increased periods of amenorrhea.

Perinatal Relating to the period shortly before and after birth.

Perineum The external region between the vaginal orifice and the anus in a female and between the scrotum and the anus in a male.

Peroxidase (as it pertains to the guaiac slide test) A substance that is able to transfer oxygen from hydrogen peroxide to oxidize guaiac, causing the guaiac to turn blue.

pH The unit that describes the acidity or alkalinity of a solution.

Phagocytosis The engulfing and destruction of foreign particles such as bacteria by special cells called *phagocytes.*

Pharmacology The study of drugs.

Phlebotomist A health professional trained in the collection of blood specimens.

Phlebotomy Incision of a vein for the removal or withdrawal of blood; the collection of blood.

Physical examination An assessment of each part of a patient's body to obtain objective data about the patient that assists in determining the patient's state of health.

Physical examination report A report of the objective findings from the physician's assessment of each body system.

Plasma The liquid part of the blood, consisting of a clear, straw-colored fluid that makes up approximately 55% of the total blood volume.

Poison Any substance that causes illness, injury, or death if it enters the body.

Polycythemia A disorder in which there is an increase in the red blood cell mass.

Polyuria Increased output of urine.

Position The relation of the presenting part of the fetus to the maternal pelvis.

Postexposure prophylaxis (PEP) Treatment administered to an individual after exposure to an infectious disease to prevent the disease.

Postoperative After a surgical operation.

Postpartum Occurring after childbirth.

Preeclampsia A major complication of pregnancy, the cause of which is unknown, characterized by increasing hypertension, albuminuria, and edema. If this condition is neglected or not treated properly, it may develop into eclampsia, which could cause maternal convulsions and coma. Preeclampsia generally occurs between the 20th week of pregnancy and the end of the first week postpartum.

Prenatal Before birth.

Preoperative Preceding a surgical operation.

Presbyopia A decrease in the elasticity of the lens that occurs with aging, resulting in a decreased ability to focus on close objects.

Preschool child A child 3 to 6 years old.

Prescription A physician's order authorizing the dispensing of a drug by a pharmacist.

Presentation Indication of the part of the fetus that is closest to the cervix and is delivered first. A cephalic presentation is a delivery in which the fetal head is presenting against the cervix. A breech presentation is a delivery in which the buttocks or feet are presented instead of the head.

Pressure point A site on the body where an artery lies close to the surface of the skin and can be compressed against an underlying bone to control bleeding.

Preterm birth Delivery occurring between 20 and 37 weeks of gestation regardless of whether the child was born alive or stillborn.

Primigravida A woman who is pregnant for the first time.

Primipara A woman who has carried a pregnancy to viability (20 weeks of gestation) for the first time, regardless of whether the infant was stillborn or alive at birth.

Problem Any patient condition that requires further observation, diagnosis, management, or patient education.

Prodrome A symptom that indicates an approaching disease.

Profile A collection of laboratory tests providing related or complementary information used to determine the health status of a patient.

Prognosis The probable course and outcome of a patient's condition and the patient's prospects for a recovery.

Proteinuria The presence of protein in the urine.

Puerperium The period of time, usually 4 to 6 weeks after delivery, in which the uterus and the body systems are returning to normal.

Pulse oximeter A computerized device consisting of a probe and monitor used to measure the oxygen saturation of arterial blood.

Pulse oximetry The use of a pulse oximeter to measure the oxygen saturation of arterial blood.

Pulse pressure The difference between the systolic and diastolic pressures.

Pulse rhythm The time interval between heartbeats.

Pulse volume The strength of the heartbeat.

Puncture A wound made by a sharp pointed object piercing the skin.

Quality control The application of methods to ensure that test results are reliable and valid and that errors are detected and eliminated.

Quickening The first movements of the fetus in utero as felt by the mother, which usually occurs between the 16th and 20th weeks of gestation and is felt consistently thereafter.

Radiation The transfer of energy such as heat in the form of waves.

Radiograph A permanent record of a picture of an internal body organ or structure produced on radiographic film.

Radiography The taking of permanent records (radiographs) of internal body organs and structures by passing x-rays through the body to act on a specially sensitized film.

Radiologist A physician who specializes in the diagnosis and treatment of disease using radiant energy such as x-rays, radium, and radioactive material.

Radiology The branch of medicine that deals with the use of radiant energy in the diagnosis and treatment of disease.

Radiolucent Describing a structure that permits the passage of x-rays.

Radiopaque Describing a structure that obstructs the passage of x-rays.

Recipient One who receives something, such as a blood transfusion, from a donor.

Refraction The deflection or bending of light rays by a lens.

Refractive index The ratio of the velocity of light in air to the velocity of light in a solution.

Refractometer (clinical) An instrument used to measure the refractive index of urine, which is an indirect measurement of the specific gravity of urine.

Regulated medical waste Medical waste that poses a threat to health and safety.

Renal threshold The concentration at which a substance in the blood that is not normally excreted by the kidneys begins to appear in the urine.

Reservoir host The organism that becomes infected by a pathogen and serves as a source of transfer of the pathogen to others.

Resident flora Harmless, nonpathogenic microorganisms that normally reside on the skin and usually do not cause disease; also known as *normal flora*.

Resistance The natural ability of an organism to remain unaffected by harmful substances in its environment.

Reverse chronological order Arrangement of documents with the most recent document on top or in the front, which means that the oldest document is on the bottom or at the back of a section or file.

Risk factor Anything that increases an individual's chance of developing a disease. Some risk factors (e.g., smoking) can be avoided, but others cannot (e.g., age and family history).

Routine test Laboratory test performed routinely on apparently healthy patients to assist in the early detection of disease.

Sanitization A process to remove organic matter from an article and to reduce the number of microorganisms to a safe level as determined by public health requirements.

SaO$_2$ (saturation of arterial oxygen) Abbreviation for the percentage of hemoglobin that is saturated with oxygen in arterial blood.

Scalpel A surgical knife used to divide tissues.

School-age child A child 6 to 12 years old.

Scissors A cutting instrument.

Sebaceous cyst A thin, closed sac or capsule that contains fatty secretions from a sebaceous gland.

Segment The portion of the ECG between two waves.

Seizure A sudden episode of involuntary muscular contractions and relaxation, often accompanied by a change in sensation, behavior, and level of consciousness.

Semicritical item An item that comes into contact with nonintact skin or intact mucous membranes.

Sequela (*pl.* sequelae) A morbid (secondary) condition occurring as a result of a less serious primary infection.

Serum The clear, straw-colored part of the blood (plasma) that remains after the solid elements and the clotting factor fibrinogen have been removed.

Shock The failure of the cardiovascular system to deliver enough blood to all the vital organs of the body.

Short arm cast A cast that extends from below the elbow to the fingers.

Short leg cast A cast that begins just below the knee and extends to the toes.

Sigmoidoscope An endoscope that is specially designed for passage through the anus to permit visualization of the rectum and sigmoid colon.

Sigmoidoscopy The visual examination of the rectum and sigmoid colon using a sigmoidoscope.

Signatura The part of a prescription that indicates the information to print on the medication label.

Smear Material spread on a slide for microscope examination.

Soak The direct immersion of a body part in water or a medicated solution.

SOAP format A method of organization for recording progress notes. The SOAP format includes the following categories: *s*ubjective data, *o*bjective data, *a*ssessment, and *p*lan.

Sonogram The record obtained with ultrasonography.

Specific gravity The weight of a substance compared with the weight of an equal volume of a substance known as the *standard.* In urinalysis, the *specific gravity* refers to the measurement of the amount of dissolved substances in the urine compared with the same amount of distilled water.

Specimen A small sample of something taken to show the nature of the whole.

Speculum An instrument for opening a body orifice or cavity for viewing.

Sphygmomanometer An instrument for measuring arterial blood pressure.

Spirilla (*sing.* spirillum) Bacteria that have a spiral or curved shape.

Spirometer An instrument for measuring air taken into and expelled from the lungs.

Spirometry Measurement of an individual's breathing capacity by means of a spirometer.

Splint An orthopedic device used to support and immobilize a part of the body.

SpO2 (saturation of peripheral oxygen) Abbreviation for the percentage of hemoglobin that is saturated with oxygen in arterial blood as measured by a pulse oximeter.

Sponge A porous, absorbent pad, such as a 4-inch gauze pad or cotton surrounded by gauze, used to absorb fluids, to apply medication, or to cleanse an area.

Spore A hard, thick-walled capsule formed by some bacteria that contains only the essential parts of the protoplasm of the bacterial cell.

Sprain Trauma to a joint that causes tearing of ligaments.

Sterile Free of all living microorganisms and bacterial spores.

Sterilization The process of destroying all forms of microbial life, including bacterial spores.

Stethoscope An instrument for amplifying and hearing sounds produced by the body.

Strain An overstretching or tearing of a muscle caused by trauma.

Streaking In microbiology, the process of inoculating a culture to provide for the growth of colonies on the surface of a solid medium. Streaking is accomplished by skimming a wire inoculating loop that contains the specimen across the surface of the medium, using a back-and-forth motion.

Streptolysin An exotoxin produced by beta-hemolytic streptococci, which completely hemolyzes red blood cells.

Subcutaneous injection Introduction of medication beneath the skin, into the subcutaneous or fatty layer of the body.

Subjective symptom A symptom that is felt by a patient but is not observable by an examiner.

Sublingual administration Administration of medication by placing it under the tongue, where it dissolves and is absorbed through the mucous membrane.

Subscription The part of a prescription that gives directions to the pharmacist and usually designates the number of doses to be dispensed.

Supernatant The clear liquid that remains at the top after a precipitate settles.

Superscription The part of a prescription consisting of the symbol Rx (from the Latin word *recipe,* meaning "take").

Suppuration The process of pus formation.

Suprapubic aspiration The passing of a sterile needle through the abdominal wall into the bladder to remove urine.

Surgical asepsis Practices that keep objects and areas sterile or free from microorganisms.

Susceptible Easily affected; lacking resistance.

Sutures Material used to approximate tissues with surgical stitches.

Swaged needle A needle with suturing material permanently attached to its end.

Symptom Any change in the body or its functioning that indicates that a disease might be present.

Systole The phase in the cardiac cycle in which the ventricles contract, sending blood out of the heart and into the aorta and pulmonary aorta.

Systolic pressure The point of maximum pressure on the arterial walls, which is recorded during systole.

Tachycardia An abnormally fast heart rate (greater than 100 beats per minute).

Tachypnea An abnormal increase in the respiratory rate of more than 20 respirations per minute.

Term birth Delivery occurring after 37 weeks, regardless of whether the infant was born alive or stillborn.

Thermolabile Easily affected or changed by heat.

Thready pulse A pulse with a decreased volume that feels weak and thin.

Toddler A child 1 to 3 years old.

Topical administration Application of a drug to a particular spot, usually for a local action.

Toxemia A pathologic condition occurring in pregnant women that includes preeclampsia and eclampsia. If preeclampsia goes undiagnosed or is not satisfactorily controlled, it could develop into eclampsia, characterized by convulsions and coma.

Toxin A poisonous or noxious substance.

Toxoid A toxin (poisonous substance produced by a bacterium) that has been treated by heat or chemicals to destroy its harmful properties. It is administered to an individual to prevent an infectious disease by stimulating the production of antibodies in that individual.

Transfusion The administration of whole blood or blood products through the intravenous route.

Transient flora Microorganisms that reside on the superficial skin layers and are picked up in the course of daily activities. They are often pathogenic but can be removed easily from the skin by sanitizing the hands.

Trimester Three months, or one third, of the gestational period of pregnancy.

Tympanic membrane A thin, semitransparent membrane located between the external ear canal and the middle ear that receives and transmits sound waves; also known as the *eardrum.*

Ultrasonography The use of high-frequency sound waves (ultrasound) to produce an image of an organ or tissue.

Urinalysis The physical, chemical, and microscopic analysis of urine.

Vaccine A suspension of attenuated (weakened) or killed microorganisms administered to an individual to prevent an infectious disease by stimulating the production of antibodies in that individual.

Venipuncture Puncturing of a vein.

Venous reflux The backflow of blood (from an evacuated tube) into a patient's vein.

Venous stasis The temporary cessation or slowing of the venous blood flow.

Vertex The summit, or top, especially the top of the head.

Vial A closed glass container with a rubber stopper that holds medication.

Void To empty the bladder.

Vulva The region of the external female genital organs.

Wheal A small raised area of the skin.

Wound A break in the continuity of an external or internal surface caused by physical means.

Index

or drug dosages is intended strictly for professional use, and because of rapid advances in the medical sciences, independent verification of diagnosis and drug dosages should be made.

IN NO EVENT WILL ELSEVIER, ITS AFFILIATES, LICENSORS, SUPPLIERS OR AGENTS, BE LIABLE TO YOU FOR ANY DAMAGES, INCLUDING, WITHOUT LIMITATION, ANY LOST PROFITS, LOST SAVINGS OR OTHER INCIDENTAL OR CONSEQUENTIAL DAMAGES, ARISING OUT OF YOUR USE OR INABILITY TO USE THE ELECTRONIC MEDIA PRODUCT REGARDLESS OF WHETHER SUCH DAMAGES ARE FORESEEABLE OR WHETHER SUCH DAMAGES ARE DEEMED TO RESULT FROM THE FAILURE OR INADEQUACY OF ANY EXCLUSIVE OR OTHER REMEDY.

U.S. GOVERNMENT RESTRICTED RIGHTS

The Electronic Media Product and documentation are provided with restricted rights. Use, duplication or disclosure by the U.S. Government is subject to restrictions as set forth in subparagraphs (a) through (d) of the Commercial Computer Restricted Rights clause at FAR 52.22719 or in subparagraph (c)(1)(ii) of the Rights in Technical Data and Computer Software clause at DFARS 252.2277013, or at 252.211015, as applicable. Contractor/Manufacturer is Elsevier Inc., 360 Park Avenue South, New York, NY 10010-5107 USA.

GOVERNING LAW

This Agreement shall be governed by the laws of the State of New York, USA. In any dispute arising out of this Agreement, you and Elsevier each consent to the exclusive personal jurisdiction and venue in the state and federal courts within New York County, New York, USA.

4

Bonewit-West: Companion DVDs for Clinical Procedures for Medical Assistants, 7th Edition

DVD RECOMMENDED SYSTEM REQUIREMENTS

Windows® PC
PC Based Pentium® 266 MMX
Windows 2000, XP or higher
256 MB RAM or higher
64 MB or higher graphics card
400 MHz or faster processor
16X DVD-ROM drive with DVD player software
Display resolution of 800 x 600 or greater
Sound card and speakers

Macintosh®
Power PC G3 300 MHZ, I-MAC, I-Book
Macintosh OS 10.2 or higher
256 MB RAM or higher
64 MB or higher graphics card
400 MHz or faster processor
16X DVD-ROM drive with DVD player software
Display resolution of 800 x 600 or greater
Sound card and speakers

1

ELSEVIER LICENSE AGREEMENT

PLEASE READ THE FOLLOWING AGREEMENT CAREFULLY BEFORE USING THIS ELECTRONIC MEDIA PRODUCT. THIS ELECTRONIC MEDIA PRODUCT IS LICENSED UNDER THE TERMS CONTAINED IN THIS ELECTRONIC MEDIA LICENSE AGREEMENT ("Agreement"). BY USING THIS ELECTRONIC MEDIA PRODUCT, YOU, AN INDIVIDUAL OR ENTITY INCLUDING EMPLOYEES, AGENTS AND REPRESENTATIVES ("You" or "Your"), ACKNOWLEDGE THAT YOU HAVE READ THIS AGREEMENT, THAT YOU UNDERSTAND IT, AND THAT YOU AGREE TO BE BOUND BY THE TERMS AND CONDITIONS OF THIS AGREEMENT. ELSEVIER INC. ("Elsevier") EXPRESSLY DOES NOT AGREE TO LICENSE THIS ELECTRONIC MEDIA PRODUCT TO YOU UNLESS YOU ASSENT TO THIS AGREEMENT. IF YOU DO NOT AGREE WITH ANY OF THE FOLLOWING TERMS, YOU MAY, WITHIN THIRTY (30) DAYS AFTER YOUR RECEIPT OF THIS ELECTRONIC MEDIA PRODUCT RETURN THE UNUSED ELECTRONIC MEDIA PRODUCT AND ALL ACCOMPANYING DOCUMENTATION TO ELSEVIER FOR A FULL REFUND.

DEFINITIONS

As used in this Agreement, these terms shall have the following meanings:

"Proprietary Material" means the valuable and proprietary information content of this Electronic Media Product including all indexes and graphic materials and software used to access, index, search and retrieve the information content from this Electronic Media Product developed or licensed by Elsevier and/or its affiliates, suppliers and licensors.

"Electronic Media Product" means the copy of the Proprietary Material and any other material delivered on Electronic Media and any other human-readable or machine-readable materials enclosed with this Agreement, including without limitation documentation relating to the same.

OWNERSHIP

This Electronic Media Product has been supplied by and is proprietary to Elsevier and/or its affiliates, suppliers and licensors. The copyright in the Electronic Media Product belongs to Elsevier and/or its affiliates, suppliers and licensors and is protected by the national and state copyright, trademark, trade secret and other intellectual property laws of the United States and international treaty provisions, including without limitation the Universal Copyright Convention and the Berne Copyright Convention. You have no ownership rights in this Electronic Media Product. Except as expressly set forth herein, no part of this Electronic Media Product, including without limitation the Proprietary Material, may be modified, copied or distributed in hardcopy or machine-readable form

Watch and Learn

with the Companion DVDs!

Use your **Companion DVDs** today to start mastering the skills and procedures you'll use as a medical assistant. The videos on these DVDs feature actual medical assistants performing more than 70 procedures from *Clinical Procedures for Medical Assistants, 7th Edition,* guiding you through each step and demonstrating proper technique.

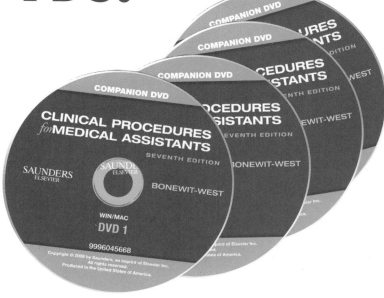

Here are just a few of the skills and competencies you'll see on the Companion DVDs:

> Measuring Oral Body Temperature — Electronic

> Measuring Temporal Artery Body Temperature

> Measuring Radial Pulse and Respiration

> Performing Pulse Oximetry

> Measuring Weight and Height

> Assisting With the Physical Examination

> Carrying an Infant

> Sterile Technique

> Administering an Intramuscular Injection

> Performing a Hematocrit Determination

> Performing a Hemoglobin Determination

> Performing Cholesterol Blood Chemistry Testing

You can also access additional resources at **http://evolve.elsevier.com/bonewit**

SEE what you've been learning about in the textbook —
Start using the Companion DVDs today!